The Modern Family Health Guide

The Modern Family

CONTRIBUTING SPECIALISTS

Harry Bakwin

Ruth Morris Bakwin

Frank A. Calderone

A. C. Corcoran

John M. Cotton

Edwin J. De Costa

Sol T. Delee

Benjamin M. Gasul

John R. Heller

Horace L. Hodes

Lewis M. Hurxthal

Aaron M. Josephson

Charles H. Lawrence

Currier McEwen

George J. Mohr

Milton M. Mosko

John B. O'Sullivan

Irvine H. Page

Carl J. Potthoff

Charles Rein

Mortimer Spiegelman

Gene H. Stollerman

Carl D. Strouse

Stanley E. Telser

Hart E. Van Riper

Samuel Weiss

VOLUME II

ENCYCLOPEDIA OF FAMILY HEALTH

Health Guide

Edited by Morris Fishbein

Formerly Editor,
Journal of the American Medical Association
Editor, *Excerpta Medica*
Medical Editor,
Britannica Book of the Year

DOUBLEDAY & COMPANY, INC.
Garden City, New York

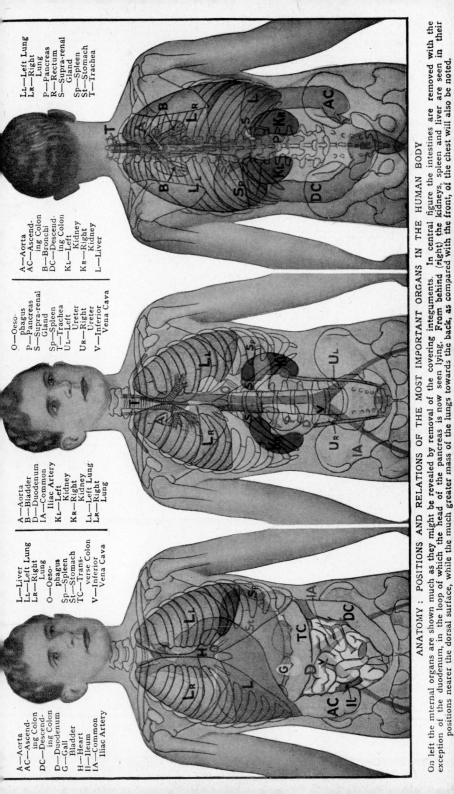

ANATOMY : POSITIONS AND RELATIONS OF THE MOST IMPORTANT ORGANS IN THE HUMAN BODY

On left the internal organs are shown much as they might be revealed by removal of the covering integuments. In central figure the intestines are removed with the exception of the duodenum, in the loop of which the head of the pancreas is now seen lying. From behind (right) the kidneys, spleen and liver are seen in their positions nearer the dorsal surface, while the much greater mass of the lungs towards the back, as compared with the front, of the chest will also be noted.

A—Aorta
AC—Ascending Colon
DC—Descending Colon
D—Duodenum
G—Gall Bladder
H—Heart
Il—Ileum
IA—Common Iliac Artery

L—Liver
L$_L$—Left Lung
L$_R$—Right Lung
O—Oesophagus
Sp—Spleen
St—Stomach
TC—Transverse Colon
V—Inferior Vena Cava

A—Aorta
B—Bladder
D—Duodenum
IA—Common Iliac Artery
K$_L$—Left Kidney
K$_R$—Right Kidney
L$_L$—Left Lung
L$_R$—Right Lung

O—Oesophagus
P—Pancreas
S—Supra-renal Gland
Sp—Spleen
T—Trachea
U$_L$—Left Ureter
U$_R$—Right Ureter
V—Inferior Vena Cava

A—Aorta
AC—Ascending Colon
B—Bronchi
DC—Descending Colon
K$_L$—Left Kidney
K$_R$—Right Kidney
L—Liver

L$_L$—Left Lung
L$_R$—Right Lung
P—Pancreas
R—Rectum
S—Supra-renal Gland
Sp—Spleen
St—Stomach
T—Trachea

ABASIA, the scientific term for lack of coordination in walking.

ABDOMEN, the oval-shaped cavity lying between the lower limit of the chest and the pelvis. It is protected at the front and sides by abdominal muscles, and in back by the bony structures and muscles of the spine. The abdominal cavity holds the stomach and large and small intestines, the liver, gallbladder, pancreas, spleen, the two kidneys, an adrenal gland lying above each kidney, and the abdominal aorta, blood vessels, and nerves which form part of the sympathetic nervous system. *See also* ABDOMINAL PAIN.

ABDOMINAL PAIN. Discomfort, cramps, or aches in the abdomen may be slight and passing or they may arise from serious causes which require medical attention.

Overeating, consuming heavily spiced foods or foods that disagree may cause stomach ache, colic, or griping pains. These can be controlled by more careful eating habits. Heavy smoking or drinking may also cause a disturbed stomach. Anxiety and nervous tension, fear and unusual emotional strain can increase the normal action of the digestive system and result in abdominal distress.

Gas in the stomach may cause discomfort. Occasional abdominal pain such as this may be relieved by hot strong tea or a cup of hot salty bouillon. Dry toast or salty soda crackers may relieve the pain or nausea which sometimes accompanies gas.

Abdominal pain which is persistent, though not severe, or which returns frequently or comes suddenly and severely usually indicates a more serious disorder. Laxatives or cathartics are therefore not advisable. Such drugs do not reach the source of the pain and only delay treatment of the disorder which may need immediate medical attention.

One common cause of pain in the abdomen is inflammation of the appendix. The chief symptom is a dull pain which begins in the center of the abdomen and gradually localizes in the right lower sector, which hurts when pressed. Laxatives must not be taken and a doctor should be called promptly if the pain and tenderness persist.

Many deficiency disorders, such as pernicious anemia and sprue, in which the body reacts to a lack of iron or vitamins, produce abdominal distress. This is also true of some transmittable diseases, including pneumonia and infectious mononucleosis. Children, particularly, are apt to have severe abdominal pain as one of the symptoms of these diseases.

An infected gallbladder will often cause abdominal distress. A gallstone blocking an outlet from the gallbladder, or any other intestinal obstruction, incites pain in this area. The presence of worms or other parasites in the intestines may also produce acute abdominal pain.

Food poisoning evokes sharp pains in the abdomen, as does poisoning by corrosive chemicals or an overdose of strong drugs.

Young children sometimes develop an intestinal obstruction known as intussusception, in which a part of the bowel is telescoped into itself. This condition causes severe, cramp-like spasms and even prostration, and requires immediate medical attention since bowel action is blocked. Adults rarely develop intussusception.

The perforation of an ulcer of the stomach or duodenum, which usually occurs without warning, produces agonizing pain in the upper abdomen and requires prompt medical care.

Because of the presence of many significant organs in the abdominal cavity, pain in this region may arise from a variety of sources. The precise location of the pain helps the physician to determine which organ is affected. To facilitate finding the exact spot the abdomen is divided, figuratively, by two horizontal and two vertical lines into nine regions.

Rt. Hypochon-driac	Epigastric	Lt. Hypochon-driac
Rt. Lumbar	Umbilical	Lt. Lumbar
Rt. Iliac	Hypogastric	Lt. Iliac

See also CRAMP; HERNIA; and Chapter 18, "Disorders of the Digestive System and Diet in Digestive Disorders."

ABDOMINAL SUPPORTS, appliances that aid in holding abdominal muscles or organs up or in place. Normal muscles should not require artificial support and are likely to weaken through nonuse if supports are constantly applied. In certain conditions, however, particularly in older people, such appliances may be helpful.

The complaint of backache, frequently heard from housewives, often is relieved by an abdominal support, which helps maintain better posture and so takes weight and stress off the spinal column. Many pregnancies, and in some cases even one pregnancy, may cause the abdominal wall to sag. Substantial overweight will relax the abdominal wall. In such instances, and after abdominal operations when the muscles have been weakened, or in abdominal hernia, a supporting abdominal belt is definitely beneficial.

In cases where pressure is required on a specific area of the abdominal wall—for example, to support a kidney which tends to sag or to secure a hernia—an appropriate pad is inserted in the abdominal belt. These supports must be properly fitted by a qualified person on the recommendation of a doctor.

ABDUCTOR, a muscle which, on contraction, draws a part from the axis of the body or of an extremity. Abductor auris, for example, is the abductor muscle of the ear.

ABLATION, removal, by excision or amputation but specifically by surgery, of a part of the body—for instance, a tumor.

ABORTION, also called interrupted pregnancy, expelling of the fetus from the uterus during the first three months of pregnancy.

Abortions may be spontaneous, as

a result of disorder in the growth of the fetus, or from some involuntary external interference, or they may be induced deliberately. Spontaneous abortions take place when the tissues which attach the embryo to the inner lining of the uterus become disconnected. Such abortions usually occur between the eighth and twelfth weeks of pregnancy because the ovum at that period is not yet firmly fixed and changes are constantly taking place in its structure and circulation. From 10 to 18 per cent of fetuses conceived are thus aborted. A miscarriage is an abortion between the third and seventh months.

Frequently a spontaneous abortion can be traced to excessive exertion or disturbance such as a bad fall. Sometimes infectious disease or disorders of the thyroid or pituitary glands may interrupt a pregnancy. In addition, poisoning by lead, mercury or zinc, vitamin deficiency, particularly of vitamins E or K, overexposure to x-rays or radium radiation may induce abortion. Abnormalities in the structure or development of the uterus or inflammation of the lining of the uterus may cause abortion. Syphilis is a common source of abortions; pregnancy in such cases is usually interrupted after the fifth month.

The first sign of a possible spontaneous abortion is vaginal bleeding or spotting, especially if this is accompanied by pain in the back or lower abdomen. Bleeding, no matter how slight, and the presence of pain should be reported to a doctor at once, and the pregnant woman should go to bed immediately. Bed rest and prompt medical treatment

may be sufficient to counteract the danger of abortion.

If the contents of the uterus are expelled, as in an interrupted pregnancy, the patient should consult her physician immediately so that he can determine whether or not the fetus and placenta have come away completely. If the abortion has been complete, further treatment may not be necessary. If some of the contents of the pregnant uterus remains, surgical scraping, or curettage, may be necessary.

ABRASION, a superficial injury to the skin or mucous membranes caused by accidental rubbing or scraping. The wound, which often feels like a burn, may bleed slightly and there may be an oozing of blood-tinged serum which soon dries and forms a crust. The affected area should be washed thoroughly, a mild antiseptic applied, and the spot covered with sterile gauze. If the abrasion is extensive, a physician should be consulted.

In dentistry, abrasion refers to the normal wearing away of the cutting edges of the teeth, or of dentine and enamel. *See also* WOUNDS.

ABRUPTIO, cleavage or tearing away—as, for example, abruptio placentae, the premature separation of the placenta.

ABSCESS, a cavity, formed by tissue deterioration, which contains pus and is surrounded by an inflamed area. An abscess may form in any part of the body when staphylococcic or streptococcic bacteria invade an area and produce a local infection. Under such circumstances white blood cells gather at the inflamed area to wall off the infection, to absorb the invading microbes and liquefy them, creating the characteristic thick yellowish pus. The surrounding area is red, swollen, and painful. The redness and heat are due to the concentration of blood around the abscess and the swelling is caused by the accumulation of pus. The pain arises from the pressure of pus upon the nerves.

As white blood cells accumulate and the mass of semiliquid contents increases, the abscess "comes to a head." When the inflamed wall of tissue encompassing the infected area thins out sufficiently on the outer surface the abscess ruptures and pus escapes. This generally brings relief of pain and swelling.

Abscesses may form in the chest, abdominal cavity, in a joint or gland. Such disorders should be treated by a physician since they may lead to extremely serious generalized infections. The sulfa drugs and antibiotics have proved effective in controlling such ailments. It is preferable to have a superficial abscess opened by a physician, rather than wait for it to burst. *See also* INFECTIONS.

ABSORPTION, the ability of the skin, mucous membrane, and other organs of the body to take in all the substances necessary to function, such as gases, fluids, and foods. Thus, the skin and mucous membranes absorb drugs applied on their surfaces, and the digestive system absorbs foods and liquids taken internally.

Fluid is absorbed mostly in the large intestine, and food almost entirely in the small intestine. The carbohydrates, fats, and proteins that make up most of the foodstuffs we eat are finely subdivided, disintegrated, absorbed into the blood and distributed by it to the rest of the body.

ABULIA, inability to make decisions and pronounced weakness of will power. It characterizes certain mental conditions, such as schizophrenia.

ACCESSORY SEX ORGANS, the auxiliaries, supplementing the reproductive organs. The epididymis is the portion of the seminal duct lying posterior to the testis. Consisting mainly of the excretory ducts of the testicles, the epididymis secretes a mildly acid fluid. The prostate, at the neck of the bladder, is a significant gland in the male which manufactures the necessary secretions to move the spermatozoa. *See also* PROSTATE; REPRODUCTIVE SYSTEM.

ACCIDENTS . . . legally an event which happens unexpectedly and without possibility of its being prevented at the moment of occurrence. Over ten million persons are involved in accidents every year in the United States. Of these, 125,000, excluding automobile casualties, result in death. One third of all childhood deaths are the result of accidents.

About 10,000 injuries occur each day in homes, many of them caused by carelessness or neglect. The bathroom has well earned its reputation of being the most dangerous room in the home. Falls in the bathtub, which cause injuries ranging from a sprained ankle to a serious fracture, are usually avoided simply by keeping a nonskid rubber mat in the tub. Mislabeled medicine bottles, strong drugs or poisons, patent medicines, even seemingly harmless drugs such as aspirin or boric acid, constitute potential dangers, especially when there are young children in the family. A special place, inaccessible to youngsters, should be reserved for all such preparations. Hazards such as highly waxed floors, rickety stepladders, and loose carpeting are responsible for falls and should be eliminated. Faulty wiring and electrical appliances that function poorly cause thousands of fires; appliances and wires should always be kept in good repair.

In the kitchen, such common household materials as floor wax, ammonia, rat and roach exterminators, and all inflammable cleansers should be kept out of the reach of children. A leaking gas line should be located and repaired promptly at the first suspicious odor. A gas flame, even a low one, burning in a room where people are sleeping, is unsafe.

The most dependable protection against accidents in the home is primarily an awareness of potential dangers. Conscious and continuous effort to recognize and eliminate such dangers can reduce the number of needless injuries and deaths. The next best protection, when accidents do occur, is knowledge of the basic methods of administering first aid. *See also* DROWNING; FIRST AID; POISONING; RESUSCITATION; SHOCK; and Chapter 26, "Medical Statistics"; Chapter 27, "First Aid."

ACCOMMODATION, the ability of the lens of the eye to change its shape when focused on objects at varying distances. For distant vision, the pupils become large, the lenses are flattened and are directed away from each other. For close vision the process is reversed. After the age of forty, when the lenses tend to harden, the ability of the eye to accommodate diminishes, and glasses are usually essential for close work.

Normal vision is acquired gradually in the process of growth. Reading small print, sewing, and other close work are especially tiring to young children and strain resulting from such efforts frequently provokes headache and pain in the eyes. *See also* EYE.

ACETANILID, a white crystalline substance, derived from aniline and acetic acid, originally used to lower the temperature in fever. Since acetanilid also relieves pain, it is used in headache remedies and mixtures sold for the relief of common aches and pains. An overdose may cause serious collapse and difficulty in breathing by interfering with the oxygen-carrying function of the red blood cells. A new derivative of acetanilid called APAP has most of the good qualities without the side effects. *See also* ANILINE; ANTIFEBRIN.

ACETEST, the commercial name for a small kit containing equipment with which diabetics can test the presence of acetone in the urine. Acetone indicates acidosis and should be brought to the attention of a physician immediately. *See also* DIABETES.

ACETIC ACID, a colorless liquid that gives vinegar its sour taste. Glacial acetic acid, which contains 99.5 per cent acetic acid, and trichloroacetic acid, a more dilute form, are used as caustics to remove warts. The more dilute concentrations of acetic acid are used to rid the hair of nits, in pediculosis (head lice).

ACETONE, a colorless volatile liquid found in small quantities in the blood and urine. Increases of acetone in the blood are dangerous for diabetics, so tests designed to detect the presence of acetone in the blood are made regularly as are the tests for sugar. *See also* DIABETES.

ACETYLSALICYLIC ACID, another word for aspirin. It is a white crystalline powder which dissolves in water and is used to relieve fever and various types of pain. It is also used locally in acute tonsillitis and pharyngitis. *See also* ANALGESIA; MEDICINE CHEST, *Pain Relievers.*

ACHE, a pain which is dull and constant, as in backache; or throbbing, as in some headaches or toothaches. Grippe or influenza is often accompanied by a dull aching pain of the bones, and muscular rheumatism is characterized by aching of the muscles.

ACHILLES' TENDON. The tendons of the gastrocnemius and the soleus muscles, which flex the ankle joints, fuse and insert into the heel bone, forming the Achilles' tendon. The term is derived from Homer's *Iliad,* according to which the only spot where Achilles was vulnerable was in one heel.

ACHLORHYDRIA, the absence of hydrochloric acid in the gastric juices. These juices secreted by the glands in the stomach aid in breaking down foods into their simpler components which can be absorbed by the blood. Complete achlorhydria is an unusual condition and occurs in only about 10 per cent of persons with stomach disorders.

The tendency to a diminution of hydrochloric acid is, however, not uncommon and to some extent is normally compensated for by digestive processes in the intestines. The condition may be treated with small doses of hydrochloric acid in water. Improvement sometimes occurs when an inert substance is substituted for hydrochloric acid, which suggests that the condition may be essentially psychological in origin.

ACHOLIA, the condition that occurs when bile cannot flow into the small intestine because of an obstruction. Bile is thus absent from the urine or feces. *See also* BILE.

ACHONDROPLASIA, more commonly known as dwarfism, is the result of an abnormal development of the embryo, which affects the growth of the bones. The torso is usually normal, but the head is disproportionately large and the arms and legs are dwarfed and curved. The majority of infants so affected are stillborn. The muscles of those who live to adulthood develop greater than ordinary strength, and mental and sexual development and longevity are not affected. The abnormal proportions of the body in this condition differentiate such people from midgets, and their normal mentality distinguishes them from the cretin type of dwarf.

ACHROMYCIN, the trade name for a new yellow-colored antibiotic similar to Aureomycin or chlortetracycline. Chemically known as tetracycline, Achromycin is produced by a process known scientifically as the catalytic reduction of aureomycin, an older antibiotic. Achromycin shows a low toxicity, has a wide range of effectiveness against bacteria, and is more soluble and more stable in an alkaline solution. Antibiotics are mixed in an alkaline solution when given intravenously. *See also* ANTIBIOTICS.

ACHYLIA, a rare condition in which all gastric juices normally produced by the glands of the stomach wall are absent.

ACID, a substance which when combined with alkalies forms salts. Mineral or inorganic acids include hydrochloric, nitric, and sulphuric acid. The organic acids include citric, lactic, and uric acids. Some acids are naturally produced in the body and eliminated by the excretory system.

High concentrations of mineral acids have a corrosive effect on human tissue, and, taken internally, cause severe burning sensations in the mouth, throat, and stomach, followed by abdominal pain and vomiting. Difficulty in breathing may develop if the larynx is involved. Generally a state of shock and collapse ensues, with a rapid feeble pulse, cold hands and feet, and clammy sweating. The antidotes for acid poisoning are liberal doses of milk of magnesia, milk, soapy water, or egg whites. Hot-water sponges and moist heat applied to the throat may make breathing easier. Hot moist applications on the abdominal area relieve stomach pains.

Burns particularly from sulphuric and nitric acids, can cause serious damage to the skin. The burned area should be washed immediately with diluted baking soda solution (4 tablespoons of baking soda in a quart of water) and then bathed continuously with the soda solution for some time. *See also* POISONING; and specific names of acids.

ACIDOSIS. *See* DIABETES.

ACNE, a chronic inflammatory disorder of the sebaceous (oil) glands of the skin, usually resulting in surface eruptions. These eruptions, caused by the overactivity and blocking of the tiny glands and hair follicles just below the skin surface, include whiteheads, blackheads, and pimples. The surrounding area becomes inflamed and develops pus, which may break through the skin or form cysts. The skin becomes toughened. The forehead, cheeks, nose, and chin are most frequently affected, though the acne may spread to the shoulders, chest, or back.

More common among boys, acne usually occurs between the ages of twelve and twenty, beginning just before puberty and ending with adulthood.

Acne is not contagious, and does not spread beyond the skin, but it may leave pitting and scarring disfigurement. Since acne affects adolescents, who are often very sensitive about their appearance, even the mildest cases should be treated as soon as the first signs appear.

Physicians stress in treatment good personal hygiene, balanced diet, avoidance of offending foods, and regular bowel habits. Mild cases are frequently benefited by washing the face with hot water and a good soap

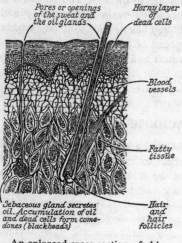

An enlarged cross section of skin tissue showing sweat glands and hair growth.

two or three time a day, using a rough washcloth or complexion brush. At night the massaging of a skin lotion or cream into the affected areas may be prescribed, with removal the next morning by the usual washing of hot water and soap. This tends to cause a mild peeling of the skin and opens plugged pores. Greases and creams, other than those prescribed by a doctor, should be avoided since they may increase the oiliness of the skin and intensify the acne. Shampooing of the scalp once or twice a week with a special lotion may also be recommended.

Many specialists advise that certain drugs and foods be avoided, such as iodides, including "iodized" salt, bromides and sedatives; chocolate in any form, nuts, cheese, shellfish or sea fish which contain iodine, oatmeal, all pork products, malted drinks, milk, eggs, spinach, and excessive amounts of fats and sweets. If a person with acne notices that foods other than those tested tend to aggravate the condition, these too should be eliminated from the diet. If woolen or rough clothing worn next to the skin aggravates itching it should be avoided. Plenty of water, sufficient sleep, and adequate exercise help keep the skin healthy. The acne areas should not be scratched, picked, or rubbed. Squeezing or irritating blackheads or pimples may spread the infection.

In some cases, a focus of infection in the teeth, sinuses, or tonsils, or a menstrual or glandular disorder may contribute to the acne, and these possibilities should be checked by a doctor.

In more stubborn cases of acne, other methods of treatment include vitamins, particularly vitamin A, vaccines, ultraviolet light, and peeling procedures. Glandular substances have been useful in some cases, and x-ray treatments, given by a dermatologist, have often been effective in extremely difficult cases. *See also* Chapter 20, "Diseases of the Skin."

ACNE ROSACEA, a skin disease similar to common acne. The face is flushed, usually about the nose, though redness may spread to the forehead and neck. Small dilated blood vessels then appear and later tiny pimples develop on the flushed areas, which are more superficial than in acne and do not leave scars. Treatment usually consists of a bland diet and the elimination of alcohol, coffee, tea, nuts, eggs, extremely hot or cold foods, and fried, highly seasoned, or rich foods.

ACONITE, a brownish-orange drug derived from the root of monkshood. Formerly it was used to slow the action of the heart, reduce temperature, and to relieve pain. It is rarely used today.

Aconite poisoning causes a tingling sensation in the mouth, burning pain in the stomach and severe vomiting, feeble pulse and slower breathing rate, and a cold wet skin. The poisoned person should be put to bed immediately, given a tablespoon of mustard in a glass of water for an emetic, and kept warm with hot-water bottles and massage. Plenty of hot coffee should be given and the doctor called immediately. *See also* POISONING.

ACOUSTIC NERVE, the eighth cranial nerve, is related to the sense of balance and hearing. Symptoms of some neurologic diseases associated with it are varying degrees of loss of hearing, ringing in the ears, disturbances of equilibrium, and dizziness or auditory vertigo.

ACRIFLAVINE, an orange-yellowish crystalline substance, one of a group of acridine dyes obtained from coal tar. Acriflavine was widely used as an antiseptic during World War I, and also in the treatment of gonorrheal urethritis, but since the development of the sulfa drugs and penicillin it is seldom used. *See also* ANTISEPTICS; GONORRHEA.

ACRODYNIA, disease that occurs in children, usually between four months and three years of age. Pain-ful red swollen hands and feet, muscular pains that make movement difficult, loss of energy, and general mental and physical sluggishness are the chief symptoms. Acrodynia is also called "pink disease" because of a rash which so colors the skin. A dietary deficiency is believed to be responsible. Acrodynia is not contagious and may persist for months, but usually clears up under medical care.

ACROMEGALY, a chronic condition in which the extremities and some soft parts of the body continue to grow after normal growth has stopped. The jaws and mouth, the nose, and the hands and feet are most often affected. The condition results from excessive action of the anterior part of the pituitary gland, which secretes the special substance, or hormone, which ordinarily brings about normal growth during childhood and youth. A related condition is giantism, in which overgrowth affects all parts of the body.

The first symptom of acromegaly is enlargement of the soft tissues, which may include the lips, tongue, ears, and nose. This is closely followed by excessive growth in associated bones, such as the lower jaw and the hands and feet. Gradually the face assumes a gross appearance, the hands become pawlike, and enlargement of the vocal cords deepens the voice. The entire body begins to show hair growth. The function of the sex glands is disturbed and, contrary to popular myth, the sexual power of the acromegalic is impaired rather than heightened.

Women who have the disease rarely bear children.

Since the symptoms of acromegaly are evident after normal growth has been reached, they can rarely be detected until postadolescence. Overactivity of the pituitary gland's growth stimulation, when it occurs in a person still in the normal growing years, produces giantism. Sometimes it stops at a point, permitting the person affected to live normally. Occasionally a single part of the body, such as a finger or toe, may grow to giant proportions. Generally, however, giantism progresses to a stage of increasing weakness and finally is fatal.

Male giants are more common than female giants. Usually the limit of such growth is well short of eight feet. However, the so-called Alton giant, named Robert Wadlow, measured more than eight feet, and some eight-footers have been recorded. Such people usually have tremendous appetites and eat enormous quantities of food.

Pituitary overactivity, with respect to growth, can sometimes be brought under control by x-ray. Sometimes surgery to remove part of the gland and eliminate the excess has been beneficial. The condition may be regulated by action affecting other glands closely related to the pituitary. Drugs, such as estrogen, act internally and depress the growth of hormone functions. Other drugs containing testosterone are also used in association with hormonal treatment.

The nervous system may be involved with growth, and changes in one or more parts of it may be responsible for certain instances of overgrowth. Sometimes great size is attained without any detectable glandular disorder. See also ENDOCRINE GLANDS; PITUITARY; and chapter 19, "Endocrine Glands."

ACTH, an abbreviation of adrenocorticotrophic hormone. The adrenocorticotrophic hormone of the pituitary acts upon the adrenal gland to produce cortisone. ACTH is not manufactured synthetically, as is cortisone, but is secured from the pituitary glands of cattle and hogs, and has been widely used in the relief of rheumatoid arthritis and of pain provoked by a variety of other diseases. The hormone is also used in a number of other conditions. See also CORTISONE.

ACTINOMYCES, a species of fungus responsible for actinomycosis, a serious disease of cattle. Meat infected with this disease is always condemned and the animals destroyed. Although rarely, actinomycosis occasionally attacks human beings. See also ACTINOMYCOSIS.

ACTINOMYCOSIS, a parasitic, infectious, inoculable disease affecting cattle and hogs and sometimes human beings. Fungi of the actinomyces, or ray fungus group, were found originally in a disease of cattle known as lumpy jaw. Actinomycosis occurs most frequently in agricultural workers and those who work around barns where cattle are kept. The infection is usually acquired by handling or chewing straw used by infected cattle, or by inhaling dust of the ray fungus.

The organisms are found in the mucous membranes of the mouth, around decayed teeth and in diseased tonsils. The head and neck are the most common locations for the disease. Actinomycosis begins as a swelling of the jaw; the skin becomes dark red with a lumpy uneven surface, and soon abscesses form which discharge pus. As long as the condition is confined to the face and neck it does not interfere with general health and there is little pain. Less frequently the disease involves the lungs or thoracic region, a result of inhaling infected material from the mouth.

The most effective treatment for this condition includes x-ray therapy and thorough surgical drainage of the abscesses, as well as use of sulfonamides and antibiotics.

ACUTE ILLNESS, ACUTE PAIN. In describing an illness the term acute indicates a relatively abrupt onset with evident symptoms and limited duration. Acute illness is distinguished from chronic illness, in which pain or discomfort are present at a less intense level for an indefinite period of time. Referring to pain, the term indicates severity and may suggest suddenness.

ADAM'S APPLE, a boxlike structure located at the entrance to the trachea, or windpipe, which encloses and protects the two vocal cords. Because of its proximity to the thyroid gland which lies independently in front of this structure, it is scientifically known as the thyroid cartilage. It is easily found in the middle of the neck, and is especially noticeable in males because of the acute angle which is formed by the junction of the two side walls. In females, the

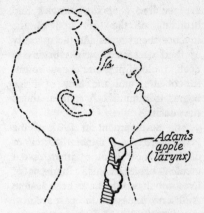

Cut away drawing showing position of the Adam's apple.

Adam's apple is less noticeable, as the angle formed by the side walls is flatter and there is extra fat in the neck.

ADDICTION, known to medical science also as pharmacopsychosis, is the habitual use of alcohol, drugs, and similar substances. *See also* DRUG ADDICTION.

ADDISON'S DISEASE. When the two adrenal glands, each of which lies on a kidney, become infected or damaged in any way the resulting condition is Addison's disease, named after a British physician who identified the disorder. Although the severity varies, the disease is always serious. The adrenal glands are so vital that death comes quickly if they are completely destroyed or removed.

Damage to the adrenal glands, whether by disease or injury, produces major bodily changes. Both salt and water are gradually lost and the total supply of fluid circulating in the blood and within the cells themselves declines. The first symptoms are feebleness of the muscles and bronzing of the skin and of the mucous membranes. As the quantity of fluid decreases, weight begins to decline, blood pressure drops, vomiting occurs, and the flow of urine begins to diminish. A state of shock may ensue.

The development in 1927 of the extract from the adrenal cortex of cattle is one of the great recent medical achievements. Hundreds of lives which would have been lost to Addison's disease in the past are now saved. Only 300 to 400 cases are reported annually in the United States. Sometimes activity of the gland is impaired without its being damaged entirely. This condition usually is given treatment similar to that for Addison's disease.

In chronic cases of Addison's disease, systematic therapy employing the cortisone group of drugs has restored patients to a state of well-being and normal living. Adrenal insufficiency to the point of crisis must be prevented, if possible. This requires careful management by the doctor, and education of the patient as to the specific part he himself can play in guarding against such crises. *See also* ADRENAL GLANDS.

ADDUCTOR, a muscle which draws a part of the body toward the median line and affects, for instance, fingers, toes, thighs, and hips.

ADENITIS, an inflammation of the lymph glands which occurs in the neck, armpit, groin, and other parts of the body. The area is generally swollen and tender.

The condition is usually a sign of infection in the affected area. A sore throat or tonsillitis may cause inflammation of the lymph glands of the neck, an infection of the arm or hand may involve the lymph glands in the armpit, and an infection in the leg might produce an adenitis in the groin. The lymph glands and lymph vessels act as a barrier against spread of these local infections. *See also* LYMPHATIC SYSTEM.

ADENOIDECTOMY, the surgical removal of the adenoids.

ADENOIDS, enlargements of the band of lymphoid tissue situated in the back of the nose where the nasal opening joins the throat. Under normal conditions the air breathed is warmed, moistened, and filtered as it passes through the nose. The adenoids, the tonsils, and the lymphoid tissue of which they are a part give additional protection by screening out infectious germs. When adenoids become inflamed or infected they enlarge, and because of their location obstruct the passage of air from the nose into the throat. Sometimes this engorgement may also obstruct the openings of the Eustachian tubes and interfere with the passage of air through the tubes into the ears. This condition is one of the most common causes of ear infection and sinusitus in children.

Infected adenoids, if untreated, usually remain enlarged and cause other disturbances. Breathing in through the mouth which remains open, and the air inspired is not filtered and warmed as in nasal breathing. Colds and other infections are common, appetite decreases, and listlessness develops. Characteristic structural changes of the face may take place.

The mouth hangs open and the upper teeth become prominent and give the face a rabbit-like, dull expression.

A child with troublesome adenoids is apt to suffer from disturbed sleep and bed wetting, and will often awaken irritable and peevish. Hearing is often impaired.

In addition, infected adenoids are usually associated with infected tonsils and the child becomes inattentive and seems dull. Therefore, adenoids which are repeatedly inflamed must receive medical attention.

Early mild cases can be controlled with antibiotics which usually will prevent more serious complications, such as deafness, kidney disease, rheumatic fever. However, the removal of diseased and enlarged adenoids and tonsils is ordinarily recommended by the doctor. The operation, though simple and short, is most effective. *See also* CHILD CARE.

ADENOMA, a form of tumor which occurs in the cellular tissue of a gland. It is usually treated according to the organ involved.

ADENOSIS, any disorder of the glands, particularly, however, one that involves the lymph nodes.

ADHESIECTOMY, scientific term for surgical removal of adhesions.

ADHESIONS, generally the cohesion of adjacent organs or surfaces which are normally separate. When tissues heal, for example, fibrous scars are formed which cause the segments to adhere to each other. Following operations within the abdomen, adhesions sometimes cause pains when pulled or stretched because fibrous tissue is not elastic.

ADIPOSIS, corpulence or obesity; an excessive accumulation, either general or local, of fat in the body.

ADNEXA, the adjunct parts of any organ. Adnexa uteri, for example, are the ovaries and Fallopian tubes, and adnexa oculi are the lids of the eyes.

ADOLESCENCE, the period in human growth between the ending of childhood and the attainment of full physical development. During this period anatomic development and glandular changes culminate in puberty, at about the age of twelve for girls and fourteen for boys. In girls, menstruation begins at this time, although it may occur a year or two earlier or later. The breasts develop, the pelvis broadens, and the body becomes more rounded, acquiring distinctive female characteristics. In boys, hair grows on the face, sexual organs mature, and the larynx enlarges, causing the voice to "break."

In both sexes the physical changes are associated with emotional and mental development. The rapid growth at this time is likely to make heavy demands on the adolescent, and adjustment to the glandular changes as well as the whole growth process is often difficult. Reactions to situations are apt to be keener and more immediate; feelings, whether of joy or depression, to be more intense than previously. The boy may become concerned that he is not growing as fast as his friends, or that his voice cracks, or by the appearance of hair on his face and body. The girl may regard with embarrassment the beginning of menstruation and its recurrence every month.

Parents, during this period, may be alarmed at what appears to be erratic growth and rapidly shifting moods in their children who want love and attention one minute and "to be left alone" the next. However, if the proper foundation of love and security has been laid during infancy and childhood, the adolescent years can be productive and rewarding for both parents and children. By gradually preparing the child for the physical changes that will take place, including giving him the necessary information about sex and reproduction, the shock of the onset of awakening maturity can be softened.

Even with understanding and sympathy, the adolescent will often still be subject to tensions, rebellion, and conflicting emotions. The period of adolescence may demand a large measure of patience and tolerance from the parents. Faced with hostile parental attitudes, the growing child may develop feelings of insecurity that find understandable but often undesirable outlets. While the adolescent may rebel against authority in the home, acceptance and approval by his group is of paramount importance to him. Few influences will shake him from conformity to teenage standards and values. The change from dependence upon parents and home to identification with his peer group is a natural step in the process of maturing.

Hero worship, romantic attachments that may ripen and wilt in rapid succession, and an intense desire for privacy are normal behavior manifestations of the adolescent.

Unless the phase becomes too intense or prolonged, authorities on child development consider that parents should not intervene since ordinarily time and growing maturity will limit or terminate it.

The proper attitudes on the part of the parents can be of immeasurable help in assuring that the period of adolescence is a significant and meaningful step toward maturity. *See also* Chapter 10, "The Problems of Adolescence."

ADOPTION. Adopting a child is often a remarkably satisfying solution for a couple who want a family and are unable to have children. However, any husband and wife considering adopting a child should give the matter thorough and mature thought; it is obviously a far more serious question than whether or not to buy a car or fur coat.

The decision to adopt a child is only the initial step. After the couple have registered with a state-licensed adoption agency, it may be months or even years before the agency is able to present them with a child to consider for their own. Every legal adoption agency makes an exhaustive examination into the husband and wife's background, economic situation, religious beliefs, personality, general home life, physical condition, mental capacity, and other areas. Children up for adoption have received an equally thorough examination. For various reasons, not every couple is eligible to adopt a child, nor every homeless child adoptable. The agency attempts to place the child in a home most mutually congenial to the prospective foster parents and to the child.

Prospective foster parents should try not to have rigid ideas regarding the type of child they would like. A couple who have decided, for example, that they want a curly-headed two-year-old girl are only impeding their chance of getting any child. The agency would like to feel that the child is desired for qualities more important than curliness of hair and, more practically speaking, the number of curly-headed two-year-old girls may be limited. Whenever possible, the agency will try to match the child and couple in as many ways as it can. Before legal adoption papers are finally taken out, there is a trial period during which the couple have the child in their home and are able to decide whether or not this is the child they want and the agency decides whether placement is suitable.

At the present time, the demand for children far exceeds the supply of adoptable children available. Because of this scarcity, there have sprung up all over the country black- or gray-market adoption agencies which financially exploit the often very intense desire of a husband and wife to have a child as soon as possible. Anyone who adopts a child through such illegal channels is taking a tremendous risk; since the black-market agencies operate outside legal standards regarding adoptability of a child and may have false or little or no information about the child, the couple could conceivably get a mentally or physically defective child. Prospective foster parents should always deal with a legal adoption agency whose primary goal is to bring together a couple and a child under the best possible circumstances.

A happier and more fortunate outgrowth of the problem of scarcity of adoptable children is the increasing number of foreign-born children who are being adopted. This possibility should be considered by couples desirous of adopting a child.

For further information, write to the U. S. Government Printing Office and ask for the U. S. Public Health Service's pamphlet on adoption, which gives all the legal requirements in the various states.

ADRENALIN, the trade name for epinephrine, is a hormone produced by the adrenal glands. It was first isolated by a Japanese scientist, Jokichi Takamine, in 1901.

This drug stimulates heart action, elevates blood pressure, constricts blood vessels, and tends to stop bleeding in wounds. When injected into the body with other medicines, it slows their absorption into the blood stream. Adrenalin is used to relax the muscles in the bronchial tubes, thus making it an invaluable aid in the treatment of severe asthmatic attacks. It is also used extensively to counteract hypersensitivity and allergic reactions. *See also* ALLERGY; ASTHMA; HAY FEVER.

ADRENAL GLANDS. Lying above each kidney is a small body called an adrenal gland, the outer part or cortex of which encloses the inner part, or medulla. The adrenals are a significant part of the system of endocrine glands which control and coordinate, by means of specialized secretions, many of the body's most essential functions.

So essential to life are the adrenals, particularly the cortex, that when they are removed experimentally from an animal it dies within a few days. Similarly destruction of the adrenals by infection or injury causes death.

The medulla produces a secretion or hormone called epinephrine, suprarenin, or adrenalin. This substance, supplied to the body through the blood stream, prepares the body physically when emergencies are encountered; breathing and pulse are speeded, blood pressure is raised, the sugar content of the blood is increased, and the muscles are temporarily strengthened. Adrenalin also relaxes the bronchial muscles and is used to relieve the symptoms of asthma and hay fever.

The adrenal cortex secretes many hormones, including cortisone, dihydrocortisone, and aldosterone. The cortical hormones are significant in the basic defenses of the body against various infections, poisons, and other invasions or threats. They are also concerned with the regulation of the supply of salt and water and the maintenance of correct blood pressure. Injury or damage to the adrenal cortex, which causes deficiency of its secretions, produces a serious condition called Addison's disease, which may be fatal, although its severity varies. *See also* ADDISON'S DISEASE.

AEDES AEGYPTI, a species of mosquito which transmits yellow fever. This insect is also called "yellow Jack" or yellow fever mosquito. If the mosquito bites a person with yellow fever during the first three days of illness, it may pick up the organisms which cause the infection in man. Once this has occurred, the mosquito retains the ability to transmit these organisms and thus the infection to other human beings. *See also* MOSQUITO; YELLOW FEVER.

AERO OTITIS MEDIA, a painful condition of the ear caused by inflammation of the middle ear. This disorder affects some people during changes of altitude—for example, when descending in airplanes from high altitudes. Symptoms like congestion and painful inflammation may be followed by temporary or permanent impairment of hearing. Relief usually follows quickly. However, if the pain continues and is not relieved by simple ordinary medication, a physician should be consulted.

Aero otitis media develops from the pressure difference of the air, which causes the eardrums to protrude into the inside. The Eustachian tube, which extends from the back of the nasal passage to the middle ear, may thus be obstructed and not open frequently enough to balance the difference in pressure between the atmosphere and the middle ear. If discomfort is caused by changes in altitude, physicians advise lusty yawning, hard swallowing, opening the mouth wide, or chewing gum. All these measures help to open the Eustachian tubes.

AEROBIC refers to the need of free oxygen or air required for life. The term is used in connection with bacteria that demand atmospheric oxygen to survive. Anaerobic bacteria live only without oxygen.

AEROPHAGIA, a condition caused by swallowing an excessive amount of air either consciously or unconsciously. It is apt to cause belching and stomach discomfort and is most common in children and hysterical persons.

AFFECT (psychology), a mood, a feeling, or an emotion as it influences a mental state or idea.

AFFERENT NERVES, sensory nerves that transmit impulses from the outside to the central nervous system.

AFTERBIRTH, or placenta, a tissue which carries nutrition and oxygen to the child, while it is in the mother's womb. Together with the umbilical cord and membranes it is expelled from the uterus after the child has been born; hence, "afterbirth."

AFTERPAINS, spasmodic cramps in the lower abdomen which resemble labor pains, though are not as severe, and may occur for two or three days after childbirth. These pains develop from the efforts of the uterus to contract to normal size again, and are stronger in women who have previously borne children. *See also* PREGNANCY AND PRENATAL CARE.

AGALACTIA, the condition following childbirth when the secretion of breast milk is absent in the mother.

AGAR, a form of seaweed, Malay type, which is used in medicine to provide bulk in the material excreted from the bowel. Sometimes drugs, mineral oil, or petrolatum are added to the agar. Also called agar-agar, the dried gelatinous substance is used in bacteriological research as a medium for breeding and preserving microorganisms.

AGGLUTINATION, a chemical reaction in which cells, such as bacteria or blood corpuscles, suspended in liquid collect into clumps when the cell suspension is treated with serum immunized against cells of the same kind and species.

AGNOSIA, lack of power of perception or recognition in one or more of the senses.

AGORAPHOBIA, morbid fear of open unenclosed places; as opposed to claustrophobia. *See also* CLAUSTROPHOBIA.

AGRANULOCYTOSIS, an acute fever-producing disease characterized by high fever, ulcerative lesions of the mucous membrane in the mouth, throat, and other areas, and a great reduction in the granular white blood cells. The disease is fairly rare, particularly in children, and occurs more often in females than males.

Excessive white blood cells called leukemia is extremely serious. Even more serious may be a sudden decrease in the number of white blood cells or their disappearance from the blood. The white blood cells are the chief defense against infection, and their sudden decrease or disappearance from the blood can lead to an overwhelming attack by dangerous germs which can cause death in a day or occasionally in a few hours.

In agranulocytosis or granulocytopenia the number of red blood cells is normal in amount, but the white blood cells may drop from 7,500 per cubic millimeter to 1,000 or even much less. Since, as a result, the white blood cells are so many fewer in number than the red blood cells, examination of one specimen after another may fail to indicate the presence of even a few white blood cells.

The exact cause of this condition is not definitely known, although recently it has become apparent that reaction of the body to various drugs or sensitivity to certain toxic agents may be responsible. Many cases have been reported in which agranulocytosis occurred after the taking of a drug called amidopyrine or Pyramidon, and also in association with various coal-tar remedies and sulfonamide drugs. Apparently the bone marrow of the body is attacked, so that it cannot form the white blood cells in the usual manner. Moreover, in some cases, the condition develops a cyclic character and at regular intervals the number of white blood cells decreases and then gradually increases.

Because the body is no longer protected against infection, one of the first signs is severe ulceration of the throat and destruction of the tissue of the gums and tonsils. Other parts of the body may be attacked, and infections of the kidneys, heart, or even the skin become apparent.

The severity of agranulocytosis is reflected by the fact that about 75 per cent of those affected die. Treatment of the disease includes—most essential—immediate rest in bed, cleaning of the infected areas, drinking fluids, and antibiotics like penicillin or terramycin to control infection which develops easily in the absence of white blood cells. Any remedies must be prescribed by the doctor, in conjunction with regular examination of the blood to indicate the progress or remission of the disease. *See also* GRANULOCYTOPENIA.

AGUE, the former name of malaria. It also describes chills associated with intermittent fever and various other conditions.

Brass founders' ague, common among brass workers, is an occupational disease with symptoms of intermittent fever. Partial ague is a painful affliction, limited to some part of the body—as, for instance, brow ague or facial ague, which is intermittent neuralgia of the brow or face. *See also* TIC DOULOUREUX.

AIRSICKNESS. *See* MOTION SICKNESS.

AKINETIC refers to loss or impairment of muscular action and power of movement from any cause. *See also* MUSCLE.

ALBINO, a person in whom melanin, the dark pigment which gives color to skin, hair, and part of the eye, is absent. The hair of the albino is platinum blond, and the skin is pink, since the blood circulating in the skin capillaries shows through the skin. The eyes have a distinctive pinkish hue because pigment is absent from the iris and the blood vessels are reflected through the pupil. Sometimes this lack of pigmentation of the eye may cause defective vision and create extreme sensitivity to light, and therefore direct exposure to the sun should be avoided by albinos. Ordinarily an albino has less energy and is more delicate than other persons. While the condition is abnormal in these respects, albinism is not considered a disease. It is hereditary and if both parents carry the albino gene their offspring are certain to be albinos. The condition, however, tends to be recessive and about one person in 10,000 is affected. When albinism is present in a family, a physician can usually estimate the chance of its recurrence in future generations.

ALBUMIN, a clear thick substance soluble in water and coagulated by heat, is one of a group of protein substances, the chief element of most animal and vegetable tissues, and the most significant part of blood serum or plasma. The largest component of egg white is albumen.

Digested foods provide proteins which are distributed by the blood to the rest of the body to sustain growth, and then absorbed in the kidneys and redistributed through the body.

Human serum albumin is a commercial preparation, used in the treatment of shock and to supplement insufficient proteins in the blood serum. *See also* PROTEIN.

ALBUMINURIA, the presence of albumin in the urine which can be easily detected by examination. It is an early sign that the kidneys are not functioning properly. Sometimes, however, albuminuria may occur temporarily as a consequence of a high protein diet or following strenuous exercise. *See also* KIDNEYS.

ALCOHOL. Ordinarily ethyl alcohol refers to a clear colorless fluid which is fit for human consumption when diluted. Alcohol is inflammable and has a characteristic taste and odor. It is obtained by distilling fermented solutions of sugar, grain, or starchy substances, or it may be prepared artificially. Whiskey, gin, rum, beer, ale, stout, wine, and brandy are some of the alcoholic beverages in common use.

Alcohol can act as a drug, a beverage, or a poison. Applied to the skin, it has a cooling and refreshing effect. In solutions of 70 per cent or over, other types of alcohol are used as antiseptics in medicine.

Small doses of alcohol are stimulating and produce a temporary sense of warmth and well-being. Alcohol dilates the blood vessels of the skin and brings an increased flow of warm blood to the skin surfaces. However, the blood in the body is cooled off by this action and body temperature drops. Alcohol also depresses the central nervous system, and acts as an anesthetic upon the cerebral cortex, which controls behavior. When a person brightens up after a drink or speaks and acts more freely than usual, he does so because the restraining influences which he usually exercises have been diminished. Moderate drinking, even as a daily habit, is practiced by many people without harmful effects. However, excessive amounts of alcohol may act as a poison and seriously damage the body.

Alcohol is quickly burnt up in the body and has little food value. The body does not have a way of storing alcohol, and excessive amounts irritate the stomach and cause chronic gastritis. Constant excessive drinking may also damage the liver, the kidneys, and other body organs. The central nervous system becomes depressed, and with continued indulgence the entire system is devitalized. Coordination of muscles and nerves is diminished, speech becomes thicker, gait and sense of balance are impaired, judgment suffers, mental changes are apparent. Constant excessive use of alcohol often leads to stupor, delirium tremens, or other manifestations of serious damage. *See also* ALCOHOLISM; DELIRIUM TREMENS.

ALCOHOLISM, poisoning by alcohol, or the severe results of prolonged and excessive consumption of alcohol. The alcoholic has a compulsive need for alcohol and can abstain only with great difficulty or not at all. Usually he is totally unable to help himself out of his situation. The causes of alcoholism are deeply rooted in the varying needs and insecurities of the individual. There is no such thing as an "alcoholic type." An alcoholic may drink steadily day after day or he may have short periods of abstinence followed by a drinking bout.

The effects of alcoholism are serious, both mentally and physically. The compulsive drinker gradually loses his desire for food and may develop dangerous malnutrition with all its varying symptoms. The liver may become enlarged, the heart damaged, and other organs affected. The central nervous system is depressed, and a steady and progressive disintegration of personality takes place.

If alcoholism continues, the person will eventually develop delirium tremens, in which he loses all sense of time, space, and surroundings and is racked by terrifying visual hallucinations. During this time, many alcoholics have seriously injured themselves in their efforts to escape from their hallucinations. The condition lasts for from three to seven days and requires emergency treatment. Afterward the alcoholic will usually revert to his usual state. Death may result from an attack of delirium tremens if hospitalization and competent medical care are not secured.

Hospitalization is desirable in treating the compulsive drinker who wishes to be cured. Physical factors are a significant part of alcoholism, and treatment includes both medical as well as psychological care. The influence of the endocrine glands, hormones, metabolism, and diet on alcoholism is being investigated. New tranquilizing drugs, such as chlorpromazine, and Miltown, when used with discretion, have been helpful, and a drug called Antabuse is sometimes used to condition the alcoholic against drinking. After the first stages of recovery have been reached, the alcoholic may respond to psychiatric treatment. Group therapy, in which victims of a common affliction meet and talk, has proved helpful.

Among the many organizations dedicated to helping the alcoholic, the best known is Alcoholics Anonymous, a group of men and women who have overcome alcoholism, and who actively help others to do so. Their sympathetic understanding of the problems of the compulsive drinker, based upon their own experiences, and their philosophy of mutual help have proved to be one of the most effective adjuncts in treating alcoholism. Alcoholics Anonymous has branches in almost every city in the United States and in many countries throughout the world.

The combined efforts of medicine, psychiatry, and organizations like Alcholics Anonymous have brought about an increasing rate of recovery in what was once considered a hopeless problem. *See also* ANTABUSE; DELIRIUM TREMENS; and Chapter 22, "Mental Illness."

ALEXIA, sometimes called word blindness, a form of aphasia in which the victim is unable to recognize or understand printed words. The difficulty may result from damage to the brain by disease or injury.

ALIMENTARY CANAL, or digestive tract of the body, is a long muscular track or tube which begins at the mouth and ends at the anus. The intestines and stomach hold, digest, and prepare food for absorption into the blood stream, and eliminate the indigestible residue. By this route the body rids itself of any excess accumulations of mineral substances.

Much of the alimentary canal consists of a series of tubes and chambers through which the food passes, and also of thousands of small glands which pour their juices into it to help break up the food and prepare it for absorption into the blood. Food enters through the mouth where it is chewed and ground to enable it to pass through the pharynx and the esophagus, and then to the stomach where active digestion begins. The stomach is lined with many glands which make the gastric juices necessary for splitting foodstuffs into their simpler components. The outer layer of the stomach consists of strong muscle fibers, which make slow churning movements during digestion. Digestion is completed in the small intestines. This coiled structure is some 20 to 30 feet long, and is entirely lined by minute, finger-like projections, called villi, which carry nutriment to the blood. Meanwhile digestive juices from the pancreas, and bile from the liver are sent to the small intestine to help break up the fats and starches and further split the protein substances. Residual matter then proceeds to the large intestine, a tube approximately 5 to 6 feet long and 3 inches wide, where it undergoes further alteration before it empties into the rectum and is eliminated through the anal canal. *See also* DIGESTION; INTESTINES; STOMACH; and Chapter 18, "Disorders of the Digestive System and Diet in Digestive Disorders."

ALKALEMIA is a condition in which there is a decrease of hydrogen concentration in the blood and an increased alkalinity of the blood.

ALKALI, derived from the Arabic word meaning potash, is a term applied to chemical substances which combine with acids to form salts, and with oils or fatty acids to form soluble soaps. One of the most common alkalies is sodium bicarbonate, or baking soda which is often taken internally to neutralize an excess of acid in the stomach. Other common alkalies are lye, ammonia, and washing soda. These are corrosive poisons and frequent contact with them, even in the dilute form of soaps and detergents, may cause skin irritations. *See also* POISONING.

ALKALINITY, the quality of being alkaline.

ALKALOID, one of a number of organic substances, some highly poisonous, which not only possess alkaline properties but contain nitrogen. It also designates a group of basic nitrogenous organic compounds, derived from plants and animals, used in such drugs as caffeine, codeine, morphine, cocaine, nicotine, quinine, and strychnine.

ALKALOSIS. A relatively high bicarbonate content in the blood or body fluids, as opposed to acidosis, incites a tendency to alkalemia. The condition is scientifically termed alkalosis.

ALLERGY, a reaction to a particular substance by a person sensitive to that substance. The condition was originally called hypersensitivity, but allergy is now the term most frequently used.

Allergy is among the most common of all human disorders. It can be caused by an innumerable variety of substances, including pollens, foods, dust, animal dander, drugs, cosmetics, toilet articles, dyes, chemicals, and fabrics. Asthma and hay fever and other major allergic disturbances affect a tenth of the population; and a much greater number of persons are subject to more limited allergies such as poison ivy, which is so common that it is rarely recognized as an allergy. Allergic symptoms may result from substances inhaled (dust, pollen, and animal dander), eaten or drunk (foods), touched (soap, wool, and cosmetics), and injected (insect bites). Sunlight and heat or cold may aggravate allergic response, as may bacteria, microorganisms, or other large parasites in the intestines.

When the disruptive substance enters the body, the body reacts just as it does when attacked by virus or bacteria. It protects itself by setting up antibodies to neutralize any further attacks. These antibodies which the body has produced attach to tissue surfaces, and when the allergen, or allergy-producing agent, again enters the body it is believed that the antibodies separate from the tissue and attack the invading substance. A very slight tissue damage results which apparently causes the release of histamines, chemical substances, which are carried by the circulation to skin and mucous membranes, with subsequent allergy symptoms.

As can be seen, two conditions are necessary to produce an allergic response. (1) The person must be first sensitized to a particular substance; he may not even notice the sensitivity. (2) A second exposure to the substance must occur, which then provokes the allergic symptoms. The reaction may be localized, if only a small area of skin is exposed to the substance, or it may be generalized, if the substance has entered the system. One part of the body may have a greater reaction than another because tissues in that part are more sensitive. The reason why a sensitivity to a particular substance exists in one person and not in another is extremely complex and a matter not entirely understood. Probably an individual structural or functional weakness is involved, a theory supported by the fact that, in some cases, allergies may be inherited. The adrenal glands probably contribute to allergic responses, and emotional attitudes also seem to be associated.

A wide variety of symptoms are caused by allergies. Since many of these symptoms are also characteristic of other disorders, in treating the condition it is necessary that the diagnosis definitely establish the cause to be an allergen. Hay fever affects the mucous membranes of the upper respiratory tract, the nose and the eyes. Asthma primarily involves the lower part of the respiratory system. Some allergies produce digestive upsets, severe headaches, dizziness, and nausea. Sometimes a skin change, as in hives, eczema, and erythema, is the only symptom.

Food allergies are relatively rare and are almost always caused by the protein in the food. Foods which most frequently produce allergic reactions are milk, eggs, shellfish, peas, and beans, and hives is the usual symptom. In infants, milk, egg white, corn, oats, wheat, and barley are most often responsible, and the allergic reaction is commonly severe eczema. A great many chemical substances can act as allergens. Although skin change is the usual symptom, cramps, ringing in the ears, nausea, sore throat, leg and arm pain, and fever may be present. Many women are allergic to face powder, lipstick, or other cosmetics. The number of substances to which persons can be sensitive is vast and it is often difficult to isolate the allergen.

To treat an allergy, the doctor compiles a detailed case history of the patient, including the first occurrence of the allergy, when it customarily appears, the patient's occupation, diet, cosmetics, clothing, habits, and many other small details. To establish what substance or substances are producing the sensitivity, the doctor may give the patient a patch test or a scratch test. In the patch test, small squares of absorbent gauze or cotton are dipped in various solutions containing suspected allergens and taped against the patient's skin, usually the forearm. In the scratch test, a minute quantity of possible allergens are placed in small scratches made on the arm. In both tests, the doctor watches for skin reaction to the different patches or scratches such as redness, blistering, or itching, which may indicate that the allergen has been isolated. Expert medical attention is indispensable in diagnosis and treatment, and the services of a dermatologist, or specialist in skin conditions, may be necessary. Basically treatment consists of locating the allergen and then avoiding the allergen, as much as possible. When other methods are unsuccessful, injections of minute amounts of the allergen may be given to the patient to increase his tolerance for the allergen, a process called desensitization. However, desensitization may have only a small or temporary effect.

Drugs such as the antihistamines, adrenalin, and ephedrine are often effective in relieving allergic symptoms, but do not cure the condition. In severe cases, the hormonal substances ACTH and cortisone may be used.

Allergies often appear to involve emotional factors as well as organic, and conversely the allergy may induce tensions which did not originally exist. The doctor must determine the place of these emotional factors in the patient's condition; sometimes all treatment for the condition fails until the psychological problems are uncovered and dealt with. *See also* ASTHMA; ECZEMA; FOOD ALLERGY; HAY FEVER; HIVES; and Chapter 21, "Allergy."

ALOES, a brownish yellow powder, obtained from the dried juice of the leaves of the aloe, a plant found in the West Indies and Africa. Aloes is used in chronic constipation for its stimulating effect on the large intestine. Large doses taken too frequently may irritate the kidneys.

ALOPECIA, loss of hair that may follow a number of different illnesses. The loss of hair may be partial or total, premature or senile. If hair falls in patches, the condition is known as alopecia areata. Alopecia cachectica is baldness as a result of general malnutrition. *See also* BALDNESS.

ALUM, a crystalline substance, colorless and odorless, which dissolves in water; an effective emetic in cases of poisoning, but seldom given internally. Although alum is strongly astringent, its use as an after-shaving styptic is not recommended. Any of the packaged stringent surgical powders which can be used in small amounts as needed and applied directly to a bleeding point are preferable. *See also* POISONING.

ALUMINUM ACETATE, an astringent used chiefly in a mild 5 per cent concentration in Burow's solution for wet dressings for minor skin disorders, boils, and in the treatment

of erysipelas. Aluminum acetate also brings soothing relief in the initial stages of sunburn.

ALUMINUM HYDROXIDE, a white, gluelike substance used chiefly to neutralize stomach acidity. In the treatment of peptic ulcer it acts as a healing agent, relieving pain and controlling hemorrhage. When the liquid preparation is not tolerable, aluminum hydroxide may be obtained in gel or tablet form, which is the dried aluminum hydroxide gel. *See also* ANTACID; PEPTIC ULCER.

ALUMINUM PHOSPHATE GEL, an aluminum salt, similar in action and uses to aluminum hydroxide gel but preferable when milder drugs are desirable.

ALVEOLI, the small air cells of the lung.

AMAUROSIS, loss of vision due to nervous disorders and not to any structural defect of the eye.

AMBIVALENCE, the coexistence within a person of opposite or conflicting feelings, such as love and hate. It refers to impulses, conscious or unconscious, that contradict each other and may be symptomatic of schizophrenia. *See also* SCHIZOPHRENIA.

AMEBIASIS, an infection caused by an organism called endamoeba histolytica. Amebic dysentery usually develops and occasionally the condition spreads to the liver, in which case amebic hepatitis follows.

The chief symptom of amebic dysentery is diarrhea, which becomes increasingly acute for three or four days and is accompanied by weakness, nausea, vomiting, and cramps, felt mostly on the right side of the body. Fever occurs infrequently. The infecting organism invades the body as tiny cysts which are able to resist both freezing and chlorine in the concentration usually used for purifying water. The amebae travel to the colon and infect the mucous surface of the wall, eventually creating abscesses of varying severity. The organisms may live in the intestines for months without producing serious consequences, and the infection may become widespread before any evident symptoms appear. Once the attacks of dysentery begin, they may recur at intervals and in the intervening periods the infected person will have various intestinal disturbances. If untreated the disease may cause anemia and emaciation. Treatment with emetine, iodine, terramycin, arsenical compounds, or new drugs like milibis usually produces satisfactory results. Amebic dysentery resembles bacillary dysentery and other acute intestinal infections. The diagnosis must be made on the basis of a microscopic examination of the infected person's excretions.

Amebic hepatitis, or abscess of the liver, involves pain, irregular fever, and tenderness of the liver. It occurs when amebae present in an intestinal infection migrate to the liver, though two-thirds of those with amebic hepatitis do not have dysentery. Abscesses are treated by surgical methods. *See also* HEPATITIS.

AMEBIC DYSENTERY, inflammation of the colon, caused by invasion of a single-celled parasite, endamoeba histolytica. It has been estimated that from 1.5 to 10 per cent of the population of the United States is infested with this parasite, which enters the body in contaminated food and drink. Amebic dysentery is more prevalent in economically poor areas and in hot climates. The number of persons infested in any area usually remains constant, but occasionally an epidemic occurs.

Symptoms of amebic dysentery may be mild, with only fatigue and depression, or may include constipation, nausea, slight appetite, gas, and abdominal cramps. When the organisms spread throughout the wall of the bowel, there is severe diarrhea with excretion of blood, pronounced weakness, prostration, vomiting, and pain on the right side of the abdomen. Usually fever is not present or only slight.

Recovery is slow and the condition may become chronic, with anemia and occasional occurrences of more severe diarrhea. When the dysentery is not cured, the organisms enter the liver and lungs and form abscesses.

Amebic dysentery is often difficult to control and it may be necessary to repeat the treatment. One method of management is to give the patient a dose of castor oil, followed by iodine-containing compounds for eight or ten days, with a diet of milk and milk products until the acute phase has passed. Aureomycin and terramycin have also proved effective. If the liver and lungs have been invaded, special drugs are given.

The organisms causing amebic dysentery are hard to destroy, and can be carried on fruit, vegetables, flies, cockroaches, and water. Careful personal and public cleanliness is the best means of avoiding the disease. *See also* BACILLARY DYSENTERY; DIARRHEA.

AMENORRHEA, absence of menstruation, either normal cessation or suppression. *See also* MENSTRUATION.

AMENTIA, subnormal mental development. It is mental deficiency, such as idiocy, which begins in infancy, adolescence, or is congenital. Amentia is contrasted with dementia. *See also* DEMENTIA; FEEBLE-MINDEDNESS.

AMINO ACIDS, organic compounds often called the building blocks of protein. They are absorbed into the blood from the digestive tract and distributed throughout the body to the tissues, which use them to build new proteins. Protein is essential to the living cells. The body uses amino acids to replace the parts of the body proteins which are constantly being destroyed or lost.

Amino acids are supplied primarily by meat, fish, poultry, cheese, milk, and eggs. They contain carbon, hydrogen, oxygen, and nitrogen, and sometimes sulphur. Their composition, as they are found in the food proteins, is the same as that of the amino acids present in the proteins of body tissues, although they have a different chemical construction. Some amino acids can be adequately manufactured from other materials in the body. Other amino acids cannot be manufactured within the body in sufficient quantity to supply the demands of growth and repair, and must be provided in the diet if the body is to survive. The supply of protein is considered adequate when the nitrogen balance of the body is maintained. The amino acids that are indispensable for the maintenance of nitrogen balance are arginine, histidine, lysine, leucine, isoleucine, methionine, phenylalanine, tryptophane, threonine, and valine.

Preparations of different amino acids are available commercially. These preparations contain the amino acids in the same proportions as are produced by the breakdown of proteins, and they are used to supplement the dietary nitrogen in readily assimilable form. They are essential in the treatment of severe protein deficiency, in conditions in which food is not assimilated normally, and after surgical operations which involve the alimentary tract. *See also* NUTRITION; PROTEIN.

AMINOPHYLLINE, or theophylline ethylenediamine, a yellowish white powder with a bitter taste generally used in conditions affecting the heart in pulmonary congestion and in the treatment of asthma. This drug may be given by slow injection into the veins and occasionally is prescribed as a rectal suppository. *See also* ANGINA PECTORIS; ASTHMA.

AMINOPTERIN, a synthetic drug, one of the so-called folic acid antagonists developed in the search for effective treatment in acute leukemia. The folic acid antagonists counteract the abnormal increase in white cells which characterizes leukemia, and aminopterin has been found to be the most effective of them. Growing experience with the use of this drug, later alternated with ACTH or cortisone, has resulted in lengthening the periods of improvements which now last as long as three years. Aminopterin is also used to treat some other forms of cancer.

AMMONIA, a highly irritating poisonous gas, easily soluble in water; forms ammonium hydroxide, widely employed in medicine and in the household. Ammonia is a strong and rapidly acting stimulant used in smelling salts for relief in cases of fainting or exhaustion. The solution and vapors are extremely irritating to the mucous membrances, and concentrated solutions will burn the tissues, as do all corrosive poisons. The antidote for ammonia poisoning is olive oil taken by mouth with large quantities of water, or weak vinegar or lemon juice in water.

AMNESIA, loss of memory, especially inability to recognize ideas represented by words.

The symptoms of amnesia are varied and of different types. Anterograde amnesia is loss of memory directly following severe shock or trauma. Auditory amnesia is an inability to recognize the spoken word. In retrograde amnesia, memory of all previous events is obliterated, and sometimes those incidents occurring after an accident are also effaced (post-traumatic amnesia). The latter is of variable duration and is a yardstick of the severity of the shock or injury.

Amnesia may be partial—as, for instance, losing one's memory for sounds, names, or colors—or it may be general with a loss of the greater part of memory. It frequently involves a sudden emotional conflict,

and memory will begin to return when the conflict is resolved. Doctors often find it difficult to decide in these cases whether or not the inability to remember is actual or simulated. If someone simply refuses to remember, the diagnosis is difficult. Cases are on record of persons who have had as many as five periods of complete loss of memory with subsequent recovery.

Occasionally one reads of a person who cannot recall his name or address. Psychiatrists believe that such persons suffer from amnesia because they have been unable to cope with certain situations which apparently were so painful that the only solution was to deny their identity.

Even in total amnesia certain habits are remembered, such as writing, walking, and reading.

AMNION, the inner fetal membrane of the sac or bag which encloses and protects the embryo. It contains the amniotic fluid which surrounds the fetus until the sac is ruptured at birth. *See also* PREGNANCY AND PRENATAL CARE.

AMPUTATION, the removal of a limb or an organ of the body, in whole or in part. *See also* ARTIFICIAL LIMBS.

AMYLASE, any enzyme which, through a reaction with water, breaks down starch into sugar.

AMYOTROPIC DISEASES, those disorders that cause degeneration of muscle. *See also* LATERAL SCLEROSIS.

ANALGESIA, insensibility to pain, may be produced by drugs known as analgesics, by anesthetics, or by nerve block. Analgesic drugs relieve pain without producing loss of consciousness. Among the milder analgesics are acetylsalicylic acid, commonly known as aspirin, and acetophenetidin, or phenacetin, both of which may be obtained without a prescription. However, recent investigations indicate that these drugs should be used with caution, and should be kept inaccessible to children.

Among the stronger analgesics, used for the relief of severe pain, are morphine, opium, and codeine, all habit-forming drugs, which should be used only under the supervision of a physician. *See also* ANESTHESIA; MEDICINE CHEST, *Pain Relievers*.

ANAPHIA, a defective or absent sense of touch, or an abnormal sensitivity to touch.

ANAPHYLAXIS, the opposite of immunity. It denotes abnormal sensitivity and susceptibility to infection.

ANCYLOSTOMA DUODENALE, a hookworm which thrives chiefly in man, though lower animals can play host to it. It is also an infestation by hookworms. *See also* WORMS.

ANDROGEN, a male hormone that produces and controls the secondary male sex characteristics, such as the beard, muscles, deep voice. The male sex hormone itself, testosterone, is the primary androgen. The secretions produced by the testes include the androgens. *See also* HORMONES.

ANDROGYNY, or pseudohermaphroditism, is the state of having congenitally malformed external genitalia resembling those of one sex while the gonads are those of the opposite sex. *See also* HERMAPHRODITISM.

ANEMIA. In a healthy body, a balance is maintained between productive and destructive blood processes. Anemia, which occurs when the concentration of hemoglobin in the blood falls below a normal level, can result from any of a number of causes. Hemoglobin is the red coloring matter whose main function in the blood is to transport oxygen through the arteries to the body's cells. It is formed in the bone marrow and is normally found in the blood in a ratio of about 16%. Anemia can be caused simply by loss of blood or it may result from a destruction of cells or from inadequate formation of cells. To treat an anemic condition, the doctor must first determine just what type of anemia it is and when this is established, correct the basic fault causing the anemia.

Anemias can follow a sudden blood loss from an injury or from internal hemorrhaging. In this case, the cells themselves are normal but reduced in number. Following a hemorrhage, the body compensates by adding fluids to the blood to restore it to its original volume. The blood is diluted by these fluids and the ratio of hemoglobin to total blood volume is lowered causing anemia. It often takes time for the body to manufacture sufficient red blood cells and other substances for the blood to become normal. Symptoms of blood loss anemia which result from the inability of the blood to carry enough oxygen include headache, general weakness, faintness, and dizziness. In more severe cases of blood loss, vomiting, intense thirst, a fast heart rate and weak shallow breathing as well as the other symptoms of shock are readily seen.

Treatment of this condition includes, of course, stopping the blood loss where such loss in evident—as in the case of wounds. Blood transfusions are sometimes given to prevent excessive dilution of the blood. In less serious hemorrhages, rest and proper diet, including iron and protein for building cells, will be sufficient to enable the body to restore the lost blood.

In a healthy body the life of a normal erythrocyte, or red blood cell is roughly 100 to 120 days. When it breaks down hemoglobin is released. To make up for this loss, new red cells containing hemoglobin are constantly being manufactured to keep the hemoglobin content constant.

In anemia caused by abnormal breakdown or destruction of red blood cells, called hemolytic anemia, large hemoglobin is released at a much greater rate then it can be replaced. This is converted by the liver into other pigments excreted in the bile. When the manufacture of bile pigments is excessive, some appear in body tissue and give the skin and whites of the eyes a yellowish cast, the symptom commonly known as jaundice. In hemolytic jaundice, the cells are so fragile that they are broken down more rapidly than usual by the spleen. Without the spleen, the cells can function properly as the spleen may have to be removed in such cases to prevent the overly rapid cell disintegration.

This condition is either congenital as in Sickle Cell Anemia or may accompany various types of systemic diseases.

An excessive breakdown of red blood cells can also be caused by allergies, poisoning, malaria, severe burns and other conditions. The treatment in each case depends on the basic underlying cause.

Nutritional anemias, which are caused by deficiencies, are characterized by defective blood formation. Most common and least severe is the type in which the amount of iron, essential for hemoglobin manufacture, is inadequate. Eighty-five per cent of the iron necessary is released from the breakdown of old cells, but some iron must be supplied in the diet. Symptoms of iron-deficiency anemia commonly include pallor, weakness and fatigue, faintness and difficulty in breathing. It is easily diagnosed by laboratory tests and responds rapidly to proper diet and rest.

Anemia in a pregnant woman is caused by an attempt by her system to care more adequately for the growing baby. Since the blood of the woman must carry food, oxygen and waste products for two beings, demands on the circulatory system are increased, which can lead to a dilution of blood, with fewer red blood cells per cubic centimeter of blood. Inadequate diet or vomiting tend to increase the possibility of iron deficiency and the doctor may prescribe iron and protein supplements to the mother's diet. Normally, a baby is born with enough iron in his tissues to last several months but if the iron supply of the mother is low, the baby will have a low reserve and develop anemia unless diet supplements of iron are given. Milk is a poor source of iron. Copper, vitamin C and other vitamins are also thought to be involved in the body process or iron utilization.

Bone marrow deficiency disease is another anemia caused by defective blood formation from decreased bone marrow formation. The red blood cell formation in bone marrow is highly complex and involves many functions of the body. In the marrow, the prospective red cells are larger than they will be when released and lack hemoglobin. Before the new cells are released into the blood stream, they shrink in size and gain hemoglobin. When something prevents normal development, or the cells are released prematurely, the result is oversized red cells. To mature properly, the cells must have a substance from the liver called the growth or maturation factor. This maturation factor is identical or closely related with vitamin B_{12}. To absorb vitamin B_{12}, the body uses a substance called the intrinsic factor, which is found in normal gastric juice. Some anemias are caused by absence of the intrinsic factor and others by a poor supply of the maturation factor.

Pernicious anemia is characterized by the disappearance of this intrinsic factor and, along with it, hydrochloric acid in the gastric juice. Therefore, vitamin B_{12} or the maturation factor cannot be absorbed and the red cells cannot mature properly. As pernicious anemia progresses, changes occur in the spinal column, with weakness and numbness of the limbs and eventually a complete loss of their control. As well as the other anemia symptoms of pallor, weakness and difficult breathing, there

may be diarrhea, nausea, sore tongue and yellow pigmentation of skin.

No treatment is known to restore the intrinsic factor and hydrochloric acid to the gastric juice. However, in 1926, it was discovered that regular amounts of liver in the diet would control pernicious anemia. Today intramuscular injections of highly concentrated liver extract, sometimes in conjunction with vitamin B_{12} and folic acid, are given instead of liver. However, this is not a cure and must be continued through the lifetime of the person.

Many other conditions exist in which absorption of material from the intestine is impaired as a result of diarrhea, excess fat in the intestine or impairment of intestinal walls. Other anemias include sprue, pellagra, infestation with fish tapeworm, liver disease, myxedema, and rare ones whose causes are unknown. Most of these conditions respond favorably to liver injections alone or with vitamin B_{12}.

Probably the most serious of the anemias are those caused by destruction of bone marrow. Cells of all types rapidly disappear from the blood stream until only a small percentage of the normal amount is left. It may be attributable to overdose of radium, X-ray, or severe infection, but usually the cause of the destruction is not known. Sometimes an improvement or cure is effected by repeated blood transfusions.

All anemias are characterized by general weakness and fatigue, since the blood cannot supply body tissue with sufficient nourishment. Treatment of anemic conditions is much more satisfactory and more rapid if it is begun before the disease has progressed far or done permanent damage and early discovery of the condition is of prime significance. Usually, diagnosis is made by a laboratory examination of the person's blood and often tests are also made of samples of digestive juice or bone marrow. After the cause has been removed, specific substances are available to bring quick relief in all but a few rare types of anemia.

ANESTHESIA, a word first used in 1846 by Oliver Wendell Holmes, means the absence of pain sensation, with or without loss of consciousness. Three forms of insensibility to pain are recognized: (1) general anesthesia, loss of consciousness; (2) regional or spinal anesthesia, lack of pain in a limited area; and (3) topical anesthesia, lack of pain on a surface area by direct application of an anesthetic agent. The concept of anesthesia is ancient and alcohol and opium were used for many centuries to relieve pain.

Nitrous oxide, or laughing gas, was discovered by Joseph Priestley in 1769; and in 1799 another Englishman, Sir Humphry Davy, noted that nitrous oxide was able to produce unconsciousness. In 1844 an American dentist, Horace Wells, tested this property by having one of his own teeth painlessly removed while he was under the influence of nitrous oxide.

Ether, which was discovered in the sixteenth century, gained prominence in 1829 when Michael Faraday discovered that it produced unconsciousness. In 1842, a Georgia physician, Crawford W. Long, used ether successfully in an operation to remove a wen; and in 1846 a Boston dentist, William Thomas Green Morton, at Harvard, demonstrated again the anesthetic quality of ether during an operation to remove a tumor of the neck performed by Dr. John D. Warren.

Chloroform was discovered by Samuel Guthrie of New York in 1831. Chloroform is rarely used as an anesthetic in the United States today because it can depress the heart and cause severe damage to the liver and kidney. However, it is still popular abroad.

Sigmund Freud first described the properties of cocaine, a drug with powerful pain-killing action, but did not go on to experiment with it. In 1884 Karl Koller of Vienna used cocaine in an operation on the eye, and it is now universally used as a local anesthetic by ophthalmologists. Cocaine proved equally effective in producing local anesthesia on the mucous membranes of the nose, throat, and larynx. The discovery that cocaine was an anesthetic provoked many experiments in its use. Dr. William S. Halsted, an American physician, produced anesthesia of an entire area of the body by injecting cocaine into the nerve supplying the area. Dr. J. L. Corning introduced spinal anesthesia, which obtained insensibility of the entire lower part of the body. Further tests produced less toxic derivatives of cocaine and led to the development of novocaine, or procaine, which soon replaced all cocaine derivatives. At present, spinal anesthesia employing novocaine has become extensively used in operations for appendectomy, and on the lower abdomen and legs.

An outgrowth of spinal anesthesia was the development of caudal anesthesia, in which the anesthetic is injected into the sacral canal. In "painless childbirth," the anesthetic is injected in small amounts, a continuous "drip injection," into the region of the coccyx and acts on nerves leading to the womb.

Improvements in the methods of administering anesthetics have accompanied the discovery of safer drugs. One of the most significant steps has been the development of the "closed system" of administration. In the past, ether was given by dropping it into an open cone held over the patient's face. In the new system of administering ether, or supplementary gases, the gas is conducted through a series of closed tubes leading into a mask fitted tightly over the patient's face. This apparatus can absorb the carbon dioxide in the air exhaled by the patient, add oxygen when it is needed to the air inhaled, and add the anesthetic gases in the necessary concentrations. Anesthesia can thus be carried on for a much longer time and with much greater safety.

New and better anesthetics have continued to be developed. Ethylene and cyclopropane are in common use in many hospitals, although they have the one disadvantage, not yet completely overcome, of being highly explosive.

Another current method of administering an anesthetic is the intravenous or basal method in which the anesthetic drug is injected directly into the blood through the vein. The amount injected can be controlled by a stopcock on the needle and the anesthetic may be given in small amounts, thus keeping the patient free from pain for a long period of time. One of the first drugs used in this type of anesthesia was evipal, a barbiturate. Another more potent barbiturate now used is pentothal sodium.

The practice of anesthesia, which entails a knowledge of the proper administration of an anesthetic during an operation, the management of the patient's respiration, the ability to apply artificial respiration when necessary, and complete familiarity with the problems of gas therapy, has become a special field of medicine. Specialists who deal solely with this field are known as anesthetists or anesthesiologists.

ANEURYSM, dilatation of an artery or vein caused when a weak spot occurs in the wall. The layers of elastic tissue that form the wall enable the vessels to dilate and contract. When they are stretched at any point, because of innate weakness, the enfeebled section pouches out and causes distention, just as in the weakened wall of a rubber tire.

This thinning out, which destroys a section of the elastic tissue, may be the result of an infection such as pneumonia, of a streptococcal or staphylococcal infection. Often physical injury to an arterial wall leaves it so weakened that an aneurysm may eventually occur. If the blood-filled sac ruptures, a serious, often fatal hemorrhage may ensue.

Aneurysms are of various types. When one of the layers of tissue of the wall of the blood vessel also becomes the wall of the sac, a true aneurysm results. False aneurysms

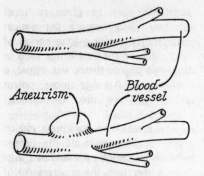

A weak spot in the surface of an
artery is called an aneurysm.

occur when the layers of the artery
are all ruptured, leaving the surrounding tissues to retain the blood.
Also the blood may force its way
between layers of the arterial wall
and separate them.

All arteries are subject to aneurysms, and a most commonly affected artery is the aorta, the large
artery leading from the heart. The
disorder may develop in a blood vessel as the result of an injury, and
even though such aneurysms are
smaller they are no less dangerous,
and may prove fatal when they
occur in the heart, brain, or other
vital organ.

Should the aneurysm become
greatly enlarged, pressure is exerted
and crowds the area in which it occurs, such as the abdominal or chest
cavity. Aneurysms may be painful,
or produce difficulty in breathing,
dyspnea, by pressing against the air
passages, or cause swelling.

New techniques of surgery have
been developed to repair the damaged
artery walls. Smaller blood vessels
are tied off and other arteries take
over their function. It is also possible
to coagulate the blood in the sac and
form a clot and thus strengthen the
walls. Plastic materials are used
around the aneurysm to prevent its
growth, giving the weakened arterial
wall opportunity to strengthen. *See
also* Chapter 12, "Diseases of the
Heart."

ANGINA PECTORIS means pain in
the chest, a symptom which accompanies any interference with
blood supply or oxygenation of the
heart muscle. Men are affected five
times as often as women, and the
symptom is seen most frequently in
the sixth and seventh decades of life,
though younger people are also affected. High-strung, sensitive, active
people are most commonly subject
to it, and in 90 per cent of cases,
arteriosclerosis, or hardening of the
arteries, is noted. Persons with diabetes, high blood pressure, rheumatic
heart disease, and anemia are more
susceptible than others to angina
pectoris.

The heart muscles, like all muscles,
depend upon the constant flow of
oxygen-rich blood into the tissues in
order to perform their required work
and sustain their health. The blood
vessels which supply the heart with
blood are the coronary vessels. Any
change in the caliber of these significant vessels, such as sudden narrowing or blockage, will seriously interfere with the flow of oxygen and
nourishment to the heart muscle.
When this occurs, pain results.

The pain of angina pectoris is
typically brief, lasting seldom more
than three or four minutes. When
longer, the cause may be something
else. The pain is just under the breastbone and often radiates to the neck
and down the left arm. Occasionally

it may move from the chest to the right arm, the stomach, or back.

In most persons, exertion or emotion precipitates the attack. Under these circumstances, the heart muscle beats more rapidly and needs a faster, richer supply of oxygen and blood. If the coronary vessels are partially blocked by fatty deposits, as in arteriosclerosis, the circulation is not able to cope with the increased demands by the heart and angina results. Angina frequently occurs after a heavy meal, because of the increased work load digestion places on the heart.

Any strong emotion may precipitate an attack of angina, especially grief, anger, or worry. It may also occur in any occupation, though less commonly to laborers because of their better muscular development. Angina pectoris is more prevalent in cities and cold climates, probably because of the faster paced life associated with northern cities.

Moderation is of the utmost importance in controlling angina pectoris. At the first sign of chest pain, the person should immediately cease what he is doing and sit down and rest. Relief of pain will often come in a few minutes. To persist in exertion after the onset of pain is extremely hazardous, and in this respect the pain is a significant symptom which informs the patient that he is overexerting himself and needs rest.

Fortunately many drugs are available which give immediate relief to those with angina pectoris or a tendency to narrowing of the coronary vessels for whatever reason. Most popular is nitroglycerine, which causes a dilation, or widening, of the coronary vessels during an attack and thus permits more blood to flow through. Nitroglycerine, taken as a small tablet slipped under the tongue during an attack, brings relief almost immediately, and seldom later than two or three minutes. Amylnitrate, a medicine which is inhaled during an attack, can also be taken. Other drugs of a similar nature may be regularly prescribed for two or three times a day to prevent attacks. No drugs should be taken without consulting a doctor, as they may have unpleasant or serious side-effects.

Relief of the acute attack, though momentarily significant, is not the entire solution to angina pectoris. The person's daily life must be regulated so as to avoid situations liable to affect adversely the circulation to the heart. Here are ten rules which are applicable to the person with angina pectoris.

1. Do not subject your heart to sudden, strenuous, or prolonged physical activity.

2. Eat regularly, slowly, and temperately.

3. Make every effort to keep your weight down, particularly after the age of forty. Angina pectoris is many times more common and serious in overweight persons.

4. Avoid physical activity for at least thirty minutes after eating a heavy meal.

5. Avoid emotional stress and strain. Plan your work so that you get sufficient rest. Avoid worry.

6. Keep your body healthy and free from infection.

7. Avoid constipation.

8. Get at least eight hours of sleep a night in a room well supplied with fresh air.

9. Keep fit with a regular moderate program of exercise.

10. See your doctor regularly for a thorough checkup.

The person who suffers from angina pectoris should not despair of his situation. It is not a disease, but a warning of danger from the heart. It is quite possible to live a fairly normal existence if the person takes proper care of himself and always heeds the warning signal of pain. *See also* Chapter 12, "Diseases of the Heart."

ANILINE, a colorless, oily liquid prepared from coal tar or benzene or indigo, used extensively in numerous industries for the manufacture of various chemicals, among them acetanilid, acriflavine, methylene blue, and other antiseptic dyes. Aniline is highly poisonous and may enter the body through broken skin or through inhalation or ingestion of the oil or its fumes or dusts, and thus lead to poisoning of the body. Acute poisoning will cause sudden prostration; blue discoloration of the lips, nose, and fingers; and may be accompanied by unconsciousness and convulsions. In case of poisoning, the doctor should be called immediately and the patient kept warm and given an emetic of a tablespoon of mustard in a glass of water. *See also* POISONING.

ANKLE, a joint between the leg and the foot, formed by the junction of the lower ends of the tibia and fibula, the bones of the lower leg, and the astragalus, or anklebone, in the foot.

Sprained ankle. Sudden twisting of the foot may stretch one of the many ligaments which connect various bones in the ankle area, and produce local bleeding, swelling, and extreme tenderness. Immediate application of cold compresses is helpful to reduce swelling, bleeding, and pain during the first twenty-four hours. Strapping the ankle with elastic bandages or adhesive tape relieves tension and mobility of the joint and hastens healing. Daily submersion in hot water and rest are also beneficial and soothing. The latest treatment includes injection of novocaine solutions for relief of pain, as well as hyaluronidase to decrease swelling, to permit earlier use of the foot.

Painful ankle. A painful ankle may occur with a sprain, fracture of ankle bones, arthritis, or gout.

Swollen ankle. Swollen ankle may occur in many conditions, especially in pregnancy, kidney disease, heart disease, and in overweight persons, because of impaired circulation. Many persons, women especially, develop swollen ankles in hot weather. *See also* JOINTS AND JOINT DISORDERS; SPRAINS.

ANODYNE, any agent that will relieve pain. *See also* ANALGESIA; ANESTHESIA.

ANOREXIA, the scientific term for loss of appetite.

ANOREXIA NERVOSA, a condition most frequently found in young neurotic women, is characterized by a pronounced aversion to food, due to a hysterical condition. In extreme cases, the loss of weight may be so great that death may ensue if the malady is not corrected in time. Both psychological and medical treatment are necessary.

ANOSMIA, complete loss of the sense of smell. It may be permanent or temporary, depending on whether or not the olfactory nerves are damaged or destroyed completely beyond hope of healing. Partial loss of the sense of smell is hyposmia, and the loss of smell in one nostril only is hemianosmia. An excessive response to odors is known as hyperosmia.

Loss of the sense of smell may be the result of a mental state, as in hysteria. In some instances of hallucination, the person imagines that he smells certain odors not actually present. Treatment of anosmia due to mental causes is difficult.

Defects of the sense of smell may be caused by dryness of the mucous membranes of the nose, by infection, injury, obstruction, deterioration of the nasal tissue, or by action of drugs. Certain diseases of the brain, brain injury, or brain tumor may also produce anosmia.

Tests to determine the presence of a sense of smell are made by releasing certain odors and noting the responses. Adjustment to the loss of a sense of smell is usually not too difficult. *See also* OLFACTORY SENSE.

ANOXEMIA, a lack of the normal amount of oxygen in the blood, due to high altitudes, low partial pressure of oxygen in anesthesia, cardiac failure, or strangling.

ANTABUSE, a recently developed drug used in the treatment of alcoholics to produce a distaste for alcohol. When Antabuse is administered to an alcoholic, extreme discomfort, severe nausea, vomiting, and flushing develop, with intolerance to alcohol. Antabuse should never be given to a person who is intoxicated, nor should it be given without the full knowledge and consent of the person. The drug is best used in conjunction with psychotherapy. *See also* ALCOHOLISM.

ANTACID, a substance that relieves acidity and neutralizes acids.

ANTENATAL denotes the time from conception to delivery.

ANTEPARTUM refers to any occurrence or condition that takes place before the baby is born.

ANTHRAX, a malignant carbuncle, is a serious infectious disease which not only attacks animals such as cattle and sheep but is also transmitted by them to human beings. The germ, found most often in the recently ejected excrement of animals or men, or in their hair or skin, is transmitted to or may enter the body through a wound, scratch, or insect bite, or through inhalation. The most frequent victims of anthrax are farmers, butchers, veterinarians, and hide workers. Anthrax of the lung is often referred to as "wool sorters' disease."

The prevention of anthrax among human beings is best achieved by protecting the animals. Failing this, obvious precautions are necessary, especially in places where men work with animals or with the products of animals. Clothing, such as overalls and rubber aprons, which protects the skin should be worn. Persons sorting hair or wool should wear breathing devices which will protect them from the inhalation of dangerous substances. Workers are advised to cleanse their hands with disinfectants when their work is done. Some precautions are merely those which any efficient industrial management insists upon: general sanitation, attention to skin lesions of workers, disinfection of dangerous wastage before it leaves the factory, and effective ventilation. Exhaust fans are particularly essential to carry away any dangerous substances which might exist in the atmosphere.

The first symptom of anthrax is painful itching. Several hours later, somewhere on the body, an inflamed pimple or boil develops which becomes hard, has a purple center, and is surrounded by a zone of red. As the boil swells, it produces a thick and bloody pus at its center, and at the same time the adjacent lymph glands swell and the veins become inflamed. The first boil is followed by many others. Eventually gangrene may develop in the infected tissue. Simultaneously the person is likely to suffer from a general weakness, together with chilliness, disinclination to eat, nausea, and a high temperature. The most serious form of this disease is anthrax of the lungs.

Serums have been developed which are useful against this malady. The sulfa drugs and other antibiotics have also been valuable, especially in the control of supplementary infections. Unfortunately, because of the rarity of the disease, the diagnosis sometimes is made too late to counteract the infection and save the patient.

ANTIBIOTICS, substances produced during the growth of molds or bacteria which inhibit or kill other bacteria that cause disease.

The search for effective and non-toxic antibiotics is unceasing. Molds and bacteria are grown and examined for antibiotic substances by bacteriologists and mycologists. Chemists then purify these substances and prepare them as concentrates which in turn are tested in animal experiments by pathologists to determine their potency and toxicity before they can be employed for human use.

Since the development of penicillin in 1942, following its accidental discovery in 1929 during an experiment by Sir Alexander Fleming, the English bacteriologist, thousands of antibiotic substances have been isolated and studied. Of these, approximately nineteen are now being used for therapeutic purposes. Among the significant ones are bacitracin and tyrothricin, and "broad spectrum" antibiotics, so-called because they are effective against many different types of infectious diseases, which include penicillin, Aureomycin, Terramycin, streptomycin, Chloromycetin, Erythroticin Kanamycin and tetracyclines. These are used in the treatment of many bacterial, viral, and fungus diseases.

Antibiotics have been employed with dramatic success in rheumatic fever, bacterial endocarditis, syphilis, tuberculosis, pneumonia, and many staphylococcic infections. However, in some instances they have produced undesirable reactions, such as diarrhea, nausea, vomiting, and abdominal cramps, and may also cause serious damage to the kidneys or other organs. When used indiscriminately, antibiotics may lead to growth within the body of new strains of previously harmless bacteria which become drug-resistant and thus expose the patient to residual infections. Most doctors believe that antibiotics should not be used in conditions, such as minor colds and sore throats, which are readily controlled by simple remedies. The patient's response to antibiotics should not be endangered or his immunity to disease decreased by the use of antibiotics for minor infections. *See also* BACTERIAL ENDOCARDITIS; MEDICINE CHEST; PNEUMONIA; RHEUMATIC FEVER; STREPTOCOCCUS; SYPHILIS; TUBERCULOSIS.

ANTIBODY, a substance, natural or artificial, introduced to serve as a protection against infections or foreign proteins in the body fluids. Antagonistic to factors which are injurious to the animal organisms, an antibody can destroy bacteria adequately and counteract poisons that cause infections. Diphtheria and other antitoxins are typical antibodies. *See also* ANTITOXIN; BLOOD TYPES; GAMMA GLOBULIN.

ANTICOAGULANT, a substance or condition which opposes or prevents coagulation or clotting. *See also* COAGULATION.

ANTIDOTE, any agent used to prevent or to counteract the effect of a poison. There are specific antidotes for different poisons; for a full discussion, *see* POISONING.

ANTIFEBRIN, or acetanilid, a drug derived from aniline by the action of acetic acid upon it. Antifebrin has been used to lower fever, but more often serves to relieve pain and is therefore one of the ingredients frequently found in headache remedies. *See also* ACETANILID.

ANTIHISTAMINIC DRUGS, synthetic substances, used to alleviate allergic conditions by diminishing the action of histamine.

Antihistaminic drugs are best known as ingredients of advertised cold remedies. The claim that colds can be avoided by taking such remedies shortly after the appearance of the first symptoms of a cold has not as yet been scientifically established. However, in combination with aspirin or phenacetin, or sprayed into the nose with camphor, antihistaminic preparations are useful in treating colds which begin with a running nose due to allergy. They also may relieve stuffiness, irritated eyes, and similar symptoms.

Antihistaminic drugs are not a cure; they may obscure the real symptoms and are occasionally harmful. *See also* ALLERGY.

ANTIMONY, a metallic crystalline substance, symbolized by Sb from the ancient word Stibium, present in many minerals. It is extensively used in the manufacture of alloy metals.

Formerly a mainstay in medical practice, salts of antimony are now less frequently used. They diminish the functional activity of the heart and the arteries, in which case they act as depressants; they increase perspiration, (as diaphoretics), and they induce vomiting, (as emetics).

Antimony is effective in cases of infestation by flukes, which are flat parasitic worms.

ANTISEPTICS, substances that hinder the growth and activity of microorganisms, or germs. Antiseptic agents differ from those which act as disinfectants, germicides, or deodorants. A disinfectant or germicide kills bacteria which cause infectious diseases; a deodorant destroys or covers disagreeable odors. Substances like chloride of lime can be used for either purpose.

In surgery, the use of antiseptics is essential, especially in disinfecting instruments and other materials used in operations. In first aid for accidental wounds and in the care of contaminated or suppurating wounds, antiseptics prevent infection from spreading in the body.

Various antiseptics may be used to disinfect a wound. Tincture of iodine is recommended in first aid. Antiseptic dyes, like tincture of Merthiolate, that can be painted on cuts and wounds are as powerful as iodine and less likely to burn or damage living tissue. Other antiseptics include Mercurochrome, saturated solution of boric acid, Metaphen, Zephiran, and hexylresorcinol solution. Hydrogen peroxide is also an effective antiseptic but should not be applied to a fresh wound because it may bring about clotting or other undesirable effects. Carbolic acid is a dangerous poison and should be used only on the advice of a doctor.

Sulfa preparations and antibiotics are effective on the skin against microorganisms, but should be used under a doctor's supervision because of possible side effects, including allergic reactions and the danger of making germs resistant to the drugs. *See also* BORIC ACID; MEDICINE CHEST; POISONING; WOUNDS.

ANTITOXIN, a substance which counteracts the effect of toxins or poisons in the body produced by harmful organisms, such as bacteria that cause disease. Antitoxins may be developed by the body itself or by the blood of an animal which has been injected with a toxin. Some of the blood is then withdrawn and the serum containing the antitoxin separated from it. This serum or antitoxin may then be injected into a person suffering from the particular infection.

Antitoxins are specific for certain infections. Each bacterial toxin may be counteracted only by the antitoxin effective against it, not by any other which may be potent against other disease-causing toxins.

Diphtheria antitoxin, specific both for curative and preventive purposes, is regarded as one of the greatest of all medical discoveries. Moreover, improved methods are now in general use. One of these consists of injection of diphtheria toxoid, a mixture of toxin and antitoxin which causes the body to develop its own antitoxin without actually suffering from the acute disease itself.

Antitoxins are also available against botulism, scarlet fever, tetanus, staphylococcal infections and snakebite. They have also been effective in erysipelas, meningitis, and epidemic sore throat. Penicillin and the sulfonamide drugs have provided such powerful chemical remedies against a number of these infections that many antitoxins are no longer used. *See also* IMMUNITY; IMMUNIZATION.

ANTRUM, a cavity or hollow space, usually within a bone. Most frequently it refers to the maxillary sinus, one of a pair of sinuses, in the upper jaw. Among others are the mastoid antrum, the pyloric and the dental antrums. *See also* SINUSES.

ANURIA, the suppression of urine by the kidneys, caused by an obstruction in the urinary tract or a lack of renal function.

ANUS, the extremity of the rectum and the outlet of the bowel.

AORTA, the largest blood vessel coming from the heart. It distributes blood to every part of the body through its system of arteries.

APHASIA, an organic condition caused by lesions in the cortex of the brain which produces loss or impairment of the capacity to use words as symbols of ideas.

APHONIA, loss of voice because of hysteria or peripheral lesion.

APHRODISIAC, any preparation or agent which stimulates sexual desire. Actually desire is mostly mental so that drugs which release inhibitions may act as aphrodisiacs. Certain substances which have an irritating effect when excreted may stimulate congestion of the sex organs. *See also* CANTHARIDES.

APOPLEXY. In apoplexy, or "stroke" or cerebral hemorrhage, an artery in the brain either ruptures and bleeds or is blocked. The victim is apt to lose consciousness and some part of the body is paralyzed, at least temporarily. Apoplexy occurs most frequently in persons whose arteries have deteriorated with age or who have high blood pressure. Age tends to bring rising blood pressure

and degenerative change in the arteries. As the proportion of elderly people in the United States increases, the proportion of people susceptible to apoplexy also increases and therefore apoplexy has become a leading cause of death. When younger persons have apoplexy it is frequently the result of a blood clot from elsewhere in the body obstructing a blood vessel which serves the brain. This obstruction has the same effect as an actual hemorrhage of blocking the flow of blood in the brain.

Apoplexy occurs in various ways. Especially with older persons, apoplexy may take place during a regular nightly sleep, with no apparent external cause. Sometimes apoplexy is associated with an emotional outburst, a sudden intense effort or acute stress. Without warning, a person may collapse suddenly. Partial paralysis is a typical consequence, regardless of the way apoplexy occurs.

Emergency assistance to a victim of apoplexy begins by putting him to bed immediately. He should lie supine and if he is unconscious be placed on his side. If he is placed on his back during unconsciouness, his tongue may fall back into his throat, interfere with breathing, and cause strangulation. A doctor should be summoned promptly.

As long as the stricken person is unconscious, fluids and foods must be given artificially; liquids will have to be injected and food injected through tubes into the veins. These measures and others are prescribed and administered by the doctor.

The extent of paralysis can be established only after the person has regained consciousness, and some-times a long period of time must elapse before the full extent of the paralysis is determined. Paralysis due to a temporary condition, such as pressure on a nerve, rather than to actual destruction of nerve tissue will disappear with recovery. The body, if adequate care is provided, tends to mend such damage and to restore power of movement lost for tem-porary reasons. A person crippled by apoplexy can be rehabilitated in most instances if the proper treatment is begun at the right time. The patient should always be handled very care-fully and gently, never abruptly pushed or jerked into position. His position must be changed every few hours in order to prevent the forma-tion of bed sores and ulcers and the skin should be kept perfectly clean at all times, including a complete bath each day. *See also* CHOREA; EMBOLISM; PARALYSIS; THROMBOSIS.

APPENDICITIS, inflammation of the appendix, more properly known as the vermiform appendix, a finger-shaped sac three to six inches long which projects from the large bowel, in the lower right quarter of the ab-domen.

Infection and inflammation of the appendix are potentially serious be-cause the infection may spread to the peritoneum, the membranous tissue which lines the abdomen. Acute peri-tonitis, or inflammation of the peri-toneum, is a grave development and may be fatal unless treated promptly.

Peritonitis may result from ap-pendicitis in at least two ways. The peritoneum is shaped to fit over the appendix, just as a glove covers a finger, and is thus in close contact with it. Accordingly infection of the appendix may spread to the peri-toneum simply by contact. More-over, if an inflamed appendix is left untreated, it may rupture or develop gangrene. In either case, masses of infected matter will be discharged into the peritoneal cavity.

These possibilities demand that the condition be accorded immediate attention by a physician. Delay often unnecessarily permits the develop-ment of complications, renders treat-ment more difficult, and may possibly endanger life. Attempts to diagnose and treat the symptoms of appendici-tis without a physician, by ascribing the symptoms to a gastrointestinal disturbance and administering a cathartic or laxative, may have seri-ous consequences. Abdominal pain should never be treated with a cathartic or laxative without the cause of the pain being first estab-lished.

Appendicitis usually begins with a sick feeling, accompanied by nausea, lack of appetite, and at first a rather diffuse abdominal soreness. Vomiting may occur, and a rise in temperature is likely. Gradually the pain tends to concentrate on the right side of the abdomen below the navel and the muscles in that region tighten when pressed in examination.

Symptoms indicative of appendici-tis can actually arise from nothing more serious than accumulation of gas or solid matter in a part of the bowel. However, ordinarily these symptoms disappear with elimination from the bowel. If they persist, the doctor should be promptly consulted. He will determine whether or not appendicitis has actually occurred. Examination of the blood will usually show abnormal numbers of white cells if the appendix is infected.

Diagnosis is not always easy because of the variety of difficulties which may manifest similar symptoms. This is especially true of the resemblance between the early stages of appendicitis and, in some cases, of early pneumonia. In early pneumonia, inflammation in the lower lungs may spread to the diaphragm, the large breathing muscle which walls off the chest and abdominal cavities from each other. Pain is present in the same part of the abdomen as in appendicitis, and is also accompanied by rigidity on touch.

Because of the danger presented by an inflamed appendix, surgery is a common and satisfactory means of eliminating the condition. Appendectomy is so completely standardized that recovery will usually be normal, if the operation takes place before the appendix ruptures.

If the appendix has ruptured, or has become gangrenous, however, the situation is much more serious. Ordinarily, in a simple appendectomy, the patient will be up in two or three days, and sent home from the hospital in a week. When complications occur, the condition demands different considerations and may involve much more time. Fortunately the antibiotic drugs such as penicillin, terramycin, aureomycin, and others control peritonitis so that death from this complication is now rare.

The precise way in which appendicitis develops is not fully understood. Doctors once believed that it was the result of food lodging in the appendix. Many appendices removed and examined were found to contain a variety of unexpected objects and materials, such as stones, hair, seeds, pins, bones, lead shot, and sometimes worms. Many other appendices, however, did not contain anything

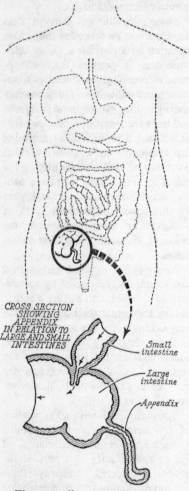

CROSS SECTION
SHOWING
APPENDIX
IN RELATION TO
LARGE AND SMALL
INTESTINES

Small
intestine

Large
intestine

Appendix

The appendix, a sac attached to the large intestine is prone to infection and often must be removed by surgery.

foreign. It is now felt that inflammation and infection are commonly caused by germs.

The structure of the appendix, with its long slender tube, narrow opening at one end only, and lining of lymphatic tissue, makes it susceptible to inflammatory swelling and the resulting closure. The organ then cannot empty its contents. An abscess forms, the swelling increases, and the accumulating infected and lymphatic matter within the tube cannot escape. The appendix may then burst or become gangrenous. Gangrene is the atrophy of the tissues locally affected.

Sudden relief after a period of pain should be considered a potential danger signal rather than a sign of improvement, for it may signify that perforation has occurred or that gangrene has begun.

Appendicitis is a significant threat to health in the United States. It ranks fifteenth among causes of death, and kills sixteen thousand persons annually. If children below the age of fifteen are eliminated from these statistics, appendicitis becomes the eighth or ninth cause of death. *See also* PERITONITIS.

APPETITE, the recurring and usually natural desire for food. A distinction must be made between appetite and hunger. Hunger pangs result from contractions of an empty stomach and are rarely felt by anyone who regularly eats adequate amounts of food. Appetite arises with the customary intervals of eating and may be influenced by numerous external and internal phenomena. Eating is one of the most firmly fixed of all habits, and appetite is usually a longing for something one wants to eat at a time when one habitually has or expects food. Ordinarily a good appetite is considered a sign of health.

Appetite, however, can become excessive or subject to distorted impulses. Occasionally people suffering from specific disorders, such as diabetes, gastric ulcers, or chronic gastritis, develop appetites out of proportion to their needs. In pregnancy or hysteria, unusual and specialized cravings may develop for particular kinds of foods, or even for injurious substances.

A close connection may exist between appetite and individual psychological experience. Children, for example, are apt to develop cravings without realizing the cause. Eating may be a form of compensation for a major loss or disappointment; or a means of securing attention from adults who otherwise might not notice the child. Some children develop unaccustomed appetite from significant new events taking place about them, such as the birth of a new baby.

A person who has duodenal ulcer seems to have a special form of appetite. His pain is apt to rise and fall with the stomach's desire for food. In such cases, eating tends to relieve the pain, at least temporarily.

Diminution or loss of appetite accompanies many disordered conditions, and is usually one of the symptoms of tuberculosis and anemia. Loss of appetite and refusal to eat anything is known medically as anorexia nervosa. Ordinarily this disease is related to some form of emotional instability and is observed more often in women than in men.

Appetite can be artificially decreased by taking such drugs as Benzedrine and Dexedrine. These drugs are sometimes prescribed for weight reduction, but should be taken only on the advice of a doctor.

Investigation indicates that small amounts of cocktails and other alcoholic drinks arouse or increase appetite, although they hinder the stomach contractions associated with hunger. *See also* ANOREXIA; and Chapter 4, "Diet and Health."

AQUEOUS HUMOR, the fluid in the front chamber of the eye, between the cornea and the lens. The transparent substance is almost totally water.

ARACHNODACTYLY, derived from the Greek words for spider and finger, a condition in which the fingers and sometimes the toes are abnormally long and thin. This abnormality has a hereditary tendency.

ARGYROL, a proprietary antiseptic drug which contains about 20 per cent silver and proteins found in egg yolk. It is used to control and counteract inflammations of membranes that are secreting or contain mucus.

ARCHES, FALLEN, are due to a breakdown of the natural arch of the foot which is an elastic spring that supports the weight of the entire body. This arch, made up of numerous bones held in place by a series of ligaments and muscles, is a curved structure resembling an arc. Flat feet, a common complaint, may be caused by the natural weakness of the arch, but usually result from certain occupations, injury, or obesity. The condition may be corrected or benefited by wearing proper shoes or arch supports, or by exercises to strengthen the muscles.

ARGYROSIS, a form of gray-blue discoloration of the skin and mucous membranes which results from deposits of silver particles. It is produced by the prolonged use of silver solutions, like silver nitrate or Argyrol.

ARM, in anatomy, the upper extremity of the body, from shoulder to elbow. Popularly, however, it indicates the arm and forearm.

ARTERIOSCLEROSIS, hardening of the arteries, a disease fairly common among older people. The walls of the blood vessels are clogged by depositions of minerals and fatty material and degenerate, losing their original resilience, and become thicker, tough, and more rigid. Arteriosclerosis represents from 25 to almost 50 per cent of all chronic circulatory disease, and is responsible for many deaths among persons living past middle age.

A healthy blood vessel can be compared to a hose made of elastic material. When the volume of liquid flowing through the hose is increased, the hose stretches to accommodate it, and when the volume of liquid decreases the hose shrinks. This is exactly what a healthy blood vessel does, stretching and shrinking to accommodate the increasing or decreasing volume of blood flowing through it. But when the walls of a blood vessel become rigid and in-

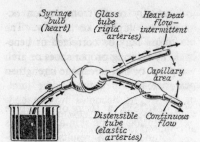

A mechanical device used to show the effect of hardening of the arteries on blood pressure.

flexible, as in arteriosclerosis, this accommodation does not take place and when increased quantities of blood flow through a hardened or sclerotic artery, the pressure within the blood vessel rises temporarily, sometimes to the bursting point. Actually the symptoms of hardened arteries develop largely from the effects of this condition on the blood pressure and the circulation of local areas of the body. Generalized high blood pressure throughout the body is not caused by hardening of the arteries, although the two conditions tend to be closely related.

The commonest symptoms of hardened arteries are drowsiness, periods of giddiness, headaches, and other manifestations of high blood pressure. Interference with circulation may cause cramps in the legs, which give them a bluish tinge. The most serious form of arteriosclerosis occurs when the blood vessels of the brain and heart are involved.

The specific causes of the hardening process within the arteries is not as yet fully understood and is the subject of much medical research. One theory, partly borne out by experimental work with animals, places responsibility on excessive consumption of fats. Another suggests that overindulgence of tobacco and alcohol somehow stimulate the condition, although this has never been proved scientifically.

Treatment for arteriosclerosis is generally limited to establishing the patient's comfort and peace of mind as much as possible, and encouraging him to take good care of himself. The patient is urged to relax and eliminate as much as possible the stresses and strains of daily living, since excitement or intense emotion may stimulate a greater flow of blood than the hardened arteries can accommodate, with the possibility of severe consequences from rupture and bleeding. A low-fat diet is often recommended, and heat treatment, either baths or exposure to hot air, has been found useful. Several new drugs are available which often prove beneficial when prescribed.

ARTHRITIS, inflammation of the joints. At least seven million people in the United States are afflicted by various forms of arthritis, causing more days lost from work than any other disability except nervous and mental diseases.

Innumerable forms of inflamed joints affect people, and only a doctor can differentiate them. Arthritis may be caused by infection, by degeneration of joint tissues coincident with overweight or old age, or by deposits of uric acid crystals within the joint space, as in gout. Arthritis may follow injury or be associated with allergy to medicine or to food. Occasionally joint pain may indicate tumor growth or inflammation of the nerves surrounding a joint.

Arthritis due to infection of a joint resulting from tuberculosis, syphilis, typhoid fever, or gonorrhea is not as common now as in former years, because treatment of these diseases is now more effective. Joint pains due to allergy to penicillin or other drugs can be relieved by simple medications with antihistamines such as Pyribenzamine, Benadryl, or Neohetramine. Inflammation due to gout is treated by drugs such as colchicine, Benemid, Butazolidin, or Anturan. When the condition is caused by old injuries, surgery may occasionally be helpful in mollifying the scar tissue responsible for the pain. Neuritis and neuralgia, mimicking true arthritis, are sometimes relieved by large doses of the B vitamins.

Arthritis in women may be related to the function of the sex glands or ovaries. In postmenopausal arthritis, which occurs after ovarian activity has ceased within the body, relief is often obtained with small doses of sex hormones.

Rheumatoid arthritis is somewhat more complex as well as more frequent than the types mentioned. While the exact cause is not known, certain factors have been established that definitely relate to the development of rheumatoid arthritis. Overfatigue, shock, injury, prolonged exposure to dampness or cold have all been thought to be associated with the development of this type of inflammation. Allergy has been postulated as a cause, as well as hormone defects. Rheumatoid arthritis often begins with pain and stiffness in a single joint months before other joints

become affected. It strikes the fingers, hands, wrists, and knees primarily, but may also affect the bones of the back and the hips. The fingers develop a typical "sausage-like" appearance in which the middle joint of the fingers becomes swollen and tender. The toes are seldom involved, as opposed to gouty arthritis in which the great toe is commonly affected. Nodules may occur under the skin in about 10 per cent of cases, usually located around the elbows, wrists, fingers, and occasionally the ankles. They vary in size from a small pea to a large walnut, appearing and disappearing without apparent cause.

Although true rheumatoid arthritis tends to be chronic, sudden complete relief of pain and stiffness may occur for months or years at a time. In mild cases the disability may be scarcely noticed, but in others the victim may become bedridden.

In older people, and in younger ones who are extremely overweight, osteoarthritis or degenerative arthritis may occur. The average age of onset of this type is between fifty and seventy, whereas rheumatoid arthritis usually strikes before forty and may affect children. In osteoarthritis the signs of inflammation are few. The symptoms of pain and disability are due to degeneration or wearing away of cartilage within the joint and, unlike rheumatoid arthritis which may affect almost any joint, the knees, back, and neck are most commonly involved. Swelling may occur in the last joint of each finger, but nodes are not found under the skin. Whereas rheumatoid inflammation tends to produce permanent de-

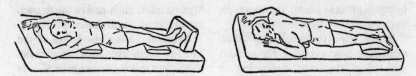

a and b. Two basic rest positions for the arthritic patient. *A* is the supine
position. *B* is the prone position.

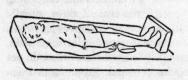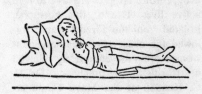

c and d. The position which the arthritic patient assumes in bed is important in preventing deformity and improving circulation. *C* is good position;
D is poor position.

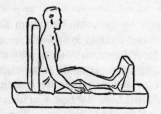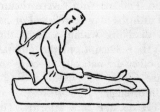

e and f. Examples of correct and incorrect sitting positions for the arthritis
sufferer.

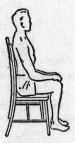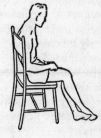

g and h. When the arthritis patient sits in a chair he should keep as upright
as he can. *G* is good position; *H* is poor position.

formity of the joints, osteoarthritis does not usually have that effect.

Many effective drugs and treatments are now available for persons afflicted with arthritis, depending on the particular type. For those suffering from rheumatoid arthritis, the discovery of cortisone has been most encouraging. With the help of this drug, former cripples are able to lead active lives. Use of this hormone, isolated from the adrenal gland, followed the observation that pregnant women often are completely relieved of arthritis during pregnancy. Dr. E. C. Kendall of the Mayo Clinic attempted to discover which element in the blood stream of pregnant women might be responsible for remission symptoms, and so cortisone was discovered. The results are often dramatic. Patients with severe rheumatoid arthritis may be relieved of pain and disability within a short time. ACTH, isolated from the pituitary, is another dramatically effective substance.

Unfortunately cortisone and ACTH do not *cure* arthritis. They do *relieve* disabling symptoms. These drugs must be taken indefinitely, always under the supervision of the attending physician. Although the drugs were originally quite expensive, newer techniques of producing cortisone may soon make arthritis treatment relatively inexpensive.

Rest is essential for the patient with arthritis. While he can continue to work, he should rest for an hour or two, preferably lying down after lunch. In severe cases, hospitalization may be necessary.

Diet may be significant. Patients are advised to eat a well-balanced, high-vitamin, high-protein diet, rich in vegetables and fruits.

Reliance is especially placed on treating arthritis with dry heat, diathermy, massage, and exercises, in order to increase circulation to the joints, which may help retard the arthritic process and keep the surrounding muscles from becoming distorted or weakened. Many arthritis sufferers get considerable relief with hot wet compresses. Aspirin, salicylic acid, and mild sedatives are also beneficial in relieving arthritic pain, especially in milder cases that do not require cortisone. People with rheumatic ailments feel better in warm dry climates, such as those of Arizona and New Mexico. Wet damp environments may aggravate the condition.

Orthopedic surgeons can do much to improve the control of deformed bones and muscles in arthritis resulting from any cause. This, plus the amazing advances made in the medical care and treatment of arthritis, should brighten the hopes of everyone who suffers from this disease. *See also* GOUT; and Chapter 24, "Arthritis and Rheumatism."

ARTIFICIAL LIMBS, known to the ancients as prostheses, which means artificial substitution for missing parts such as legs, arms, and dentures. Improved prosthetic techniques have always followed wars. Today the stumps of limbs are being effectively used by salvaging the functions of the remaining muscles in the stump to manipulate the artificial replacements.

Many materials are suitable for the manufacture of artificial limbs. Wood, especially willow, has excellent qualities and is generally used. Aluminum, or duralumin has the advantage of lightness and is therefore preferable for weak and elderly people. Much work is being done with plastics but as yet is still largely in the experimental stage. The U. S. Army uses fiber in artificial limbs. The straps, belts, and foot coverings are made of leather, although it has certain disadvantages.

In artificially replacing a lower limb, the ankle and knee, and particularly their sockets, are especially important. The socket determines the gait. The amputee must learn to use the artificial limb effectively, which involves control of his thigh and hip muscles.

Because of its intricacy, the artificial arm is used less than the artificial leg. The type of replacement depends to a large degree upon the occupation of the amputee. Some find the peg arm, a stable jointless short arm, best since it can be fitted with a hook which gives great lifting power. The voluntary-control hand can hold a pencil and other small objects, and many utility appliances can be worn for special occupations, depending on the needs. A recent development is a hook operated by a chest or arm muscle. Through an operation known as cineplasty the control muscle is brought outside the body and covered by skin, and the device is then managed by contracting the muscle. Artificial hands that are purely cosmetic and without any functional purpose are also available.

ARTIFICIAL RESPIRATION. *See* ASPHYXIA; RESUSCITATION.

ASBESTOSIS, a lung disease which occurs among workers who inhale dust and other materials from asbestos, a complex calcium magnesium silicate. Inhalation of asbestos fibers produces fibrous changes in the lungs which represent an attempt of the tissue of the lung to wall off the foreign substance.

Asbestos contains about 41 per cent iron oxide. The lungs react particularly to silica and develop silicosis. Workers with asbestos also develop warty growths, called asbestos corns, on the skin. *See also* INDUSTRIAL HEALTH; and Chapter 5, "Occupational Health."

ASCARID, a type of long cylindrical parasite worm which sometimes infests the intestines.

ASCORBIC ACID, or vitamin C, a white or slightly yellowish crystalline powder, soluble in water, is an organic compound found in citrus fruits and juices, fresh green leafy vegetables like kale and broccoli, potatoes, cantaloupe, tomatoes, and strawberries. Ascorbic acid is essential to the proper development of teeth and bones and the walls of capillary blood vessels. It is an aid in resisting infection and its absence leads to the once dreaded scurvy. Vitamin C is significant in infant diet, and is usually added two weeks after birth. Children may need a supplementary form of this vitamin, but only on recommendation of a doctor. An adult male requires 75 mg. daily. *See also* VITAMINS.

ASEPSIS, the absence of disease-producing bacteria. A wound is aseptic if it is cleansed and in a germ-free condition. *See also* ANTISEPTICS.

ASPHYXIA, suffocation, coma or unconsciousness caused by deprivation of oxygen which results in accumulation of carbon dioxide and fixed acids. When breathing stops, no matter what the cause, oxygen must be supplied artificially or unconsciousness will take place, followed shortly by death.

The causes of asphyxia or suffocation are many, the most frequent being electric shock, gas poisoning, heart attacks, brain injuries, smoke, and drowning. Babies occasionally suffocate in their cribs.

Many industries and nearly all cities and towns have first-aid teams which can handle cases that require artificial respiration. Many different machines have been developed to aid resuscitation, and they are available at most fire departments, police emergency services, and hospitals. Ambulances are equipped with emergency apparatus to give aid to the victim of asphyxia at the earliest moment as well as during the ride to the hospital for further treatment. However, time must not be lost waiting for equipment to be brought to an asphyxiated person. Artificial respiration should be started immediately. Few people survive after their lungs have gone without a change of air for more than twelve minutes. In drowning, this time is reduced to four minutes.

A person who has drowned should be placed immediately in a horizontal position, back up, abdomen down, head turned to one side and resting on one hand to keep sand or water out of the mouth and eyes. If the body can lie slightly inclined downward on a slope of twenty to thirty degrees, elimination of fluid from the throat and the breathing tubes will be facilitated. Then alternate pressure and release on the chest is applied, forcing air in and out of the chest. Artificial respiration must be kept up, regardless of time, until medical help arrives.

A form of artificial respiration known as the back pressure-arm lift was formerly recommended by the American National Red Cross and was adopted in the armed services and other organizations. Here the victim is placed face down in a prone position, with arms overhead and bent at the elbows, one hand upon the other, and the head turned to one side so that the cheek rests on the hands. The rescuer, on one or both knees at the victim's head places his hands on the victim's back, with thumbs just touching, and the heels of the hands just below a line running between the victim's armpits. The rescuer rocks forward slowly, elbows straight, until his arms are almost vertical, exerting steady pressure upon the back. Next the rescuer rocks backward slowly and slides his hands to the victim's arms, just above the elbows, which are raised until resistance is felt at the victim's shoulders. Then the arms are dropped. This completes a full cycle, which is repeated twelve times a minute.

Most recently recommended is mouth to mouth artificial respiration, and when available use of a tube through which air is blown and exhaled. This tube also keeps the tongue out of the way.

Everything possible must be done to keep the asphyxiated person warm, because failure to do so may result in shock, which in turn may be responsible for death.

Linesmen working on electric wires are shocked and asphyxiated frequently and a special technique has been developed to meet such an emergency. As the shocked linesman is probably hanging by his safety belt, the rescuer pushes the victim's head forward and circles the waistline with his arms, placing one open hand on the abdomen and then grasping the first hand with the fingers of the other to insure a firm grip. Pressure is applied on the abdomen inward and upward, then completely released. The cycle is repeated, making about eighteen to twenty pressures a minute.

Rescuscitation should be attempted for long periods of time, with the hope that the period during which the person has been without air is less than has been originally estimated. *See also* RESUSCITATION.

ASPIRATION, the act of breathing; may also indicate the removal of fluids or gases from a cavity by suction.

ASPIRIN. *See* ACETYLSALICYLIC ACID; MEDICINE CHEST, *Pain Relievers.*

ASTASIA, inability to stand in a normal manner because of lack of coordination. Astasia-abasia is a symptom of neurosis in which the affected person is apparently unable to walk or stand normally and seems to collapse when he tries to walk or stand.

ASTHENIA, lack of vitality and loss of strength which creates a general weakness. *See also* EXHAUSTION; FATIGUE.

ASTHENOPIA, weakness of the eye muscles and of visual power due to overuse or to errors of refraction.

ASTHMA. A disorder of the upper respiratory tract involving the lungs and the bronchi, characterized by wheezing, coughing, choking and shortness of breath. Asthma is a symptom and not a disease; therefore remedial measures involve locating, isolating and eliminating the cause rather than treatment of the condition itself.

About half the incidence of asthma is due to allergy-irritation of the bronchi by specific allergens breathed into the respiratory system. The balance of the asthma cases are brought on by specific infections in the bronchi. The allergens causing allergic asthma are the same as those which are responsible for hay fever, and include pollens, organic dust, house dust, feathers, and so forth. The reason that these allergens should affect the lungs and bronchi rather than the nasal passages as in hay fever is not known. Allergic asthma begins most often between the ages of twenty and forty, while asthma caused by infection tends to occur in older people, although it can occur at any age. The disorder is generally equally divided between men and women. In both types of asthma the mucous membrane of the bronchial tubes swells and the air passages are partially closed.

A sudden asthma attack is apt to be more frightening than it is dangerous. The affected person finds himself suddenly unable to fill his lungs, and then when he has struggled to gasp in a partial breath is unable to expel it. The person in an asthma attack may bend over slightly to aid his breathing efforts. In prolonged or especially severe attacks, there may be evidence of cyanosis—the blueness of the skin that indicates that the blood had been unable to pick up sufficient oxygen from the lungs. Attacks rarely last for more than a few hours and are often of much shorter duration, although often the condition will persist for a much longer time in milder form with a slight wheezing noise evident in the sufferer's breathing.

The tests for the antigen involved in allergic asthma are very similar to those performed in the search for the causative factor in hay fever. The timing of attacks is carefully charted to ascertain whether they occurred after any one action of the sufferer, such as visiting in the area of a dust-producing factory, or after eating a particular food. Often the antigen is found simply by this method. If it is not, skin tests of possible culprits are made and the subsequent treatment will involve avoidance of the particular substance or substances responsible.

Treatment of the acute serious attack is usually by injection of epinephrine, or adrenaline. This is always prescribed and almost always administered by a doctor. For those people subject to frequent, compara-

tively mild attacks, the physician will often prescribe the inhalation of adrenaline by use of a nebulizer or atomizer.

Often, people who suffer from allergic asthmatic attacks will outgrow the tendency—however, this is by no means always the case. The asthmatic must learn to avoid the cause of his condition and to control it when it appears.

See also ALLERGY; BRONCHITIS; HAY FEVER.

ASTIGMATISM, faulty vision which results from irregularity in the curvature of one or more refractive surfaces of the eye. When the eye is at rest, and parallel rays are focused exactly on the retina the seeing tissue at the back of the eye, vision is said to be normal. The human eye is farsighted when the rays of light focus in front of the retina, or nearsighted when the rays of light focus behind the retina. When parallel rays of light coming into the eye are focused at different meridians, or angles, the eye has astigmatism. Astigmatism is usually due to a change in the curvature of the cornea, or outside membrane of the eye, sometimes with some shortening or lengthening of the diameter of the whole eyeball.

Occasionally astigmatism is caused by defects in the curvature of the lens of the eye. The exact origin of these anatomic differences is not known beyond the fact that the shape of the eyeball varies in different people so that a tendency for astigmatism appears in members of the same family. The shape of the eyeball itself is inherited. However, injury, inflammation, or operative procedure on the cornea of the eye have been known to change the curves and produce astigmatism. Apparently, too, pressure on the eyelids may distort the eyeball and cause astigmatism.

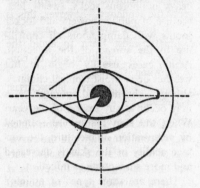

A chart of the mechanism of astigmatism showing the four planes of distortion due to curving of the eyeball.

Probably every eye has some astigmatism. However, many people do not have it enough to warrant special attention. In other cases, astigmatism causes blurred vision which necessitates corrective eyeglasses to properly focus the rays of light on the retina. When the degree of astigmatism is great, the acuteness of vision diminishes for both distant and near objects.

The specialist who examines the eyes is likely to suspect astigmatism when the eye cannot see the line of letters numbered 20 at a twenty-foot distance with the aid of spherical lenses. A simple test is made with the astigmatic dial, a clock with lines radiating to each of the hours. If the person is unable to see all of the rays with equal clarity, astigmatism is responsible. The lines that are seen more distinctly and the lines seen

least distinctly indicate the principal meridians. By the amount of blurring, the eye specialist can determine the areas in which curvature of the lens needs correction. *See also* EYE.

ATABRINE, known as quinacrine hydrochloride in the U. S. Pharmacopoeia, was developed during World War II as a substitute for quinine, used in the treatment of malaria. *See also* QUININE.

ATAXIA, disorganization of muscular coordination so that movement can be controlled only partially. It is a symptom rather than a malady.

One of the best known ataxias is St. Vitus' dance, in which an abnormal nervous system, perhaps as a result of streptococcus infection, causes constant sharp twitching of various parts of the body. Another ataxia is multiple sclerosis, in which sections of the nervous system degenerate and form scar tissue, which causes partial paralysis, among other symptoms.

Parkinson's disease, also known as shaking palsy and paralysis agitans, manifests itself in trembling and loss of power in the muscles. Locomotor ataxia, characterized especially by muscular disorganization and disordered sensation, is the result of infection of the spinal cord by syphilis. Several other special ataxias are known, including that which affects children suffering from cerebral palsy.

Any symptoms, such as loss of control over certain muscular movements or unusual involuntary movements in the muscles, should receive the immediate attention of a doctor, preferably a neurologist, a specialist in nervous disorders. Although the condition may be temporary, a major disturbance of the nervous system is a serious condition. The doctor will know which ataxia is involved, and often, if the condition is a degenerative one, he can take measures to retard or even stop its advance.

Some particular ataxias are hereditary and make repeated appearances in the same family. Such ataxias, the result of a localized developmental failure in some part of the nervous system, may affect not only muscular movement but also the sense of sight, touch, hearing, taste, and smell.

In cases of cerebral palsy, lack of coordination, most commonly associated with generalized muscle weakness, is notable. Treatment consists of muscle-strengthening and coordination exercises. *See also* CEREBRAL PALSY; LOCOMOTOR ATAXIA; MULTIPLE SCLEROSIS; PARALYSIS AGITANS; and Chapter 23, "The Neuromuscular and Neurological Disabilities."

ATELECTASIS, complete expansion or partial collapse of the lung. It may be present at birth or result from diseases of the lungs or bronchi. It is a condition in which the air is lost from the small alveoli, or air chambers, in the lungs, giving the lung a contracted, solid appearance when viewed with the x-ray.

ATHLETE'S FOOT (tinea pedis), a ringworm infection or dermatophytosis of the feet, is a superficial fungus disorder. It is not restricted to athletes, but is found in all age groups and in both sexes, although it occurs more frequently in men. Usually the infection occurs where skin surfaces meet, such as between the toes, and, more rarely, the fingers, groin, and under the arms. Tight, ill-fitting shoes, heavy nonporous socks, sweaty feet, the use of public showers and locker rooms with damp floors all contribute to the spread of the infection. Acute cases usually begin in hot weather or in moist tropical climates, although chronic and sporadic cases may occur at any season of the year. When the skin tissues are softened by perspiration or moisture, the surface acidity of the skin is decreased and more susceptible to infection.

There are three types of athlete's foot, determined by the kind of fungus which attacks the skin, and the manner in which the tissues react. In the acute, weeping, highly inflamed stage, little blisters appear singly or in patches between the fourth and big toe, with scaling, cracking, and oozing of the skin, which may spread to the undersurface and sole of the foot. The more chronic form, intertriginous, begins with a crack in the skin between the fourth and big toes, and formation of loosely clinging dead skin beneath which can be seen red shiny raw tissue. The dry scaly form, hyperkeratotic, is a pronounced thickening of the skin. All three types may spread to cover a portion or the entire surface of the sole.

Cracked, peeling, or sodden skin, or blisters and scaling of the feet may not always be due to a fungus infection. These may be contact dermatitis, a reaction of the skin to shoe dye, to certain chemicals in rayon or nylon stockings, or merely the result of constant friction from ill-fitting shoes or stockings. This condition requires different treatment from athlete's foot.

Treatment of athlete's foot depends upon the type of infection present. Do not use any advertised remedy indiscriminately. If the condition is the result of allergic sensitivity, these remedies may not only be ineffectual but may actually lead to more serious secondary infections. The diagnosis should be made by a physician, who may take a scraping of the infected area for microscopic examination and cultures of the suspected material. Patch tests are also made in some cases to determine whether or not a sensitivity to dyes or chemicals in the footwear causes the condition.

The fungi responsible for athlete's foot are normally found in the dead, superficial layers of the skin, so that a continuous possibility of reinfection exists. When the skin is moist and warm for a long period of time, the fungi again become active. Contact of the bare feet with organisms picked up around swimming pools, shower baths, or locker rooms may also stimulate growth of fungi. The fungi produce allergens which cause an eruption on the feet. The eruption itself may not be severe, but the allergens enter the blood stream and are carried to other parts of the body; people sensitive to the fungi or their products then develop secondary eruptions on the hands or elsewhere. This type of eruption, known as dermatophytid or "id" eruption, usually disappears after the primary infection is treated.

A universal method of controlling athlete's foot is not known. However, the toes must be kept clean and dry at all times, and friction in that area avoided. Dusting the feet freely with foot powder each day and after baths helps keep the area dry. Sandals or perforated shoes and highly absorbent cotton socks permit the evaporation of sweat, and help absorb moisture between the toes. Small cotton wads inserted between the toes help to absorb perspiration. Paper slippers or bath clogs worn in public bathing places lessen contact of bare feet with the fungi. These simple precautions are effective in controlling athlete's foot and in eradicating milder cases.

In acute cases with reddened, blistering, weeping skin, the use of wet compresses once or twice a day, with mildly astringent agents such as saturated boric acid or Burow's solution diluted in twenty parts of water, is beneficial. When the acute inflammation subsides, a calamine lotion may be applied. In the acute stage, the use of antiseptics or advertised remedies may be harmful. Some leading dermatologists believe that once the more acute phase has subsided under suitable treatment, prolonged therapy with a simple mild foot powder is usually enough to control the symptoms of athlete's foot. They all caution that indiscriminate self-treatment of the infection with prepared ointments may lead to more serious inflammation.

For the chronic stages, the treatment usually suggested is to soak the feet in a diluted solution of potassium permanganate for half an hour daily, and then to remove the crusts, scales, and dead skin. A sodium propionate ointment may be applied overnight and removed the following morning, and the feet dusted with a 15 per cent calcium propionate talcum powder. *See also* CONTACT DERMATITIS.

ATROPHY, the normal or abnormal shrinking of an organ or cell which has previously reached mature size. Degeneration of tissue sometimes accompanies pathological atrophy.

ATROPINE. *See* DEADLY NIGHTSHADE POISONING.

AUDITORY NERVE, one of the sensory nerves which influence hearing and control equilibrium.

AUREOMYCIN, a yellow crystalline substance, the trade name for chlortetracycline, one of the newer antibiotics. *See also* ANTIBIOTICS.

AURICLE, either of the two upper chambers of the heart which receive blood from the veins. The left auricle admits the blood from the lungs and the right auricle from general circulation. An auricle is also any appendage shaped like an ear, and refers, too, to the projecting part of the external ear. *See also* BLOOD; CIRCULATORY SYSTEM; HEART.

AUSCULTATION, the detection and study of sounds produced by the lungs, heart, and other organs to help determine their physical condition. The listening device is the stethoscope.

BACILLARY DYSENTERY, an acute infection of the large bowel, caused by bacilli, rod-shaped bacteria, called Shigella, after the Japanese doctor who first identified them. They enter the body in contaminated food or water. The symptoms of the infection include diarrhea and cramps, and it normally runs its course in about ten days and is rarely fatal.

Epidemic bacillary dysentery prevails most frequently when large groups of people are crowded together without adequate sanitation— for example, in armies or refugee camps. World War II was the first war in which sanitation was sufficiently developed to prevent such epidemics in the field.

Sulfonamide drugs are usually effective against the invading bacteria, but if the bacilli develop resistance to sulfa, other antibiotics or drugs may be used. Prevention involves not only identification and isolation of all cases but also of carriers, persons in whose bodies the organisms live without producing in them the usual symptoms of the disease. These persons, particularly if they have an occupation such as cook or waiter, may spread the bacilli.

The symptoms of bacillary dysentery are not unlike those of amebic dysentery, cholera, typhoid and paratyphoid fevers and the diarrhea due to infection by Salmonella, another rod-shaped organism which may get into food. Special tests and examinations are therefore essential to determine the particular bacteria present in each case. *See also* AMEBIC DYSENTERY; DIARRHEA.

BACILLI, one of the main divisions of bacteria, have a characteristic rod shape. They include a large proportion of the most significant bacteria. Bacilli of one type or another are responsible for tuberculosis, diphtheria, typhoid fever, leprosy, plague, tetanus or lockjaw, and other diseases. Bacilli are also involved in the decomposition of dead organic substances, in acid fermentation, and in various processes of wine making. *See also* Chapter 7, "The Process of Infectious Diseases and Immunization of Children."

BACKACHE, like headache, a symptom rather than a disorder and, similarly, may originate from a multiplicity of causes. (Lumbago and low-back pain are words meaning no more than that the back aches.) Because of the complex structure of the human backbone, it can be subject to a great variety of disorders. Its vertical position, which enables man to walk vertically and perform tasks impossible for animals, throws a burden on the spine which most creatures are spared.

Back pain and back ailments may be closely related to occupations in which the spinal structure is required to absorb more stress than it can tolerate. Continued heavy lifting or prolonged standing on the feet impose unusual strains and have a perceptible effect on the body, even during a single day, and may be responsible for back pain. For example, a traffic officer who stands on hard pavement all day without rest will often lose a full inch in height between the beginning of his work and bedtime. Eight hours' rest permits the spine to spring back to its full normal length and the inch is restored.

Backache may result from infection, overstrain, disruption of some part, injury or failure to function

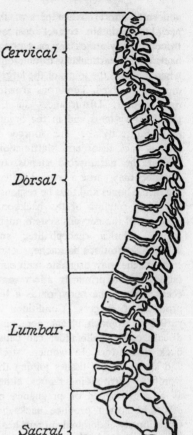

The five major classifications of the bones in the spine.

properly in any part of the complicated spinal system. The structure of tissues of the back may have been defective from birth. Perhaps one or more of the many parts of the back have been injured or strained. Occasionally a slight difference between the length of the legs will put the whole body off balance and require abnormal effort on the part of the back to maintain correct position. Infection may attack any part of the back and is particularly troublesome when it affects the joints or the largest muscles involved. Tumorous growths may appear. Disturbances in the glandular systems and in the organs may indirectly be the source of serious back disorders. Malfunctioning of the parathyroid glands, for instance, may cause a general softening of the bones and thus be responsible for a fracture of the backbone. Diseases of the nervous system, meningitis, sciatica, encephalitis, and others also produce backache.

Backache may originate with conditions which primarily affect some other part of the body, or as a by-product of surgery. Conditions as varied as stomach ulcers, gout, and disease of the gallbladder can cause back discomfort. In women, stress and strain on the tissues joining the womb to surrounding tissues, either as a consequence of pregnancy or otherwise, often produce backache. Occasionally abdominal surgery heals in such a way that scar tissue develops in a place that becomes troublesome to the back. Finally, some cases seem primarily to have a psychological basis.

In treating backache, the doctor first endeavors to establish the specific condition involved and its sources. Sometimes this is simple to do, but frequently it includes extensive tests, x-ray studies, and collection of the fullest possible medical history of the patient as well as complete information of the conditions of his work and daily activities.

Excess weight, flat feet, and other structural conditions can and should be controlled. Frequently braces which support and rest a long irritated tissue will bring relief from backache. Warmth and gradually increasing degrees of massage and exercise are also often helpful. For acute or chronic backache due to strain in the lumbo-sacral region (low-back pain), rest on a flat, rather hard surface is beneficial. Boards can be inserted between the mattress and springs to insure a nonsagging sleeping surface. As long as it does not have too much "give," the bed need not be too hard. Those who suffer from postural backache will obtain definite relief from sleeping on a flat surface and by improving their posture.

Some of the many products sold to alleviate the pain of backache do afford a temporary relief. Persistent back pains, however, are a sign of a deeper disorder and the doctor should be consulted. *See also* SLIPPED DISC; SPINAL CORD.

BACKBONE, another term for spine. *See* SPINE.

BACTEREMIA, blood poisoning, the presence of bacteria in the blood. When the body's natural defenses around the site of an infection have been temporarily disorganized, bacteria may enter the blood stream. Such an invasion is called bacteremia. Symptoms are chills, heavy sweating, or general collapse.

Bacteremia is especially severe when caused by the entrance of staphylococci into the blood stream from abscesses in the skin or bone. The migrating bacteria may set up new abscesses at distant points in the body, in the deeper tissues or in the lungs. A physician should be called promptly because time is of the essence in controlling such a situation. Infections of this type can usually be controlled with antibiotics. Before the introduction of the newer drugs, especially penicillin, fatalities were numerous. The best means for preventing bacterial invasion is to care for all wounds adequately and immediately, and to get medical attention without delay for infections of the skin, tonsils, mouth, and ears. *See also* PYEMIA.

BACTERIA, one-celled organisms, scientifically classified as members of the plant world. They reproduce by fission; that is, each splits, producing two completely new organisms. Bacteria constitute one of the basic and largest classes of microorganisms. The term bacteria is preferable to the more popular name, germ, which indefinitely indicates almost any invisible, disease-causing organism. Although innumerable kinds of bacteria are known, only a few can live within the human body, and many of these are not harmful. However, other bacteria, known as pathogens, can produce such diseases as tuberculosis, diphtheria, tetanus, typhoid fever, and pneumonia.

The French scientist, Louis Pasteur, was one of the first to investigate the relationship of bacteria and other microorganisms to human and animal disease. Subsequently another scientist, Robert Koch, developed specific standards for proving that specific germs cause certain diseases. Koch's rules are: (1) the germ must be located within the body of the person or animal suffering from the disease. To verify the presence of the germ, swabs are taken of the infected area, such as the throat or ear. (2) The organisms, if grown in another body, must be able to produce a similar illness, or, if grown in a laboratory culture medium, more of the same organism capable of causing the same disease.

Bacteria are extremely sensitive to the conditions under which they live, which renders them relatively susceptible to complete control. For instance, they do not survive a high degree of heat or a lower heat sustained over a longer period, especially when moisture is associated with it. Consequently surgical instruments can be cleansed thoroughly of bacteria by fifteen or twenty minutes of boiling. Complete dryness, however, renders it impossible for bacteria to live, which is the reason that wound dressings are kept as dry as possible. Sunlight retards some bacteria and destroys others. Again, some germs, called aerobic, must have air to live; without it they die. Others, known as anaerobic, can live only in the absence of air.

Disease-causing, or pathogenic, bacteria harm the human body by the poisons or toxins which they produce. Some of these are excreted while others are held within the bacterial cell until it is destroyed. One of the protective measures of the body against infectious disease is the production of antitoxins which counteract these bacterial products. In addition the body produces other substances which prepare the bacteria for easier attack by the protective white cells of the blood, which also leads to the disintegration of the bacteria.

Bacteria usually abound wherever any moisture is present within the human environment, and protection against dangerous bacteria is a matter of selective measures rather than an attempt to avoid them entirely, which would be impossible. Eating and cooking equipment must be kept thoroughly clean for the elimination of bacteria. The hands should be washed before eating, especially after prolonged soiling or contact with anything in which dangerous bacteria are likely to live, such as human or animal wastes. Likewise bathing should be frequent.

The significance of these measures was established by a study at a midwestern university. The results proved that the effective laundering and drying of ordinary underwear cuts the bacterial count to one thousand or less per square inch, and the number rises to 400,000 per square inch in a single day's wear; that is, the numbers of bacteria present multiply 400 times, and reach 10,000,000 per square inch after underclothing is worn a week without washing.

Since Pasteur's basic discovery in the nineteenth century, medicine has developed a formidable array of specific weapons against bacteria, in addition to cleanliness, clean water supplies, and adequate sewage systems. Antiseptics like iodine and alcohol are available to clean wounds and instruments, and immunization procedures ward off many of the worst infectious diseases, such as diphtheria, lockjaw or tetanus. In addition the antibiotic drugs, like penicillin and the sulfas, are effective against a wide range of bacterial infections. The best protection is prevention, which means maintenance of clean conditions in and about the body. *See also* BACILLI; INFECTIONS; INFECTIOUS DISEASES; IMMUNIZATION; and Chapter 7, "The Process of Infectious Diseases and Immunization of Children."

BACTERIAL ENDOCARDITIS, an infection of the membranes of the heart cavities, which often attacks people who have had a previous heart disease. This condition also accounts for about 2 per cent of all organic heart disease, usually affecting young adults, although persons of every age group may have it.

Two forms of bacterial endocarditis are the acute and subacute. The acute form strikes suddenly and may cause death within a few days unless treated immediately. The subacute type comes on slowly and may also cause death within a year or so unless medical treatment is begun promptly. About 30 per cent of the cases end fatally, from various causes such as cerebral embolism and cardiac failure, in spite of treatment with the new antibiotics.

A characteristic sign is fever, especially with the acute form, although intermittent fever is usual in the chronic type. Anemia is also a symptom; as is embolism, which may disrupt circulation in acute cases, and in some instances cause nodes to appear in the skin of the fingers and toes. Fingers may also take on a clubbed appearance. Other complications include involvement of the lungs and kidney. Effective treatment of almost all cases of bacterial endocarditis consists of the use of one or more of the various antibiotics, such as penicillin or erythromycin, over varying periods of time.

For people who have heart defects and who may be susceptible to bacterial endocarditis, special care should be taken in dental or surgical treatment to prevent the possibility of its development. Such persons should be given large doses of penicillin or other antibiotics before any operation. *See also* ANEURYSM; and Chapter 12, "Diseases of the Heart."

BACTERICIDE, any substance able to destroy bacteria.

BACTERIOPHAGE, the name applied to a virus when it infects bacteria. *See also* VIRUSES.

BACTERIOSTATIC denotes the power of stopping the growth of bacteria.

BALANITIS, inflammation of the foreskin and the tip of the penis.

BALANTIDIASIS, or Balantidial colitis, an infection by a species of protozoa, unicellular bacillus, called balantidium. It is characterized by diarrhea and dysentery.

BALDNESS, or alopecia, loss or absence of hair. According to one authoritative estimate, nearly 300 million dollars a year is spent on alleged remedies and treatments for baldness. Occasionally good results seem to occur from these remedies, usually because hair, in many types of baldness, returns regardless of treatment or lack of it. This type of baldness and spontaneous regrowth often follows infectious diseases accompanied by fever, including pneumonia, typhoid, and influenza. Serious hair loss sometimes follows childbirth and surgery. In all these conditions, normal hair growth returns without help.

Bald or balding persons often wonder if there is anything that can be done to remedy their condition. The medical, and only reliable, answer at this time is that not much can be done. However, some hope for the future is held out; solution awaits the time and money needed for more thorough investigation.

Hair remedies and treatments for baldness are as old as civilization. The first known written medical record, the Ebers papyrus, contains a remedy for loss of hair. This prescription has among its ingredients fats of the lion, hippopotamus, crocodile, goose, serpent, and ibex.

Aristotle stated more than two thousand years ago that men and not women are usually afflicted by baldness, and today's medical science confirms this observation. Baldness seems not only to be largely restricted to males but appears also to be actually a male disease. According to Drs. Peter Flesch and Fred Urbach of the University of Pennsylvania, "Male sex hormones circulating in the body stimulate the sweat glands to produce a surplus of sebum which increases baldness." Attempts to counteract the effects of the male sex gland have not been successful, and neither have experiments with the female hormone, estrogen, in hair creams and lotions. Dermatologists agree that the use of estrogen in baldness may be dangerous and is thus ill-advised.

The only explanation scientists give

for the fact that many men do not suffer from baldness while so many others do is that baldness is largely hereditary. Most popular beliefs about baldness are untrue and exploited by quacks. Dry brittle hair, dandruff scales, thinning of hair in the crown and temples, tight and itching scalp actually do not cause baldness. Nor is it encouraged by wearing hats, tight or otherwise.

Excessive falling of hair is rarely a symptom of true baldness, as has been pointed out, but more often a sign of a physical disorder which a physician should attend to. Some illness usually precedes the condition known as "patch" or "area" baldness. It may be due to any of a variety of maladies, and may clear up when the patient has recovered from the illness that caused it.

If dandruff were a cause of baldness, most people would be victims of it. Dandruff, the flaking of the scalp, is apparently a normal process and, in the opinion of most doctors, is not harmful to hair. Yet while the chances are great that most cases of dandruff are the simple kind, a rarer type, seborrheic dermatitis, cannot be disregarded. It is caused by an infection of the glands in the scalp, and produces thick scales which provoke soreness and itchiness and may result in serious loss of hair. For control of dandruff, preparations of selenium, such as Selsun, are now available in ointments, lotion, and other forms. *See also* ALOPECIA; HAIR.

BANDAGE, a strip of material, usually of gauze, muslin, or flannel, in rolls of varied width, used to secure dressings, to immobilize a part, to check hemorrhage and to support an injured member or to apply pressure.

BARBER'S ITCH, scientifically sycosis, an infection of the bearded areas of the face and neck, may be caused by a fungus, *tinea barbae,* by a germ, such as staphylococcus, *sycosis barbae* or *sycosis vulgaris.*

Tinea barbae, which affects the chin and jowls and rarely the upper lip, is a severe inflammation, resulting in boggy little lumps and deep-seated sores that contain pus. At one time the infection was often spread by the use of contaminated shaving articles and towels in barber shops, but state laws which govern sanitation in barber shops have to a great extent controlled this problem. All shaving equipment must be sterilized after use, while barber's itch is being treated. Antiseptic lotions, fungicides, and ointments are helpful in reducing the inflammation. The disease is curable. If neglected, it may leave disfiguring scars; but if it is treated promptly, and the doctor's instructions followed carefully, it improves rapidly.

Sycosis barbae, sometimes caused by an infective discharge from the nose, begins with red sores around the hair follicles. The sores tend to become grouped and form pus. The condition most frequently attacks the upper lip, though it may involve the entire bearded area. The skin usually burns and is painful.

Early treatment prevents destruction of the roots of the hair and the resulting scarred and distorted skin. If the skin is inflamed, hot, saturated, boric acid dressings may be applied daily. The infected hairs are sometimes removed with a forceps until the skin seems to be healed. Soothing lotions or ointments are used at night, care being taken not to apply anything that would irritate the skin. X-ray therapy has been found beneficial in some cases. Shaving may be continued throughout the duration of the infection, but the razor should be dipped in alcohol before it is used; and a shaving cream used that does not require a brush.

BARBITURATES, derivatives of barbituric acid used in medicine as hypnotic and sedative drugs. Sedatives, or hypnotic drugs, are a valuable requisite to medicine. They can help break the cycle of insomnia in some cases, and restore the sleep pattern in others. Often they help to induce sleep when nervous and physical exhaustion has set up such a pattern of irritability that the person needs to relax for a long time. The inability to sleep can surely increase tension, making sleep exceedingly difficult. Sedation may be essential as the initial step to restful slumber.

Barbiturates are usually taken by mouth. Around barbituric acid, various pharmaceutical concerns have arranged diverse chemical groupings. Their main difference lies in absorption and elimination, onset and duration of action. In the United States, the most commonly known barbiturates are pentobarbital, (Nembutal), secobarbital (Seconal), amobarbital (Amytal), and phenobarbital (Luminal) which is the most slowly absorbed and longest acting.

Small doses of these barbiturates evoke drowsiness by depressing the functions of those parts of the brain related to mental activities. Therefore, physicians often prescribe these drugs to help patients with ulcers to relax and thus overcome contributing causes such as worry and anxiety.

Only in large doses do barbiturates have any value as analgesics. Some quick-acting barbiturates, such as pentothal sodium and evipan sodium, have been found effective as anesthetics during short operations because they rarely have any aftereffect.

In spite of newer drugs, long-acting barbiturates like phenobarbital remain a medical adjunct in epilepsy, in which the cerebral motor cortex is abnormally active. Barbiturates are effective because they not only produce a hypnotic effect but also slow down the activity of that segment of the brain which induces movement. Phenobarbital drugs also elicit calmness in patients in whom conditions of abnormal motor activity are produced by overactive thyroid glands.

Unfortunately barbiturates are too often subject to abuse. The physician with a patient who is psychologically disturbed endeavors to direct his treatment toward the eradication of the fundamental cause of the disturbance in preference to treating the symptoms by a long-term prescription of barbiturates. Barbiturates should serve only as a temporary bridge.

Taken frequently over a long time, and in large doses, barbiturates are harmful. As in the case of alcoholism, it is not easy to say when proper use of such drugs ends and improper use begins. Dr. Harris Isbell of the U. S. Public Health Service says that many people use 0.2 grams without any apparent ill effects. This equals two 1½-grain capsules, or one 3-grain "block-buster." Much more than this amount will cause various degrees of mental and physical impairment. Four times this quantity taken for only a few months will produce a dependency that may give the user withdrawal symptoms similar to those an addict goes through when the drug is removed, according to Dr. Isbell.

F. Leslie Hart, chief of the Boston District U. S. Food and Drug Administration, says of the habitual use of barbiturates, "From a purely physical viewpoint we feel that barbiturates are worse than narcotics. The habitual victim has difficulty thinking, cannot perform even simple calculations, loses the power to judge distances, becomes infantile, weeps easily and eventually has a desire for death."

According to both state and federal laws, barbiturates are not to be sold without a doctor's prescription and there cannot be any legal refilling of a prescription without specific orders from a doctor. Unfortunately the ways in which these laws are violated are numerous, and the frequent and tragic misuse of drugs which the medical profession considers useful must be curbed.

Barbiturate poisoning may be mild, moderate, or severe. About 1,500 deaths are caused yearly in the United States by the acute form, which is the most common. Women are more subject to excessive doses of barbiturates than men. Some time ago, the U. S. Public Health Service investigated 547 nonfatal cases; 407 women took an overdose of the drug to 140 men. Of these cases, 254 were accidental and 293 were attempts at suicide. In addition, poisoning may result from a pronounced sensitivity to the drugs. Drowsiness induced by a small dose may pass into a coma after an overdose.

The symptoms of acute barbiturate poisoning resemble, to some degree, those of alcoholic intoxication. Among the numerous mental symptoms are moral deterioration, aggressive outbursts, slurring of speech, and impairment of mental activity. A reeling gait, because of uncontrolled muscular action, rapid beating of the heart, disturbed digestion and vision, and, in severe cases, exceedingly slow and shallow respiration are other signs.

Mortality, which is at present about 8 per cent in all cases of barbiturate abuse, is highest in older people and in those with a weakened physical condition. Care should be exercised not to give barbiturates to people with liver and kidney disorders, since the liver is actively involved in destroying toxins and the kidney in excreting them.

New sleeping pills, nonbarbiturates, have recently been developed. Chemists are on the threshold of developing a whole new category of hypnotic drugs safer than the powerful habit-forming barbiturates and still strong enough to induce sleep. The promising new leads have come from animal experiments with a chemical called tertiary amyl alcohol. This substance, known since 1890, seems to meet some of the requirements for the long-sought-for ideal hypnotic drug in that it is not habit forming, and does not have some of the disagreeable aftereffects associated with barbiturates. Compounds of this drug produced satisfactory results. *See also* TRANQUILIZING DRUGS; POISONING.

BARIUM SULPHATE, a compound formed by barium and sulphuric acid, used as a pigment and as a filler in such products as paper and rubber. It is also invaluable in taking roentgenograms of the stomach and intestines, because, when taken by mouth, it renders those organs opaque to x-rays, and subsequently the drug passes unchanged through the gastrointestinal tract. Barium sulphate should be carefully distinguished from barium sulphide and sulphite, which are poisonous.

BARLOW'S DISEASE. *See* RICKETS; SCURVY; VITAMINS.

BASAL GANGLIA, groups of nerve cells, situated internally in the brain substance. They control inherited basic emotions and deter muscles from certain movements which would occur if this area of the brain were injured.

BASAL METABOLISM. Metabolism is the conversion of food into energy in a living body. Basal metabolism is a measure of the chemical changes involved in the body at rest. The basal metabolic rate measures the speed at which basic, constant processes within the body are taking place and, in particular, how much oxygen a person uses in a given time. A normal male between the ages of 20 and 50 produces 38 to 40 calories of heat every hour for every square meter of body surface, or about 1 calory per kilogram of body weight. This figure does not vary with height, weight, or general body size in healthy men. The basal metabolism indicates whether or not heat is produced at a greater or smaller rate than is normal for most people in developing energy from food and oxygen.

When a basal metabolism test is made, the person rests after arising in the morning, without having had any breakfast, and breathes from a tank containing a measured amount of air. The rate at which the oxygen in that air is consumed indicates the level of the basal metabolism. A range of 7 plus to 7 minus, relative to the average, is considered normal. Some persons, however, have rates as low as 25 minus without ill-effect on their health. Children who are active and growing have a noticeably higher rate than the average. Various factors cause the basal metabolic rate to be greater than normal. Intense emotions, such as fright or rage, speed up the metabolism, as do certain diseases, such as hyperthyroidism.

Lowered basal metabolism is noted in such bodily states as sleep or undernourishment. It is also found in persons who are anemic, have certain nervous disorders or thyroid deficiency. Inadequacy of either the pituitary or the adrenal gland may have the same effect, while excessive action by either can raise the basal metabolism.

The basal metabolism of a pregnant woman remains at its usual level until the last two or three months before birth. Then the rate in this period will represent the combined metabolism of both mother and child.

In contrast to physical exertion, mental exercise has little effect on the metabolism. According to one authority, half of a salted peanut would provide all the extra calories needed to support a full hour of intense mental concentration.

BASEDOW'S DISEASE. *See* EXOPHTHALMIC GOITER; GOITER.

BCG VACCINE. The letters BCG indicate the bacillus first noted by Calmette and Guerin, two researchers of the Pasteur Institute. It is a vaccine used as a means of increasing resistance to tuberculosis, which is spread chiefly from one person who has it to those who have not.

The vaccine is made from a bovine strain of tubercle bacilli, weakened by growth on potato glycerin and bile for several years. The supporters of BCG vaccine point out that it has been successfully used on many millions of children and adults all over the world. *See also* IMMUNIZATION.

BATHING, the total or partial immersion of the body in a medium such as air, vapor, sand, or water, in order to cleanse, soothe, stimulate, heat, cool or irritate it.

Bathing habits of people vary according to their habits and living conditions. The routine use of soap for cleansing is recent. In ancient times, people oiled the skin, and sometimes cleansed themselves with a sweat, or Turkish steam, bath. Soap cleanses the skin by breaking up or emulsifying the oily secretions and then dissolving them. Thus the layer of grease is removed and the accumulated dirt along with it.

For cleansing the body, a moderately warm bath or shower—from 95° to 100° F.—with soap is best, with thorough washing of portions of the body likely to perspire and acquire odor. Usually the best cleansing soap is ordinary white soap which is easily rubbed into a lather. A soft washcloth helps to cleanse parts of the body difficult to reach. The soap lather should be thoroughly washed from the body with plenty of water since soap left on the skin may irritate it. Brisk rubbing with a towel stimulates circulation and will not injure ordinary skin. However, patting dry with a soft towel is better than rubbing the body if the skin is delicate.

Persons with extremely dry, sensitive, or itching skin may irritate the condition by excessive numbers of hot soapy baths; in many cases, a mild cleansing and oiling is sufficient.

Cool baths conduct heat away from the body and are often recommended to lower the temperature in fever. Hot water causes dilation of the superficial blood vessels and such excess stimulation causes profuse sweating. In taking a hot-water bath, the temperature should be about 98° at the start and then be increased to 115°. Remaining too long in a hot bath may lead to exhaustion and even collapse. A quick cold shower or bath, often called a tonic bath, is stimulating because of the sudden change in temperature which produces an immediate contraction of the blood vessels. After the tonic bath, rubbing the body vigorously with a rough towel adds to the stimulation. A cold shower or bath does not agree with many people, and there is no evidence that it is particularly healthful or that it will harden the body against catching colds. *See also* HYGIENE; SKIN.

BED AND BEDDING. The bed, the mattress, and the pillows should be designed to give proper support as well as comfort in health and in sickness. The mattress should usually be rather hard to give back support. Many good beds, springs, and coverings are available. In the case of long illness, a hospital bed is preferable, for it permits the head and feet of the patient to be raised or lowered, is of correct height for the person giving nursing care, and can be easily moved from place to place on its casters. During illness, the bed should be placed where the opening of the door does not cause a draft. If the windows or door are open, a screen should be placed before the bed. For tall patients, a chair can be used to extend the bed. Kitchen chairs tied together and placed against the side of the bed will safeguard the patient against falling out of bed.

The mattress should be covered by a rubber sheet as well as a draw sheet to protect it when using a bedpan or giving a bed bath. A draw sheet which extends from the patient's shoulder to the knees can easily be removed when soiled.

Cotton sheets should be of sufficient length and width so that they can be carefully tucked in on the sides and at the bottom of the bed. Wool blankets, warm but lightweight, are preferable.

The general condition and the type of disease from which the patient is suffering will determine the number of pillows on the bed, and the advice of the physician should be followed. Pillows should be thin and light, and frequently shaken and aired in a shady place.

If the patient is bedridden, the task of making up the bed becomes more difficult. Whenever possible, the patient should be moved into another bed beside his own bed. If the patient can be moved, he should be assisted to a footstool or chair next to the bed. If this is not possible, and the bed must be made up with the patient in it, follow these directions. Remove the blankets, pillows, and top sheet. Cover the patient with the blanket and loosen the bottom sheet and the draw sheet. Roll the patient onto his side, on the right side of the bed, and push the soiled sheets toward the patient, so that they are next to his back. Smooth the mattress pad and rubber sheet, making sure that they are not wrinkled or creased. Spread the clean sheet the length of the bed, and fold the half of the sheet on which the patient is lying next to his back on top of the sheets which are to be removed. Then begin at the foot of the bed to tuck the sheet under the mattress, being sure to make a square corner at the foot and head of the bed. Put half of the draw sheet on, tucking it under the mattress and leaving half of it free for the other side of the bed. Then help the patient roll over onto the clean sheets, and proceed to make the other side of the bed in the same manner. First remove the soiled sheets. Smooth out the rubber sheet and mattress pad. Then tuck the bottom sheet and draw sheet under the mattress. Place the top sheet over the blanket, remove the blanket, and tuck the sheet in at the foot of the bed. Replace the blankets, tucking them in at the foot, and change the pillow cases and replace the pillows on the bed.

A bedridden patient may best be shifted with the aid of soft pillows, air cushions, blankets, or similar materials to hold him in a different position.

BEDBUG, a common domestic insect pest; small, wingless, and light brown in color. Although it feeds on the blood of human beings, it is not, strictly speaking, a human parasite. It comes to the human skin only for its food and may, in the absence of human beings, feed on other warm-blooded animals. The bedbug lives in the crevices of bedsteads, floors, walls, wallpaper, and furniture. Usually it is carried from house to house on clothing and bedding, but it may also travel from one dwelling to another in search of nourishment.

Several insect bites resemble one another, but bedbug wheals, swollen inflamed areas surrounding central puncture spots, may be distinguished from those of mosquitoes because they seem to be limited to one area and to follow a track.

Aside from constituting a nuisance and secreting a mildly unpleasant odor from their glands, the species, *cimex lectularis,* common to the temperate zone, may also be the carrier of such diseases as kala azar, European relapsing fever, and, according to certain experiments, plague and tularemia.

Because their area of operation is limited, bedbugs seem to be minor pests compared to mosquitoes, yet are sufficiently prolific and hardy to defy nonchemical attempts at extermination. A bedbug can live as long as six weeks without any nourishment. The female lays 200 eggs from three to four times annually, in batches of approximately fifty. The larvae hatch in from one to three weeks, grow slowly, and mature in six weeks to six months; the young moult five times at intervals of eight days leaving characteristic shells. Usually a 5 per cent spray of DDT, or one of the better exterminating preparations on the market, will be efficient.

BED SORES. A bed sore is a degeneration of skin at a particular spot, which exposes underlying tissues and invites infection. At first glance, it may seem rather insignificant but actually, in a bedridden paralytic or aged person, bed sores are potentially so serious that nurses and doctors must continually guard against them. They are much easier to prevent than to treat.

Those persons most susceptible to bed sores are the chronically sick and the people affected by specific disorders of the nervous system. Protracted pressure on a particular area of skin, especially such as occurs from lying in one position too long, is the immediate factor.

Once established, a bed sore causes degeneration of tissues in the area involved, and ultimately leads to ulceration. Expert medical care for such condition is imperative to prevent extensive damage in the area of the ulcer.

The weight of a human body, no

matter what its position, presses against the body's outer surface unevenly. Standing, the heels get most of the pressure; and sitting, the buttocks, the lower end of the spine, the upper parts of the hip bones and the thighs receive it. Lying down, the areas bearing the greatest pressure will depend, again, on the exact posture, but will usually include the shoulders, buttocks, and thighs.

Tissues that are not healthful tend to break down when subjected to more than 1½ to two pounds per square inch for any length of time. An average man weighs approximately 150 pounds, and the weight is usually focused in some of the spots indicated. The risk of tissue damage and resulting bed sores in a bedridden patient is obvious.

Bed sores may be prevented by frequent shifts of the position in bed, by changes of type of gown or bedclothes materials to eliminate irritation to the skin, and by keeping the skin in the best of care. Normally, as research studies on sleeping people have proved, the body almost automatically shifts posture every few minutes. One of the special dangers involved in paralysis and chronic, debilitating illness is that the person affected is either unable or too weak to turn alone. In such cases, one of the major responsibilities of the person caring for the patient is to do it for him. Different kinds of props and pillows can be used to help.

Another special problem arises with paralyzed people when control over their basic excretory functions is lost. In such cases, constant care is essential to remove soil and moisture from the skin. Skin that is wet, or even damp, is much more easily damaged by friction or pressure than dry skin.

In general, bathing and suitable care of the skin are among the most important preventives against bed sores. Powder, to guard against excess dampness, and alcohol are particularly useful.

Bedclothes should be clean and free of particles of food or other wastes. They should be soft and unstarched. Sheets should be smoothed out and wrinkling and bunching corrected frequently.

Reddening of the skin in one area, which disappears if lightly pressed, is the danger signal, warning of a potential bed sore. Such spots should receive prompt and thorough medical attention. Powerful disinfectants, which many people are inclined to apply thoughtlessly to a developing sore, may increase the existing damage rather than help.

BED WETTING, urination during sleep after the age of three, by which time normal bladder control is ordinarily expected to be established.

Bed wetting is an early childhood habit that is not easy to control. In the adult, urination is regulated by two nerve centers; one, involuntary, in the spinal cord and the other, which in turn controls that in the spinal cord, in the brain. The newborn infant releases urine automatically and the act is regulated from the spinal center in accordance with the need to empty the bladder. As the child grows and is gradually trained, the brain becomes involved in the conscious control of urination and eventually regulates it during sleep.

Some children acquire this control earlier than others, but the average time is two years. If, however, this habit has not been well established by the end of the third year, medical attention is warranted.

The causes of bed wetting vary greatly. Physical reasons alone are often responsible, such as infection, inflammation, or faulty nutrition. A doctor will always examine a child thoroughly at the outset to determine whether or not such a factor is involved. Bed wetting may also be of nervous or emotional origin, and a large proportion of cases are of this kind. In such instances, attempts to control the problem directly are unavailing. Improved psychological adjustment is indicated and is the principal hope of curing bed wetting. Punishment is likelier to work in reverse, to reinforce the habit rather than break it.

Some young children urinate in their clothes during the waking hours, largely because they are too interested in what they are doing to bother to go to the toilet. The preferred solution to this problem is to explain the situation to the child, help him to remember, and praise him for adequate continence. Here again, punishment accomplishes little or nothing.

The following methods will facilitate bladder training:

1. Give the child plenty of water during the day, but no water or other fluid after 5:00 P.M.

2. A bit of fruit may be given if the child complains of thirst at bedtime.

3. Get the child out of bed to go to the toilet at 10:00 P.M. Awaken him sufficiently to permit him to urinate thoroughly and consciously.

4. When he awakens, get the child to the toilet without delay. Bed wetting often occurs a few minutes after the child's sleep has ended, if he does not get to the toilet promptly.

5. When diapers are finally omitted during the day, omit them also at night, but protect the bed adequately.

6. In "dry" suppers, omit milk, water, or cocoa for drinking, and do not serve milk with cereal or with dessert. Cook foods with milk when possible. Whole-grain cereal and bread are preferable.

If it is necessary to take the child to the toilet a second time at night, note the time when the bed wetting occurs, and then plan to awaken him a few minutes before that time. The interval between the first picking up and the second can be regulated to aid the child's progress. *See also* CHILD CARE; and Chapter 9, "Child Care and Training."

BEE STINGS. The injection of bee poison by a bee into the skin is a bee sting. A blister and a surrounding area of redness appear immediately, but usually all symptoms disappear within twenty-four hours or less. But some people have such a sensitivity to the venom that the symptoms are exceedingly dangerous and have been known to be fatal.

The poison injected by the bee is composed of acid and alkaline materials and a substance much like histamine, which is a chemical released into the blood stream by allergies. Ultrasensitive people can be desensitized by being injected with small amounts of bee poison over a period of time, thus building up a resistance to it.

The bee stings by inserting a sharp, fine, horny needle with two barbs into its victim. The needle with its barbs remains anchored in the skin. The bee, in its efforts to get away, presses on the sac containing the bee venom and the pressure empties it into the skin of the victim. Research has proved that this bee venom is a virulent poison, that it affects the heart and destroys the red blood cells, lowers blood pressure and contracts the muscles of the heart and intestines.

A person who has had multiple bee stings or is known to be sensitive should immediately rest, and the action of the heart and kidneys must be carefully watched. If the blood pressure falls too rapidly, and such symptoms as swelling of the body or collapse appear, a physician should be called. He must also be consulted promptly if the sting is on the tongue or in any other very sensitive place. He can give relief by injecting or applying locally such antihistamines as Benadryl, Pyribenzamine, or Neohetramine.

Generally, and especially in the case of children, the stinger should be removed with tweezers, if possible. For relief of itching, a paste of baking soda, well-diluted ammonia, or soothing lotions may be applied. Vinegar is beneficial in stings of wasps, hornets and yellow jackets. The wounds of insect bites should never be scratched.

BELCHING, the eructation of sour substances, including acid of the stomach, air, or gas. People who eat too fast swallow air and then belch it back.

Belching has become a recognized part of baby care and has brought a new word into our language, burping. In nursing, especially with the bottle, the baby swallows quantities of air. As the small capacity of his stomach does not allow for air bubbles, these cause pressure and pain. The process of assisting the baby to bring up the bubbles is called "burping the baby."

In cases of cancer of the larynx, when the larynx is removed, belching is necessary so that the patient can learn to speak by the esophageal method. To help him acquire this skill, the patient is encouraged to drink carbonated water. It brings air into his mouth and thus he can cause it to vibrate against the roof of the pharynx.

BELLADONNA. *See* DEADLY NIGHTSHADE POISONING.

BELL'S PALSY, paralysis of the muscles of one or both sides of the face. Rarely are both sides affected, nor is any other organ of the body involved. Charles Bell, a Scottish physician, first described the condition early in the nineteenth century, but its cause is still not definitely established. Drafts or overexposure to cold have been alleged as causes of this condition, but this belief also has not been proved.

A mild pain in the eye, ear, or face often precedes Bell's palsy. The paralysis develops so abruptly that frequently the person affected realizes it only by a feeling of numbness and stiffness on one side of the face. Within a few hours the eye on that side seems to be more widely open than the other eye. It cannot be closed and waters excessively. The mouth is drawn over to the side of the face and speech is impaired. Eating is disturbed, chewing or swallowing is difficult, and taste is dulled. Sensitivity to sound may also be abnormal.

Milder cases generally clear within a month or two, and in about 85 to 90 per cent of the cases complete recovery ensues. In the more severe cases, in which severe paralysis has occurred, improvement is much slower and more limited. Taste may be lost on the front two-thirds of the tongue, and muscles which remain affected after many months are apt to be permanently weakened. In such instances, muscular movement, such as blinking the eye, may be accompanied by a twitching of the corner of the mouth or of the muscles of the neck.

Patients with Bell's palsy are cautioned to keep the eyes protected at all times against dust or foreign bodies, since sensation is lost during the active stages when the eyelids cannot close. Physicians recommend a drop of mineral oil in the eye, morning and evening, to keep it clean. To prevent permanent sagging of the facial muscles, physiotherapy and facial massage at frequent intervals are advised until the muscles begin to indicate resumption of their normal functions. Splints have been devised to support the sagging tissues, and electric stimulation may be used during this period although it should be discontinued as soon as the muscles show signs of recuperation. Cortisone seems to be effective in shortening the duration of the palsy and in making recovery more complete. Surgery is sometimes tried in more stubborn cases, but the results have not been uniformly successful.

BENADRYL, an antihistaminic drug which opposes the action of a substance called histamine which is released into the tissues by allergy or sensitivity. It is used in allergic conditions like hay fever, asthma, urticaria, contact dermatitis, erythema, rhinitis, drug sensitization, serum reactions, and irradiation sickness. It has also been used to relieve motion sickness.

"BENDS." *See* CAISSON DISEASE.

BENZEDRINE, the trade name for amphetamine, a potent stimulant usually taken orally in tablet form, and rarely injected. This drug has a powerful action on the brain, in addition to its ability to cause physiological changes similar to those produced by action of the sympathetic nervous system. In a milder form, Benzedrine parallels the effect of cocaine. This drug is prescribed by physicians as a stimulant and to cut down appetite in obesity. An amphetamine produces a sensation of well-being so intense that the user is not interested in food. This property of the drug has led to its utilization in weight-reduction programs, sometimes promiscuously, without a physician's direction.

The abuse of Benzedrine has become common among alcoholics, barbiturate addicts, and thrill seekers who turn to the amphetamines for the delusive sense of well-being and confidence that they cannot find for themselves. Among the symptoms of overdose and of chronic poisoning are nervousness, apprehension, tremors, insomnia, hypertension, and dilatation of the pupils of the eyes. Hallucinations and delusions of a paranoid type may be a psychotic consequence.

BERIBERI, a deficiency disease resulting from an inadequacy of vitamin B_1 or thiamine in the diet. This condition was first brought to public attention in countries with limited diets, where the population subsisted on polished rice. In 1897 Dr. Eijkman, a Dutch physician in Java, observed forms of neuritis and paralysis among chickens fed on polished rice, and found that they were absent in chickens fed on whole rice. Shortly thereafter, a British doctor in Malaya noticed the same symptoms among human beings subsisting mainly on white rice.

As polished rice is the main article of diet in the Orient, incidence of beriberi is greatest there. The bran of the rice grains contains sufficient thiamin, but this bran is often thrown away with the outer portion, which also contains the protein and fat. Such deficiency in a milder form also exists in Western countries because of inadequacies in the diet. Typical symptoms include waterlogging of the heart and disturbances of sensation in the extremities.

Beriberi attacks the gastrointestinal tract and causes changes in the nervous system. Manifestations of this disease are multiple neuritis, paralysis, progressive edema, inflammation of the nerves, collection of fluids in the legs, changes in the adrenal glands, mental deterioration, and heart failure. In addition, there is a tingling and numbness in the portions of the body reached by the nerves affected, tenderness of the muscles, wasting of the tissues through secondary infections, fever, and general weakness and disability.

Beriberi was once prevalent in the Far East and parts of Brazil, Newfoundland, and Labrador, and also on ships making long voyages. Since the cause of the disease has been discovered, it is now rare. Nevertheless, it is possible that a relative deficiency of thiamine in the diet may produce a mild form of the disease.

Occasionally invalids on greatly restricted diets suffer from a deficiency of thiamine. After surgical operations on the bowel, in cases of chronic diarrhea, ulcers of the stomach, chronic alcoholism, or after long infectious diseases, signs of thiamine deficiency may appear. Food faddists, living on incomplete diets, may show a moderate form of beriberi, and chronic alcoholics, who stop eating during their periods of drinking, often manifest the same symptoms.

BICEPS usually refers to the large muscle on the front of the upper arm. The name is derived from the fact that it has two heads, one long and one short, which are attached to the shoulder blade at two different points. On muscular people, these two heads unite and swell out into a single large muscle. When this muscle contracts, it bends the forearm toward the upper arm and is therefore used in all lifting and pulling motions. Another bicep muscle in the human body is located at the back of the thigh.

BICHLORIDE OF MERCURY, a compound of two equivalents of chlorine with mercury; highly poisonous when swallowed. In a weak solution it is a germicide. Taken internally it produces serious inflammation of the kidney and a general poisoning of the peripheral nerves, with paralysis of the limbs. *See also* POISONING.

BICUSPID, a tooth with two cusps, or points. An adult with a full set of teeth has two bicuspids between each canine and first molar, eight in all. The bicuspid is often called premolar. *See also* TEETH.

BIFOCAL, a system of lenses with double focus. Those who need different glasses for near and distant vision can have the proper lenses combined in a single pair of glasses. The smaller lens, for near vision, is placed below the center of the larger lens, which is for distant vision. These are called bifocal lenses and are said to have been invented by Benjamin Franklin.

BILE, a bitter, bright golden-red fluid, manufactured in the liver and excreted into the intestines. Its function is the digestion of fat and its absorption from the intestines. It stimulates movements of the intestines, prevents fermentation of the contents, and serves as a disinfectant. Bile is essential for the absorption of vitamins A, D, E, and K, and is also known to have a mild laxative effect in its salt form.

The amount of bile secreted daily by a healthy liver varies from twenty to thirty ounces; a diseased liver may not secrete bile properly. Although secretion of bile is continuous, it is more active directly after meals. Whenever there is an interval in the digestive process, bile accumulates in the gallbladder, a bag-shaped organ that projects from the tubes that carry bile from the liver to the intestines. When required again, bile is poured into the intestines. The necessary stimulus to the renewed flow is given by the passage of the acid contents of the stomach over the intestinal orifice of the common bile duct.

Bile consists of water, bile salts, a little fat, which in part is lecithin, and pigments. Cholesterin is another ingredient, which appears to be a fatty substance but is actually an alcohol. Together with other elements found in bile, cholesterin is the basis of formation of gallstones in the gallbladder or the biliary ducts. Passage of these stones through the ducts is connected with painful spasms known as biliary colic.

Any obstruction of the flow of bile into the intestines results in the absorption of the secretion into the blood, and jaundice occurs when it accumulates there. *See also* DIGESTION; JAUNDICE; LIVER.

BILHARZIASIS, a disease caused by a parasite, Schistosoma haematobium, a genus of trematode worms, which gets into the human body, principally when people swim in contaminated waters. The intermediary host of this worm is the fresh-water snail. The condition has previously been a tropical disease, and apparently originated in the Nile Valley thousands of years ago. When the parasite gets into the skin, it produces an inflammation. Then the eggs get into the human bladder and other hollow organs of the body, where ulcers and inflammations occur. Certain specific drugs, like emetine and those of antimony, will eliminate this parasitic blood fluke from the human body. Repeated infections in the intestine, however, will cause ulcers and bleeding. The worst form, which is severe and which may lead eventually to death, is the Asiatic variety.

BILIOUSNESS, in popular usage, a condition of digestive disturbance accompanied by headache, nausea, constipation, thick tongue, and other similar complaints. The word is scientifically a misnomer and rarely encountered in medical literature. It goes back to the time, centuries ago, when illness was interpreted in terms of "humors," of which bile was considered the worst.

The amount of bile in the body actually has little or nothing to do with whether or not a person is "bilious." Symptoms that accompany "biliousness" are due to one or more of many different specific causes. If the disorder is serious and demands treatment, the doctor must determine the cause in order to prescribe correctly. The term "bilious" does not convey any pertinent information except to suggest the presence of certain symptoms. Excessively rich food, migraine, eye strain, glaucoma, brain tumor, or other conditions may provoke the symptoms. Liver infections, by ameba or organisms of malaria may be the source of the trouble. Hardening of the liver from various causes is another possibility. Severe infections induce destruction of liver cells. The liver has a safety factor of unusual size—in fact, seven times as large as necessary for minimum requirements—but even this margin can be endangered by persistent abuse through eating and drinking. The person who suffers from "biliousness" usually has discomfort and loss of well-being without particularly severe pain. He is easily tired and disinclined to work. The symptoms often disappear at midday when the person develops an increased appetite.

Sufferers of "biliousness" will feel more comfortable if they avoid rich foods such as pastry, chocolate, candy, and eat more protein-rich food. Alcohol should be omitted. Glucose, taken either by mouth or injected, will provide relief.

BILIRUBIN, orange-red crystals or powder which constitute the main pigment of bile. The crystals are normally present in feces or excrement and are also found in the urine in cases of obstructive jaundice. Bilirubin is sometimes injected into the veins as a test of liver function. *See also* BILE.

BINET-SIMON TEST. The Binet-Simon test is a method of testing the mental capacity of children. In 1908, after experiments with large groups of school children, the French psychologist, Alfred Binet, introduced the first systematic intelligence test. A revised form of Binet's scale was issued in 1911 in collaboration with Theodore Simon. The method provides groups of questions and problems, suitable for the mental age of the subject. On the basis of these tests and a standard developed for normal subjects, a psychologist can quickly determine whether or not a child is advanced, retarded or normal in relation to his own age group. The original Binet-Simon tests have been the subject of many more recent modifications. *See* I.Q.

BIOPSY, the removal and examination, usually under a microscope, for diagnosis of material from the living body. This material may be removed by means of a needle, punch, sponge, or other instrument. Surface biopsy involves the microscopic study of cells which have been scraped from the surface of suspected areas. This technique is frequently employed when examining for cancer of the uterus or bowel. Scrapings are also studied, including those from the stomach, intestines, or other tissues.

BIRTH CERTIFICATE, the written, authenticated record required by law of the birth of a child, whether at home or at the hospital and reported by the doctor or the midwife to the local registrar or the Bureau of Vital Statistics. The birth is placed in a permanent record and a certificate is issued to the parents. A name for a boy or girl should be picked beforehand so that the certificate is complete and accurate. If a child dies during birth, an immediate certificate is demanded. This certificate must contain not only a statement of the cause of death, but also any secondary causes which have been noted.

The birth certificate is of great importance on many occasions. Proof of parentage is required when a person applies for citizenship, a government position, passport, entrance to school or college, and on many other occasions. Therefore, a birth certificate or a certified copy should always be on hand. As the birth certificate is so significant throughout life, some certified copies should be made with the original. If a certificate is not received by the parents in due time, the delay should be checked with the local Board of Health.

If any person does not have a birth certificate and if he knows where and when he was born, he should write to the city clerk in the place concerned and on payment of a small fee obtain a copy of his birth certificate.

BIRTH INJURIES. Hazards to the well-being of an infant while it is still in the womb of the mother may result from an injury or disease during pregnancy. Other dangers may develop during the birth itself, or just after birth. The brain of the baby may remain undeveloped, or birth injuries may be of varying degree. In some instances, delivery is hastened to safeguard mother and child, or forceps applied to the baby's head before it appears at the opening of the birth canal, methods which can, in some cases, cause birth injuries.

Even a normal birth subjects the skull and brain of the baby to much possible trauma. In the case of premature births, the chance of injury is even greater. The softer bones of the premature baby do not protect the brain as well as the harder ones of the full-term infant; thus intracranial injuries are more frequent. So many factors are involved that physicians find it difficult to diagnose certain afflictions as being due to birth or postnatal injuries. Such traumas of the brain at birth are responsible for at least one-third of all infant fatalities during the first two weeks of life.

Bleeding into the brain is a frequent cause of immediate disturbances in the newborn infant, or even of death. A tendency to these intracranial hemorrhages in the newborn will increase the peril of even the slightest injury to the baby as well as to the pregnant mother. While fractures of the skull of newborn babies are rare, pressure on the skull occurs with consequent contusions and cerebral injuries not accompanied by hemorrhages. Irreparable damage to the brain may be the result of a premature separation of the placenta, or twisting of the cord and an inadequate oxygen supply. Birth injuries may bring about chronic lesions or alterations of functional capacity. Varying in the degree of severity, they include congenital faulty development of the external gray layer of the brain, cysts and hardening.

Birth injuries have various symptoms, such as suffocation, irregular and curtailed breathing, feeble cry, pallor or excessive redness, stupor and inability to suck. Involuntary muscular spasms and convulsions may also be observed, as well as dilated eyes and irregular pupils because of bleeding of the retina. In some cases, positive symptoms from hemorrhages cannot be discerned. Diagnostic signs may be as obscure as lack of appetite, inability to gain weight, a slight increase of the size of the head or one or perhaps a few convulsive seizures.

Persistent injuries of the brain, re-sulting from birth casualties, produce some types of neurological disturbances such as paralysis of one side of the body or of muscles and limbs with a characteristic rigidity. Birth injury is one of the causes of the paralysis, due to a lesion of the brain, commonly called cerebral palsy.

Difficulties during delivery are responsible, too, for damage of the spinal cord. As the tendons of the spinal column of the newborn baby are elastic, the slightest twisting or stretching may result in serious dislocation. Damage to the skeleton may not be apparent and yet such injuries can have a direct effect on the spinal cord and its membranes. A complete breaking of the cord may follow in the wake of a severe mishap. Here, too, however, hemorrhages provoke the most serious consequences. The damages of the spinal cord may be of different degrees of severity, and the neurological symptoms may thus vary in the few infants who survive such birth injuries. *See also* CEREBRAL PALSY.

BIRTHMARK (nevus), a congenital skin blemish or circumscribed area of pigmentation. Birthmarks include pigmented moles and skin discolorations brought about by blood vessels, as, for instance, "strawberry" marks. Some birthmarks develop years after birth, but the skin defect is there from the beginning, from the formation of the skin in the fetus. Nothing can be done to prevent birthmarks. Immediately after birth, these marks may be small and insignificant, but they may gradually grow larger and more prominent by the time the child is a few weeks or months old.

Then they may stop growing or, in some cases, even disappear. Yet it is impossible to foresee whether or not a spot will cause symptoms.

The strawberry birthmark is produced by a mass of blood vessels which collect in a cluster near the surface of the skin. It may be deep scarlet color if deep below the skin, or bluish if more superficial. Pressure on such a birthmark makes it colorless, in proportion to the blood forced from the blood vessels. A survey made in 1955 by a surgeon proved that without surgery or other treatment ordinary strawberry birthmarks often disappeared or became inconspicuous as the person grew older.

Another type of birthmark, of a pale blue or gray color, is characterized by more cellular tissue and less fluid, and is less spongy than the strawberry blemish. Its color cannot be pressed out, since it contains a smaller amount of blood vessels.

The port-wine birthmark, another type of skin blemish, is a collection of small blood vessels with various amounts of pigment deposited from the blood into the skin. Not much can be done for these, but fortunately they rarely enlarge. Treatment with ultraviolet rays may, in some instances, effect complete disappearance. If the blemishes are large and unsightly, they can be covered with one of the several cosmetic preparations available.

Usually skin lesions of the birthmark type are treated with the electric needle, frozen with carbon dioxide snow, cauterized with heat or various chemicals like carbolic or nitric acid, removed surgically, or treated with radium. All these methods have merit when properly used in the right case.

Recently a "plastic planing" device has been successfully applied. The marks are actually scraped or planed away with a surgical device like an emory wheel, allowing the growth of smooth new skin. Another modern method is to inject the blood vessels in such growths with various chemical substances that cause a slight inflammatory reaction inside the blood vessels which eventually results in scarring and obliteration or disappearance of the birthmark. Such methods are exceedingly delicate, but in most instances successful when carried out under proper conditions by an experienced physician.

BIRTH, MULTIPLE, the birth of more than one offspring at the same or approximately same time, with all having been conceived at the same time.

Twins occur about once in every 90 births, triplets once in 10,000, quadruplets once in 750,000 and quintuplets once in many million births. Seventeen quintuplet births have been reported in the United States in the past hundred years, and 71 authenticated quintuplet births have been reported throughout the world. As is most often the case, few of the infants survived. Sextuplet births have been reported on five occasions, without survivals. Twins are extremely common among Negroes, and least common in Orientals. Frequency of twins seems to be related to heredity factors in both parents, and is more often seen in women past thirty who have had large families. If a woman has had one set of twins, she is ten times as likely as other women to have another set.

Twins may develop from one egg, in which case they are identical in sex, appearance, and mental capacity; or they may arise from the fertilization of two separate eggs, the more common type, in which case they may not necessarily be of the same sex and will resemble each other no more than ordinary siblings. Identical twins occur about 25 per cent of the time, while fraternal twins occur in 75 per cent of the cases.

Twins are frequently born early, 80 per cent within three weeks of term and less than 50 per cent reaching the ninth month. Although the size of each baby is apt to be smaller than those of normal birth, the combined weight often considerably exceeds the weight of a singly born baby.

Because complications of pregnancy occur more often with twins, women expecting multiple births should cooperate closely with their physicians as regards weight gain, frequent rest periods, and other hygienic measures.

Perhaps the most famous of all multiple births are the Dionne quintuplets in Callander, Ontario.

BISMUTH, one of the elementary bodies, a hard white crystalline metal with a reddish tint. Its derivatives are used chiefly in medicine as contracting agents for the mucous membranes and as sedatives, antiseptics, and neutralizing substances for the stomach and the bowels.

Bismuth subcarbonate, for ex-

ample, may be employed by the physician in food poisoning, in case of chronic gastritis, and for vomiting in indigestion.

Compounds of bismuth with arsenic were once used in the treatment of syphilis, but have been replaced by the newer drugs, especially penicillin.

BLACKWATER FEVER, a tropical disease which occurs almost exclusively among members of the Caucasian race, and is limited in the United States to the South. Apparently produced by small intracellular parasites in the blood, it is infectious and often fatal. Among the symptoms are irregular fever, chills, vomiting, jaundice, and labored breathing, with nephritis as a complication.

BLACK WIDOW SPIDER, the female of a common American variety; it gets its name from its shining black body and its habit of devouring its mate. Its bite is exceedingly poisonous. This notorious spider exists in a wide area, extending all the way from Canada to Chile, and is easily recognized by the scarlet hour-glass figure on its belly. It is about half an inch long; the male is considerably smaller.

The black widow is one of the few spiders whose fangs, through which the venom is discharged, can actually penetrate the human skin. The first evidence of such penetration is a sharp pain and a swelling and redness in the bitten area. Dizziness and weakness are soon felt, with a trembling of the legs and frequently stomach cramps. Other symptoms may include inability to urinate, reduction of the heart beat, a feeble pulse, and difficulty in breathing and speaking. Delirium may also occur. In some instances the bite has been known to cause death.

After the patient has been placed in bed, the physician will often inject medication into the veins to reduce the pain. Ordinarily, immune serum will then be administered.

The black widow should be avoided and never disturbed. Her web is frequently found in caves, under rocks, and at the base of posts or lumber piles. Insecticides are effective in destroying the spiders in these areas.

BLADDER, urinary, a hollow muscular organ which serves as a reservoir for urine. *See also* BLADDER DISEASES.

BLADDER DISEASES. The term bladder designates two organs of the body: the urinary bladder, a sac which receives urine from the kidneys and holds it temporarily until voided; and the gallbladder, a similar structure which stores a supply of bile, manufactured by the liver for use in digestion. The term bladder used by itself usually refers to the urinary bladder.

The kidneys deposit urine in the bladder at the rate of about thirty drops a minute through two tubes, the ureters, each about a foot long and a fifth of an inch in diameter. The passage through which urine is excreted from the bladder and from the body is the urethra, a tube about eight inches long in the male and an inch and a half in the female.

The urinary bladder and the urethra are susceptible to a number of diseases and accidents. Either one may become inflamed or infected. New and abnormal growths may occur in or on the bladder, it may form stones, or it may be bruised or ruptured.

Inflammation of the bladder is known scientifically as cystitis. It can occur in either acute or chronic form and from many different causes. Cystitis is much more common in the female because the shortness of the urethra affords invasive organisms easier access than in the male. An inflamed bladder is almost always related to a previous infection, above or below the bladder, in the urinary tract, or to an obstruction. Infection in the bladder alone, without infection elsewhere, is a rarity.

A common source of infection is an obstruction to the normal flow of urine, such as tends to occur in elderly people or anyone of advanced years who is bedridden. An enlarged prostate gland may affect a male in a similar way. Sometimes the offending factor is bacteria introduced on a catheter which has not been properly cleaned. Older men who must be catheterized frequently practically always develop some cystitis.

Symptoms of cystitis are undue frequency of urination, a burning sensation when voiding, and sometimes the appearance of blood in the urine. Persistent desire to void after retiring therefore calls for careful medical investigation. Bladder infection usually is not accompanied by fever, and a normal temperature is not an assurance that an infection may not be present.

Diagnosis of a bladder inflammation usually demands a number of tests which include examinations of the urine taken at various times over the full 24-hour period, especially for the presence of bacteria, pus, or solids. Frequently dye stuffs are used to determine the body's ability to excrete fluid. In addition, the condition of the prostate gland will be sought.

One of the remarkable achievements of modern medicine is the development of an extraordinary instrument, the cystoscope, to aid in making such a diagnosis. Through this, the doctor can actually look at the inside of the bladder. The cystoscope, a long tube with a light at its end, is passed into the bladder through the urethra. Fluid is then injected into the bladder by way of the tube, distending its walls temporarily for purposes of the examination. The tube and its light then are turned in different directions and a system of mirrors which are part of the cystoscope are so focused as to enable the physician to see the presence of infection inside the organ. Sometimes inflammation is indicated by abnormal changes in the wall of the bladder and growth can usually be seen with this instrument. The cystoscope can be used to administer drugs and for other treatment of infections of the bladder.

New methods for combatting bladder infection represent a vast advance over what was formerly available. These include penicillin and other antibiotic drugs, the sulfas, Mandelamine and Furadantin, and others. They are administered both by mouth and by injection, through which they reach the bladder by way of the blood stream. Some drugs are injected into the bladder itself, for direct application to an affected area.

Cystitis in chronic form may result from an initial acute attack, but may be caused also by stones or tumors. Occasionally older men contract it as the result of retaining urine in the bladder for a long time, especially if the urine decomposes.

The most critical infection that may affect the bladder is tuberculosis, which usually accompanies tuberculosis of the kidney. Some of the new drugs have considerable effect on this disease. When tuberculosis affects only one kidney and the other is found with certainty to be sound, the diseased kidney often is successfully removed.

Stones in the bladder, formed either within the bladder itself or passed into it from the kidney, although not uncommon are not encountered as often as in the past. Men are twenty times more susceptible to stones in the kidney than women because men in general are much more prone to disorders of the bladder. In part, difficulties which older men have with the prostate gland, an organ lacking in women, are responsible. The stones may be tiny or range in size to that of an egg, and symptoms encountered are similar to those of cystitis.

The newer advances in medicine offer a variety of ways to care for stones in the bladder. Diagnosis is much quicker and more certain than was possible in the past. The cystoscope, aided by x-ray, reveals stones unmistakably where formerly the doctor had little to guide him except the patient's general symptoms or accidental occurrence of stones in the urine itself.

Generally the x-ray is used to detect stones anywhere in the urinary tract. The patient is given a substance that is opaque to x-rays, and the subsequent photograph will disclose the exact location of the stone. The cystoscope is also used for this purpose and can even go beyond the bladder into the ureters. Other instruments inserted into the bladder sometimes are used to crush stones which then can be removed in pieces through the tube. Occasionally surgical removal of the stones may be necessary. In women, often a stone may be extracted by dilating the relatively short urethra.

A variety of tumors may affect the bladder. Most common among these is the papilloma, noncancerous, which especially seems to attack workers in aniline factories. Considerable pain, often accompanied by blood in the urine, is manifested, and chronic cystitis may develop. Treatment is similar to that of cystitis, followed by removal of the tumor or treatment by radiation. Abnormal bladder growth may be removed with instruments inserted through a cystoscope, thus eliminating surgery. The size of the tumor or nature of the repair needed for the wall of the bladder determines the specific procedure. *See also* URETHRA; URINATION; URINE.

BLASTOMYCOSIS, or Gilchrist's disease, an infection caused by a yeastlike fungus. It is found chiefly in the central regions of North America, and is more common in men than in women.

The infection, which usually starts on the exposed parts of the face, neck, or extremities, consists of large, purplish, thickly crusted ulcers. While the infection is confined to the skin, the general health of the patient remains good. Often, however, the lungs become infected, and the disease then bears a striking resemblance to tuberculosis. The symptoms are fever, loss of weight, night sweats, and cough, and the sputum frequently is bloody. Correct diagnosis is made by finding the fungi which cause the disease either in the sputum or in the discharge from the ulcerous material.

Management of blastomycosis includes the use of potassium iodides, the newer stilbine drugs, and x-ray.

The South American variety of this condition is best treated with sulfonamides.

BLEEDING. *See* HEMORRHAGE; WOUNDS.

BLEPHARITIS, a contagious inflammation of the edges of the eyelids that most often affects children, especially following an illness. Small infected blisters form at the roots of the lashes. These may lead to ulcers, then scars, which change the direction of the lashes, turning some of them inward against the eyeball. Sometimes the entire edge of the lid is distorted inward or outward. If not eliminated, the condition will eventually make the affected area red, thickened, and covered with scales.

Because faulty vision may prolong the disease, the eyes should be examined promptly so that glasses can be prescribed if necessary. The general health and sanitary habits of the child should also receive careful attention, not only for his own welfare but also to protect the rest of the family from infection through use of the same towels or bedding.

In severe cases, sulfa or penicillin drops may be prescribed by the physician. Boric acid compresses and drops may also be desirable. Recurrence frequently calls for repeated and persistent treatment.

BLISTERS, small bladder-like cavities under the skin containing watery material. Blisters may be the result of an infection, such as eczema, herpes, impetigo, or chicken pox, or they may be caused by injuries, such as pinching, chafing, burning, or scalding. Anyone who does much walking should make certain that his shoes are well fitted, large enough so that they do not pinch his feet but not so large that they produce irritating friction between the leather and the flesh. A vigorous walker often hardens his feet before an excursion with some appropriate medication, such as a solution of alum. After a walk, the feet should be washed and rested.

Painful blisters may also result from sunburn. To prevent this, yellow petroleum jelly, olive oil, or cold cream may be applied to the skin before going out into the sun for any length of time. A number of commercial preparations are available which are designed to filter out some of the ultraviolet rays. If blisters occur as a result of exposure to the sun, they are treated as any

other burn with soothing medications or creams. Severe sunburn can be dangerous as well as painful, and should be treated by a physician.

Blisters are sometimes deliberately induced as a counterirritant in the treatment of such ailments as lumbago, sciatica, and pleurisy. For this purpose, a mustard plaster is used.

In time, most blisters dry up without special treatment. Those which burst should be washed with soap and water and covered with a sterile dressing. If a large blister is opened, this is done near the outer margin with a sterilized needle. After pressing gently to eject the fluid, a sterile dressing should be applied. *See also* BURNS; SUNBURN.

BLOATING, a swelling or accumulation of fluid brought about by any cause.

BLOOD, the opaque red fluid which flows through the blood vessels, is the transport medium of the body, bringing to all the tissues the food and oxygen they need for growth and repair. It distributes the secretions, or hormones, manufactured by the important glands of the body, to the organs where they are needed to carry out their special functions. It removes the waste products from the tissues, transmits the carbon dioxide to the lungs where it is liberated and the remaining materials to the kidneys from which they are then eliminated from the body. Blood helps to maintain the body at a uniform temperature and keeps the other body fluids in a state of equilibrium. When the body is invaded by disease, the blood is the first line of defense against the infection by the action of its white cells and other substances, antibodies, which it transports to the involved site. Another of its functions is to prevent any increase in acidity or alkalinity within the body.

The blood is made of a light, straw-colored fluid, or plasma, in which are suspended the red blood cells, or erythrocytes, the white blood cells, or leukocytes, and the platelets, or thrombocytes. The red cells are biconcave, disclike bodies, so small that a drop of blood the size of a pinhead contains about 5 million cells. Formed in the red marrow of the blood, the average number of red cells in man is about 5,000,000 per cubic millimeter; in women it is about 4,500,000. About 95 per cent of the red cells is a red iron-containing pigment called hemoglobin which gives the cells and the blood a bright red color. The iron makes it possible for the hemoglobin to combine with oxygen in the lungs, which is then distributed in the body. When the hemoglobin picks up the oxygen, the color is a brighter red than when it returns to the heart after circulating through the body, having deposited its oxygen in the body tissues. The active existence of these red cells is normally about 120 days, and as they are broken down they are immediately replaced by new cells from the bone marrow. When the old red cells are destroyed they undergo a highly organized breakdown. The iron from the hemoglobin is stored in the liver, passed into the general circulation, and then used again in the production of more hemoglobin. The remaining substances are changed by the liver into bile pigment and most of this is excreted in the stools or urine.

The white cells are complete organisms within themselves, each cell being a small mass of protoplasm containing a nucleus, while the red cells lose their nucleus before leaving the bone marrow. The white cells consist of several varieties of colorless cells, which are classified into two main groups: the granulocytes, which contain granules, and the agranulocytes, which do not. The white cells have the specific function of fighting disease. Normally, in the adult, there are about 5,000 to 10,000 white blood cells per cubic millimeter of blood. In the infant this amount is almost doubled. The cells are usually almost spherical in shape, but they vary in size, some being somewhat smaller than the red cells, others larger. They move about freely in the blood stream, rapidly when necessary. They decrease in number when the body is at rest, and increase during activity. When infection develops in the body, the white cells greatly multiply in number, and are immediately propelled to the affected tissues where they engulf and digest the bacteria or other foreign material. This process, phagocytosis, of devouring a smaller cell or germ is carried out by the white cells known as phagocytes. The term means to eat cells. In pneumonia, for example, as many as 60,000 white cells per cubic millimeter have been found in the blood. One of the first symptoms in appendicitis is the abnormal increase in the white cell count. This property serves as one of the most reliable indications of infection and helps to confirm diagnoses in infectious diseases. The formation of pus is due not only to diseased tissues and bacteria but also in large measure to the white cells which have been caught in the infected area.

The blood platelets are colorless, disc-shaped or irregular bodies, much smaller than the red cells, averaging about 300,000 to the cubic millimeter of blood. They serve primarily to clot any minor tears in the small blood vessels or capillaries, clumping together at the site of injury and acting as a block until the tissue heals. Although plasma deprived of platelets will also clot, the platelets are generally found at the site of the injury, where they release a substance called thromboplastin, which initiates the clotting process.

Plasma, the fluid portion of the blood, is composed of approximately 90 per cent water, 7 per cent of various proteins, and a fraction of various kinds of salts and other raw materials needed by the body. The proteins include albumin, globulin, fibrinogen, and prothrombin, and these, together with the salts in the plasma, are of the greatest significance in maintaining a normal water balance between the fluid in the tissues and the fluid in the blood. They have a strong attraction for water and are able to hold water molecules to replace the water lost to the tissue fluid. When the protein in the blood is decreased, the water balance is upset and more fluid escapes from the plasma to the tissues, causing swelling, or edema, as is sometimes seen in cases of kidney disease. The albumin is largely responsible for keeping the blood volume constant. The fibrino-

gen is acted upon by another chemical compound or enzyme called thrombin, and is converted into fibrin, which is essential to blood clotting. This enzyme is derived from another protein in the blood plasma, the prothrombin. The various mineral salts carried in the plasma are also essential for the proper functioning of the organs. Even slight changes in the salt content of the blood may induce improper functioning of some of the tissues; those primarily affected are the nervous and the muscular tissues.

Among the significant contributions made in the war on disease is the use of gamma globulin as an aid in the treatment of measles and other infectious diseases and the effective action of fibrin foam, a derivative of fibrinogen, as an aid in treating hemorrhage. The use of blood plasma and blood transfusion to control shock, particularly on the battle fields during World War II, served to sustain life until adequate surgical treatment could be obtained, and was responsible for saving countless lives. *See also* BLOOD TYPES; HEMOPHILIA; LEUKEMIA; and Chapter 13, "Diseases of the Blood."

BLOOD BANK, exactly what its name implies: a depository for blood or blood derivatives. The first blood bank in the United States was established in Cook County Hospital, Chicago, in 1937. Blood storage has now become a significant adjunct to most hospitals. Blood of the various types, O, A, B, and AB, given by donors, is stored so that victims of accidents, patients after surgical operations, and sufferers from certain diseases can be quickly supplied with new additions of blood.

Blood plasma instead of liquid blood now also is widely stored. It keeps for long periods and does not require typing. By addition of water to the powder, plasma is promptly available. In a few diseases of the blood, however, plasma cannot be used. *See also* BLOOD TRANSFUSION.

BLOOD POISONING. *See* BAC-TEREMIA.

BLOOD PRESSURE, measured in two levels, is the degree of pressure exerted by the heart and arteries to keep the blood circulating in the blood vessels throughout the body. The maximum level, the systolic pressure, records the force exerted in the arteries with each heartbeat or contraction to propel the blood out of the left ventricle of the heart into the aorta, the large artery. The minimum level, the diastolic pressure, records the relaxed phase of the heart, between beats. This pressure indicates to the doctor the condition of the small blood vessels or arterioles —that is, their ability to contract and keep the flow of blood constant throughout the body. This pressure is maintained at a constant level, since each heartbeat forces into the large artery an amount of blood equal to that which escapes more gradually from the arterioles into the capillaries.

The systolic and diastolic pressures are recorded by means of a sphygmomanometer, a word from the Greek, meaning measurement of pulses. The instrument consists of a broad rubber cuff covered by a long cloth sleeve and two rubber tubes leading out from the cuff through the cloth. One of the tubes is connected to a small rubber bulb which inflates the cuff and has a control for the inflow and escape of air; the second tube is attached to the pressure gauge, which contains a column of mercury and is graduated from 0 to 300 millimeters.

To record blood pressure, the rubber cuff with its cloth cover is wrapped around the upper arm. Usually the brachial artery of the left arm is used to measure pressure. The examiner places his stethoscope on the artery, at the bend of the elbow, and inflates the cuff by squeezing the bulb. This produces pressure on the artery, which causes the mercury to rise in the sphygmomanometer, and the sound of the pulse can be heard through the stethoscope. The examiner continues to inflate the cuff until the sound can no longer be heard. Then he gradually releases the pressure on the bulb until the sound is heard again. At this point the height of the column of mercury in the sphygmomanometer indicates the systolic pressure. The examiner then permits the bag to deflate gradually until the sound suddenly becomes faint or cannot be heard at all. The height of the column of mercury at this point records the diastolic pressure. *See also* BLOOD PRESSURE, HIGH; BLOOD PRESSURE, LOW; BLOOD PRESSURE, NORMAL; CIRCULATORY SYSTEM; HEART; and Part III, "Your Heart."

BLOOD PRESSURE, HIGH (hypertension), the state of blood pressure beyond the normal limits. One cause of hypertension is the narrowing, or constriction, of the smallest branches of the arteries throughout the body. This tends to slow the flow of blood through the tiny vessels, and causes the heart to pump harder in order to keep the blood circulating throughout the body. The increased resistance in the arterioles is indicated on the device for measuring blood pressure by a rise in the diastolic pressure; and the increased pumping force of the left ventricle of the heart is indicated by a rise in systolic pressure. Hypertensive disease affects about 5 per cent of the adult population.

A simple elevation of blood pressure may be due to a variety of causes, all of which increase the systolic pressure and are classified as systolic hypertension. Persons who are excitable may show a rise up to 50 millimeters above normal level when the blood pressure is taken, and this may indicate only a reaction of extreme anxiety. In such cases, a few hours of quiet rest will bring the blood pressure down to normal. In older people whose arteries have lost their elastic quality, the heart must pump more forcibly, with a resulting rise in the systolic pressure, but without appreciable change in the diastolic pressure. A high systolic pressure is frequently the result of decreased elasticity of the arteries, as in some types of rheumatic heart disease, which causes heart block; in hyperthyroidism, which causes the thyroid gland to function excessively; and in arteriovenous aneurysms. These conditions are not considered true hypertension, but are significant as indications of an underlying disease.

True hypertension, or diastolic hypertension, due to a narrowing of the arterioles, is rare in persons under thirty-five years of age, and then usually is a hereditary manifestation. As a rule hypertension is found in persons past forty, though many persons who first discover a mild hypertension at forty to fifty years of age may have had an elevated blood pressure for many years previously. The disease is more prevalent in persons between sixty and seventy years of age, and occurs more often in women, but more seriously in men. Usually these cases follow a mild uneventful pattern. Hypertension also is found more frequently in patients with diabetes mellitus.

Since hypertension is prevalent among the people of Europe and North America, it has been called a disease of civilized life. Inhabitants of tropical and subtropical countries and of the Orient rarely develop this condition. Whether or not the variation is due to the difference in climate or diet or to less strenuous living conditions in those countries is not known. When nonoccidentals move to western countries they too develop hypertension.

Although the body build does not seem to be significant in hypertension, obesity does constitute a serious factor. Overweight increases the amount of work the heart must perform, and a loss of weight is often accompanied by a fall in blood pressure. The person with high blood pressure is frequently a high-strung person who reacts tensely to the everyday problems of living, and is apt to suppress hostilities, aggressions, and fears. These inner conflicts establish a nervous reaction which may become localized in the tiny blood vessels and eventually cause high blood pressure, just as tensions in some persons may cause ulcers of the stomach. Although hypertension is not a hereditary disease, the tendency or predisposition to the disease is stronger in some families than in others and, not infrequently, the condition will be found in more than one member of a family.

In true diastolic hypertension, the cause is definitely known in only a small percentage of cases and in these is generally attributed to kidney disease. Acute glomerulonephritis, a kidney disorder often seen in children and young people following a streptococcal infection, results in high blood pressure. Most of those affected recover completely. The toxemia of pregnancy, which usually occurs after the sixth month, involves the kidneys and is associated with high blood pressure.

Chronic pyelonephritis and congenital polycystic kidneys have also been found in association with hypertension. In all cases in which kidney disease is suspected as an underlying cause, the urine is examined for abnormalities at regular intervals. When infection or degeneration of a kidney causes hypertension, particularly in persons under fifty years of age, the removal of the kidney by operation sometimes results in lowering the blood pressure to normal.

Hypertension may also be caused by tumors of the endocrine glands, or by certain nerve cells. The adrenal glands, which are a part of the endocrine apparatus, are located over each kidney and secrete the hormone adrenalin into the blood stream. Adrenalin raises the blood pressure and when a tumor develops in the adrenal area an excessive amount of adrenalin is secreted. Surgical removal of the tumor lowers the blood pressure to normal. A tumor of the pituitary gland, another endocrine gland, located just below the brain, may also induce hypertension. Occasionally tumors arising in certain nerve cells of the sympathetic nervous system will produce a sustained type of hypertension. Surgical removal of the tumors reduces hypertension. The increased occurrence of hypertension during the menopause in women and the climacteric in men is also attributed to endocrine causes, although the mechanism involved is not clearly understood.

Another form of true hypertension, a narrowing or stricture of the aorta, found in children and young people is coarctation of the aorta. Some children are born with the disorder, which results in a high blood pressure in the arms and a low pressure in the legs. This condition is cured by surgery.

The specific causes of high blood pressure are known in only about 20 per cent of all cases involving hypertensive disease. In these cases, high blood pressure is called "essential hypertension," which also has the characteristic narrowing of the arterioles throughout the body with the consequent resistance in these tiny vessels to the flow of blood, and the rise of blood pressure necessary to keep the blood circulating in the body. The course of essential hypertension and the complications that accompany it are practically identical with that of diastolic hypertensions due to known causes. When the ailment progresses slowly over many years, it is noted as benign, or mild.

Benign hypertension may exist for many years without any evidence to suggest its presence other than a moderate elevation of blood pressure. A person past forty may see a doctor because of headache, dizziness, failing vision, or noises in the head, expecting to be told that the discomfort is due to high blood pressure. Actually the elevation of blood pressure may not be great, and it may vary from one visit to the next; such changes are of little significance. In many instances, persons with high blood pressure remain well for years without showing any apparent change in health. The complaints are not due to the hypertension, but rather to some of the complications associated with hypertension.

Once the presence of the disease is definitely established, a thorough, inclusive examination is essential to evaluate the complications and determine the progress and severity of the hypertensive condition. These complications may not appear for years, but when they do the organs most frequently affected are the heart, eyes, brain, and kidneys. The examination, therefore, is directed toward a search for signs that indicate an insufficient flow of blood to any of these organs, or that suggest the possibility of disease of any of these organs.

When the arteries which feed the heart, the coronary arteries, become narrowed, a person may experience a temporary pain, angina pectoris, on exertion. Or he may be subjected to a more serious attack, coronary thrombosis, which is accompanied by shortness of breath, particularly at night, and other manifestations of shock. Hypertension may also cause an enlargement of the heart which results from the exertion of the heart muscles pumping against the resistance of the arterioles. Eventually this disorder will also cause heart pain and shortness of breath.

When the arteries in the brain become hardened, personality changes appear, with emotional instability, failure to concentrate, and forgetfulness, especially of recent events. This is particularly true of older people who have developed cerebral arteriosclerosis. Temporary weakness, unsteadiness in walking, and noises in the ears are symptoms which may precede a cerebral hemorrhage or clot in one of the arteries, which causes a stroke or apoplexy. The less serious cases of stroke cause paralysis of one side of the body with, occasionally, an interference in speech. The paralysis usually disappears entirely or partially within a period of months.

In benign, essential hypertension, the function of the kidney is generally never seriously impaired unless the condition is associated with an underlying kidney disease.

Examination of the blood vessels in the retina of the eye often helps the doctor to determine the condition of the blood vessels in cases of hypertension. The eye is the one place in the body where the arterioles can be seen directly with an ophthalmoscope, a mirrored instrument used to examine eyes. These arteries show varying degrees of spasms or narrowing in the early stages of hypertension, and often indicate the presence of arteriosclerosis. The retinal arterioles also indicate a generalized arteriolar disease, but do not indicate the specific degree of involvement of any particular vessel.

High blood pressure is frequently accompanied by hardening, sclerosis, of the arteries throughout the body. This process is called arteriosclerosis, one of the commonest disorders of advanced age. Usually the first indication of its presence is a clotting of a larger artery, or thrombotic occlusion. This may develop into cerebral thrombosis, angina pectoris, or coronary thrombosis.

In this country, about 15 to 20 per cent of deaths in people over fifty is caused by the immediate or remote consequences of hypertension. This has tended to obscure the fact that, of itself, hypertension is a relatively harmless disorder, which may not provoke symptoms or disability for many years. People with hypertension can, if no unforeseen complications develop, live out their lives normally. Extensive studies have shown that such persons have survived as long as forty years after a diagnosis of hypertension was made. The outlook is somewhat less favorable in men than in women, and in patients who have an existing kidney disorder.

In the course of treating a hypertensive person, the doctor is mindful of symptoms or complications involving other organs. He observes any changes in his patient due to high pressure. A rise or fall in blood pressure is not as significant as examination of the eyes, size of heart, electrocardiograms, degree of kidney function, and other physical measurements which give the doctor information.

In cases of hypertension, both physical and psychological factors are significant. Most doctors feel that an overconsciousness of blood pressure makes some people lead lives of excessive concern and even semi-invalidism. While the prevention of anxiety may not alter the course of the hypertension itself, it makes a great difference in the person's attitude and outlook on life. Too often people have been invalided merely from overawareness of their high blood pressure rather than from the physical effects of the hypertension. Hence, the re-education of those people with high blood pressure is essential so that they may carry on normal lives. They should learn to discuss themselves and their problems objectively, as individuals rather than as medical cases. This will not only permit a greater insight into the situation but will often result in relief from anxiety.

The general fear of hypertension is one of the great obstacles to minimizing an anxiety reaction. Yet this can be overcome when one knows how blood pressure normally varies, not only from time to time but from person to person, with every exertion or emotional experience. That the definition of normal blood pressure has been broadened is significant and encouraging.

Many persons with milder degrees of hypertension need not even be subjected to dietary restriction unless they are obese. They can follow the activity pattern of normal living, avoiding only overwork, overexertion, and excesses.

Overweight in people with hypertension is a liability and the frequency of incidence of illness and death is directly proportional to the amount of extra weight. A suitable low-calorie diet, usually high in proteins and low in fats, starches, and carbohydrates, should be selected and continually supervised by a doctor.

The use of a low-salt diet for hypertension has been effective in reducing the blood pressure in many cases, often bringing it to normal levels. Since most natural foods, such as milk and meats, and many prepared foods, such as bread, contain a considerable amount of salt, adherence to this type of diet was difficult until recently when many salt-free foods became available. In addition, planning a low-salt diet has been simplified by publications which are available to the public. A pamphlet, "Food for your Heart," published by the American Heart Association may be obtained from them for a few cents. Low-salt diets should be undertaken only on the advice and under the supervision of a doctor since some salt in the diet, particularly during hot weather, is required to prevent sodium depletion, the so-called low-salt syndrome.

A surgical operation on the sympathetic nervous system has been devised for treating hypertension. The nerves in this system, in a chain on either side of the spine, carry the impulses from the brain which cause the tiny arterioles to become narrow. When these nerves are cut, the narrowing process is halted and blood pressure drops. Sympathectomy has

been in use for fifteen years. Some persons improve dramatically after the operation, but many are not helped at all, and to know beforehand just which patients will benefit is difficult. It is a major operation and is done in only a few medical centers throughout the country. Another major operative procedure now being tried is radical bilateral adrenalectomy, which involves removal of the adrenal glands. These glands are useful in the general metabolic action of the body, and it is still too soon to know whether or not the operation is effective in reducing symptoms of hypertension, and to know what are the aftereffects of removal of the glands.

New drugs for the treatment of hypertension are designed to paralyze the sympathetic nerves in an effort to accomplish what surgical procedure does in cutting these nerves. Development of new drugs is making operation much less frequent. Among the most frequently used drugs are Apresoline, Hexamethonium and Hydergine. In some cases, these remedies are prescribed in combination. All are extremely potent and should only be taken under the direct supervision of a doctor. Two other drugs, taken by mouth and widely employed, are rauwolfia serpentina, which slows the pulse rate and seems to relieve anxiety and temporary elevations in blood pressure, and veratrum viride, which tends to dilate the blood vessels and slow the pulse rate. In addition to these potent medications, a new drug widely used is chlorothiazide called Diuril. Among the milder sedatives which prove helpful during periods of emotional stress are

BLOOD PRESSURE, NORMAL

phenobarbital, chloral, and the bromides (not containing sodium). *See also* BARBITURATES; Part III, "Your Heart."

BLOOD PRESSURE, LOW (hypotension). Approximately 25 to 30 per cent of the population has primary hypotension, arbitrarily described as pressures falling below 110 millimeters of mercury for the systolic level, and below 70 millimeters for the diastolic.

When a known cause cannot be found for the low pressure, it is called primary, or essential, hypotension. Many normal men and women have blood pressure in this range. Symptoms cannot be attributed to this type of low blood pressure, and actually it is compatible with a greater than average life expectancy.

Hypotension which sometimes develops in the course of a serious disease is known as secondary hypotension. Among such diseases are acute infections, heart failure, Addison's disease, malnutrition, Simmonds' disease, circulatory shock from hemorrhage, trauma, hyperinsulinism, or other causes. Persons with secondary hypotension are weak, tired, and occasionally complain of dizziness and faintness. In general, despite the drop in blood pressure in these cases, the body manages to maintain a sufficient blood supply for its needs. As recovery from the original cause progresses, the blood pressure becomes normal.

Another type of low blood pressure, postural hypotension, as the name implies, is associated with change of position. Usually, when a person stands up, the blood pressure rises, in response to the energy exerted for this motion. In some cases, however, the blood pressure drops and causes faintness. Many normal people feel a slight dizziness when they change position suddenly, because the flow of blood to the brain is thus suddenly slowed and the brain tissue is sensitive to a lack of blood and oxygen. However, in postural hypotension the change in position provokes blurred vision, weakness, and fainting, and on lying down consciousness returns. Such persons should get up gradually from a recumbent position, wear an abdominal binder or special elastic stockings, or use blood-pressure stimulating drugs as prescribed by the doctor. *See also* Part III, "Your Heart."

BLOOD PRESSURE, NORMAL. People vary in their response to external stimuli such as heat or cold, and also in their blood pressures. Transient deviations from the normal in any person are caused by such everyday activities as digestion, change of posture, exercise, and emotional stimulation. The degree to which the pressure is raised depends on the intensity of the stimulus and the individual response.

At birth the blood pressure is about 75 millimeters systolic and 40 diastolic, or, as it is usually written, 75/40. This rises gradually and at adolescence is about 100/60, and between the ages of twenty and forty it is 120/80. The rise continues slowly and at the age of sixty is around 145/90. After that the diastolic pressure remains fairly stationary, although the systolic may become somewhat higher. However, these figures represent the average, and a difference of 10 per cent or more in either direction is still within normal limits.

In the past, people over forty were believed to have limits of normal blood pressure around 150 systolic and 90 diastolic, regardless of age or sex, and many people with supposedly high blood pressure remained in good health. In 1952, Dr. Arthur M. Master and his associates undertook a study of the blood pressure of more than 50,000 men and women of varying ages. It was found that the limits of normal blood pressure are much greater than the figures previously accepted, and that they vary with age and sex. It was also observed that blood pressure gradually increases with age; at sixty-five most normal men may have a systolic pressure up to 170; and normal women, up to 175. The diastolic pressure may range between 100 and 110. In some cases a systolic pressure as high as 180 and a diastolic pressure of 110 seemed to be normal. Another significant observation was that with an increase in weight there was a progressive increase in blood pressure, regardless of age or sex.

Wide variations exist in the so-called normal blood pressures at different ages. Blood pressure which falls in the outermost limits of normal does not in itself constitute a disease. Many factors combine to keep the blood pressure within normal limits—for instance, the exertion of the heart muscles as they pump the blood through the body, the degree of elasticity of the arterial walls as the blood flows through them, and the resistance encountered by the blood in the smaller blood vessels. Since all these may influence blood pressure, they must be carefully considered before an elevation of blood pressure is considered significant. *See also* Part III, "Your Heart."

BLOOD TRANSFUSION, the transfer of blood from a donor to a recipient; one of the most widely used procedures in medical treatment. When severe hemorrhage has resulted in a great loss of blood, a transfusion will restore the circulating blood volume and the red blood cells which provide oxygen and food to the body tissues. Blood transfusion is an invaluable supporting treatment for surgical shock, to replace an excessive loss of blood at childbirth, or in such conditions as leukemia. In some cases, even when the circulating blood volume is normal, transfusion is used to replace a deficiency in one of the constituents of the blood, thus providing red cells in cases of acute anemia, or in hemophilia, which is due to the lack of a specific clot-promoting factor in the blood plasma.

The first recorded transfusion is believed to have been performed between two dogs by Richard Lower in England in 1665, and soon after it was tried in France. However, the results in human beings were so disastrous that a law was passed in France forbidding transfusions. Not until the turn of this century, when Karl Landsteiner began his study of the blood groupings, was progress made in this field. For many years, only direct transfusions were given, because no means of keeping fresh blood from clotting were known. However, in 1914, Luis Agote of

Argentina found that sodium citrate served this purpose, and by this discovery an incalculable number of lives were saved during the First World War. Richard Lewisohn of New York's Mt. Sinai Hospital developed practically the citrate method.

Since that time methods have been perfected for obtaining and storing human blood for future use. Blood banks for emergency use have become a part of many hospitals.

All blood which is to be used for transfusions is obtained under the most exacting sanitary conditions, completely free from germs or other contaminating influences. Blood donors are meticulously screened to rule out infectious diseases, and given tests for the presence of syphilis before their blood is used. *See also* BLOOD BANK; BLOOD TYPES; HEMORRHAGE; LEUKEMIA; and Chapter 13, "Diseases of the Blood."

BLOOD TYPES. The existence of human blood types was established by Karl Landsteiner in 1902 when he began a study to determine why fatalities occurred following some blood transfusions. He discovered that the cause was an incompatibility between the blood of the donor and that of the recipient. From this observation came the Landsteiner classification, the ABO blood groups, which classifies blood into four types, A, B, AB, and O, and the recognition of which blood groups can be safely mixed.

Type O blood can give to all blood types, but can receive only from type O. AB blood type can give to only AB, but can receive from any group. Thus type O is sometimes called the universal donor and type AB the universal recipient. Type A can give to types A and AB and receive only from types A and O, and type B can give to types B and AB, and receive only from type B or O. The ideal blood transfusion utilizes the same type of donor and recipient blood. In this country, 85 per cent of the population belongs to groups A or O, and type AB is rare. The distribution of blood types varies considerably with geographical population. Blood types are inherited.

As a safety measure, before a patient receives a whole-blood transfusion, the compatibility of his blood with the donor blood is checked by a cross-match test. Small samples of red blood cells and sera of the two bloods are combined and examined under a microscope for signs of incompatibility or clumping.

If incompatible bloods are mixed, the red cells of the donor blood are rapidly destroyed, liberating free hemoglobin into the patient's circulating blood. The free hemoglobin breaks down and may be excreted through the kidneys; if the urine is acid the newly formed pigment which has resulted from the destruction of hemoglobin cannot be absorbed by the kidneys and is deposited in the tubular cells of that organ. This causes kidney failure, with eventual death. The practice of cross-matching bloods before transfusions has virtually eliminated deaths from transfusion.

Highly significant in transfusions and obstetrics are Rh blood groups, which were first recognized in 1940 by Landsteiner and A. S. Weiner.

The Rh factor, a substance present in red blood cells, was uncovered during experiments with rhesus monkeys; thus the name Rh for rhesus. Subsequently this factor was related to unexplained accidents in transfusion, including hemolytic disease of newborn infants, characterized by disintegration of red blood cells. Eighty-five per cent of white persons have Rh positive factor, indicating that the red cells are agglutinated by antirhesus serum; the other 15 per cent are Rh negative, since their cells are not agglutinated by antirhesus serum.

When an Rh negative person receives Rh positive blood, he will develop particular antibodies. If the Rh negative person later again receives Rh positive blood, a hemolytic anemia may result. This anemia appears in newborn infants most frequently when the mother is Rh negative and the father is Rh positive. It will occur only when the mother has had previous direct contact with Rh positive blood, such as in transfusion or by bearing an Rh positive child. Treatment involves giving the infant transfusions of Rh negative blood, and in severe cases the infant's blood is almost totally replaced by Rh negative blood of the correct type. Blood banks keep on hand large supplies of Rh negative blood.

Laboratory tests can reveal this sensitization, and the physician can then take measures to avoid or diminish accident to mother and child. A mother-to-be whose tests show she might give birth to an Rh positive child must receive careful medical attention. Only one in 40 or 50 cases of mating between an Rh negative woman and an Rh positive man results in hemolytic anemia. *See also* ANEMIA; CROSS-MATCHING OF BLOOD.

BLUE BABY, a baby born with a congenital structural defect of the heart, which results in constant recirculation of some of the dark or venous blood without its prior passage through the lungs to pick up oxygen, thus giving the skin, lips, and nails a bluish look. Since 1945, many such infants have been saved by an operation developed by Drs. Alfred Blalock and Helen Taussig at Johns Hopkin University. Before that time, little could be done for the condition except to keep the child at rest and free of infection. Life expectancy was low.

Such defects occur frequently when the prenatal opening between the two pumping vessels of the baby's heart, the ventricles, which normally closes at birth, fails to close. In addition, distortion of the major artery leading away from the heart, and of the artery leading from the heart to the lungs, throws an abnormal load on one of the ventricles. Blood which has been oxygenated by the lungs and has taken on the characteristic color associated with arterial blood is mixed with the bluish blood from the veins, which should have gone to the lungs but did not.

By joining two arteries, the Blalock-Taussig operation increases the flow of blood to the lungs so that a greater proportion of the baby's blood receives oxygen. This ends the blueness of the skin and the breathlessness associated with the condition. Short of violent athletic competition, such children are thereafter able to live normally active lives. *See also* CYANOSIS; and Chapter 8, "Congenital Heart Disease in Children."

BLUSHING. *See* PIGMENTATION.

BODY. The human body consists of trillions of cells, organized into tissue, which are organized into organs and the organs into systems. The body is formed by systems.

The histological basis of the body structure cells are the physiological visible units of the body of organisms. They vary in function, shape, size, and structure.

Tissues are masses of cells. All tissues are composed of various kinds of cells which are again combined with varying quantities of intercellular substances. In the epithelial tissue, which composes the glands and skin, the intercellular substance merely forms a cementing link for the cells; but in various connective tissues, those of bone, fat, and cartilage, it comprises the bulk. Degrees of hardness depend on the solidity of the intercellular substance and the differences in its structure. It is soft and jellylike in the mucous membranes, hard because of mixture with lime salts in bone, and firmly massed in cartilage. Besides epithelial and connective tissues, the muscle, nervous, and vascular tissues are represented by blood cells.

Different types of tissue have different forms of cells, but within each type the cells are the same. The connective tissue is the most widely distributed tissue; in its different forms, such as fibrous, elastic, cartilage,

bone, and in combination, it comprises the body's supporting framework.

Organs are the different structures adapted for definite functions in the body and are apparent even in the lowest forms of life. They form, for example, the difference between living beings and minerals, which are inorganic. In human beings, the organs are more nervous and their functions more varied. Anatomic organs, like the eye, stomach, heart, and limbs, are combinations of lower-ranking organs which again are composed of unit organs, the cells.

The real essence of organization in the body organism is division of performance. Division prevails, but the parts are ruled by a whole. The function of an organ may be impaired and yet the organism can survive, because the balance possesses the capacity of adjustment.

The origin of tissues, as well as of organs, is in the elementary layers of the embryo. Why some cells develop to form one kind of tissue and others another kind is still a matter of conjecture.

Some organs are undeveloped, others rudimentary and useless structures, as, for example, the appendix. This is probably due to disuse. Organs may degenerate and still appear in a rudimentary form in the embryo, but later disappear or remain useless. Incomplete development will occasionally result in imperfect structure of organs.

The human body consists of ten distinct systems: the nervous, skeletal, digestive, circulatory, respiratory, reproductive, excretory, muscular, endocrine, and lymphatic.

Physiologically and anatomically all human beings have the same kinds of systems, organs, tissues, and cells. Individuals of the same race have the same body structure. Pronounced differences in structure are subject to factors such as heredity, activity, health, and deformities. *See also* BONES; CELLS; NERVOUS SYSTEM; and separate organs; and Chapter 3, "The Body and How It Functions."

BODY LICE, (pediculus humanus), small wingless insects, ectoparasites, carriers of disease and producers of irritating dermatitis. The louse is one of the commonest of the insects that attack the hairy parts of the human body. Wherever large numbers of people congregate, as in the armed forces, concentration camps, or jails, delousing techniques have to be developed to cope with the pest. Not only must the body be rid of the louse, but its eggs (nits) must also be eliminated from clothing. For the latter purpose, live steam is generally used.

The louse is a carrier of typhus. It becomes infected by ingesting the blood of a diseased person.

For the eradication of lice infestation of the hair, a mixture of half a pint each of kerosene and olive oil is recommended. This mixture is rubbed into the scalp, and the hair then covered with a piece of muslin for from two hours to overnight. Care must be taken to keep the hair away from contact with flames. When the muslin is removed, the hair and scalp should be washed with soap and hot water and rinsed well with clear water, and the procedure repeated as often as necessary.

To remove the nits, the hair must be wet thoroughly with hot vinegar, and a fine-toothed comb used. This should be repeated daily, making sure that the hair is thoroughly dry before the individual goes outdoors. *See also* CRAB LICE; LICE.

BODY ODOR (bromidrosis, or fetid perspiration), the excretion of sweat with an unpleasant odor. The eccrine and apocrine are the two types of sweat glands in the body. The apocrine glands are found only in certain sections of the body, such as under the arms, and they produce a secretion often regarded as unpleasant. Women have twice as many apocrine glands as men.

Sweat with the accompanying offensive odor is usually excreted from certain parts of the body, such as the armpits, feet, and occasionally other regions. Persons who have bromidrosis must pay particular attention to personal cleanliness, and bathe once or even twice a day, using plenty of soap. Special soaps are available but they do not appear to be any more effective than ordinary soap. Deodorants and antiperspirants may be used on parts of the body where perspiration is likely to be excessive. Checking perspiration under the arms or other parts of the body is not harmful. After the lotion has been applied, an antiseptic dusting powder may be used on the skin.

For excessive perspiration of the feet, the doctor may prescribe a regular bath with a 1 per cent solution of liquor formaldehyde. This is an exceedingly active chemical substance and should not be used except on the advice of a physician. When it is applied to the skin, persons sensitive to it may have eruptions.

Chlorophyll preparations advertised as controlling body odors have proved disappointing. Combined with other substances, they simply mask odors.

Extra excretion of sweat may be associated with nervousness. Proper treatment will help control abnormal perspiration. In some instances, the application of x-ray by competent specialists has been found useful. *See also* Chapter 11, "Feminine Hygiene."

BOECK'S SARCOID, a chronic disease characterized by benign tumors resembling flesh. It is usually an ailment of young adults, but sometimes of older people. Skin, eyes, lungs, and bones of the feet and hands are especially affected. The cause of Boeck's sarcoid, named after a nineteenth-century Norwegian physician, is unknown, and a specific treatment has not as yet been found. Cortisone has been used with great success in treating the condition, but relapses are frequent.

BOILS. *See* FURUNCLES.

BONE BANK. Until 1946, when bones were needed in orthopedic surgery, they were usually taken from the patient's own body. In many cases this procedure resulted in weakened limbs, subject to easy fracture. Following an idea of Dr. Philip D. Wilson of New York City's Hospital for Special Surgery, bone banks have been established at many hospitals. Small chips for filling cavities, and larger bones are preserved in deep freeze, to be grafted, after thawing, in the operating room. They are taken originally from amputated limbs, from deceased people, or from those undergoing orthopedic surgery. The thawed bone which is grafted does not itself grow, but stimulates growth of the healthy bone to which it is united.

BONES, the solid elements of the body. Without a bony skeleton, the human being would collapse into a heap of tissues and organs, be completely unable to move and extremely vulnerable to injury. In addition to acting as a framework, bones often play a crucial role in the protection of organs. The skull, for example, protects the soft tissue of the brain; the spinal column shields the spinal cord; the pelvic bones help guard the kidneys and other organs of the abdomen against damage; and the ribs help avert injury to the lungs and other organs of the chest. With the aid of muscles attached to them, bones also make movement possible.

Bones are a part of the connective tissue system, one of the most widespread systems of the body. Generally, this system consists of collagenous or fibrous tissue or both, but bone also contains mineral matter which gives it hardness.

Bone originates from small, irregularly shaped cells called osteoblasts, which are believed to come from the connective tissue system. During the early stages of bone formation, these cells manufacture a soft substance which forms around them and into which animal material, called ossein or gelatin, and minerals, mainly calcium phosphate and calcium carbonate, are later deposited to impart the stony quality. About one-third of the weight of bone is the animal material; the rest is mineral. In the childhood disease rickets, which is caused by a deficiency of vitamin D, the bones lack adequate mineral material and are relatively soft. The long bones of the legs bend under the weight of the trunk, and other bone malformations occur, depending upon the degree of softening. Vitamin D is essential to the metabolism of calcium in the human body.

Bone difficulties can accompany old age. Osteoporosis is characterized by a general decrease in bone mass with resulting strains on the skeleton. Usually a thinning of the long bones in the legs develops, sometimes with spontaneous fractures. The cause is a reduction in osteoblast activity so that new bone is not laid down at a rate needed to replace worn bone. Osteoporosis may also occur earlier in life, as a result of metabolic disturbances such as diabetes, overactivity of the adrenal glands, or as a consequence of vitamin deficiencies, particularly vitamin C, or starvation.

The growth of bones in childhood and adolescence determines the height and body structure of the person. This is usually hereditary, but is often influenced by diet. Frequently improved nutrition results in offspring who have attained heights several inches above those of their parents. In some instances, disturbance of the glands which regulate growth may cause either giantism or dwarfism. The anterior portion of the pituitary gland, a gland located at the base of the brain, is particularly involved with the growth of long bones, and may undersecrete, causing dwarfism, or oversecrete, producing giantism. Either condition should be treated by an endocrinologist, a physician who specializes in glands and their secretions. Dwarfism can be treated by the administration of pituitary extract. Undersecretion of the thyroid gland, which causes cretinism, in which the mental and physical growth of the child is stunted or slow, can be corrected by administration of thyroid extract.

The number of separate bones in the human body is generally given as 206. Up to the age of twenty-two, the number of bones in men differs from that in women, because of the changes that take place in the joining together of small bones to make up larger ones. While every bone has a name, bones are classified into four types, according to their shape, These include the long bones, such as those in the arms and legs; the short bones, such as those in the fingers; the flat bones, such as the shoulder blades and skull bones; and the short and irregular bones, like those of the wrist, ankles, and spinal column. Bones which are both long and flat, like those of the wrist, breastbone, and lower jaw, are classified as mixed bones.

The three most significant characteristics of bone are hardness, strength, and lightness. While minerals produce hardness and animal and mineral matter both contribute strength, the hollowness, such as in the long bones and spongy bone tissue, found in many places, accounts for lightness.

The cavities of all bones in the body are filled with marrow, which in the bones of the young and in spongy bones of adults is red. Red marrow is considered a valuable breeding place for red blood corpuscles. Marrow in adults generally is yellow. Marrow consists of connective tissue interlaced with a network of small blood vessels. In the meshes of this network are various kinds of cells, including red and white blood cells, connective tissue, and fat cells. An examination of bone marrow tissue has become an advantageous technique for the diagnosis of many disease conditions, pernicious and other anemias, and ailments such as hypersplenism, leukemia, and lymphoma.

Externally bones are smooth and are covered with a tissue called the periosteum, a tough fibrous structure which gives support to the ligaments, tendons, and muscles attached to the bone. The periosteum also admits blood vessels and nerves to the underlying bone, and, in case of a fracture, helps produce callus to protect the injured area. If the periosteum itself becomes badly damaged, the bone beneath may die because it receives nourishment from that covering.

Bone is assured the good blood and lymph supply which it requires, just as other tissue of the body does. Some of the blood vessels are in the marrow or center of the bone, others pierce the periosteum through holes, the foramina, and enter a system of canals called the Haversian canals, which branch their way to the bone cells, enabling the blood vessels to carry the nutriments needed for growth and repair of the bones. Bones, however, sometimes become diseased as a result of infectious material being carried from other areas of the body through the blood vessels in the Haversian canals. Tuberculosis is among the most common of the bone infections. Nerve cells, too, branch through these canals and produce sensations of pain in event of injury to the bone. Inflammation of the periosteum, or osteomyelitis, an inflammation of the deeper bone tissue, usually due to infection, also produces much pain. Growth, however, does not cause pain, and if a child complains of pain in the bones or joints, it should not be dismissed as "growing pains" but investigated by a physician.

The function of a bone chiefly determines its shape and substance. If fundamentally needed for leverage, as in the legs and arms, the bones are long; for flexibility, as in the spine and fingers, the bones are usually short and irregular; and for protection, flat, as in the skull. The spinal column is constructed so as to supply both rigidity and strength, since it has to support the entire body with the exception of the lower limbs and also supply flexibility for bending, turning, and twisting. The spine is also designed to absorb the shock of violent movement and impact. To do this, twenty-four bones called vertebrae have been shaped to fit together in a way that permits strength and mobility. Two small bones, the sacrum and the coccyx, at the end of the spinal column are fused into a single bone.

Bone must be both hard and strong enough to withstand the weight and pressure to which it is continually subjected, the strain from the pull of muscles and tendons, and the accidental blows it receives. Bone building does not end with maturity. Childhood is the period of the greatest growth in size, strength, and shape of bone, but bone building is a daily process which continues throughout a lifetime. The diet of everyone, not only young and growing children, should include ample mineral-containing foods, proteins, and vitamins. Children need a larger amount of calcium and phosphorus-containing foods, such as milk and cheese, and adequate vitamin D. Older people also require milk, though the period of intense bone growth is over, and a pint of milk daily is advisable. Necessary amounts of vitamin C, vital to connective tissue health, should be assured.

Although the bony structure has amazing tensile strength and flexibility, it can and frequently is pushed or shocked beyond the straining point. A closer knowledge of the structure might help people avoid distressing injuries. For example, a joint is an area where one bone joins another or where bones "articulate." These joints are classified as movable, slightly movable, and immovable. Most joints are movable and of several distinct types: the ball-and-socket joints, such as that of the hip; the hinge joints, such as that of the knee; the pivot joints, such as that of the skull which rests on the spine; and gliding or sliding joints.

The ends of bones in movable joints are usually enlarged and fit each other so well that force is needed to dislocate them. The ends of bones articulating with one another are covered with cartilage which replaces the periosteum. The cartilage is covered at the end with membrane, except at the place where the bones articulate, called the synovia, which secretes a fluid that keeps the joints lubricated at all times. This fluid prevents the friction that inevitably results when parts move on each other and keeps the cartilage and the bone at the end from wearing down. In osteoarthritis, a disorder which in some degree afflicts most people over sixty-five years of age, a wearing down or fraying of the cartilage, and sometimes even of the bone tissue beneath, often occurs. This is not the same disease as rheumatoid arthritis, which is a general disorder of the collagen tissue of the body, often symptomatized by swelling in the joints.

Cartilage is tough, smooth, and elastic and forms a covering for all movable joints. Each spinal vertebra, for example, has circular pads of cartilage at the end. It is next to bone in hardness and is found elsewhere in the body where hard tissue is required, as at the tip of the nose, ears, and windpipe.

The types of injuries, outside of fractures, which are most likely to afflict bones and their joints involve tendons and ligaments. Tendons tie muscle to bone, and ligaments are tough bands of fibrous tissues that bind the articulating bones together. Sometimes ligaments form a circular band, a capsule, that surrounds the joint and attaches to the periosteum and the bone beneath. Ligaments do not have the ability to contract, but are slightly elastic and bear much of the brunt of injury in case of sprains and dislocations.

In a sprain, for instance, a tearing of the binding ligaments occurs with swelling caused by ruptured blood and lymph vessels and an increased secretion of synovial fluid. In a dislocation, however, the articulating ends of the bones are displaced. The ligaments are usually badly torn, the blood vessels at the joint severely injured, and the muscles around the joint are frequently in contraction because of the pain. This muscular contraction adds to the difficulties of getting the bones back into place. Injury to the nerves may also occur, and swelling and the degree of deformity in the joint will depend on the extent of the injury.

Crippling injuries to and malformations of the bones, joints, and muscles are cared for by medical specialists called orthopedic surgeons. These doctors can make bone grafts to replace damaged areas, transplant bony tissue and create new sockets for the ends of bones which have been injured or destroyed by disease. A number of bone banks have now been established throughout the country, from which bone tissue can be drawn for grafting. By their work and skill and ingenuity, the orthopedic specialists have done much to free human beings from pain and suffering. They have repaired the crippled in great numbers and restored to useful activity many people who would otherwise have been permanently disabled. *See also* CARTILAGE; FRACTURES; OSTEITIS; OSTEOMYELITIS.

BOOSTER DOSE, "shot" of vaccine given some time after the original immunization to maintain the immunity against certain diseases. The added injection of a particular vaccine will greatly stimulate the formation of antibodies at a time when the concentration of antibodies may be at a low level. *See also* IMMUNIZATION; chapter 23, "The Neuromuscular and Neurological Disabilities."

BORAX, chemically known as sodium borate, a colorless transparent powder or crystal. Soluble in water, borax is used medicinally as an antiseptic, for stomatitis, an inflammation of the mouth, and as an ingredient of various preparations used on the skin.

In weak solutions, 1 pound of borax to 25 or 30 gallons of water, sodium borate effectively destroys larvae of flies on plants and animals. In an overdose, borax is a depressant poison, 30 grams of which have been fatal.

BORIC ACID, a substance of colorless scales or crystals or a white crystalline powder, possessing the properties of a weak acid. Soluble in water, it is used externally as a mild antiseptic. For example, diapers may be rinsed in a saturated solution of boric acid in the case of intertrigo or "diaper rash." Because of its action in deterring the growth of germs, a small amount of boric acid is an ingredient of many protective and soothing dusting powders.

Boric acid eyewash soothes irritated membranes of the eye and inflammation of the eyelids, or conjunctivitis.

It is also extensively employed as an antiseptic first-aid dressing for burns, local inflammations of the scalp, in the care of babies' ears, and as a throat spray and mouthwash.

Taken internally, boric acid is poisonous and can cause death. It should always be plainly and distinctly marked in the medicine chest, and should be kept out of the reach of children. *See also* POISONING.

BOTULISM, the most severe and dangerous of all food poisonings, which occurs as a result of eating canned and preserved foods which have been contaminated by the germ Clostridium botulinus. This organism produces a toxin or poison of extraordinary power, so great that one part of it in ten million will kill a mouse. The symptoms occurring in human victims of the disease are due to the toxin rather than to the presence of the organism itself.

The toxin attacks the nerves, induces weakness and paralysis, including difficulty in swallowing, talking, and seeing. Death, which finally results from respiratory failure, has occurred in 65 per cent of cases in the United States, although the death rate in Europe is much lower.

The bacillus Clostridium is an inhabitant of the soil in every country in the world and is therefore a potential contaminant of everything grown in soil where it exists. In the United States, the danger develops when contaminated farm products, especially string beans, corn, spinach, asparagus, beets, and apricots, are preserved and canned by inadequate methods, and the germ survives, produces its toxin, and poisons the food in the can or jar. The amount of toxin produced depends on the character and chemistry of the food in question, its acidity, the presence of sugar, and the quantity of heat applied to it. In Europe, preserved sausage meats and similar products, such as fish pastes, have been implicated most frequently.

The foremost problem about the bacillus Clostridium is that its reproductive spores survive treatment that ordinarily disposes of microorganisms. Six hours of boiling does not destroy them, nor does six minutes' exposure to steam pressure at fifteen pounds. The toxin itself is fortunately much less resistant and is rendered harmless by six minutes of boiling.

While it is ordinarily safe to regard commercially canned foods as safe, and an outbreak of botulism from this source has not occurred for some time, the same cannot be said for home-preserved products, which are processed under less rigid standards. All home-canned foods should be boiled for six full minutes before being even tasted. One exception is those packed in brine, which renders a food reasonably safe. Cold salads of home-canned fruits or vegetables have been involved in several outbreaks of botulism, which could have been due to the use of containers or foods or both which were not sterilized under pressure. This omission permitted the survival of the spores.

Speed in summoning the doctor and securing treatment, which will consist primarily of administration of one or more antitoxins that have been developed, is a matter of life and death to the victim of botulism.

Damage suffered from the toxin cannot be repaired. All that can be done is to arrest the progress of the poisoning, and assist with secondary measures. *See also,* FOOD POISONING.

BOWEL, the portion of the digestive system which extends from the stomach to the anus, and includes twenty-three feet of small intestine, five feet of large intestine, and the rectum which is about six inches long.

The small intestine occupies most of the intestinal cavity, where it lies in coiled loops that can move about. The first portion, fixed to the posterior abdominal wall, is the duodenum, and the ducts of the liver and pancreas open into it. The rest of the duodenum is divided into the jejunum, about eight feet long, and the ileum, which is twelve feet long.

Digestion takes place in the small intestine by means of secretions of pancreatic juice from the pancreas, bile from the liver, and juices secreted by the intestine. These secretions are alkaline and are responsible for the splitting of proteins and the digestion of carbohydrates and fats.

Four hours are usually required for the food to be prepared in the small intestines. Then it moves along at the rate of an inch a minute. The intestinal walls have muscles, and the food is passed along by waves of muscular action. The bowel contracts immediately behind the bolus, or food mass, and relaxes in front of it. Besides this forward movement, the intestine regularly constricts, twenty to thirty times a minute, churning the food as it mixes with the digestive juices. The absorption of the food

takes place almost entirely in the small intestine. At the juncture where the small intestine opens into the large intestine, a valve permits the contents to pass at regular intervals.

The large intestine, about five feet long, includes the ascending, transverse, and descending colons. It handles the indigestible material which remains after the food has given the body its requirements. Food remains in the large intestine from ten to forty-eight hours, and its movement occurs periodically at intervals of about eight hours.

The contents of the bowel pass into the rectum, where a mechanism is localized to indicate that material is ready to be expelled from the body. The desire to empty the bowel is a reflex, initiated by pressure on the walls of the rectum by the waste material or feces. At times, emotional disturbances may generate the reflex, as, for example, is often the experience of combat troops when they first come under fire.

Any obstruction of action in the intestines is serious. A disorder may occur when one section of the bowel is drawn inside another section. This may be the result of a tumor, of indigestible material being impacted, or by the pushing of a portion of the bowel into a rupture. Such an obstruction causes severe pain and demands immediate attention by a physician. Since almost any acute condition of the abdomen may simulate intestinal obstruction by producing pain and vomiting, diagnosis must be meticulous. If actual obstruction exists, operation is usually necessary. *See also* INTESTINES; and Chapter 18, "Disorders of the Digestive System and Diet in Digestive Disorders."

BOWEN'S DISEASE, named after Dr. John T. Bowen, an American physician, a skin affliction believed to be of a cancerous nature. It occurs as circumscribed, horny elevations of the skin, as small as pinpoints or as large as peas, and may not damage adjoining tissues for long periods.

BRACHIAL, a term relating to the arm. Brachial arteries, for example, extend along the inner side of the upper arm, and brachial glands are the lymphatic glands in the armpit.

BRACHYDACTYLY, based on the Greek *brachy* meaning short, and *dactyly* meaning condition of fingers, a term denoting abnormally short fingers and toes.

BRAILLE SYSTEM, a form of printing for the blind, wherein letters and characters are represented by raised dots or points punched in paper and elevated above the surface, so as to be easily recognizable to touch. It was perfected in 1837 by Louis Braille, a French teacher of the blind. Somewhat modified, it is now used universally. Books and periodicals in Braille can be obtained in most public libraries.

BRAIN. The human brain is a large mass of nerve tissues contained in the skull, connected to the spinal cord, and surrounded by three layers of tough membranes called the meninges. The brain cells, with the spinal cord, are interwoven into a complex relay system which collects, stores and sends out sensations and information.

Over the centuries as man evolved toward his present state, man's brain has developed and grown. Each area of the brain is responsible for the control of a particular part of the body, or for a particular group of sensations or impulses.

Just within the cranial cavity and continuous with the spinal cord is the lower brain stem which controls the muscles and the sensory organs of the head. Above the lower brain stem is the part known as the midbrain where eye movements and a number of involuntary muscular reflexes are controlled. The cerebellum, which is the second largest single section of the brain, grows out behind the midbrain. Its function is to coordinate and integrate the action patterns from throughout the nervous system, and thus is responsible for smoothness of action. A disturbance in the cerebellum results in spastic, disjointed movements and lack of muscular coordination.

The hypothalmus is located directly above and in front of the midbrain. This group of cells regulates, among other things, sexual functions,

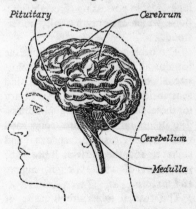

The major areas of the brain.

body temperature, sleeping, and aggressions. The hypothalmus is intimately connected with the pituitary gland and the other endocrine glands. The thalmus, which is involved with the emotions and with the integrations of basic patterns, and the paleocortex grow out of the brain stem above the midbrain and are continuous with the largest and most complex of the brain's parts, the neocortex or cerebrum.

The neocortex, which is divided into two hemispheres, is made up of a thin layer of cells and a subsurface mass of interlacing fibers. It represents altogether about 70 per cent of the total nervous system. The surface is intricately folded to provide a maximum of surface space and the approximately seven billion nerve cells that make up the entire mass of the neocortex are interconnected in an almost unbelievable manner. Each of the cells has about 5,000 connections, or synopses, with other cells, and it is believed that every cell is connected at least indirectly to every other cell in the whole cerebrum. The cerebrum is divided into five lobes, each possessing special functions, which are only partially understood.

The occipital lobes are responsible for the ability to differentiate color, size, shape, motion and distance, and thus to identify an object. An injury to these lobes can cause blindness. The temporal lobes are concerned with hearing, smell, speech and balance, and the parietal lobes with sensations of taste, weight, shape, and texture.

The frontal lobes are the site of some of the most complex intellectual abilities, such as reason, emotion, and judgement. Furthermore, in back of the frontal lobes is a group of large cells, the motor cortex, which is involved with complicated voluntary muscular movements, including speech. If these cells are destroyed, a total loss of these voluntary movements results. The frontal lobes have numerous connections with the other lobes and the thalamus. Here feelings and emotions combine with other associations, and this combination of feeling and knowledge determines most voluntary actions. Thinking, imagination, reasoning, and judgement all evolve as the sensory and emotional associations grow more complex. The manner in which these higher capacities are used constitutes personality and a disease in the frontal lobes produces distinct personality changes, errors in judgement and weak emotional control.

As can be seen, the human brain is a highly complex and fascinating organ. Much remains to be learned of its intricate functions and activity.

BREAST, one of the paired mammary glands on the front of the chest. They are composed of fatty tissue and glands capable of producing milk and are ordinarily much more developed in women than in men. At the center of each breast the milk glands fuse into a single outlet, the nipple, also more developed in the female. Since the growth of the breasts depends largely on production of female hormone, they may become larger in some young boys before puberty, and also in men who develop hormone-producing tumors. The female breast is usually much larger during pregnancy, because of heightened production of female hormone and increased production of milk glands.

Breast cancer is perhaps the most frequent female cancer and for this reason every woman should know how to detect early symptoms within her breasts. The most common sign is a small lump. Other symptoms are pain, bleeding from the nipple, or ulcerations which do not heal. Not all lumps in the breast are cancerous, however, and many, perhaps most, are due to small clumps of fibrous tissue called fibromas; to small cysts which are collections of fluid; or to harmless clusters of glandular tissue called adenomas. The nipple may bleed in cases of bruising or because of harmless glandular development. A doctor should be consulted in all cases, however. If the condition seems suspicious, a small piece of tissue is removed from the breast and thoroughly studied under a microscope by experts. This procedure, known as biopsy, is usually performed in a hospital.

Men rarely develop breast cancer. However, any lumps in the male breast should be carefully studied. The small infant may develop a swelling under the breast shortly after birth. This is harmless and usually due to accumulation of the mother's sex hormones in his system. Older boys sometimes develop hard lumps under the nipple which may disappear spontaneously after puberty. Occasionally this condition is associated with tumors of the testicle. Such cases, known as gynecomastia, should be seen by the doctor immediately. Fatty deposits in the breasts of some men due to obesity also imitate this disorder.

Infection of the mother's breasts may occur after childbirth, and is characterized by high temperature, and redness and pain in the breast. This condition is successfully treated with penicillin or other similar drugs.

The nursing process after childbirth depends on hormones from the pituitary gland which help produce actively secreting glandular structures. Generally milk begins to flow within a few days of birth, though it may begin sooner. At first, the milk, yellowish and cheesy, is a protein-rich substance known as colostrum. Finally this gives way to true milk, a thin bluish white secretion. Opinion favoring breast feeding fluctuates. However, it seems best for new mothers to try to breast feed their babies. Allergies are fewer in such babies and infants usually do much better in general on mother's milk. Some belief prevails, too, that breast cancer may be lower in women who nurse their babies.

The size and shape of a woman's breasts depend on fatty tissue rather than glands, and thus women with larger breasts do not find it easier to nurse their babies than do those with smaller breasts. Many products are sold to help women increase the size of their breasts. Hormones are used but in general are best avoided, because of the dangers of stimulating a cancerous process. There does not seem to be any completely safe or desirable way to increase the size of the breasts. *See also* CANCER; FEEDING, BREAST; MASTITIS; PREGNANCY

AND PRENATAL CARE; and Chapter 6, "Prenatal Care and Childbirth"; Chapter 17, "Cancer."

BREATHING. *See* ASPIRATION.

BROMIDES, compounds of bromide, a poisonous, caustic, nonmetallic element, with another element. Among others, bromides of potassium, calcium, iron, ammonium, and sodium are used in medicine. Bromides generally have a sedative effect and allay nervous tension. For more than half a century, bromides have been employed in the control of epileptic attacks and other spasmodic afflictions. More recently, however, safer and more effective sedatives and anticonvulsants, such as phenobarbital and dilantin, have been found. Some people are as allergic to the basic bromine as they are to some other drugs and may develop skin rash, boils, inflammation of hair follicles and other inexplicable symptoms during the course of a disease.

Taken over a long period, bromides have a cumulative effect. When the level gets too high, bromide intoxication, or bromism, occurs, with such symptoms as headache, coldness of the extremities, drowsiness, apathy, delirium, hallucinations, and pallor of the skin.

Blood tests for bromide intoxication, have been developed in the laboratory and are relatively simple. Once the condition is discovered, it can be eliminated by continuous baths and doses of salt.

BRONCHIAL TUBES. *See* BRONCHIECTASIS; BRONCHITIS; BRONCHIAL PNEUMONIA; PNEUMONIA; and Chapter 15, "Respiratory Diseases."

BRONCHIECTASIS, a chronic enlargement of the major or minor passages which carry air to and from the lungs; it usually produces an accumulation of infected mucus, consequent violent coughing, and markedly offensive breath. The cause may be an acute infection such as tuberculosis, pneumonia, or bronchitis, a protracted asthmatic condition, or a foreign body in the main air passages.

In the violent bursts of coughing characteristic of bronchiectasis, the person discharges large amounts of purulent mucus, sometimes as much as a quart a day. In severe cases, he may have to maintain a position in bed or in a chair that will help in draining the mucus from within the chest. Severe attacks of fever, increased spitting, loss of weight, and sometimes night sweats and bleeding from the lungs are other manifestations of bronchiectasis. Inflammation and scarring eventually render associated areas of the lung useless and threaten the rest of the body with further infection.

Patients are often so depleted by the disease that normal activity becomes impossible. Anemia is a frequent complication. Rest, proper food, fresh air, and sun are usually the basis of treatment. Penicillin and sulfonamide drugs are useful, especially in early stages of the disease. If bronchiectasis becomes chronic, some form of surgery is often necessary. Air may be injected into the cavity around the lung to collapse it and give it rest, or a phrenic nerve may be severed. In some cases, a part or all of the lung is removed. *See also* LUNGS; and Chapter 15, "Respiratory Diseases."

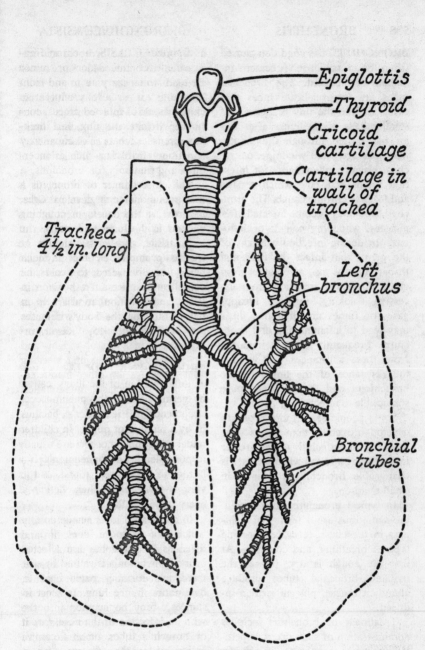

Epiglottis

Thyroid

Cricoid
cartilage

Cartilage in
wall of
trachea

Trachea
4½ in. long

Left
bronchus

Bronchial
tubes

The breathing tract.

BRONCHITIS, the condition caused when the bronchial tubes become inflamed or infected. The bronchial tubes are large delicate tubes that carry air into the tiny branches and smaller cells of the lungs after this air has passed through the mouth, nasal passages, and windpipe, or trachea. Usually inflammation or infection begins as a cold which persists and leads to chronic cough. The bronchial tubes may become infected after measles, whooping cough, or influenza, or during infection with any of the germs that infect the nose and throat. Viruses may also cause bronchitis. Bronchial irritation from excessive smoking, inhaling noxious gases or fumes and irritating dusts may lead to inflammation and bronchitis. Frequently chronic irritation from these substances will weaken the resistance of the lining of the bronchioles and they become more susceptible to infection by germs.

Some people seem more prone to develop bronchitis than others. The tendency to bronchitis seems greater in the spring and fall when weather is changeable. Bronchitis is common in small children.

In typical bronchitis after a cold, the symptoms are a feeling of tightness in the chest, fever, a wheezing type of breathing, and coughing. At first the cough is dry, but as the irritated bronchial tubes produce abundant mucus, phlegm is then induced.

Treatment of bronchitis includes administration of such drugs as penicillin to combat infection, if it exists, and also medications to loosen the phlegm within the bronchial tubes to permit easier breathing. The use of a vaporizer in the bedroom at night is often recommended, since moist air tends to loosen phlegm and make breathing easier. Adults with bronchitis should avoid contacts which further irritate the bronchial lining membranes, such as smoking and occupations involving inhalation of dusts and fumes.

The chief danger of bronchitis is that pneumonia may develop. Other hazards are the development of pus pockets in the lungs and scarring of lung tissue. Bronchitis should be treated promptly by the physician when first discovered, to avoid such complications. Rest, fresh air, sunshine, and nutritious food are essential in building the body's defenses. *See also* Chapter 15, "Respiratory Diseases."

BRONCHOPNEUMONIA, a type of inflammation of the lungs, caused by germs such as the pneumococci, streptococci, Friedlander's bacillus, or by a number of others. In children under three, pneumococci are usually responsible. Bronchopneumonia is a hazard to life all year round, and its various forms claim their victims at every period of life.

In contrast to lobar pneumonia, in which one or more lobes or large divisions of the lobes are affected, bronchopneumonia is caused by scattered pus forming patches of inflammation in the lung. In most instances, bronchopneumonia begins with an infection of the nose, throat, or bronchial tubes, or as a complication of another disease such as whooping cough, measles, influenza, or a common bronchitis. As a secondary disease brought about by a variety of organisms, it may affect all age groups, but as a primary disorder bronchopneumonia occurs only in children under three years of age.

The aged often become victims of bronchopneumonia because of their tendency to accumulate mucous material in the lungs. As the power of the lungs to repair themselves has diminished, small areas of degenerated tissue are affected and the accumulating material must be expelled from the lungs. The continued inhalation and coughing results in disturbances such as bronchopneumonia.

The disease may not start as abruptly as other types of pneumonia. Symptoms like fever, coughing, and shortness of breath gradually become worse. The temperature lowers step by step with recovery.

Such drugs as the sulfanilamides and antibiotics are most frequently used in the treatment, and the response is best if the invading organisms are susceptible to them. *See also* PNEUMONIA; and Chapter 15, "Respiratory Diseases."

BRUCELLOSIS. *See* UNDULANT FEVER.

BRUISES, injuries, sufficiently severe, to the surface of the body which do not break the skin. If the skin breaks and bleeds, the wound is called a laceration. Bruises are usually caused by bumping against hard or sharp surfaces, by falls, or by blows.

The characteristic discoloration that follows injury to the small blood vessels in the tissues beneath the skin or, at times, to infiltration of blood into the muscles is a hematoma. As a blood clot forms, the skin becomes dark and when the pigment material is absorbed, the area becomes bluish, then brownish, and finally yellowish.

Some people bruise much more easily than others, probably because their blood vessels are more permeable or fragile, permitting blood to escape with greater facility. In other instances, hematoma may develop because the blood itself does not contain enough of the substances that permit prompt clotting. Some women bruise more easily during menstruation. Obese and anemic persons are more susceptible to bruises than others.

Most bruises heal without attention. Cold applications or heat by hot compresses or electric pads give relief if the bruise incites swelling or pain. Massage is not advisable. Some bruises require attention because of possible complications beneath the skin under the bruised area. A bruise of the larynx, for instance, may have many complications, such as pain when swallowing and speaking, shortness of breath, hoarseness, and even suffocation, and prompt attention by a physician is imperative. An injury of the scalp is also significant because of a possible skull fracture. There have been cases in which the only symptom of a ruptured liver was a slight bruise on the surface of the body.

In severe cases the injured part should be rested, and if much swelling occurs in an arm or leg, absorption of blood can be promoted by elevating the limb or application of heat. If a secondary infection invades the blood clot, a serious condition can result. Usually the blood in the clot beneath the skin is readily absorbed, but if the pressure of the clot menaces nearby parts of the body, the physician may remove the accumulated material. When muscles are injured, blood infiltrates them, the muscle fibers swell, and the resulting lumps may be so large that a physician must make incisions to remove the clot. *See also* CONTUSION.

BUBO, a painful inflammation or swelling of a lymphatic gland, which usually develops in the groin, especially after venereal infections. An abscess caused by injury or irritation, not by infection, is a "sympathetic" bubo. *See also* LYMPHOGRANULOMA VENEREUM.

BUBONIC PLAGUE, an acute infectious disease caused by bacteria transmitted by the rat flea. It is characterized by enlargement of the lymphatic glands and toxic symptoms of great severity. The mortality rate is high. *See also* PLAGUE.

BULBAR, in medicine, a term pertaining to the medulla of the brain. Formerly the medulla oblongata, the lower part of the brain stem, was called a bulb.

BULBAR POLIOMYELITIS. *See* POLIOMYELITIS.

BUNION, a painful swelling and overgrowth of bone on the foot. The deformity usually affects the large toe, the joint becoming swollen while the tip of the toe is forced outward against the other toes. Occasionally a bunion will occur on the top of the foot. The skin is usually thickened. Bunions are often caused by poorly fitted footwear; and properly fitted shoes, perhaps padded, will usually help to relieve the discomfort. Complete relief, however, is brought about only by surgical removal of the bunion together with a part of the overgrown bone beneath it.

BURNS. A burn is a searing of the flesh which can be caused by many agents—from hot steam to the sun's rays. Each year over 6,000 fatal burns occur in the United States and burns are a common cause of death in young children. Burns involving over one-third to one-half of the body are often fatal, especially in children.

Burns are classified into three groups and in all cases symptoms and treatment are somewhat similar. (1) First-degree burns involve only reddening of the skin and usually require only cleaning with soap and water and the use of a soothing ointment. (2) Second-degree burns include blistering of the skin as well as superficial burning. (3) Third-degree burns cause destruction of the tissue. Second- and third-degree burns are best treated by promptly covering the burn with warm, wet compresses until the doctor arrives. Wet saline compresses are beneficial. In larger burns, gauze permeated with petroleum jelly is used to keep the area clean and free from infection as well as to prevent excess loss of fluid in the injured area. To counteract shock, which in severe burns may be fatal, the victim should lie flat without a pillow, have his clothing loosened, and be kept covered with a light blanket until the doctor arrives. *See also* SHOCK; and Chapter 27, "Safety and First Aid."

BURSA, a small fluid-filled sac which serves as a cushion against friction among joints that move upon each other. For example, a bursa lies between the heel bone and the Achilles' tendon. *See also* BURSITIS.

BURSITIS, an inflammation of a bursa; one of the most frequent rheumatic ailments. A bursa is a small sac situated between joints that move on each other, a kind of lubricating part around them. An inflamed bursa contains calcium deposits in a semisolid state. Bursae in any of the joints may become inflamed. Most frequently, however, the shoulder is affected; bursitis of the elbow and above the knee is less frequent.

Ordinarily bursitis is extremely painful in both the acute or chronic form. It may appear suddenly, following chilling, strains, blows, or infection. Frequently bursitis results from excessive use of a joint, as, for example, in playing tennis, or prolonged standing or stretching. Chronic bursitis may be a consequence of acute bursitis or it may be a chronic manifestation from the beginning.

The symptoms of acute bursitis are always a sharp pain and discoloration at the spot where the inflammation is located. In some cases, limited swelling is present and the inflamed bursa can be felt. In chronic bursitis, swelling and tenderness fluctuate and progress with intermittent pain, brought on perhaps by changes of weather or excessive use of the joint.

Sometimes acute bursitis heals without any treatment. The inflamed bursa may drain itself, through rupture. Resting the afflicted part, however, is always imperative. Hot or cold applications, whichever the patient prefers, are often soothing, and exposure to the sun may help relieve chronic recurrent pains. Most physicians do not recommend massage under any circumstances. If the pain does not subside with such usual palliatives as aspirin, analgesic drugs, or even codeine, morphine or other narcotics may be prescribed by a physician. Sometimes he will irrigate the bursal cavity by needle or by incision and drainage.

Cortisone and ACTH have been successful in relieving severe cases of bursitis, but these drugs must be used for long periods. Deep x-ray therapy often brings good results. *See also* BURSA.

BUTTOCKS, the two fleshy parts of the posterior part of the body on which one sits; they are formed by the glutei or buttock muscles.

BUTYN, a trade name for butacaine sulphate, a substitute for cocaine as a surface local anesthetic for mucous membranes and eyes.

CAISSON DISEASE, also known as "the bends," compression air disease, and diver's palsy, a condition caused by a too rapid return from high to normal sea level atmospheric pressure. The nitrogen in the body appears in the blood as nitrogen bubbles which obstruct the circulation. Caisson disease is limited to certain occupations, occurring mostly in divers and tunnel workers who work under high atmospheric pressure and then are subjected to rapid reduction of air pressure.

Principal symptoms of Caisson disease are pain in the legs or abdomen, dizziness or staggers, and itching of the skin. Partial or total insensibility, paralysis of face, arms, and legs on one side of the body, paralysis of the lower part of the body, and pronounced nervous symptoms may also develop. The first sensation, a feeling of pressure in the eardrums, is often relieved by swallowing.

Experience has shown that recompression of the worker, followed by slow decompression overcomes the symptoms of Caisson disease. If, however, the symptoms are not promptly relieved, the worker is placed in a high-pressure chamber or tunnel where he remains for a long period of time (this is known as the "overnight soak"). Afterward he receives gradual decompression.

CALAMINE, zinc carbonate, pulverized and cleansed. In compounds it is used externally as an astringent and dusting powder. As a soothing protection, calamine lotion is applied in cases of sunburn, insect bites, acne, and other skin irritations.

CALCIUM, a silver-white, soft metal which occurs only in combination with other elements. It is present in spring and river waters and in plants and the bodies of man and animals.

The body of the average person contains significant amounts of thirteen minerals. Of them all, calcium is present in the largest amount and is one of the most essential. It is present in and vital to the health of every known tissue and cell in the body. It is a significant element in building strong bones and teeth.

Research on the nutritional value of minerals in food, conducted by the Chemistry Department of Columbia University, led to the conclusion that "Diets with low calcium content have a harmful effect on well-being and health of far greater significance than hitherto supposed." The encyclopedic yearbook published by the United States Department of Agriculture under the title *Food and Life* states positively, "In spite of the fact that knowledge of effective measures for the prevention of calcium and other mineral deficiencies is at hand, there is abundant evidence that a considerable proportion of the general population of all ages does not receive adequate amounts of calcium."

A calcium deficiency may be involved in the cause of so-called degenerative diseases—those diseases involving a loss in the power of functioning of any part of the body— such as hardening of the arteries, some allergies, disorders of the heart, kidney, and blood vessels. The U. S. Department of Agriculture publishes lists of foods rated as excellent or good in calcium richness, which can be used as a guide in helping to assure an adequate supply of calcium in the diet. Listed as *excellent* are: broccoli, buttermilk, cabbage, chard, cheddar and Swiss cheese, clams, dandelion greens, kale, milk in all its forms—whole, skimmed, evaporated, condensed, and dried—molasses, mustard and turnip greens, watercress, and yeast. Listed as *good* are: almonds, artichokes, all kinds of beans including dried, kidney, string, and snap, carrots, celery, cottage cheese, crabs, cream, eggs, endive or escarole, dried figs, lettuce, lobsters, maple syrup, oysters.

If foods were listed in the order of their significance, milk in its various forms, excepting butter, would lead the list, followed by green, leafy vegetables.

To insure a good supply of calcium during pregnancy and eliminate leg cramps, physicians frequently prescribe calcium in different compounds as a dietary supplement. *See also* NUTRITION; VITAMINS.

CALCIUM-PHOSPHORUS RATIO. A particular balance between calcium and phosphorus must be maintained within the body so that healthy tissue evolves from strong bone cells. Therefore, both calcium and phosphorus are essential in the diet.

CALCULUS, a stone, or concretion of mineral salts, which forms most frequently in the cavities of the body which act as reservoirs for fluids. Often the stone takes its name from the cavity in which it grows—for example, kidney stone or gallstone. Calculi may develop in any tissue in which calcium or other minerals are deposited.

The calculus usually takes its mineral content from the fluid in which it is found. Its nucleus, however, may be a small blood clot, a bit of dried mucus, or some other foreign body which may have entered the cavity.

The stone ordinarily does not become evident until it begins to pass out of its cavity. Then it may produce a severe pain, called renal colic if the calculus is a kidney stone, or biliary colic if it is a gallstone. *See also* BLADDER, DISEASES OF; COLIC; GALLSTONES; KIDNEY.

CALLUS, generally any area of hardened, thickened skin caused by friction, pressure, or other irritation. It is also new tissue which forms where a fractured bone heals.

Most calluses—for example, those on the palm of the hand—do not cause trouble and do not require medical attention. But in other locations calluses may cause pain. For instance, when pressure is exerted on a heavily thickened callus on the foot at a point where it is caught between the shoe and the prominent bones beneath the ball of the foot, treatment may be necessary. Paring off the outer layers of the hardened skin with a sharp knife or file is the usual way, but chemicals also are sometimes used. In severe cases, relief is secured by inserting a protective device within the shoe or by changing the area of weight bearing.

Great care must be taken not to damage the delicate tissue beneath the callus by cutting too deeply. Diabetics and persons suffering from any arterial disease must *never* try to treat corns or calluses themselves. It is better to prevent calluses by making certain that shoes are properly fitted, by avoiding continued pressure irritation, and by taking sensible care of the feet. *See also* FEET.

CALOMEL, mercurous chloride, a white, almost tasteless and insoluble powder. It was formerly commonly used as a purgative. It has also served as an antisyphilitic, an intestinal antiseptic, and as a kidney stimulant.

CALORIE, the unit by which the energy value of food is measured. Specifically it is equivalent to the amount of heat required to raise one cubic centimeter of water one degree Centigrade. Foods vary widely in their caloric contents. For instance, a pound of butter will supply a vastly larger number of calories than a pound of lettuce. By checking the number of calories consumed against the energy output charted for a person's age, height, weight, and occupation the doctor can determine whether or not the person eats too many, too few, or sufficient calories for his daily needs. If too many, the excess is stored as fat in specially provided cells in the body. If too few, the body draws either upon its fat deposits or tissues to make up the deficit and the person will show a weight loss. If caloric intake and energy output balance, weight tends to remain stable. *See also* NUTRITION.

CAMPHOR, a volatile oil with a characteristic aromatic smell. It is obtained naturally from a tree native to eastern Asia, and artificially from turpentine oil activated by hydrochloric acid. It is a mild irritant and cooling antiseptic when applied to the mucous membranes and the skin.

Camphorized ointments and oils aid the relief of nasal congestion, but must not be used for infants or small children. In acute inflammations of glands, camphor has been beneficial as a cooling pain reliever.

Occasionally camphor is used by injection to stimulate the circulation of the blood, in the treatment of painful diarrhea, vomiting, and as a medicine to induce perspiration. *See also* POISONING.

CANCER, a disease characterized by abnormal and often unpredictable growth of cells. Cancerous growths are also disposed to invade normal healthy tissues which can be destroyed or even replaced by their wild growth. Nerves may be affected, causing pain; blood vessels may be broken open by the invading growth, causing hemorrhage; and structures such as lung tissues, the arteries, kidneys, or bladder may be obstructed by infiltration of cancer tissue. Every part of the body is susceptible to cancerous growths, though some organs, such as stomach, bowel, lung, and the sexual organs, seem more frequently involved.

Accumulations of rapidly growing cells may form a lump known as a tumor, but not all tumors are cancerous or dangerous. Many, such as fibromas, clumps of scar-type tissue; adenomas, clumps of harmless glandular tissue; warts, fatty tumors, or lipomas do not invade normal tissue and do not lead to serious consequences. They are benign or harmless growths or tumors. Groups of cells which invade normal tissue and destroy healthy cells are malignant. Growth may be rapid or slow, but usually is progressive; that is, the cancers do not stop growing once they originate.

Some cancers remain in one location; others tend to spread through the blood stream or lymphatic stream throughout the body. These "pilgrim-type" growths, metastases, in general represent a more serious type of cancer.

The exact cause of cancer is unknown. Some scientists believe that persons are born with abnormal cells and that these remain quiescent throughout life or until some factor starts them growing. Others believe that chronic irritation of a certain group of cells may lead to cancerous changes. Cancer of the lip is common in pipe smokers and lung cancer in cigarette smokers. Some specialists feel that irritation from the sun may lead to skin cancers, common in farmers and outdoor workers. Chemicals also may induce cancer. The sex hormones are related to cancer development, especially of the breast or reproductive system. Because wives of circumcised men rarely develop cancer of the cervix, some experts believe that the uncircumcised male may harbor a cancer-producing secretion under the foreskin. A relationship may exist between failure to breast feed and breast cancer. Heredity is probably significant, but just how is not yet known. Cancer is probably not contagious; nevertheless, experiments utilizing our knowledge of viruses are being made to confirm this.

Kinds of cancer. Doctors classify cancer according to many factors: the type of tissue involved; the speed of its growth; the portion of the body involved; and sometimes even according to the chemical changes that take place within the tumor.

Some cancers are easily seen or felt, such as breast and skin cancers; some can be detected or suspected by rectal or vaginal examination and by introduction of instruments into the stomach; some by x-ray, by blood or urine tests, and by other techniques.

Certain cancers—for instance, breast cancers—are found predominantly in women; lung and mouth cancers are more common in men.

The symptoms of early cancers are often barely noticeable; therefore, everyone should have a complete and thorough medical checkup at least once a year, and oftener if abnormal symptoms occur. Lives are needlessly lost because cancer is diagnosed much too late for the doctor to achieve successful treatment. Often the symptoms are caused by a harmless condition, but delay in treatment can be hazardous.

Any of the following symptoms should be checked promptly by a competent physician.

Mouth. Any sore in the mouth, or anywhere for that matter, that lasts more than a few days without healing should be reported.

Larynx. Hoarseness that persists for more than a week, and for three weeks at the most, should be suspected. By examination of the vocal cords, the doctor can determine whether or not they are inflamed or irritated, or affected by tumors of a benign or malignant nature. Removal of the growths and examination of the specimen under the microscope will aid in making the diagnosis.

Breast. Any discomfort, pain, thickening, dimpling, or lump in a breast of a man or woman that does not disappear within a week, and any discharge from the nipple, bloody or otherwise, demands immediate attention. Delay can be perilous. If the doctor demands surgical removal of the lump for expert examination, this should be done without delay as only by microscopic examination of tissue can definite diagnosis be made.

Stomach. Stomach cancer seldom causes pain. Ordinarily early signs include loss of appetite, diarrhea, appearance of black material in the stools, regurgitation, or difficulty in swallowing food. Generally these symptoms point to conditions less serious than cancer, and the doctor can make correct diagnosis by using x-ray and other techniques.

Female organs. Prolonged, irregular, or unusual bleeding, especially after the age of thirty-five or between periods, should always be investigated promptly.

New aids to cancer diagnosis. Cancer may be diagnosed in many different ways, some simple, others complicated. Most significant is a detailed history of the onset and nature of the patient's symptoms, followed by a thorough examination. When suspicious growths are noted on the skin, in the breasts, or within the reproductive organs, the doctor may take a piece of tissue for examination under the microscope. This is known as biopsy. The cancer cell, when viewed under the microscope, is different from the normal cell. In some cases, changes in the cells may be difficult to detect, even by experts.

Among the most recent medical discoveries is the Papanicolaou test for cancer. In this test, scrapings taken from the surface of the cervix of the uterus or from the walls of the vagina are treated with certain chemicals. The tissues are then placed under the microscope, where careful examination can usually rule out or indicate the presence of early cancer

changes. The test can be used on the sputum of presumed lung cancer, and also on stomach secretion when cancer in that organ is suspected.

Tissue from within the body can be removed for analysis by curettage, as in the uterus when the uterus wall is scraped. Investigation may be performed by bronchoscopy, in which a long tube is inserted into the lung structure to remove tissue; by gastroscopy, done with a stomach tube; or proctoscopy, in which a long telescope-like instrument is inserted into the rectum. These instruments used for detecting cancer are often provided with a light so that the operator can actually look into the organs.

X-ray is invaluable in detecting cancer. To aid in finding stomach or rectal cancer, barium, a white substance, is introduced into these organs and helps x-rays detect any tumors by outlining them. Occasionally substances may be injected into the blood stream which outline the kidneys or other organs.

Blood tests for the detection of cancer, except for cancer of the blood, are being studied extensively, but as yet none of the tests has been accepted.

Is cancer caused by a germ? Some scientists are inclined to feel that cancer may be caused by a virus, a form of living growth too small to be seen under the microscope. Already there seems to be evidence that certain substances like viruses can cause cancers. A factor that passes through the mother's milk in mice has been found capable of causing cancer in other mice. However, this finding is not applicable to human beings.

Another technique that has aroused interest is the attempt to grow tumors in yolk sacs of developing chicks. Here certain viruses are grown and distinguished from one another. Success has been reported in growing transplants from breast cancer on yolk sacs of chick embryos. This may not prove that viruses cause cancer, but rather that cancer cells can grow on a suitable medium if transplanted. At present experiments are being conducted on human beings by inoculating volunteers with deadly cancer cells. The results may have far-reaching effects on our knowledge and treatment of cancer.

Hormones, particularly sex hormones, may stimulate cancer growth. These include the female hormone, estrogen, and the male hormone, testosterone. Estrogens in large amounts may stimulate growth of breast cancers while they may delay growth of male cancers, notably prostate cancers. The male hormone may actually help to stop the growth of female breast cancer, and conversely stimulate prostate cancer.

Is cancer hereditary? Studies on animals indicate that the tendency to develop cancer seems stronger in some families than in others, although there does not seem to be a true inheritance. In some families, cancer apparently will develop in certain circumstances. Therefore, when any cancer is common in one family, members of the family should avoid taking sex hormones and overexposure to x-rays or to other chemicals or irritants.

Cancer-stimulating substances are thought to include coal tars, x-rays, excessive exposure to the sun, viruses,

and hormones. Mechanical irritation, such as tight girdles or collars and friction on a mole on the skin may be harmful. Rough teeth and improperly fitted dentures may, by causing irritation, lead to cancer of the mouth, as may pipe and cigarette smoking.

Cancer of the blood usually manifests itself by anemia, fatigue, loss of weight, and shortness of breath. The diagnosis is made by examining the blood and a specimen of tissue taken from the bone marrow.

Treatment. Surgery has always been one of the most effective ways to remove cancers. By the removal of localized growths, the patient may be completely cured. Approach to treatment may be varied, and may not, in some cases, even include surgery. X-ray, or radium treatment is employed successfully in many types of pelvic cancer. Chemical therapy includes hormone treatments of breast and prostate cancer, and also drug management of the leukemias, blood cancers. Often a combination of surgery, x-ray, and drugs is used.

Most exciting of recent approaches to treatment is the use of radioactive isotopes. The isotopes are chemicals having radioactivity combined with a chemical element. Since these chemicals are likely to go directly to one tissue of the body, they concentrate in that organ and destroy abnormal tissues there. Cancer of the thyroid has been successfully treated by using radioactive iodine. Iron, sodium, potassium, chlorine, bromine, calcium, strontium, sulphur, carbon, and hydrogen have all been subjected to experiments in controlling growths in various parts of the body. Radioactive phosphorus has also been applied externally to warts, moles, and other growths on the surface of the body, and in some instances with apparent success.

The nitrogen mustard chemicals, developed for use in warfare, have been helpful in destroying cancer cells of the blood. These drugs are used effectively in Hodgkin's disease, chronic leukemia, and in other forms of blood tumors.

Much remains to be learned about cancer, and much will depend on the cooperation of patients in promptly reporting to their doctor any suspicious signs. Regular yearly checkups aid in early detection of cancers. *See also* Chapter 17, "Cancer."

CANKER SORE, usually a small ulceration on the inside of the mouth, lips, and cheeks, which may appear from a variety of causes. Sometimes the cause stems from the nervous system; often the sore is a manifestation of a sensitivity to certain substances taken into the body; and frequently it is due to a virus infection such as a cold. Whenever canker sores appear persistently, a medical study should be made for some functional disturbance, including an examination of the blood to determine the status of the clotting elements in the blood stream. Tests should also be made for sensitivity to various foods, and the fillings in the patient's teeth examined, since it has been shown that dissimilar metals used as fillings in the same mouth may create electrical currents sometimes associated with the appearance of cankers in the mouth.

CANTHARIDES, popularly called Spanish fly, a bitter-tasting powder made from an insect known scientifically as Cantharis vasicatoria. The active principle in the drug is cantharidin, which is marketed in many forms, such as cantharidin plaster, blistering fluid, cantharidin ointment, and tincture of cantharidin.

The drug should be used only when prescribed by a doctor, and the utmost precaution should be taken to prevent it from entering the mouth, the eyes, or other sensitive areas.

Cantharidin is never used before the condition of the patient's kidneys has been checked, since the drug is easily absorbed through the skin. It must not be applied to any part of the body on which the patient is likely to lie, since the heat and perspiration result in blistering. Furthermore, it is dangerous when applied to paralyzed arms or legs. Such reputation as it has as a stimulant to sexual desire is without any good evidence.

Cantharides is intensely irritating to the kidneys and should never be taken internally. In the treatment of children, the aged, or the weak it should never be used, even externally, for any purpose.

Symptoms of cantharidin poisoning may be intense pain in the alimentary canal, in the stomach and kidneys, or in the urinary organs. Vomiting and diarrhea ordinarily occur, and a persistent desire to urinate is noticeable. The pulse is usually weak and slow and collapse is not unlikely. *See also* BLISTERS.

CAPILLARIES, the smallest branches of the arterial tree; fine, filament-like vessels through which blood pumped by the heart through increasingly smaller branches of the arterial tree finally passes by osmosis, an exchange of substances, to the cells of body organs and tissues. They are the minute structural elements which connect arterial circulation with venous circulation and which carry deoxygenated blood back to the heart. *See also* BLOOD; CIRCULATORY SYSTEM.

CARBOHYDRATES, organic substances which contain carbon, hydrogen, and oxygen and are stable, easily digestible sources of calories or nutritional energy. They belong to the class of nutriments represented by sugars, starches, celluloses, and gums. Foods with large carbohydrate content are sugars, jams, jellies, preserves, syrups, molasses, honey, cocoa, chocolate, candy, grains, grain products, and farinaceous substances. Nuts, although they contain a larger proportion per weight of protein, and an even greater proportion of fats, are also substantial in carbohydrate content. All dairy products, fruits and vegetables have carbohydrates in varying amounts. Dates and figs are especially rich in this nutriment, and potatoes, parsnips, and most lentils are also plentifully supplied with carbohydrates. *See also* NUTRITION; and Chapter 4 "Diet and Health."

CARBON DIOXIDE, a colorless odorless gas, a molecule of which consists of one atom of carbon in combination with two atoms of oxygen. It is one of the end products of the cellular metabolism of proteins, carbohydrates, and fats, all of which are carbon-containing compounds. It is given off by the body during that phase of respiration known as exhalation. The oxygen taken in during inhalation passes through the walls of capillaries lining the lungs, combines with the iron in the red blood corpuscles, is carried to the heart and from there distributed by the arterial system to all the cells of the body. In these cells, together with other substances, it enters into the chemical reactions essential to life. The carbon dioxide, among other waste products which result, passes through the cell walls into the venous blood supply, back to the heart, and from there to the lungs where it is exhaled. Although residual amounts in the blood stream are essential for normal body function, carbon dioxide in sufficient concentration can cause death. Generally the amount of this gas contained in the atmosphere is less than .03 per cent. In an unventilated room crowded with people, the concentration might rise dangerously. An atmospheric concentration of about 25 per cent is said to be lethal, but symptoms of a rising carbon dioxide concentration, such as headaches and drowsiness, would set in much earlier. In cities, carbon dioxide concentration is increased by the combustion of carbon-containing compounds in transportation, heating, and industrial processes. Fortunately urban atmospheres are continuously refreshed by winds which carry oxygen-laden air to the city and dust and carbon dioxide-laden air from it. The presence of green plants also helps decrease the carbon dioxide content of atmosphere, since plants predominantly inhale carbon dioxide and exhale oxygen during the process of photosynthesis. This takes place during sunlight; and at night, like the human being, the plant takes in small quantities of oxygen for its cellular metabolism and gives off some carbon dioxide as waste. Throughout a twenty-four-hour period, however, the plant removes much more carbon dioxide than oxygen, and gives off much more oxygen than carbon dioxide.

CARBON MONOXIDE, a colorless odorless gas, a product of the incomplete combustion of carbon. It is extremely poisonous. It burns with a pale blue flame to form carbon dioxide. Carbon monoxide may develop when coal oil, charcoal, gas, or kerosene are burned in a poorly ventilated room. A frequent source of carbon monoxide is from the exhausts of automobiles. In the open air, the gas quickly becomes carbon dioxide, but in a closed garage a running motor may produce enough carbon monoxide to kill in a matter of minutes.

Carbon monoxide invades the blood stream through the lungs, unites with the hemoglobin in the red blood corpuscles so that they cannot carry oxygen to the cells of the body, and asphyxiation ensues. The blood of victims of carbon-monoxide poisoning is a bright cherry red.

Early symptoms of carbon-monoxide poisoning include yawning, headache, nausea, dizziness, ringing in the ears, and abdominal pains. Gaspy breathing and unconsciousness quickly follow. The victim should get fresh air immediately, and he should be kept lying down and warm. A physician should be called promptly, and inhalations of oxygen or of oxygen-carbon dioxide mixture administered. Pure oxygen accelerates the release of carbon monoxide and frees it from the blood about four times faster than simple inhalation of air. If the breathing of the victim is gasping or has stopped, artificial respiration should be given at once.

If the carbon-monoxide poisoning is serious, the victim should be taken to the hospital as soon as possible for treatment which may include blood transfusions. Since the nerve cells are involved in the poisoning, temporary or permanent damage can be done to the brain, with serious disturbances of vision, hearing, speech, and memory.

Because carbon monoxide cannot be seen or smelled, danger of poisoning is especially insidious. Care should be taken that rooms in which fuels capable of producing carbon monoxide are being burned are properly ventilated, and that a car motor is not kept running in a closed garage.

CARBUNCLES, painful infections of the skin layer below the surface, accompanied by the production and discharge of pus and dead tissue, and tending to affect the general health. A carbuncle may be distinguished from a boil by its greater severity and depth and especially by its having several openings instead of one.

The first symptom of a carbuncle is a painful hard lump which develops under a tight and reddening skin. Several pus-discharging openings later appear in this surface. Eventually the entire mass will tend to separate itself, leaving an open sore.

Carbuncles appear most frequently on the face, neck, and shoulders. They particularly afflict persons who suffer from diabetes or Bright's disease. In such people resistance to invasive microorganisms which set up infection is lowered.

The severity of the infection can often be diminished at the outset by means of x-ray treatment, sulfa drugs, or penicillin. The immediate pain may be relieved by the application of hot compresses. These increase the flow of blood, thus strengthening the defensive forces in the infected area.

When the accumulation of pus becomes considerable, the carbuncle should be opened and drained by a physician. Unless special precautions are taken during this operation the protective wall, which the tissues have built to seal the infection from the rest of the body, may be broken down, thus permitting the infection to spread.

To avoid a repetition of this painful and exhausting experience, the person should have himself tested for diabetes and Bright's disease which predispose the body to this type of infection. The person should pay increased attention to the state of his general health; the body must develop resistance against such invasion. *See also* FURUNCLES.

CARCINOGENS, substances or agents that cause the development of cancer of any type—for example, certain tar or coal products.

CARDITIS, an inflammation of the heart, a manifestation and significant part of rheumatic fever. Internal carditis or endocarditis is the inflammation of the valves of the heart and membranes which line it. Pericarditis is the inflammation of the sac which encloses the heart. *See also* BACTERIAL ENDOCARDITIS; ENDOCARDITIS; PERICARDITIS; and Chapter 12, "Diseases of the Heart."

CARMINATIVE, an agent which relieves flatulence and colic.

CAROTENE, a chemical precursor of vitamin A, is a yellow pigment found in green and yellow vegetables such as carrots, sweet potatoes, yellow corn, and string beans. It can be extracted in a chemical laboratory and is converted in the animal body into vitamin A. *See also* VITAMINS.

CARPAL BONES, the eight bones of the wrist. On the back of the hand, five metacarpal bones connect the fingers with the wrist.

CARSICKNESS. *See* MOTION SICKNESS.

CARRIER OF DISEASE, the agent which transmits a communicable disease. It can be any of a vast number of things—air and dust, nose and throat secretions, sputum, clothing, insects. For example, certain mosquitoes carry malaria, dengue, and filariasis. Disease-producing bacteria cannot penetrate unbroken skin and must enter by means of wounds, scratches, abrasions, or a natural opening of the body. *See also* BACTERIA; INFECTIOUS DISEASES.

CARTILAGE, a white, semi-opaque connective tissue characterized by extreme smoothness, elasticity, and toughness. It covers the ends of the bones where they meet to become joints. Circular discs of cartilage lie, for example, between each layer of bone in the spine, acting as cushions or shock absorbers for these bones and for the strain to which the spinal column is subjected. Cartilage covers the movable joints of the legs, arms, and fingers, giving smoothness and resiliency to their movements. It is also found in other parts of the body, such as the tip of the nose, eyelids, ears, and the windpipe.

CASCARA, a drug usually derived from the bark of a tree native to Mexico, and also from certain shrubs. Because of its effective action on the colon, cascara is widely used as a laxative. Usually cascara is prescribed in the form of an aromatic extract. Cascara sagrada, the bark of California buckthorn, is especially useful in cases of chronic constipation.

CASEIN, the principal protein in milk. In milk, a liquid precursor, caseinogen, is present rather than casein itself. Converted into solid casein, for instance by rennet, a ferment in the stomach, it is the basis of curds or cheese. When milk is drunk slowly, its casein content becomes a light and flaky mass of curds in the stomach, rather than an indigestible dense body. This action is significant for children, older persons, or invalids. Casein is not only high in nutritive values, but also has many industrial applications in the production of plastics, paints, and adhesives.

CASTOR OIL, a pale yellow oil, expressed from the seeds of the ricinus or castor oil plant. It is an effective and prompt purgative and one of the oldest household remedies for constipation. It is likely, however, to be followed by costiveness and is therefore seldom used in chronic constipation. Castor oil is also used to counteract the effects of acid splashed in the eye.

The medicinal uses of castor oil have been recognized for centuries. It is mentioned in Egyptian papyri as an ideal purgative and as a stimulant for hair growth. The Incas of ancient Peru believed that castor oil possessed spiritual powers and used it to exorcise demons.

CASTRATION, the removal of one or both testes or ovaries, with a consequent deficiency of the endocrine hormones, testosterone and estrogen. It is one of the oldest surgical operations and was well known in earliest antiquity. Male foreign captives were castrated to prevent a mixing with foreign blood. Castration was sometimes a ritual which eliminated sexual desire so that an ascetic life could more easily be led. Among the self-imposed emasculates were Origen and St. Francis. At various times in history, especially in oriental countries, boys were castrated to become eunuchs. Later young male sopranos in church choirs were castrated so that their voices would not change. Castration as necessary medical surgery, too, was applied in cases of injury or disease. A castrated male was not always considered inferior; in fact, as in ancient Persia, he was sometimes highly esteemed and given important court positions.

Castration may be performed at almost any age. However, its effects are much more pronounced when performed before puberty. Removal of the testicles after puberty is accompanied by fewer symptoms because the body is fully developed. The early loss of testicular functions by injury, inflammation, or surgery results in definite characteristics. Castrated males, though often tall, are narrow-chested and effeminate, shy, gentle, placid, and lacking in endurance. Their voices are soft and highly pitched. While not necessarily bald, they do not have any hair on the face, armpits, and pubic areas. Obesity, especially layers of fat on the hips, are common and pronounced breasts not unusual. Some of the secondary male sex characteristics do not change, however, if the operation is performed after the age of sixteen.

When the testicles are diseased or severely injured, castration is sometimes essential—for example, in cases of cancer of the prostate. Castration does not have any effect on sexual capacity, even though it has a pronounced one on sexual urge, and it does not prevent or increase susceptibility to mental breakdown. Castration must be differentiated from sterilization. Sterilization is not mutilating and does not interfere with sexual physiology; only the procreative capacity is eliminated.

Animals are usually castrated to make them plumper and more gentle, as well as to restrict capacity of reproduction. In females, castration, or spaying, consists in removing the ovaries, and is medically termed an oophorectomy.

CATARACT, opacity producing loss of transparency of the lens of the eye; if the lens becomes entirely opaque, sight is lost. A cataract may be present at birth, and in young people it may appear as a result of injury. However, most cataracts occur in persons between the ages of fifty and seventy and are due to the gradual degeneration of the tissues of the lenses. To some extent, a tendency to this degeneration may be hereditary. Although the disease may show itself at first in only one eye, in almost all instances it will eventually appear in the other also. The process is gradual and "ripeness" or full opacity may take two years to develop.

Among the earliest symptoms of cataract are red eyelids, unexplainable daytime headaches, small specks seen constantly before the eyes, and gradually worsening vision. These or similar symptoms should be called promptly to the attention of a physician skilled in treatment of eye disorders. Temporary eyesight can be maintained by frequent changes of glasses.

Physicians generally agree, however, that the only effective treatment for a cataract itself is an operation. Such an operation restores good vision to approximately 97 persons out of a hundred. The surgery, relatively simple, is followed by the prescription of so-called cataract glasses, which contain biconvex lenses to replace the clouded natural lenses that are removed. *See also* EYE.

CATARRH, a term which was formerly used for inflammations of mucous membranes, especially those of the nose, throat, and the air passages. A cold with secretions—as a "running nose," for example—was popularly called a catarrh.

CATHARTICS, drugs or medicinal preparations that will relieve constipation and cause an evacuation of the bowels. Cathartics stimulate the muscular activity of the intestines and promote the flow of liquid to the bowels, thus flushing the alimentary canal. If the cathartic is especially strong, it is called a purgative. If it is mild, it is called a laxative.

Elimination of waste is a natural process, assisted by coarse foods, water, exercise, and laxative material in the diet such as fruit juices, vegetables, whole wheat, honey, and oatmeal. Most people can eliminate waste materials without artificial stimuli. The frequency of defecation—emptying the bowel—is not significant in most cases. If the use of cathartics appears to be frequently necessary a physician should be consulted. The habitual use of cathartics irritates the bowels, weakens their normal movement, and results in irregularity of elimination. The incidence of hemorrhoids, for example, is high among those who habitually use cathartics. In obesity, the prolonged use of cathartics is not only ineffectual but harmful.

Cathartics of any kind should never be taken when abdominal pain is present. This pain may be the first sign of a beginning appendicitis, and if an abdominal pain persists or appears to be exceedingly severe, medical treatment is imperative. When the appendix is inflamed, cathartics may increase the irritation and peritonitis may occur as a result.

In many cases, such inflammation of the membrane which lines the interior of the abdominal cavity is fatal.

Mineral oil and mineral oil modified with various substances are among the mildest of the cathartics currently used. Mineral oil is a lubricant which relieves constipation by mixing with the material in the bowel, softening it, and permitting easier passage along the intestinal tract. It is not fattening, as are other oils, because it is not absorbed by the bowels. The usual dose is one or two tablespoonfuls. Sometimes mineral oil is modified by the addition of agar, a form of seaweed, or by psyllium seed or other mucilaginous materials which swell when water is added and increase the bulk of waste material, thus preventing possible leakage of the oil from the anus, the excretory orifice of the body. However, too much mineral oil may interfere with the absorption of vitamin A. Mineral oil is also modified by the addition of strong laxative material like cascara and phenolphthalein. Cascara is a plant laxative made from the bark of a tree and is also available in the form of extracts and aromatic mixtures. Phenolphthalein is a laxative widely used as the basis of most advertised laxative remedies. This substance, which is a coal tar derivative, acts on the large intestine as a purgative. Some people are especially sensitive to phenolphthalein and in these cases its use will cause eruptions of the skin.

Other methods of relieving constipation are glycerin suppositories, enemas, and castor oil, an old household remedy. A tablespoon or two of milk of magnesia taken occasionally is considered a safe cathartic. Saline cathartics such as Epsom salt (magnesium sulfate), sodium sulfate, etc., are active cathartics, especially useful in inflammatory infections and as blood purifiers in cases of poisoning. *See also* CONSTIPATION; MEDICINE CHEST; and names of specific cathartics.

CATHETER, a flexible or rigid tube used to drain fluid from various cavities of the body, especially when the normal outlets do not function properly. The tube may be passed gently through the nose to the Eustachian tube which communicates with the ear, for example, or through the penis or vagina into the urethra which connects with the urinary bladder. A catheter should never be forced into or through any cavity.

Persons who use a catheter without professional assistance should remember that absolute cleanliness is essential. Before use, a catheter made of rubber or metal can be sterilized by being boiled in water for several minutes. If it is made of silk or some other material which could be damaged by boiling, it may be soaked in an antiseptic solution prescribed by the doctor. The hands of the person who passes the catheter should also be clean. When the catheter is to be passed through the urethra, the end of the penis or the outer surface of the vagina is ordinarily washed before the instrument is inserted. If difficulty is encountered in this process, an appropriate lubricant may be employed.

After use, the catheter should be thoroughly cleansed with soap and water. Grease may be removed with denatured alcohol. The catheter should be carefully dried and returned to a clean container. A worn catheter should be replaced.

CAUL AT BIRTH. Caul is a popular term for the sac in which the child lies during pregnancy. Part or all of this fetal membrane may be brought forth in labor, preceding the child. A caul at birth has sometimes been considered by superstitious people to be a sign of good luck.

CAUSALGIA, a sharp burning pain, sometimes a symptom of injuries of the nerves, particularly the sensory nerves supplying the palms and soles. The disturbance may be associated with many vasomotor, digestive, and dermal changes in the affected parts.

CAVITIES. *See* DENTAL CARIES.

CECUM, a portion of the bowel on the lower right side of the abdomen. It is the large blind pouch located at the junction of the large and small intestine. The appendix branches off the cecum.

CELIAC DISEASE, an ailment which affects children under five years of age, most frequently between the ages of two and three. In celiac disease, the child is unable to digest and utilize fats, starches, and sometimes sugars. Sensitivity to gluten from wheat or rye grains was recently established as the cause of this inability. The child becomes weak and undernourished, anemic, and his growth is stunted. Sometimes the stomach is swollen, as in starvation. Since the child is not well, he may be irritable, sullen, and behavior problems result as a consequence. Usually he has little appetite and even when obviously hungry will often refuse food. Conversely he may eat voraciously, with no gain in weight. Severe diarrhea is almost always the most telling symptom and stomach cramps may accompany it. Most of these symptoms are common to other conditions, and only a doctor can determine if celiac disease is the cause.

Celiac disease is ordinarily treated by a special diet. Fats, such as butter, cream, fried foods, and ice cream, and foods containing wheat or rye grains are excluded from the diet. Sugar tends to increase the amount of gas and to provoke diarrhea, and natural sugars, as are found in fresh fruits, are best tolerated. Protein foods can usually be eaten with no ill effect, and so milk protein, egg white, lean meat, fish, liver, and protein-rich vegetables constitute part of the diet. Of special benefit is a milk preparation which is high in protein but low in milk sugar and fat. For a time bananas were considered beneficial and banana diets were prescribed. However, now it is felt that any benefit derived from bananas is due to the fact that bananas replace gluten in the child's diet. Vitamin B complex supplements are also given.

CELL, a mass of protoplasm containing a nucleus; it constitutes the basic unit of life. *See also* BLOOD; BODY.

CELLULITIS usually refers to a diffuse inflammation of connective tissue. However, any inflammation of the cells of the body, at any point, can be called cellulitis. This disease may be caused by various bacilli, such as streptococci, staphylococci, or pneumococci.

CEREBRAL denotes anything that is related to the cerebrum, the chief portion of the brain. For example, the cerebral cortex, also called "gray matter," is the outer part of the cerebrum where most of the cell bodies are located. The cerebrum is divided by a deep groove into two cerebral hemispheres. These cerebral hemispheres are representative of approximately 70 per cent of the nervous system.

Illnesses associated with brain injuries are denoted by the addition of the word "cerebral," as, for example, cerebral dysrhythmia which is epilepsy, and cerebral palsy or paralysis due to hemorrhage. *See also* BRAIN.

CEREBRAL ARTERIOSCLEROSIS. *See* SENILITY.

CEREBRAL HEMORRHAGE. *See* APOPLEXY.

CEREBROSPINAL MENINGITIS. Meningitis, as such, is not a definite disease but an inflammation of the meninges, the membranes of the brain and the spinal column. The invasion of the cerebrospinal column by microorganisms such as pneumococcus, staphylococcus, or streptococcus is usually responsible, but various viruses also cause meningitis.

Cerebrospinal meningitis, also called spotted fever and cerebrospinal fever, is a sporadic or epidemic form of meningitis caused by a germ, the meningococcus. This disease is characterized by inflammation of the cerebrospinal meninges.

While the cause of cerebrospinal meningitis is not yet fully established, medical scientists believe that it is spread by contact with germ-laden droplets, produced by coughing and sneezing, from the nose and throat of infected carriers. The incidence of the disease, which most frequently affects children and adolescents, is highest in winter and early spring. In its epidemic form, cerebrospinal meningitis sometimes occurs in overcrowded, unsanitary surroundings. Epidemics in schools are much less frequent than generally believed.

The onset of cerebrospinal meningitis is sudden, and has many characteristics of the common cold, such as chills, headaches, and pains in the neck and limbs, often accompanied by vomiting and prostration. Stiff neck is one of the most characteristic symptoms of cerebral meningitis. It develops within thirty-six hours and renders movement of the head extremely painful. The victim ordinarily will be sensitive to noise and light, and his face may be either pale or cyanotic.

Fatalities from cerebrospinal meningitis have been greatly reduced by chemi- and bio-therapeutics, including sulfa drugs and penicillin. Thus, while still serious, it is no longer feared as it was in the past. The duration of cerebrospinal meningitis is variable, but recovery is now usually rapid. However, in some cases, consequences such as behavior changes, muscular weakness, and disturbances in vision and hearing may develop.

Anyone who suspects that he has come in contact with an infected person should be examined by a physician immediately so that sulfa and antibiotic treatment can be given, if necessary. *See also* MENINGITIS.

CEREBRAL PALSY, a long-term, nonfatal, neuromuscular disease of the central nervous system. It is usually caused by damage to the brain. Once injured, the brain does not heal without scar tissue and areas are destroyed and cannot function. Thus far cerebral palsy cannot be prevented or cured, but research in causes and prevention has progressed greatly, and much can now be done for the afflicted child if treatment and training are begun early.

The crippling that results from cerebral palsy is a physical complication, but its cause lies in the original brain damage, with different degrees of physical disability, impairment, and mental retardation. Spasms, lack of coordination, weakness, tremors, rigidity, and difficulty in seeing, hearing and speaking can be observed in the patient.

While cerebral palsy is not synonymous with mental deficiency, a large proportion of afflicted children, estimated at 50 to 70 per cent, are mentally retarded to some extent, and the disease is significant in an overall consideration of the problem of mental deficiency. The brain of the child with cerebral palsy may be damaged before birth or during infancy. Various factors may cause the brain damage, such as faulty brain-cell development of the child in the mother's womb, disorders such as kidney disease, convulsions in the mother, incompatibility of the Rh-blood factors of mother and child, or childhood infections with accompanying high temperatures.

Weight at birth seems to be involved in cerebral palsy incidence, because of more protracted and difficult labor. As older women generally have heavier babies and boys are frequently heavier at birth than girls, the disease occurs more frequently in male babies born to older mothers. The risks are particularly great during breech deliveries and in premature babies since the skull of a premature baby is so mobile that damage to the brain can easily occur. Since a greater number of premature babies now survive than formerly, the incidence of cerebral palsy is steadily increasing.

Treatment varies according to the cause and severity of the disease. In mild cases, the child may receive muscle training and other special treatment and live a relatively normal life. Braces are employed to support weak muscles and prevent their shortening. Training in muscular movements, relaxation, and speech therapy are also essential. Any treatment of cerebral palsy requires great patience and must be supplemented by common-sense management of individual cases. *See also* BIRTH INJURIES.

CEREBROSPINAL FLUID, a clear watery fluid, secreted by the capillary blood vessels in the small cavities of the brain. It is contained in the space between the arachnoid membrane, the middle of the three membranes covering the brain and spinal cord, and the pia mater, the vascular membrane enveloping them. The cerebrospinal fluid acts as a cushion for the brain and spinal cord, as well as a conveyer of the waste of metabolism.

CEREBRUM, the frontal and upper part of the brain, consisting of two hemispheres or separate halves. The nerve endings believed to control thought and judgment are centered here. In human beings this organ is by far the largest part of the entire brain. Because of its vital functions, the word "cerebrum" is often used as a synonym for the brain itself. This term should not be confused with cerebellum, the smaller rear portion of the brain which governs muscular movements. *See also* BRAIN.

CERVIX, the entrance or mouth of the womb. It is situated deep within the female sexual passageway and resembles a small hollow cylinder about two inches long and one inch wide. Following ejaculation by the male, the spermatozoa travel through the canal of the cervix into the uterus and Fallopian tubes, where fertilization may take place should an ovum be present. During pregnancy, this canal is tightly closed by a thick plug of mucus which prevents infection from entering the womb. At the beginning of labor, this plug is discharged as the "bloody show" which heralds the onset of labor in most women. During labor, the opening in the cervix, normally the width of a pencil, is gradually stretched to permit the child to pass through. This is known as dilation and is accompanied by the familiar labor pains. After delivery, the cervix quickly shrinks to its normal dimensions.

The cervix is one of the most significant tissues in a woman's body.

It may be affected by infections, inflammations, or cancer. Fortunately the physician is able to see this tiny organ clearly with the aid of a small instrument known as a speculum which separates the walls and tissues of the vagina. Early treatment of disorders of the cervix is always essential.

Infections of the glands within the cervix are especially common after childbirth. Symptoms include profuse irritating discharge from the vagina and occasionally oozing of blood, especially after sexual relations. These infections may be treated with vaginal creams and suppositories, by painless treatment in the doctor's office, or with douches of prescribed medications. Sometimes a badly infected cervix may require surgery or cauterization. Cauterization involves burning away infected tissue with chemicals or electrical current.

Raw areas, erosions, may occur after delivery, and cause oozing of blood and irritating discharge. Their treatment is similar to that of infections. Treatments should be continued until the cervical infection or erosion is completely cured, for malignancy may develop in later years unless infections are entirely eradicated.

Fleshy warts which often grow on the cervix and sometimes cause bleeding are best removed by simple surgical measures. Cysts on the cervix may provoke bleeding or watery discharge. Treatment varies and is usually performed in the doctor's office.

Cancer can occur on the cervix and constitutes one of the most common types of cancer affecting women, especially after forty. Symptoms vary from none at all to bloody or irritating discharge. To verify his diagnosis, the doctor will take a small bit of suspicious tissue from the cervix for examination under the microscope. Should cancer be present, treatment includes complete surgical removal of all the internal female structures, and often the use of x-ray and radium. Only the doctor can decide which combination is best. Results in early cases are excellent. For this reason, all women over thirty-five years of age should have an internal examination every six months. *See also* CANCER; and Chapter 17, "Cancer."

CESARIAN SECTION, the surgical operation by which childbirth is accomplished when normal delivery is either dangerous or impossible. Each year, approximately 150,000 births occur in this manner, comprising 4 per cent of all deliveries. The operation was done in early times, and received its name from a law in the days of the Caesars stating that all pregnant women dying before giving birth be so delivered in hopes of saving the unborn child. Tradition has it that Julius Caesar was delivered this way, but this is refuted by the fact that Caesar's mother lived years after his birth.

Formerly, because of uncontrollable hemorrhage and infection, the operation was extremely hazardous, but today, in skilled hands, the risk is about the same as that in simple appendectomy. The technique of Cesarian section consists of entering by incision the abdomen and uterus in which the child develops during pregnancy. Once a woman has had one Cesarian section, future pregnancies are usually delivered by this operation, but occasionally normal delivery is possible. *See also* PREGNANCY AND PRENATAL CARE.

CHAFING, the irritation which results when two delicate skin surfaces persistently rub against each other, or when a foreign substance rubs the skin. The skin becomes red and painful and is often raw and moist. Chafing occurs most frequently under the armpits, in the groin, between the buttocks, below the breasts, in the folds of the skin, and also between the fingers and toes where it may be mistaken for a finger infection. Such an irritated area is a fertile place for germs or fungi.

For simple chafing, the treatment may consist of drying the skin thoroughly after bathing and applying a suitable dusting powder, zinc ointment, or cold cream, or one of the newer protective ointments. Cleanliness is important. Primarily essential, however, is the removal of the irritant which originally produced the lesion. This may mean more carefully fitted shoes, a larger, looser garment, or possibly a loss of weight. Sometimes a flat gauze bag filled with talcum powder and placed between the rubbing surfaces is soothing. *See also* ECZEMA.

CHAGAS' DISEASE, (American trypanosomiasis), a tropical ailment found prominently in South and Central America. It is transferred to man by parasites, in the excretions of a blood-sucking bug which usually bites the human lips. In the human body these flagellate protozoans change into intracellular forms which infest the cells of the brain and heart, and therefore the symptoms of Chagas' disease resemble those of heart disease. Tissues are destroyed and the victim is incapacitated. A cure has not yet been found, and the fatality rate is high. Antibiotics have proved ineffective in Chagas' disease.

CHANCRE. The first visible symptom of syphilis is a sore, known as a chancre or hard chancre. The chancre usually develops from three to five weeks after exposure. It appears at the point where the spirochete has entered the body, which is ordinarily on the genital organs. Since it is possible, however, to contract syphilis without sexual contact, the chancre may occasionally appear in some other area, such as the mouth. If syphilis is treated in the primary, or chancre, stage, it can be cured with the use of antibiotics.

The term soft chancre, also known as chancroid, designates an inflammation of the genitals caused by an entirely different microorganism from that responsible for syphilis. The soft chancre, a yellow sore, discharging pus, appears a day or so after exposure. Unless the person is confined to his bed, so that his movements can be restricted to a minimum, the soft chancre may become an abscess. Swelling may also develop in the glands of the groin. Chancroid yields readily to treatment with proper hygiene and the use of antiseptics. Since syphilis may be involved, a physician should always be consulted. *See also* CHANCROID; SYPHILIS.

CHANCROID, a lesion in which the chancre, or sore, is soft, in contrast with the syphilitic chancre which is hard. It involves the genitalia and is usually of venereal origin. Chancroid was a fairly common disease in ancient Rome and is mentioned by several Roman historians. Early English writers sometimes referred to the disease, calling it the "groyne bump" or "Winchester goose," a name derived from the city of Winchester, where the disease was apparently widespread, and from the awkward gooselike walk of the victim.

The disease starts with an ache in the groin and inflamed glands. These swollen glands gradually gather into a painful poison-filled mass, called a bubo. Eventually the bubo bursts and the poison drains out. In many cases, the bubo remains open for weeks, and during this period the person may experience so much pain and discomfort that he is unable to walk.

Chancroid is a disease of uncleanliness, and is most common in dirty poverty-stricken areas where hygienic conditions are almost impossible to maintain. Its incidence is high in seaports and cities and towns with large transient populations.

Chancroid is caused by the streptobacillus of Ducrey and its incubation period is two to fourteen days after sexual intercourse. Treatment varies from washes and salves to caustics, electric cautery, and surgery. Sulfonamides are now an effective treatment, and antibiotics like streptomycin have also been successfully used.

CHAPPED SKIN, a roughened, reddened, irritable condition caused by loss of the natural oils in the skin. It occurs especially when the air is dry or when the skin is exposed to irritants such as cold hard water and harsh soap. Some persons are particularly susceptible to chapping because their skin glands do not respond to climate changes.

To prevent painful irritation of the skin, the use of soap and water during the winter months should be kept to a minimum. For personal use, mild oils may occasionally be used instead of soap and water, and fats in the skin replenished with cold creams, or lotions and creams, available in stores, which increase the moisture content of the skin. Rubber gloves or similar protective gloves may be used for household tasks.

The use of harsh soaps should be avoided. Hard water may be softened with washing soda or borax. A soft towel should be used to dry the hands; never a hot fire or an electric air drier. Lips, especially vulnerable to chapping because their sensitive surface is frequently moistened, may develop ugly painful breaks in the skin which are easily infected. A precautionary measure is to apply cold cream or petroleum jelly to the lips before going out into the cold. Chapped skin can be minimized if the home is properly heated, and overheat and excessive dryness avoided. A pan of water kept on the floor in each room will add moisture to the air through evaporation.

Despite all precautions, some chapping of the skin will occasionally occur. When this happens, the affected area should be protected from infection just as a wound is protected. Cracks in the skin may be treated with a mild ointment such as cold cream and then covered with clean gauze. If the irritation is prolonged, a physician should be consulted. *See also* CHILBLAINS; FROST-BITE; SKIN.

CHEMOTHERAPY, the prevention or treatment of certain infectious diseases by various chemical agents which act as antiseptics in the body or inhibit invading parasites without producing serious toxic effects on the patient.

CHEST, or thorax, starts just above a dome-shaped muscle called the diaphragm, ends at the shoulder blades, the clavicles, and is surrounded by a cage of flexible bones, the thoracic cage. This cage is formed by twelve pairs of flat bones, the ribs, which are attached to twelve pairs of spinal vertebrae in the rear. The ribs curve frontward, the first seven pairs connecting to the breastbone, the sternum, while each rib of the next three pairs is attached to the one immediately above by cartilage. The last two pairs of ribs are floating, or unattached, in front. In the chest cavity, slightly left of center, is the heart with blood vessels going to and from it, the lungs, the bronchi, bronchioles, and a section of the windpipe. The food pipe, the esophagus, which starts in the lower part of the neck, extends the entire length of the thorax, joining the stomach just below the diaphragm.

Breathing is controlled partly by the chest muscles but chiefly by the diaphragm. When the diaphragm lowers, the space in the chest

cavity increases. Pressure is consequently greater outside the thorax than inside, and air rushes into the lungs. This is inhalation. In effect, a partial vacuum is created by the movement of the diaphragm, so that when the diaphragm is raised, the space inside the thorax decreases. Pressure is then greater inside than outside, and gas and water vapor are pushed out of the lungs. This is exhalation. The diaphragm also separates the organs of the abdomen, such as the liver, pancreas, and duodenum, from the chest cavity. *See also* Chapter 15, "Respiratory Diseases."

CHICKENPOX, one of the most common as well as one of the most acute contagious diseases of childhood. It is characterized by a superficial eruption of flat transparent blisters which appear in successive crops on different parts of the body. Chickenpox develops most often in winter and spring, and the age group five to six is particularly susceptible. The condition is seldom seen in persons over twenty.

Chickenpox is caused by a virus, and is medically known as varicella because its rash resembles the rash in mild cases of smallpox, or variola. The infection is spread in the air, from the patient's nose, mouth, and blisters, and by contact. The contagious period is usually about fourteen days, starting about two days before the rash appears. One attack of chickenpox normally confers permanent imunity.

The infection usually begins with a slight fever, headache, listlessness, and loss of appetite. In a day or two, tiny red patches, about the size of a pinhead, appear on the back and chest. Within a few hours, blisters filled with clear liquid begin to develop in the center of the pocks, surrounded by a reddened area of skin, and continue to appear for three or four days. The rash may spread to the face, scalp, hands, and feet. The fluid turns yellow in a day or so, then a crust forms. The crust begins to peel off in the next five to twenty days. During this period, troublesome itching develops, and the chief difficulty is to restrain the child from scratching and incurring further infection.

Chickenpox is usually mild and does not require special treatment. If itching is severe, the doctor may prescribe a calamine lotion or some other drug to relieve it. The child's fingernails should be cut short, and the fingertips and nails scrubbed often and thoroughly with soap, water, and alcohol. As long as fever is present and new blisters continue to appear, the child should be kept in bed and isolated, especially if other young children who have not had the disease are in the house.

As with other virus diseases, body resistance is lowered, and the child should be protected against possible complications, especially secondary infection. The scabs should be kept clean and free from irritation, and should be allowed to loosen and fall off naturally. Forcible removal of crusts may leave permanent scars. Diet should be especially nourishing, to build up the body and encourage more rapid healing. *See also* Chapter 7, "The Process of Infectious Diseases and Immunization of Children."

CHIGGERS, the larvae, or young, of certain types of mites. Depending for survival on other organisms, they frequently attach themselves to the skin of human beings. Although they do not actually burrow under the surface, they do introduce into the skin a substance which produces severe itching. Red blotches develop on the skin and are soon followed by blisters.

Anyone who plans to enter a tropical or wooded area should protect himself against this pest by sprinkling flour of sulphur on his undergarments and stockings, or by rubbing sulphur foam on the skin. Leggings are also a useful protection against chiggers.

Those who encounter chiggers should wash the skin carefully with soap and water. This treatment is more effective if the lather is left on the skin about ten minutes. Thereafter one of the many anti-itch preparations can be applied. This treatment will lessen the discomfort from itching until the lesions have gradually healed.

CHILBLAINS, an inflammation of the skin and of the tissues under the skin caused by cold; appears most often on the toes, fingers, ears, or nose.

The initial inflammation is followed by a burning or itching sensation, after which the area ordinarily becomes swollen and dark red. This color, as well as the characteristic chilled feeling, is due to a reduced circulation of blood in the area.

Those susceptible to chilblains should take protective measures. Warm clothing and carefully fitted warm shoes and gloves should always be worn during the winter months. Regular and vigorous exercise, such as walking and skating, is also advisable. Vulnerable areas of the body should be briskly massaged every day to encourage circulation of the blood. Regular doses of cod liver oil, as well as a healthful diet, are helpful, and general good health should be maintained.

Treatment of chilblains often includes painting the inflamed areas with a tincture of iodine. Zinc ointment is also beneficial. If blisters form, every effort should be exerted to prevent them from bursting, since healing is likely to be slow because of the condition of the affected area. If they do break, a stimulating ointment should be applied. A lotion composed of hydrogen peroxide and warm water in equal parts is useful for washing the sores, especially if they are discharging pus. *See also* FROSTBITE.

CHILDBIRTH. *See* PREGNANCY AND PRENATAL CARE; and Chapter 6, "Prenatal Care and Childbirth."

CHILD CARE

Structure and Growth. The average infant weighs about seven pounds at birth, girls generally weighing about half a pound less than boys, and Negro babies often weighing more than white. It is not unusual or abnormal for a child to weigh eight or even ten pounds. Babies born weighing less than five and a half pounds are classified as premature, regardless of how long the pregnancy has lasted, and require special care. Most babies will double their birth weight at six months of age and triple it at a year.

Length at birth is generally between nineteen and twenty-one inches and by the end of the first year the baby will have grown an additional ten inches. The baby's head and chest circumference should be equal at birth. Thereafter, the head size grows rapidly, increasing two and a half inches in circumference by the end of the first year. The bones of the skull are soft at birth and often the skull is misshapen from the effect of labor and may be molded right after delivery. An odd-shaped head should not cause alarm; within a few weeks the skull will assume a normal contour. Since the bones of the baby's skull are soft and easily molded into an incorrect shape, the infant should not lie in one position too long during the first year. He should lie on the left side after one feeding, on the right side after another, and be encouraged to sleep on both stomach and back. Fontanelles, the two soft spots in the skull, are places where the skull bones have not yet fused. The spot toward the back of the head usually fills in by the fourth month, and the spot in the front by the eighteenth month. Special care of the spots is not necessary, but they should not be disturbed.

PROGRESS CHART

One year

Weight: boys 21.5 pounds; girls 20 pounds

Height: boys 29.5 inches, girls 29 inches

Teeth: six by end of the year

Speech: Babbling; may say three to five words.

Two years

Weight: boys 28.4 pounds; girls 27.8 pounds

Height: boys 33.1 inches; girls 32.7 inches

Teeth: sixteen

Speech: vocabulary of 100 to 500 words; two-word sentences.

Three years

Weight: boys 33.5 pounds; girls 31.5 pounds

Height: boys 36 inches; girls 35.6 inches

Teeth: twenty

Speech: 500 to 1500 words; uses pronouns.

Four years

Weight: boys 36.4 pounds; girls 35.1 pounds

Height: boys 38.6 inches; girls 38.4 inches

Teeth: twenty milk teeth

Speech: makes complete sentences; 500 words added.

Five years

Weight: boys 41.4 pounds; girls 40.2 pounds

Height: boys 41.7 inches; girls 41.3 inches

Speech: articulation nearly perfect; shows an interest in rhyming.

Six years

Weight: boys 45.1 pounds; girls 43.6 pounds

Height: boys 44 inches; girls 43.4 inches

Teeth: twenty-four, four of which are permanent

Speech: articulation perfect; inflection of nouns and verbs almost perfect.

Learning to walk. Some children will begin to creep about the seventh month, while others sometimes wait until as late as the tenth or eleventh month. By the end of the first year the child should easily be able to pull himself into the standing position and to walk holding on to something. Usually he can walk at about eleven months if someone holds his hand. Walking unaided usually starts at about twelve to sixteen months. Of course, some children progress faster than others, but about 40 per cent of children can walk at a year, and 67 per cent at fourteen months. Occasionally, if the child is fat or has been ill, he may not walk until the end of the second year. Sometimes a slippery floor or crowded play area, or ill-fitting shoes discourage the child from walking. Occasionally muscle disease, rickets, or nerve damage may be involved but this is rare. Parents should be patient with the child who is reluctant to start walking. Urging him to walk before he is ready can only make him insecure. Letting the child play with other toddlers will encourage him to imitate them and try to walk himself.

Seeing and Hearing. At birth, babies can distinguish between light and dark, but they are not able to fix their attention on any object until about two weeks of age when the eyes can focus on light. Usually, at four weeks, the child can look at something and at two months follow a moving object with his eyes. During the first few months, difficulty in focusing correctly the delicate eye muscles may cause the eyes to look crossed. Parents should not be alarmed since this difficulty normally disappears soon.

Babies recognize noises and voices soon after birth, but are unable to distinguish specific sounds for two or three months. An infant of two or three months enjoys listening to music and often will stop crying if the radio or phonograph is turned on softly.

Babies do not have a developed sense of taste as a rule and can usually distinguish only between sweet and sour foods.

The first six years. The most rapid growth period in a child's life is the first four months. At one month, the baby will look at a person near by, hold objects placed in his hand. His eyes can follow a moving object and he can hold his chin up when lying on his stomach. Whether or not the child really smiles, or just has a gas bubble in his stomach, is difficult to say, but at two months he definitely smiles when he sees his parents and persons who give him attention or when he feels contented. The two-month-old baby will coo, hold up his chest when prone, and turn his head away from bright lights. He turns toward a spoken voice and sometimes is frightened by loud noises.

At three months the baby can hold his head steady and may laugh. He can roll over, so it is not safe to leave him unprotected on an open bed. He gurgles and grasps objects. He may prefer his mother or whoever takes care of him to anyone else.

A four-month-old baby loves to study his hands, fingers, and objects around him. His attention is easily distracted by the world around him and feeding time may become a problem.

By five months, the child will sit propped, and recognize and be afraid of strangers. He will begin to scratch and to put toys in his mouth.

By the end of the sixth month, the child may sit briefly without support, reach for things he wants, and pound on furniture. He will probably love to watch himself in the mirror, and will stretch his arms to go to his parents or those he likes.

When he is seven to eight months, the baby will play peek-a-boo, pick up small objects, and often stand, if held. He may pull his mother's hair, and can wave good-bye.

In the last four months of the first year, the child will begin to recognize his own name and names of persons around him. He can open boxes, play with appropriate toys, walk alone or by holding on, notice other babies, and repeat simple words.

Speech is a significant means of testing development of the child. At the age of one year, a child can say a few simple words.

Dr. Arnold Gesell, child psychologist, states that at two years of age the child should be able to fold paper, name familiar objects such as keys, pennies, and watches, listen to stories, look at pictures, and attempt to describe his own experiences. He will ask for things by their own names and begin to make sentences of about two to three words.

According to the Stanford-Binet tests, at three years of age the child of average intelligence will be able to point out his mouth, nose, and eyes and repeat two numbers, but not consecutively. He will look at a picture and pick out four or five objects meaningful to him such as a boy, dog, tree, or car. Most children do these things quite easily, and failure to accomplish these simple tests may necessitate special training.

At four, the child should know his sex, and be able to name three familiar objects shown to him, such as a spoon, book, and pencil, and to repeat three nonconsecutive numbers.

At six, the child should know whether it is noon or evening, and to define the use of a fork, chair, knife, or table.

Crying. Physiologists recognize the value of crying for the new baby. Crying helps ventilate the baby's lungs, forcing out old air and replacing it with fresh air. The thrashing about of arms and legs associated with crying helps develop the body musculature. Also crying is the only way a baby can indicate his needs, whether it be food, sleep, a change of diapers or love, to those around him.

Most of the time a baby cries because he is uncomfortable, and parents should check for wet or soiled diapers or an open safety pin. The child may be too hot or cold. Often crying may indicate fear or anger. A new baby enjoys being in command and if he learns that he can control adults by crying he will continue to do so. Always be sure when the baby cries that he is comfortable, dry, and has had enough to eat.

Thumb sucking. Practically all babies, some more than others, suck their thumbs. In moderation, thumb sucking does not do any harm and interference with the eruption of teeth will ordinarily not happen unless the habit continues past two years of age. Thumb sucking may indicate that the child is hungry or unhappy. It frequently occurs among babies who are weaned too soon, thus depriving them of the pleasurable satisfying practice of sucking. Artificial devices to prevent thumb sucking, such as arm splints or bitter preparations on the thumb, should not be used. It is better to try to find out the reason why the baby sucks his thumb. He may need more love and security. His hand should not be pulled out of his mouth, and the parents should avoid appearing upset about the habit. Ordinarily the child will discontinue sucking his thumb before the habit is prolonged enough to harm him.

Bed wetting. Children usually learn bladder control during the daytime some time during the end of the second year. Nighttime control may not occur until the third or even fourth year, but ordinarily it is accomplished by the end of the third year. If persistent bed wetting continues beyond four years of age, consult the doctor.

Bed wetting may arise from emotional reasons, such as insecurity or jealousy of a new baby in the family. It can also occur if parents are too vigorous and rigid in insisting on early toilet training. Best results are obtained if the parents are understanding, patient, and do not push day or night toilet training and do not make a fuss about occasional accidents.

When the child is young, the bladder empties automatically, without any control from the brain. Gradually the brain becomes involved so that the child is able to control his urine when awake. Nighttime control does not require much help from parents and if they are patient the child will eventually discipline himself.

In helping the child to keep dry at night, the following points should be remembered. (1) Water, milk, or other fluids should not be given to him after 5 P.M., unless he insists on a small drink to quench thirst. If the child complains of thirst at bedtime, or to delay going to bed, he may be given a piece of apple or orange. (2) Some parents awaken the child at ten o'clock to permit him to empty his bladder. If the child does not wake easily or has trouble going back to sleep, this practice should be avoided. (3) Protect the bed with a rubber sheet or have the child wear two diapers at night. (4) The child should be taken to the bathroom when he awakens. (5) The evening meal should be somewhat dry, and milk as a beverage or on cereals or puddings omitted. However, milk is, of course, to be given regularly throughout the day and used in foods when possible.

Bowel control. Bowel control is easier to teach than bladder control. The following points will help the child learn to control his bowels. (1) Do not begin bowel training until the child can sit comfortably by himself, at about the age of eight or nine months, although some authorities suggest much later. (2) The child may be placed on the toilet two or three times during the day at about the time he usually moves his bowels.

This may be following meals and just before bedtime. (3) Soiled diapers should be promptly changed. (4) Do not leave the child on the toilet seat for more than a few minutes at a time, and do not permit the child to play with toys while on the seat. (5) Undue fuss should not be made over moving his bowels, or failing to do so.

Many mothers, because of excessive modesty, teach the child all sorts of tricks to indicate that he wishes to go to the toilet. Often strange gestures and queer words are used. The child should learn from the beginning the commonly accepted words used for this normal function.

Exercise. Babies need exercise as much as adults do, though often of a different kind. Kicking and moving about vigorously is really strenuous exercise for a baby and time should be allowed every day for unrestrained activity. All his clothes should be removed, the child placed on the bed or a thick blanket on the floor in a warm room and then permitted to kick and move about freely. Someone should play with the baby.

Exercise is essential in all stages of childhood, but violent play is to be avoided, especially just before eating. Be sure the child is dressed suitably for the temperature with clothing that is loose and unconfining.

Care should be taken in exercising the small baby not to push him into activity for which his body is not ready. The baby will indicate when his muscles are ready to perform such actions as sitting or standing. Playpens are good places for babies to learn to stand and move about without danger when they cannot be closely watched.

Bathing the baby. Many hospitals today hold baby care classes for parents, either before or after the birth of the child, which include instructions for bathing a baby. Most babies should not have a soap-and-water bath until the umbilical cord falls off. Until then their bodies are washed with cotton balls dipped in bland baby oil. The bath is given in a warm room with a temperature about 98°, and drafts guarded against. It should only take a few minutes, and afterward the baby should be dried thoroughly, but without vigorous rubbing, with an absorbent towel. If the child's skin is exceptionally delicate, a handful of table salt to a gallon of water helps to lessen irritation. As the child grows older, a warm bath just before bedtime may help promote more restful sleep.

All the bath equipment and change of clothing should be assembled before the child is undressed. The head and neck of the baby must be supported during his bath. It is neither necessary nor advisable to wash the baby's mouth or clean his ears and nasal passages with a cotton-tipped stick. Any discharge from these areas should be reported to the family doctor.

If the scalp develops a slight irritation, overactivity of the sweat and fat glands may cause caking or "cradle cap," a type of dermatitis. This caking is caused by a mixture of fat and secretion with layers of skin and dirt. Warm oil or petroleum jelly rubbed on the scalp, which helps to soften this condition, followed by a bland-soap shampoo will eradicate the difficulty.

After the bath, powder may be used but it is not essential. If used, care must be taken to keep the powder out of the child's reach, and not to spray it about since irritation in the lungs can be caused if too much powder is inhaled. The use of oil on the baby's body is also not necessary.

Breast feeding. The best possible food for the infant is its mother's milk, particularly during the earlier months of life. For unknown reasons, many women today are unsuccessful in nursing their babies, but fortunately many excellent substitutes are now commercially prepared which resemble mother's milk. The new mother should not feel disturbed or guilty if she is unable to nurse her baby.

Babies can derive benefit from breast feeding for about six months or even as long as nine months. When the baby cannot get at least half his food supply from his mother's breast, it is advisable to begin weaning. Most babies require weaning by the fourth to sixth month.

All mothers should make every effort to breast feed their babies, since breast-fed infants have a much lower incidence of infection, and seem to develop a little faster. In only rare instances does the milk of the mother fail to agree with the child. Occasionally diarrhea occurs if some element in the mother's diet disagrees with the child, but this can easily be detected and corrected in most cases.

Diet for nursing mothers. A common belief persists that a mother who wants to produce sufficient good rich milk for her baby should eat plentifully, drink excessive amounts of milk, cocoa, or even beer. This is not true; many women who have done this have become unpleasantly fat, disgusted with nursing, and inclined to discontinue. Actually the diet for a nursing mother is little different from that of any healthy adult woman, with about an extra quart of fluid, half of which is whole milk, each day. The diet should be about 2500 to 3000 calories, which usually does not lead to any increase in the mother's weight. The nursing mother should avoid taking substances such as strong laxatives which deplete her body's fluid resources, or stimulate the kidneys, such as excessive amounts of coffee or tea.

The theory that a nursing mother should avoid gassy or sour foods such as cabbage, salads, and raw fruits is also without foundation, unless, of course, she herself is allergic to a particular food. Fried foods may be eaten when a woman is nursing, but it is best to avoid chocolate since many people are sensitive to it. The best flow of milk results from regular nursing of the baby because the sucking action actually stimulates the formation of milk in the mother.

The diet of the nursing mother should contain about one quart of milk each day, some butter, four eggs a week, two green vegetables daily, and fresh fruit every morning, particularly oranges or tomatoes which are rich in vitamin C. Butter provides vitamins A and D; to provide a full supply of these vitamins the mother may take cod liver oil as directed by her doctor. The milk drunk daily may be whole, or nonfat

dry milk if she is overweight. If she doesn't wish to drink milk, it may be used in food such as ice cream, custards, or cocoa drinks.

Mothers often worry about taking medicine, fearing that it will appear in the breast milk and harm the baby. Actually few drugs will do this, but if in doubt consult the doctor.

Secretion of milk begins a few days after the baby is born. In some cases, the breasts may leak fluid during the last few weeks of pregnancy. During the first few days, the flow is usually scanty but becomes more profuse by the end of the first week if nursing is frequent and the child is hungry enough so that he sucks vigorously. The first secretion of milk is actually not milk, but a cheesy protein-rich substance known as colostrum which appears about the third day and is nourishing for the baby. Later the true milk begins and is pale bluish white in color, resembling skim milk. This color is normal and does not mean that the milk is weak.

By the end of the first week, the average mother should have no difficulty secreting a pint of milk daily. This gradually increases and by the sixth month she is producing a quart of milk daily. The amount produced usually parallels the demands of the baby. Complete emptying of the breasts at nursing time is desirable to encourage good milk production. Nursing from both breasts at each feeding is recommended until maximum production is established. Then alternate the breasts to avoid overproduction.

Mature milk which is secreted by the mother after the first month is about 87.5 per cent water, 1.25 per cent protein, 7.5 per cent sugar, and 3.5 per cent fat. Breast milk is considerably sweeter than cow's milk, though somewhat lower in protein. It is also much more digestible and breast-fed babies are less apt to regurgitate or have gastrointestinal upsets. Through the mother's milk they also receive protective antibodies against disease which are not found in cow's milk. If the mother's diet is insufficient, the milk will be poor in quality. Vitamins should be taken by the nursing mother to enrich the milk.

Smoking does not affect the milk, and alcohol may be taken in moderation while the mother is nursing since it does not pass into the milk except in small amounts.

Hygiene during nursing. The nursing mother should keep in good physical condition and eat properly, and allow for a good night's sleep with a rest period in the midafternoon and, if possible, before nursing periods. Worry and overfatigue are to be avoided.

The size of the breasts does not seem to be linked to supply of milk and women with smaller breasts often produce the most milk. Determining in advance whether or not a mother will be able to nurse her baby is not possible. Certain women should not nurse, however. These include those women who are not in good health, those who have active tuberculosis or other infections, those who have had arduous labors, and those who have previously had tumors of the breast or breast infection. If the breasts become infected while nursing, it should be discontinued.

Premature babies thrive on mother's milk, but often their sucking power does not permit nursing. In some hospitals the mother's milk is drawn off by a breast pump and then fed to the baby with an eye dropper or small tube until it is strong enough to nurse by itself.

If the baby begins vomiting or fails to gain weight, the mother probably should stop nursing. However, she should consult the doctor first. Failure to nurse one child need not imply that future attempts will be unsuccessful.

Frequency of feeding. Babies are usually given their first feeding about twelve to twenty-four hours after birth. The feeding is started at about four-hour intervals. If the mother does not have milk, sugar-and-water solutions may be fed to the baby.

Although opinion as to how often to feed the baby varies, most doctors seem to favor a three- or four-hour schedule. During the first few days it may be necessary to nurse the baby more often but the interval should not be less than two hours. In short time, most babies seem to wish to be fed every four hours and by the sixth week sleep through the night and do not wake up to be fed. Babies should never be awakened just to feed them unless their sleep pattern becomes set in such a way that the entire household is upset. One theory favors letting the baby get hungry before feeding him, since usually he will not only nurse more vigorously but also take more at each feeding. Generally, after being fed, the baby will sleep for several hours. When he awakens he may be wet or need to expel gas and cry, which does not necessarily mean that he has not received enough to eat.

Nursing should take place in a quiet surrounding. The mother should lie down on her bed or sit in another comfortable position during the feeding. Prolonged nursing is not desirable and may lead to irritation of the nipples and not more than ten or fifteen minutes should be allowed for nursing. Studies show that the food obtained after the first six to eight minutes is hardly sufficient to be significant. Breast-fed babies develop strong sucking powers and can empty the breast rapidly. Mothers should be sure to "burp" the baby about halfway through the feeding. Once the baby is on a regular feeding schedule, it is desirable to try to maintain it, except in unusual cases.

Overfeeding and underfeeding. If and does not rest or sleep, the the baby seems fretful after nursing mother's milk may be insufficient. In such cases, the doctor will prescribe a supplementary formula to be given after the regular nursing period.

Most babies stop nursing when they have had enough and seldom does a nursing baby overfeed. Occasionally, however, a baby getting too much milk too fast may vomit or regurgitate, or have an upset stomach afterward, but this is rare. If it does occur, the nursing time should be shortened.

It is not advisable to weigh the baby before and after the feeding to see how much milk he gets; this is not only bothersome but may also disturb the mother unnecessarily. The behavior of the baby after the feeding is the best indication of whether or not he has received the proper amount. After nursing, hold the baby for a few minutes until he is ready to sleep. If he sleeps satisfactorily for two or three hours, he has had enough to eat.

Cow's milk. Generally the formula for babies is based on cow's milk, which should be pasteurized to remove harmful bacteria and purchased from a reliable dairy or market. In country homes where milk is obtained directly from cows, the milk must be boiled immediately after being drawn, then strained through cheesecloth into thoroughly boiled and sterilized bottles, cooled promptly, and placed in the refrigerator. In cities, these precautions are not necessary since milk is produced and pasteurized under the supervision of a health department. Heating milk does not remove any nutritional factors but does kill bacteria which may cause infections with streptococci or transmit tuberculosis, typhoid, diphtheria, or scarlet fever. Heating also helps to increase the digestibility of cow's milk. Because the vitamin C in the milk, essential to the child, may be destroyed by heating, it is customary to begin giving the child diluted orange juice or vitamin drops at two weeks of age.

Directions for feeding a baby with cow's milk should be obtained from the doctor. Cow's milk varies in composition from human milk, but in the formula must simulate breast milk. Ordinarily the baby cannot digest plain cow's milk until he is six months old and should receive it only upon suggestion and supervision of the doctor.

Preparing the baby's formula.

When preparing the formula, all equipment needed should be washed thoroughly and boiled daily. The top of the bottle or can containing the milk must be washed with hot water and soap and rinsed thoroughly. Mix and measure the ingredients in sterilized containers, wash and boil the bottles to contain the formula, and close with sterilized rubber nipples. Individual bottles for each feeding are preferable to one large bottle from which the milk is measured. To provide for accidents, such as breakage or contamination, make one extra bottle. It is usually easier to make the whole day's supply in advance, preferably in the morning. After the feedings are prepared, the formula should be placed in the refrigerator. Nipples should be made of thin rubber, washed and boiled daily, and rinsed after use to extend their life.

Before feeding the baby, the mother should wash her hands well with soap and water. The bottle can be warmed by placing it in a pan of water on the stove. To test the temperature, shake a drop or two of the formula on the inside of the wrist. It is best to let a spray of milk run out until the drops fall one by one. In some cases, the holes in the nipple may need to be enlarged, which can be done by heating a pin over a flame and plunging it into the top of the nipple.

Cleanliness in the care of the baby's feedings is essential when he is young to protect him against serious infection. Sterilization is not essential after six to nine months, but the equipment should continue to be carefully cleaned before use.

Changes in the formula should be made only on the advice of the doctor because the baby's stomach and digestive system are extremely sensitive. If the baby seems healthy and continues to gain weight, there is ordinarily no need to change the formula. If he fails to gain weight, or if diarrhea or constipation occurs, the doctor may prescribe a new formula with an increase or decrease or adding or elimination of some ingredient.

A baby's weight gain is not always continuous. If he drinks greedily and rapidly, cries for more, or gets fretful long before feeding time, he probably needs more food. But the baby may be crying for other reasons and the mother should be sure that underfeeding is the reason before increasing his food, or overweight may occur. At one time, fat babies were considered the healthiest babies but this idea has been disproved and in fact the opposite may be true. The baby should never be deliberately overfed. He can handle so much food a day and beyond his limit will become upset and nauseated.

Water requirements. In relation to his weight, an infant needs about three times more water than an adult. His output of heat is greater and his body metabolism requires more water. Therefore, he occasionally ought to receive a bottle of lukewarm water. In winter, especially in dry apartments, he may awake fretful, with a dry throat, and need a few swallows of water to quench his thirst. The total fluid intake, including milk, water, and juice, of a growing baby should be about three ounces per pound of his weight, and a little more in hot or dry climates.

Feeding with spoon and cup. Food or a few drops of juice or formula on a spoon may be given to the infant when he is just a few weeks old. This will prepare him to use a spoon for solids later. At first he may appear to spit out the food because he cannot control his tongue. To prepare the baby for drinking from a cup, let him sip his daily orange juice from a small glass. Some babies do this easily, others find it difficult. By the sixth to ninth month, many babies can drink successfully from a cup. If, during the first few attempts, the baby shows any reluctance to drink from a cup, further attempts should be discontinued for a few weeks. Even if he cannot drink from a cup by one year, the parents should not be alarmed. He will learn to do this by imitating those around him, and forcing will only disturb him.

Solid foods. At the end of the first month, most babies can begin to take solid foods mixed with formula or water. The baby may begin with bran, rice, or oat cereal; avoid cereals containing wheat until he is nine months old. The foods should be given in small amounts, thinned with formula or water so that the baby can swallow them more easily. After the cereals are well established in his diet, vegetables are tried one by one, carrots, peas and string beans first. It is usually cheaper and more convenient to purchase the vegetables already cooked and strained and ready to eat after a slight warming. At three months, the baby can begin to eat fruit; at four to five months, meat. When the baby is seven or eight months old, if he has teeth, he may begin on the junior foods, which are coarser and must be chewed slightly. They should not be given until the baby's teeth appear and he is able to eat the food without fuss. A new food should be introduced in a small amount, only a teaspoonful, and then increased according to the baby's appetite. A boiled potato may be given when the child is seven months old; crackers, zwieback, dried bread or toast added when the teeth appear. Substances eaten by the baby may appear in the bowel movements, and this should not cause alarm. By ten or eleven months, the baby may eat many of the easily digested foods that the rest of the family are served, if they are cut up or chopped.

Schedule for the one-year-old child. When the child is a year old, he will be eating approximately as follows.

Upon arising, he should have from 7 to 8 ounces of milk. About 8:30 he receives breakfast of cereal, fruit and, if the doctor recommends it, egg yolk.

At noon, the baby should have 4 to 6 ounces of vegetable or meat broth, or one egg, or as a third possibility some scraped or chopped meat. To this may be added some white vegetables, such as 2 tablespoons of potato or rice, and from 2 to 4 tablespoons of a green vegetable, such as string beans, peas, or spinach. He may also drink more milk.

In the evening, around six, he should have cereal and milk, and also a cracker or small piece of toast, and 1 or 2 tablespoons of cooked fruit, which has a slight laxative quality.

Babies thrive best on a strict daily schedule. Occasionally exceptions must and should be made in his daily routine, but they should be kept to a minimum.

Self-feeding. At the end of the first year, babies ordinarily show an interest in self-feeding and can pick up pieces of carrot, potato, or toast. Actual self-feeding should be accomplished by the end of the second year. Rarely is there need to feed a child after this time. The child should eat a variety of foods at mealtime, and the mother see to it that the diet is well-balanced and the food attractively prepared. The child should drink water several times between meals, but soft drinks and candies should be avoided.

Most pediatricians recommend that food be given at regular intervals, and removed if not eaten in a reasonable time, about twenty minutes, and the child not given more food until the next regular meal. Coaxing the child to eat does little good and should be avoided.

Cleanliness. The child should have a complete bath at least twice a week after the first year and preferably one every day, before bedtime. Washing the hands should be encouraged during the second year. The child, if he plays as he should, is likely to get dirty and disheveled. The mother should not badger the child to remain clean, although it is wise if the mother teaches the child to clean up following play and meals.

The young child's hair should be shampooed about every three or four days, according to the season, and oils need not be used afterward.

Cleanliness will become more habitual if it is made easy—the soap and washstand within easy reach, the mirror low enough for the child to see himself, and the towel readily available. This does not mean that child-size bathrooms are necessary, but perhaps it might require a steady firm stool or box on which the child can stand. It helps the child if one of his parents washes or brushes his teeth at the same time as the child, since children love to imitate and learn best this way.

Feeding the older child. At one year of age, the child will probably be able to eat some of the foods that the family is eating, unless he has an allergy to one of them or does not have enough teeth to chew his food well. Eggs should be taken easily in all forms by one year. While egg yolk is started at six months, egg white should not be given until the end of the first year.

Cod liver oil. In the United States, cod liver oil or vitamin compounds in liquid form are practically universally given to children daily. Cod liver oil contains large amounts of vitamins A and D, which prevent or help cure rickets. In rickets, softening of the bones occurs due to failure of the body to use properly the mineral substances calcium and phosphorus. Vitamin D is the essential material involved in utilization of these minerals and so should be added to the diet in plain or mint-flavored cod liver oil, or through other vitamin preparations. Vitamin D is created by the body from exposure to sunshine in the summer, so most children do not need supplements at that time; but they are essential in the winter. At one time 50 to 80 per cent of children developed rickets; their bones did not grow properly and their muscles were flabby. Now milk is often fortified with vitamin D and additional vitamins are also given. Cod liver oil in straight form is also prescribed by some doctors.

Sleep for the baby. Newborn babies with good digestion and good appetite, plus proper foods, will usually sleep about nine-tenths of the time. Gradually they require less sleep, so that by the age of six months they sleep only about fifteen hours a day; from then until they are six, about twelve hours; from seven to ten years, eleven hours a day; from eleven to fourteen years, ten hours a day. Nine hours of sleep are needed by older teen-agers. Up to six years, a child should also have a nap during the day, lasting from 45 minutes to an hour and a half.

A baby should sleep in a room that is darkened and away from routine household noises. Hunger, pain, sudden noises, flashes of light, and sudden changes in temperature will awaken a small baby. The child will sleep soundly if he is warm, but not overly warm, well fed, and in a quiet darkened room. A baby often tends to wake up at a slight sound, and so the mother should not rush into his room every time he whimpers, even at night.

A baby should be put to bed at a reasonably early hour, usually around six o'clock, and not kept up late, unless for a good reason. Frequently an overtired child has difficulty going to sleep and will be cranky and irritable the following day.

The mattress on which a baby sleeps should be firm, but soft enough to be comfortable. The child should be lightly covered and his room comfortably warm, but not hot. In good weather, the window may be open enough to permit fresh air to circulate freely. Pillows are not necessary until the third year.

In nice weather, naps may be taken out-of-doors as early as two weeks of age; in winter, not until six weeks. If it is inconvenient to put the baby outside, he can be placed in his carriage next to an open window, with the door of the room shut to avoid draft. In cold weather, cold cream applied to the baby's face will protect its delicate skin.

Clothing. Most mothers dress the baby too warmly, and as a result the child perspires excessively and may kick off his covers and then become chilled. There has been much discussion whether or not a baby should wear cotton, wool, silk, rayon, or mixtures of these fabrics. Cotton is usually not warm, since it carries off heat rapidly. However, it can be easily boiled or sterilized and is useful for diapers and summer clothes.

Because it conducts heat poorly, wool is a warm material, but it is somewhat irritating to the skin and is often difficult to launder. Wool must be washed with lukewarm water and mild soap since boiling or hot water and strong soap harden and otherwise harm its fibers.

Silk is not a warm material and some babies are sensitive to it. Rayon, too, is not particularly warm and must be washed with some care.

Sleeping bags. The sleeping bag is very useful for the baby. Correctly sized and constructed, it is loose enough to permit plenty of motion and warm enough to prevent loss of heat. Also, it cannot be kicked off during sleep. Care must be taken that the sleeping bag fits loosely, particularly around the wrists and neck, and that it is long enough to permit the baby to stretch. Materials used may be sheeting, canton flannel, French flannel, or light blanketing, the choice depending upon the season.

Protective pants. Protective pants, made of various materials such as rubber, plastic, and rubberized silk, are a great convenience. To avoid skin irritation, they should be replaced by dry ones when the baby's diaper is changed. Washing immediately prolongs the life of the pants. If the child has irritated buttocks, avoid continuous use of the pants. They should fit loosely around the legs and waist. The pants themselves do not cause irritation; nevertheless, they retain both the heat given off by the body and the urine, which may produce irritation. Protective pants save time and money by cutting down on the amount of diaper changes necessary; however, the mother must be careful not to leave them on too long without changing the diaper.

Care of the baby in hot weather. In summer, babies require more fluids and should be offered plenty of water to drink. The need for solids diminishes and the baby may seem less hungry. Since fats produce heat, the baby's diet should contain less fat than during the winter.

In hot weather, if the baby vomits or has loose stools, all food must be stopped immediately and boiled skimmed milk substituted for the formula. If the symptoms cease, the formula may be given again in weakened amounts until full strength is attained. When older children have stomach upsets, fluids—juices, weak tea, skimmed milk, clear soup—only are to be given.

During the summer, a baby can be clothed in very thin cotton underclothes and diapers. He will need more clothing early in the morning and late in the afternoon. A cotton sunsuit is sufficient clothing for a hot day. The baby's clothing should be a little lighter in hot weather than an adult's.

If the baby's skin is moist in hot weather, he is probably wearing too many clothes; and if his lips, fingers, and toes are cold, he needs more clothing.

Frequent baths are comforting to the baby in hot weather. The bath water should be tepid, not cold. One teaspoonful of baking soda to a pint of water soothes and helps cool the skin. After the bath, the baby may be powdered lightly. Cornstarch is as good as any other powder.

Exposure to sun. Moderate exposure to the sun is not dangerous to the baby's eyes or skin. In summer, the baby may take a nap in the sunlight in the morning or late in the afternoon, avoiding the extreme of heat at midday. Exposure to sun should be gradual, beginning with just a few minutes and increasing to about half an hour in direct exposure. A child may become ill or sunburned if exposure to sun is excessive. Various lotions are available which help to prevent an excessive reaction to the sun.

Traveling with the baby. Travel is not recommended or desirable for a very young baby. But short trips are often possible when the baby is slightly older and, if adequately planned in advance, can be done with a minimum of difficulty.

Car beds are obtainable and can be placed in the back seat of an automobile or taken on a train, bus, plane, or ship. They provide a comfortable resting or sleeping place for the baby. Extra diapers, fresh water, and canned formula or evaporated milk should be taken along in case of emergency. Refrigeration for the baby's formula bottles is sometimes possible on trains and other public transportation. If refrigeration is not available, a thermos bottle is a handy container for juice, formula, and other drinks for the baby, or an ice container may be used to keep the drinks cold.

Travel will be less taxing for the mother and child if it is done at a time when the roads or the transportation system is least congested.

The child's teeth. Development of teeth differs among children, as do the time of eruption and the reaction to teething. Even very healthy children may become fretful, sleep poorly, and refuse meals during teething periods. Teething often causes drooling of saliva, and looseness of bowels and slight fever. The doctor should be consulted; he may prescribe some medication to ease the baby over the teething period. Eruption of the child's teeth usually proceeds as follows: the two central lower teeth during the sixth to ninth month; the four upper central teeth during the eighth to twelfth month;

the other two lower central teeth and the four front double teeth during the twelfth to eighteenth month. Altogether twenty teeth are in the first set. Most children have six by the end of the first year, although it is not unusual for a child not to have any teeth the first year. The rest of the teeth come between the eighteenth and twenty-fourth month, except the four back double teeth, which usually appear between the twenty-fourth and thirtieth month, but may come even later.

Because the teeth begin to form before the child is born, the pregnant woman's diet should be nutritionally adequate, including sufficient vitamins, minerals, especially calcium which is found in milk, and fresh vegetables, eggs, cooked fruits, cereals. Calcium supplements are often recommended.

To build healthy teeth, adequate food materials are essential in the child's diet, especially calcium and phosphorus, and the vitamins A, C, and D. The diet should include a sufficient quantity of milk each day, or its equivalent in butter or cheese, and eggs, leafy green vegetables, and fresh fruit. For growing babies, the diet is often supplemented by cod liver oil. Milk and cheese are the best source of calcium. Foods rich in vitamin A are eggs, butter, carrots, and other vegetables. Vitamin C is abundant in citrus fruits, and D is found in fortified milk, in cod liver oil, and in most vitamin preparations.

Many physicians feel that coarse foods strengthen the jaws and help to harden the gums. When a new tooth is coming in, coarse foods serve as a resistance against which the gums may work to permit the teeth to cut their way through. Heredity is also significant in determining the type and quality of the child's teeth.

Special mouth care is not essential during the first two years. Some time in the beginning of the third year the child may be shown how to use a toothbrush by having him imitate the actions of the older person. During his third year the child should see a dentist, who will note any difficulties and plan for future care.

The sick child. Since children are not as articulate in drawing attention to their needs as adults, most mothers soon learn how to detect the first signs of illness. The child who is listless, drowsy for no apparent reason, flushed, and breathing with difficulty is obviously in need of medical attention. A child who looks and acts well and has plenty of energy probably is well. The child should get regular checkups at frequent intervals during the first two years, and after that twice a year. Most communities have public health services where a child may receive a checkup without charge if a private pediatrician cannot be consulted. Medicine should never be given to a child unless ordered by a physician. Unused portions of medicine should always be destroyed after the illness for which they were prescribed has been cured. If, months after an illness, the child develops what seems to be the "same" condition, under no circumstances should he be given the original prescription unless ordered by a doctor.

The child in the hospital. If a child must be hospitalized, for an operation or a protracted stay, there are a number of things to know and to be done which can help the child through the experience. The child should be intelligently prepared for his stay in the hospital. Confidence in the doctors and nurses should be established by suitable explanations; visits to the child planned as periods of happiness rather than of worry. The child will reflect his parents' attitudes so it is important that they appear hopeful, confident, and encouraging throughout the entire experience. The homecoming should also be carefully planned.

Prevention of infection. Some diseases can be prevented by inoculation or vaccination, including smallpox, diphtheria, whooping cough, scarlet fever, measles, typhoid fever, tetanus, and poliomyelitis.

Although smallpox is rare nowadays, every child should be vaccinated against it, and in most parts of the country this is mandatory before the child can be admitted to school. The child may be vaccinated when he is from three to six months of age. Ordinarily vaccination is not done during the summer months, and it should be postponed if the child is not well or if other children in the family have infectious diseases.

Vaccination is best performed on the outer side of the upper arm. Although many parents of baby girls demand vaccination on the thigh, this is not always a safe technique because of difficulty in keeping the area clean and free of infection.

Usually, after a week, a small pimple forms at the site of the vaccination and in a few days the area around the vaccination may swell and become black and blue. This is the normal process of a vaccination and should not cause alarm. The vaccination must be kept dry until the crust falls off. To prevent scratching the area, the child may wear a long-sleeved shirt day and night. Occasionally the vaccination will not "take," and must be repeated. Smallpox vaccination is usually repeated at age six, just before the child enters school, and again at the age of twelve.

For protection against diphtheria, toxoid is given in three doses, once a month, starting at the age of three months. Booster injections should be given at eighteen months and again at the age of three or four. Whooping cough vaccination is usually given at the same time.

Polio vaccination should be given when the child is six months old, repeated two weeks to a month later and again in about six months. Inoculations against other illnesses, such as measles, scarlet fever, and typhoid fever, can be given as the need arises according to the physician's judgment of the individual case.

Hygiene for the sick child. If the child has an infectious disease, all unnecessary draperies, carpets, pictures, and other articles such as books and toys should be removed from the sickroom before the child is put into it. Occasionally, in a serious illness, objects with which the child has been in contact must be destroyed. Hardwood or metal pieces of furniture are preferable for the sickroom rather than stuffed furniture, because they are easier to clean. When possible, the child's room should be near the bathroom to lessen the amount of work.

The person who cares for a child with an infectious disease should wear a washable smock over her clothing. She should also wear a cloth mask and wash her hands thoroughly after leaving the child.

A large paper bag is useful at the side of the sick child's bed. In this can be placed soiled towels, used gauze, cotton, and other sickroom items. The entire bag and its contents can then be conveniently disposed of daily. If the infection is contagious, it is best to burn the waste.

The sick child should be dressed in a loose-fitting, easily washable garment and the room should be well ventilated, although free from unusually cold drafts. Bathing the sick child is preferably done by a careful sponge bath rather than immersion in a tub. After the sponge bath, the child may receive an alcohol rub, or, if he is too young for this, talcum or cornstarch may be patted over his body. If the child has much fever, cold cream or petroleum jelly applied to the lips helps to overcome dryness and crusting.

Fever. A fever usually indicates that the child is ill, although occasionally a slight variation in temperature is not a sign of illness. Every parent should know how to read a thermometer and both rectal and oral thermometers should be on hand in the medicine chest. A small child's temperature is best taken with a rectal thermometer. The normal range is between 99° and 100° when taken rectally (usually one degree higher than an oral temperature). To be certain of a correct reading, the thermometer must be shaken down well and left in position for three to five minutes. After use, it should be washed in lukewarm, not hot, water, rinsed with alcohol if possible, dried, and put away in a safe place.

A variety of disorders may cause elevations of temperature in children. Simplest and most common is the ordinary cold, which may give a high temperature. A sore throat, stomach upset, or infection will cause fever, as will the onset of the common childhood diseases, scarlet fever, measles, whooping cough, or chicken-pox. When the temperature is above normal, the doctor should be consulted and no home treatment, such as laxatives or enemas, should be given until they are prescribed.

Many feverish babies feel better after a sponge bath with lukewarm water. Ice-cold rub-downs or alcohol should not be given to babies under two years of age. Occasionally the doctor may order a cool-water enema for a high temperature, or prescribe a small dose of aspirin. These treatments are soothing, but usually do not cure the cause of the rise in temperature. The doctor should always be consulted about what to feed the sick child. In most instances a poor appetite follows a high temperature and parents should not force the child to eat. Fluids may be encouraged, but solids are to be avoided during the first few days of the illness.

The common cold. The most frequent illness in babies is the common cold. It is usually not serious, even when the temperature is elevated, but because of the danger of the cold's developing complications such as pneumonia, bronchitis, or ear infection, the doctor should be called promptly. The best way to avoid contracting colds is to avoid exposure to persons with colds. Other factors, such as chilling, poor nutrition, and fatigue are probably also significant in making the child more prone to the cold. The child with a cold is more comfortable in a moist environment. This does not mean a damp room, but rather a properly humidified room.

Enlarged tonsils and adenoids seem to make children more susceptible to sore throat. If the tonsils are found to be infected, the doctor should decide whether or not they should be removed.

Babies may have tub baths in winter, but the room in which it is given should be warm and free from drafts. A brisk, gentle rub-down afterward is also helpful. Preferably the bath is given at night, just before the baby goes to bed.

Use of vaccines to prevent colds is as yet not established as effective. Nose drops may be prescribed to clear the nasal passages and permit easier respiration. At the first sign of a cold with nasal drip, cough, or rise of temperature, the child should be put to bed, and his food intake lessened. If the child runs a fever, of more than 102°, the doctor should be called.

Hernia. Frequently a child is born with a weak spot in the muscles of the belly wall or groin. This condition is commonly known as a rupture or hernia. Swelling is caused when the intestines or other tissues are pushed through the weak spot in the wall. Often the spot appears around the navel in newborn babies.

When the child coughs, cries, or strains, the rupture is seen more easily because of the increased pressure within the abdominal cavity. Usually the lump disappears on lying down. Operation is not immediately necessary in these instances and often the doctor may just tape the navel hernia for a few months in the hope that scar tissue will seal over the defect. Hernias in the groin are less likely to disappear without surgery.

Tonsils and adenoids. Apparently tonsils serve to take care of infectious germs. The tonsils frequently become inflamed, swollen, and infected in children, and may cause pain on swallowing, earache, difficulty in hearing, breathing, or talking, and high temperature. The organism which causes most tonsillitis, the streptococcus, is similar to the organism that leads to rheumatic fever, erysipelas, scarlet fever, and other disorders. Penicillin is effective in curing tonsillitis in most cases and removal is not always necessary unless sore throats are particularly recurrent or resistant to penicillin, or the tonsils are enlarged.

The child with tonsillitis should remain in bed. If he is able to gargle, salt water will help to shrink the throat tissues. An ice collar and aspirin may give relief of pain. The doctor may use injections of penicillin or pills to help cure the infection, or he may prescribe other medicines such as Terramycin, Achromycin, or one of the other antibiotics. These drugs must never be administered without a doctor's orders. Because of the serious nature of complications from neglected tonsillitis, the doctor should be consulted if the parents suspect the child has a sore throat.

The adenoids lie in the cavity behind the nose. Like the tonsils, they are prone to infections. When they are enlarged or infected, breathing and talking is difficult and the child's voice has a nasal twang. Typically he keeps his mouth open at all times. Eventually this may even lead to a change in facial expression; the upper lip is shortened and turned out, the lips are thickened, and a line between the cheeks and lips is formed as a result of the narrowing of the dental arch of the upper jaw.

Infections of the ear may follow adenoid infection and, if neglected, can lead to permanent deafness. Enlarged adenoids should be removed; this may be done at any age. Usually further trouble will not be encountered after tonsils and adenoids are removed, but in 10 to 15 per cent of cases they grow back and a second operation may be required.

Care of the ears. The ears do not require special care. Syringes should not be used to wash out the ears, nor should cotton-tipped sticks be employed to remove wax or other objects. When a small child has a pain in his ear, he will usually indicate his discomfort by putting his hand to his ear or by crying when the ear is touched. Infections of the ear frequently follow infectious conditions in the nose or throat and acute infectious diseases.

When the doctor examines the child with a painful ear, he routinely takes the temperature, which is usually quite high, even in simple ear infections. Next he will look directly into the ear canal with a special instrument, the otoscope. If infection is present, and the condition warrants, the doctor may make a small opening in the eardrum to release accumulations of fluid or pus. Otherwise, simple antibiotic treatment may be all that is required. Relief of pain is usually prompt following drainage or other therapy. Sometimes the pain of earache may be relieved by ear drops prescribed by the physician. Such treatment should not be used unless a doctor has seen the child.

Before the introduction of penicillin, ear infections often caused more or less permanent deafness. Mastoid infection too was frequent. In mastoid infection, severe pain and tenderness are noted in the mastoid bone which is just behind the ear. Opening the mastoid bone to free it of accumulated pus, the so-called mastoidectomy, was a common operation in children twenty-five years ago, but is relatively rare today.

Puncture of the eardrum by the doctor to release pus is not a dangerous procedure. If it is done early, hearing will not be impaired because the eardrum will heal promptly and hearing be as good as before. Puncture of the eardrum is far less dangerous than postponing the operation too long.

Cuts and bruises. Little children frequently suffer cuts, bruises, burns, and similar injuries to the skin which can possibly become infected. In such instances, first aid given at home is of the greatest significance in preventing complications from simple injuries. Many different antiseptic substances are available to kill germs located on the skin around a skin injury. The area affected should be washed immediately with plenty of soap and water. A suitable antiseptic may then be applied, but a clean cut usually requires only a finger-bandage such as the Band-Aid. Children often object to iodine solutions or alcohol because of the burning sensation, and other non-burning antiseptics may be used.

Occasionally a bruise to the fingertips may result in a painful swollen area of blood clot under the nail. The doctor should be called. Most likely he will make a small nick in the nail to permit free drainage and relief from pain. This should never be done by anyone but a physician. Bruises which are painful often can be relieved from pain by cold compresses.

Convulsions in babies. Babies have convulsions much more frequently than adults. The nervous system of a baby is so sensitive that frequently an infectious disease or high temperature will give rise to a convulsion or extensive shaking. In ordinary convulsions, the child loses consciousness and becomes rigid. Then there may be a spasmodic jerking of the face and of the arms and legs. It may be difficult for the parent to differentiate between a simple convulsion and one due to epilepsy. In only about one-fifth of convulsions in children is the cause epilepsy. Convulsions should be promptly reported to the doctor. During a convulsion, the child should be placed gently on his side. Usually the child will sleep following a convulsion.

See also BED WETTING; COLIC; EYE; FEEDING, BREAST; HEAD BANGING, HEAD ROLLING; IMMUNIZATION; THUMB SUCKING; and Chapter 7, "The Process of Infectious Diseases and Immunization of Children"; Chapter 9, "Child Care and Training."

CHILL, a sensation of cold, accompanied by shivering and usually with teeth chattering, throbbing, and trembling. It is frequently a prominent early symptom of acute infection. Any severe chill during a fever is a danger signal and a doctor should be called at once.

A chill results from an increase in the chemical activity going on in the body and therefore a rapid rise in the production of heat by the body. The ultimate result of a chill is increased body temperature. A person with a chill is usually quiet, lies doubled up, has a pale cool skin and sometimes "goose flesh," due to the constriction of the superficial blood vessels under the skin which is sometimes so great that the skin appears blue. A mild chill can usually be controlled to some degree by the person; however, a severe chill cannot. Warm blankets and clothing, hot drinks, hot-water bottles, and electric pads will help relieve the discomfort of the person with chills.

A chill can be induced in patients by injecting certain nonspecific protein substances. It can also be prevented by drugs which act as sedatives and as controls of body temperature. The action of these drugs, which are known as antipyretic and antifever drugs, is to depress the activity of the center in the brain which controls chills and shivering.

The chill is being studied to gain further knowledge as to its cause and significance. Many physicians feel that a chill is often of real importance in helping to overcome a disease since it raises the body temperature through muscular movement. *See also* FEVER.

CHIROPRACTIC, a therapeutic system based on the theory that the bones of the spinal column, by pressing on the spinal nerves, cause an interruption of the normal function of the nerves. The result of this pressure is said to be eventual damage to the tissues. Extensive medical investigation has failed to show any scientific foundation for this system. Chiropractors are nevertheless licensed to practice in most states. Practically all chiropractors are in the United States.

CHLOASMA. *See* LIVER SPOTS.

CHLOROFORM, trichloromethane, a heavy colorless liquid with a typical ether smell. Chloroform is best known as an anesthetic, and has been used for that purpose since 1847 when Dr. James Simpson, an Edinburgh gynecologist, dissatisfied with ether, discovered the narcotic qualities of chloroform. It became fashionable as an anesthetic in childbirth when Queen Victoria permitted its administration during the delivery of her seventh child.

Too large quantities and habitual use of chloroform may result in poisoning, injuries to the liver and kidneys, a condition of transient albuminuria, albumin present in the urine, and other diseases. *See also* ANESTHESIA.

CHLOROSIS, a form of anemia, characterized by a large reduction of hemoglobin in the blood, but with only a slight diminution in the number of red cells. Some decades ago, chlorosis, or "green sickness," was common among girls and young women, but today it has almost completely disappeared because of increased knowledge of the place of iron in the diet. The symptoms of this iron deficiency are a greenish color to the skin, and menstrual and gastric disturbances.

CHOLECYSTITIS, the scientific name for inflammation of the gallbladder. *See also* GALLBLADDER; and Chapter 18, "Disorders of the Digestive System and Diet in Digestive Disorders."

CHOLECYSTOGRAPHY, roentgenography, x-ray diagnosis, of the gallbladder after it has been made visual by substances not transparent to the x-ray.

Gallstone attacks have characteristic symptoms, yet differences in related symptoms and severity of pain often makes a definite distinction from other diseases difficult. The introduction of cholecystography has been a great advance in the diagnosis of gallstones.

CHOLELITHIASIS, a condition associated with calculi, stones in the gallbladder or in a bile duct. *See also* GALLBLADDER.

CHOLERA, an acute infection which chiefly involves the small intestine. The main symptoms are severe, constantly flowing diarrhea, vomiting, collapse, cramps in the muscles, and suppression of the flow of urine from the kidneys.

Cholera spreads most rapidly in moist warm climates. From time immemorial it has existed in India, from where at one time it spread throughout the world, probably traveling along caravan routes into Europe and along water trade routes.

The cause of cholera was described some fifty years ago by the German researcher, Robert Koch. A germ, the comma bacillus, gains entrance into the body through polluted drinking water. The organism then gets into the bowel where it causes acute infection. Cholera spreads in much the same way as typhoid fever does, the germs escaping from the body along with material that is vomited or passed from the bowel.

To prevent the spread of cholera, the cholera patient must be isolated. Material that is passed from the patient must be destroyed by fire. Only food that has been cooked, and boiled, or preferably chlorinated, water should be used by people in an area where cholera exists. The food and water should not be permitted to stand for any length of time since they may become recontaminated. Those who live or travel in cholera-ridden areas can be partially protected against this disease through vaccination with a serum made from the killed bodies of the specific cholera germs. The incidence of cholera among inoculated people has been low.

About five or six days after a person has been infected with cholera, a severe diarrhea begins, with violent purging, and eventually practically pure mucus and water are passed. Then vomiting begins, followed by collapse. The skin loses its elasticity, the muscles cramp, the eyes are sunken, and the voice is feeble. As more and more water is lost, the thirst becomes intense, the pulse becomes rapid and weak, and the blood pressure falls. The face becomes sunken and the skin develops a blue, cyanotic tinge, as the blood gradually loses its oxygen. As the patient's condition improves, the reverse of the process occurs.

Whenever large amounts of fluid are lost from the body, danger of death from acid intoxication ensues. Therefore, the chief step in the treatment is restoration of the fluid. Large quantities of normal or physiological salt solution are given to the patient by injection into the veins. Delay may be fatal, and frequently it is necessary to give one or two quarts of this solution, every six or eight hours, for two or three days. The acidosis may be overcome by giving large doses of sodium bicarbonate. Usually the person with cholera is content to remain in bed. Warmth is sustained by blankets, hot-water bottles, and electric pads. The physician can help to control the vomiting by prescription of proper remedies.

In the United States, cholera has ceased to be a serious problem, although it still occurs in many other parts of the world.

CHOLESTEROL, a fatty substance, a basis for hundreds of chemical processes in the body. Animal meat, cream, butter, and eggs contain large amounts of cholesterol and its presence in excess amounts in the blood stream is believed by many medical investigators to be responsible for a type of arterial hardening known as atherosclerosis. In this disease, cholesterol plaques in the inside wall of arteries cause the wall to thicken and roughen. Ultimately the flow of blood through that portion of the artery is restricted, or a piece of the roughened wall may tear away and block the flow of blood to those tissues served by the artery. When this occurs in the arteries that supply the heart muscle with blood the condition is called coronary thrombosis.

Dr. John Gofman and his associates at the University of California have proposed that a definite correlation exists between severe coronary heart attacks and excess blood cholesterol. Other medical investigators have produced atherosclerosis in animals by feeding them diets high in cholesterol. Certain heart specialists advocate a low-fat, low-cholesterol diet to prevent or control coronary heart disease, but others believe that since the body produces its own cholesterol, dietary restriction of it will not help appreciably. Investigations indicate that factors other than the existence of excess cholesterol may be responsible for arterial hardening. These may involve the body's ability to metabolize the cholesterol, or its ratio to other substances, such as protein and phosphatides, in the blood stream, the size and number of the cholesterol molecules, and the effect of exercise on the amount of circulating cholesterol. In one experiment, Dr. Frederick J. Stare of Harvard University's School of Public Health reports a definite correlation between exercise and a reduction in certain types of cholesterol molecules.

CHONDROMA, a slowly developing tumor growing from tissues or cartilage. In the chest this tumor tends to spread toward important organs. Generally benign, chondroma may recur after removal by surgery.

CHOREA, more familiarly known as St. Vitus' dance, a disease of the nervous system which causes involuntary twitching of various parts of the body. Children prior to puberty are most often affected.

Unlike many diseases of the nervous system, St. Vitus' dance normally lasts a relatively short time, often no more than twelve weeks. Sometimes relapses occur, and in other instances the disease may endure for one or two years, although not usually.

Chorea is believed to be the result of a general streptococcus infection which in some apparently indirect way, perhaps through toxic substances developed by the germs of the infection, strikes at the brain and the nervous system. Children may develop a temporary, habitual twitch from imitating the movements of other people, but this is completely different in origin and in character from the involuntary twitching that is seen in St. Vitus' dance.

The onset of the disease, which often accompanies rheumatic fever, may appear as a generalized illness with fever, vomiting, and headache, along with dizziness and weakness. The first disturbances of bodily movement are often mistaken for clumsiness of the child. However, the true nature of the ailment soon becomes apparent.

When fully developed, the movements are rapid, of short duration, and distinctive; none exactly duplicates any that preceded. Muscular

coordination becomes difficult and approximately 25 per cent of the cases are so severe as to disturb the speech function. The child becomes irritable and restless, and his memory, attention span, and emotions may be mildly disturbed.

The treatment of chorea, a disease implicating the whole system and not just isolated parts, begins with prolonged bed rest of three to six weeks at least. Because of the close relationship to streptococcus infection, the child should be kept under close observation. Any infection of the throat, in the tonsils or adenoids, in the teeth or elsewhere should be eliminated quickly and the child kept in bed. Both in streptococcus infections and in chorea attention must be given the heart, which may be particularly affected. The use of penicillin or sulfa is recommended by the American Heart Association to prevent streptococcal infection and to protect against a recurrence of rheumatic fever.

Baths and sedative drugs directed at alleviating the symptoms of chorea are frequently quite helpful. Both heat and drugs striking at the infection itself are often beneficial, but neither are specifically effective.

Convalescence of the patient with chorea should be gradual, with a nutritional diet assuring plenty of vitamins and minerals. Exercise and play should be resumed in moderation and under supervision, but the child must relax and not overdo. *See also* ATAXIA.

CHORION, the outermost of the fetal membranes which covers, nourishes, and protects the developing ovum. Later it becomes the fetal part of the placenta.

CHROMOBLASTOMYCOSIS, a rare skin infection caused by a fungus which grows on plants and trees in warm humid areas. Only a few cases have been reported in the United States, but the disease occurs more frequently in South America.

The infection usually starts on the feet or legs. The skin turns purplish red and develops colored, warty, cauliflower-like growths. X-ray, used externally in combination with appropriate drugs, has successfully disposed of the fungus and the growths. A potential danger, however, in any such disorder is that the offending organism will reach the lung or some other vital part where it may cause death.

CHRONIC signifies long-continued or of long duration. A chronic disease is prolonged, often slowly progressing and never completely cured —as, for example, chronic bronchitis or chronic arthritis.

CHRYSAROBIN, an orange powder, derived from the bark of a Brazilian tree, which stains the skin a deep brown. It is used to treat psoriasis, and is also effective in fungus infections called dhobie itch and gym or jockey itch, involving the skin of the groin, perineum, and perianal regions.

CILIA, fine, hairlike appendages which cover the surface of mucous membranes, the moist sensitive lining of the respiratory tract. The cilia are filtering organisms, a protective measure to keep harmful particles out of the lung. They move upward and downward, and through the more pronounced upward movement, mucus, dust, and other infectious particles are swept and propelled toward the mouth, so that they are not breathed into the lungs. Eyelashes are also cilia, and protect the eyes from foreign particles.

CIRCULATORY SYSTEM. The heart pumps the blood through a "pipeline" of closed tubes or vessels. This pipeline forms two major circular routes in the body, the systemic circulation and the pulmonary circulation, with the heart acting as a central pump. The circulatory system, with its major and minor routes, reaches every cell in the body, bringing the blood with its life-sustaining products from the organs where they are manufactured to the tissues where they are needed. It also carries away the waste products to other organs in the body, where they are broken down and either converted to be used again or excreted as waste. In addition, the circulatory system takes care of the more active organs by bringing them an increased flow of blood, whereas those organs which are less active, or temporarily at rest, receive less blood.

The heart is divided into a right side and a left side. Each side is further divided into two chambers an auricle and a ventricle. The auricles are the collecting depots for the blood, while the ventricles pump the blood out of the heart into blood vessels.

In the systemic circulation, the blood is pumped from the left ventricle into the aorta, or large artery, passing through a series of smaller arteries which branch from it, then continues through the arterioles, or smallest arteries, which end in a fine network of tiny vessels called the capillaries. The capillaries transfer the blood, with its oxygen and nutriment, to the various tissues of the body and then conduct it from the tissues into the venules, or tiny veins, on through larger veins until it finally reaches the inferior vena cava, one of the two great veins on the right side of the heart. From here, it passes into the right auricle, and thus completes the systemic circle. The blood, venous blood, dark in color, which enters the right auricle, has deposited most of its oxygen, and has picked the carbon dioxide from the tissues.

Before the blood can resume its systemic flow, it must secure a fresh supply of oxygen. The right ventricle now pumps the blood through the pulmonary artery into the capillaries of the lungs, where it deposits its carbon dioxide and gathers up the new oxygen. This blood, now a bright red, is arterial blood which then enters the pulmonary vein, flows into the left auricle from which it enters the left ventricle, and is then ready to start on its route through the body again. This circuitous routine is the pulmonary circulation.

In addition to these two major circulations, some of the blood stream from the systemic circulation is diverted by the capillaries of the stomach and intestinal tract to the portal vein and is carried to the liver, which acts as a storage depot for blood. Here some of the impurities are removed and excreted into the digestive tract, and the blood is returned through the hepatic vein to the superior vena cava of the heart. This system is the portal circulation. Another accessory circulation from the systemic feeds blood to the kidneys and is called the renal circulation. The coronary arteries, veins, and their capillaries supply the heart itself with oxygen and nutriments and remove waste material, and constitute the coronary circulation. The brain and head are served by the two carotid arteries which bring the blood supply, and also by the jugular veins which carry away the blood and waste materials.

The circulatory pipeline consists of the three types of blood vessels described: the arteries, the veins, and the capillaries. The capillaries connect the ends of the smallest arteries to the beginnings of the smallest veins. Valves inside the heart and also in the veins keep the flow of blood continuous and in one direction. In the veins they are spaced at various distances, opening toward the heart, so that the flow cannot go backward. The valves control the rate of the flow and its distribution through the body. The final control of the blood flow is exerted by the capillaries, which are so small that the blood cells can pass through only in single or double file.

The walls of the capillaries are a thin layer of fine platelike cells, endothelium, which are dovetailed to form a membranous network where the blood deposits its nutriment, oxygen, and other substances needed by the body tissues, and from which it picks up the gases and other waste products. Those tissues which are not reached easily by this interchange receive their nutriment from the liquid constituents of the blood, which also filter through the capillary network and carry food and oxygen to the tissues. This clear fluid which filters out of the capillaries is the tissue fluid. The capillaries are found throughout all tissues and organs of the body, and are more numerous, where the body organs are most active. Over a million capillaries may run through a square inch of muscle tissue, and if all the capillaries were joined in a single tube it would stretch for thousands of miles.

The walls of the arteries must be thick and strong to accommodate the stream of blood within them which is pumped by the heart under great pressure. They consist of three layers, the endothelium, or fine inner layer; the middle layer, on which the strength and caliber of the vessel depends, which is a thick coat of strong muscle fibers and heavy elastic tissue permitting expansion and contraction of the artery; and the outside coat, or adventitia, a thick layer of connective tissue which gives the vessel elasticity and enables it to act as a reservoir for the blood flow, and at the same time prevents the blood from oozing into the tissues.

The walls of the veins are structurally similar to the arteries, but they are thinner and their diameter is much larger since the flow of blood through the veins and into the heart is under less pressure and slower in rate.

In the course of normal routine, and more so in disease, much strain is placed upon the structures that constitute the circulatory system. As cells deteriorate, new cells replace them.

Fortunately not all the cells wear out at the same time, and the process of replacement continues throughout life, so that a steady balance is maintained between the removal of worn-out cells by the circulating blood and the regeneration of new cells. *See also* CORONARY THROMBOSIS; EMBOLISM; HEART; LYMPHATIC SYSTEM; and Chapter 12, "Diseases of the Heart."

CIRCUMCISION, is the surgical removal of the loose fold of the skin, the foreskin, which covers the head of the penis.

Circumcision was originally a religious rite in ancient Egypt and among Hebrews, Mohammedans, South Sea Islanders, and American Indians. The Book of Genesis interprets circumcision as a blood covenant, and it is still practiced as such among some Jews.

Today the operation is still recommended by many doctors as a routine hygienic measure, or to diminish the possibility of contracting venereal diseases. With improved sanitary conditions, permitting frequent bathing and washing, circumcision as a sanitary measure is probably not as significant as it formerly was.

The best time for the operation is before the infant is ten days old, when it represents a minor procedure. Circumcision should always be done under strictest surgical or aseptic conditions. Proper repair of the tissues after the extra skin has been removed is essential. If the doctor's instructions regarding protection and cleansing of the wound are carefully followed, complications are rare.

Circumcision is recommended

when the foreskin is unusually long so that it retains urine which might cause infection. Inflammation and irritation under the foreskin are also associated with various nervous manifestations.

CIRRHOSIS, a chronic progressive disease, essentially inflammatory, with a pathological hardening of tissue brought about by an increase of connective tissue elements. The lungs, ovaries, heart, or stomach may be affected with cirrhosis, but it occurs more often in the kidney and liver.

Cirrhosis of the kidney, chronic interstitial nephritis, is a chronic inflammation of the connective tissue elements of the kidney. Cirrhosis of the liver, the most frequent type, is usually a disease of adults but may occasionally occur in younger people, and is three times more common among men than women. It involves a scarring or hardening of the liver, produced by an overgrowth of the connective tissue elements to the neglect of the true hepatic cells.

Heavy consumers of alcohol are often victims of cirrhosis, but moderate drinkers may become affected. The disease may also be caused by bacterial infection, particularly from bacteria of the colon, infectious cirrhosis. *See also* LIVER; and Chapter 16, "Common Disorders of the Liver and Gallbladder."

CITRIC ACID, a tribasic acid occurring in the juice of many fruits and in various animal tissues. It appears as translucent crystals or a white crystalline powder, soluble in water, and is employed as an acid flavoring and in effervescent drinks. Citric acid has an alkalizing effect, but is with-

out vitamin value and is not an effective substitute for citrus fruits.

CLAUSTROPHOBIA, an intense fear of being in a confined area. *See also* AGORAPHOBIA.

CLAVICLE, or "collarbone," the curved bone which extends from the top of the breastbone out to each of the shoulders. Because the two clavicles are thin and small and support much weight they are frequently and easily broken. While mending, a small bony disfigurement is likely to occur, unless the person will lie motionless on his back, without a pillow, so that the two parts can remain in perfect adjustment to each other until they have completely grown together. *See also* FRACTURES.

CLEFT PALATE, a congenital defect, due to failure in fusion of embryonic facial processes, which results in a fissure through the palate. This cleavage, starting in the soft palate, may extend forward all the way across the bony roof of the mouth and even reach to the upper lip, resulting in harelip.

A person with this deformity is abnormally susceptible to inflammations in the area of the palate. Speech is difficult, as well as sucking, drinking, and chewing. Food being swallowed will frequently go through the roof of the mouth into the nostrils, and special feeding techniques become necessary.

A cleft palate can usually be corrected by an operation in which the tissues in the roof of the mouth are loosened and then fitted together. This operation is sometimes performed as early as the third month, or as late as the third year. If done before the child begins to talk, undesirable speech habits can be prevented. Even after a successful operation, however, some physical defect may remain. New techniques employing braces or plate or other prosthetic devices, along with intensive training, can significantly benefit persons with cleft palate. *See also* HARELIP; LIPS; PALATE.

CLIMATE, the average weather condition of an area over a period of years, as indicated by the temperature, rainfall, barometer, and other measurements. The connection between climate and health is a subject which has interested people for centuries. Greek and Roman physicians recognized that malaria affected persons living in low marshy areas, but they believed the cause of malaria was sleeping in night air. Hippocrates, the father of medicine who lived in the third century B.C., wrote, "If there be no rivers and the water that the people drink be marshy and stagnant, the physique of the people must show protruding bellies and enlarged spleens." He did not know that the protruding belly and enlarged spleen are results of malaria, prevalent in marshy areas. In his book *Air, Water and Places*, he notes that ". . . the inhabitants of a region that is mountainous, rugged, high and watered, where the changes of the seasons exhibit strong contrasts, are likely to be of big physique, with a nature well adapted for endurance and courage." This is the first recorded recognition that the Temperate Zone is a region conducive to human well-being.

More recently, persons with "consumption" or tuberculosis went to dry, high-altitude areas in an attempt to cure their illness. However, today it is felt that climate is not important in treating tuberculosis, and emphasis is placed on drugs, food, rest, and competent medical care.

Persons with rheumatic conditions frequently feel better when they are not exposed to cold and dampness. Research on rheumatism has shown that changes occur in the composition of the body tissues, including the blood, when there are changes in barometric pressure. Changes in blood supply to the joints are associated with sudden changes in temperature. While climate cannot cause rheumatic conditions, it may lower the resistance so that a rheumatic inflammation results.

For years the belief has been prevalent that dampness, cold, and drafts are associated with colds and pneumonia. However, statistics seem to indicate that, unless a person has a tendency to respiratory ailments, inclement weather does not cause such illnesses. For example, students at Stanford University at Palo Alto, California, have about as many coughs and colds as students at Harvard University in Massachusetts, despite the fact that the California climate is mild and the Massachusetts climate rigorous. However, persons whose resistance is generally low will be more susceptible to inflammation of the nose, throat, and sinuses during cold weather, and will benefit by a change to a warm dry climate.

Persons with heart disease do not do well at high altitudes, because of increased difficulty in getting oxygen for circulation.

Generally a mild climate is most beneficial to those persons with chronic diseases, and a specialist may propose that a change of climate be made to relieve their symptoms. But it is wise to check with a physician before assuming that another climate will be more beneficial. *See also* HAZARDS OF COLD.

CLINITEST, a commercially available kit by means of which persons having or suspecting a diabetic tendency may check the extent of sugar in the urine. *See also* DIABETES.

CLITORIS, the organ in women which resembles, in miniature form, the penis of the male. This small tubelike body is located in the angle at the top of the vulva, the external sex organ of women. Like the penis, the clitoris is composed of tissue which becomes engorged with blood, and hard and erect during sexual excitement. *See also* REPRODUCTION SYSTEM.

CLUBFOOT, a deformity of the foot, present at birth or caused subsequently by muscle paralysis or injury, in which the heel or the ball of the foot or one edge of it does not touch the ground.

In three-fourths of the cases noted at birth, the heel and inner edge of the foot are raised. This condition occurs once in every thousand births, and considerably more than half of those affected are male children. Also, in more than half the deformity occurs on only one side.

Treatment must be started at the earliest possible moment. The later therapy begins, the longer it will take to remedy the deformity. Children under a year can be treated in twenty-three weeks, whereas those of six years or more require almost forty-two weeks. One of the signal achievements of modern medical science has been the development of treatment for club foot.

The doctor, usually an orthopedist, will outline a routine of the manipulations of the parts involved to get them into the correct position and then make the position secure with one or more of the devices designed especially for the purpose, such as adhesive bindings, plaster casts, or braces and splints. After the proper position has been firmly established, special exercises, shoes, massage, and other measures which may be beneficial will be prescribed. Active treatment often continues for several months, and follow-up supervision is necessary for years.

Manipulation alone may not be satisfactory. Then surgical rearrangement of the affected tissues and parts becomes necessary.

The cause of clubfoot is unknown. Heredity is suspected by some persons, because approximately 5 per cent of cases occur in families in which the deformity has appeared previously; others believe that an incorrect position of the child before birth is responsible.

COAGULATION, the formation of a coagulum, clot, or curd as in blood or milk. When bleeding is present, threadlike fibers called fibrin are produced by a substance in the blood, the fibrinogen. These fibers trap white and red blood corpuscles which form a clot. Contraction of the fibrin squeezes out the liquid portion of the blood, the serum, and a crust develops. The system of clotting is counteracted by agents, including heparin and other anticoagulants, which keep the blood fluid. The power of coagulation of the blood varies with different persons. In people with hemophilia, a hereditary disease, the clotting is so retarded that they bleed profusely from minor wounds and may even bleed to death.

Formation of a blood clot in a coronary artery may obstruct the flow of blood to the heart muscle and produce coronary thrombosis. The incidence of clotting may be increased when the person is under stress. A blood clot blocking an artery of the brain, usually where a weak spot has resulted through arteriosclerosis, is able to produce some conditions of rheumatic heart disease. Coagulation of blood in the lower body regions can cause serious complications if particles of the blood clot reach the lungs and obstruct the major blood vessels.

In 1917, Dr. Jay McLean of Baltimore succeeded in isolating heparin, and since then dicumarol, Tromexan, and other anticoagulants have been developed and the administration of anticoagulants has become a significant medication. *See also* CORONARY THROMBOSIS; EMBOLISM; HEMOPHILIA; MENORRHAGIA.

COCAINE, an alkaloid derived from the coca bush, in use for centuries. Inca priests in Peru, for example, were aware of its anesthetic effect and chewed coca leaves in an attempt to improve their physical endurance.

Medically it was first used as an anesthetic in eye operations in Vienna in 1884. Cocaine is now employed as a local anesthetic. It produces temporary insensitivity to pain when applied to the surface of mucous membranes or injected by hypodermic needle.

Cocaine is habit-forming and poisonous, and should never be used in any way except when prescribed and administered by a physician. The amount of cocaine required to poison varies greatly; some people react unfavorably even to small doses. New synthetic compounds have been developed which are similar to cocaine but less toxic. *See also* DRUG ADDICTION.

COCCIDIOIDOMYCOSIS, also known as desert fever, San Joaquin fever, valley fever, or the bumps, a disease with pulmonary symptoms caused by one of the fungi, coccidioides immitis, which thrives in the dry dusty areas of the San Joaquin Valley and in the southwestern states. During World War II, thousands of servicemen stationed in camps throughout this area became ill with coccidioidomycosis after inhaling the tiny invisible particles of spore-laden dust. Spores may also enter the skin through open wounds.

The first symptoms, which resemble the symptoms of tuberculosis, are generally chills, fever, headache, general malaise, night sweats, and coughing. These symptoms usually subside after a week or two and small bumps may then appear under the skin, which also disappear in time. In severe cases, x-rays show changes in the lungs and occasionally thinwalled cavities which may persist for years.

Recovery from a simple lung infection is usually rapid and complete even without treatment, but in cases where deep lung cavities have developed, surgery may be indicated.

The growing prevalence of coccidioidomycosis has made it a public health concern. About 90 per cent of the people living in these arid regions have had the infection within a ten-year period as a result of inhaling the spores of the fungus. Droughts in this area add to the disease hazards. Residents or visitors who show signs of a chronic infection resembling any of the serious respiratory diseases should have chest x-rays and skin and blood tests.

COCCYX, from the Greek meaning "shaped like the bill of a cuckoo," the last bone at the lowermost end of the spine.

CODEINE, an alkaloid derived from opium and closely allied in chemical constitution to morphine. Though weaker, its action is similar to that of morphine, and it is used medically to diminish sensitivity to pain.

COD LIVER OIL, the partially destearinated fixed oil, obtained from the fresh livers of cod. The liver of the cod (and also of the halibut) is one of the richest sources of vitamin A and D, and cod liver oil has been known for many years as an effective treatment for malnutrition. Mild cases of rickets improve quickly with cod liver oil. Diets which do not contain enough fat-soluble vitamins are a basic factor of sinusitis in children, and cod liver oil is recommended by many physicians as an effective preventive measure against this infec-

tion. Every growing baby and child should have cod liver oil or its equivalent in vitamins A and D, and nursing mothers are advised by physicians to take it regularly. The amount of cod liver oil usually recommended is a teaspoonful daily of the more concentrated preparations, or two teaspoonfuls of the less concentrated. However, since today more and more foods are being vitamin-enriched, the diet usually does not need to be supplemented by cod liver oil. *See also* CHILD CARE.

COFFEE, a beverage made by an infusion or decoction from the roasted and ground or pounded seeds of a shrub, small tree, or other species of the madder family. Although coffee has no nutritional value, taken in moderation it does have some distinct pharmacological worth.

In his *The Romance of Medicine,* Dr. Benjamin Lee Gordon describes its discovery. "For centuries the coffee plant was looked upon as a useless weed until one day a Turkish herdsman noticed that some goats in his charge which were feeding on the coffee beans became unusually playful and hilarious. Being curious to know the reason for their peculiar actions, he picked some coffee beans and parched them in the sun; when he reached home he brewed them and drank the beverage. To his surprise, after taking a cupful of the beverage he felt greatly stimulated without any bad effect. On the following Friday, the Mohammedan Sabbath, he treated his guests with this stimulant and they experienced the same effect. Henceforth, coffee became a national drink among Mohammedans all over the world, who use it in a strong and syrupy way."

An average cup of coffee contains about one grain of caffeine, an alkaloid which stimulates the brain, kidney, and circulation. It increases the force and beat of the heart and the flow of urine and thus helps cleanse the body of metabolic end-products. This action has made coffee valuable in cases of edema or dropsy, conditions in which fluid accumulates excessively in the tissues. In these cases, it is vital to increase the heart rate so that more blood is pumped into the blood vessels, thus promoting greater flow through the kidneys with elimination of fluid.

Generally a cup of coffee after dinner may have a good effect on the digestion since it increases the gastric juice. However, an excess of coffee can easily have toxic effects, such as rapid pulse, nervousness, irritability, and insomnia. In some persons, too much coffee may even bring on attacks of dizziness and faintness, or palpitation from an overaccelerated heart rate and force. The amount of coffee that can safely be drunk varies among people. Although Voltaire is said to have drunk more than fifty cups of coffee a day, for some people a few cups a day may be excessive. People should discover what is the correct amount for them.

Tests made in 1955 by the American Medical Association established that a cup of regular ground coffee has almost twice as much caffeine as a cup of instant coffee, and a cup of regular decaffeinated coffee has about one-third the amount of caffeine as a cup of regular ground coffee.

COLCHICINE, a water-soluble, pale brownish alkaloid derived from the meadow saffron which has been used as an efficient pain reliever in gout for more than a hundred years. However, it has proved of little value in other types of arthritis and rheumatism. *See also* GOUT.

COLD. *See* COMMON COLD.

COLD CREAM, a mixture in an ointment of petrolatum, lanolin, and rosewater, which is useful for soothing dry, inflamed, or irritated skin, and also for removing cosmetics. *See also* COSMETICS.

COLD SORE. *See* HERPES SIMPLEX.

COLIC, the abnormal and violent contraction of certain internal muscular tissues. Intestinal colic is caused by a sudden contraction of the intestine. When the bile ducts contract abnormally, biliary colic results, and renal colic is caused by a tightening of the tube, the ureter, which passes between the kidney and bladder. Alternate contraction and relaxation is the normal behavior of these organs, and pain occurs only when this contraction becomes spasmodic.

Intestinal colic is the most common. The pain is noticed usually around the navel, and is often accompanied by a clogging or loosening of the bowels. If the cause of pain is doubtful, cathartics and laxatives should be avoided but an enema may be given if necessary. A simple chill, infected food, or a nervous condition are a few of the many possible causes of colic. Colic may be easily confused with a serious disorder, such as appendicitis. If the pain does not respond promptly to simple treatment, such as an electric pad or a hot-water bottle, or bicarbonate of soda, a physician should be called.

Intestinal colic, produced by gas, is commonly seen in infants. Often this condition results from the air taken in with the child's milk or food. Occasionally, however, it may be generated by the fermentation of food in the bowels. Regardless of the source, this gas can often be relieved simply by placing the baby across one's shoulder after every feeding and tapping it lightly on the back until it "burps." If the pain persists or is severe, a doctor should be consulted.

A special type of stomach colic, afflicting adults, which involves spasmodic contractions of the large bowel, is known as mucous colic. The pain occurs characteristically after meals, and is located chiefly in the right section of the lower abdomen. Such symptoms should be carefully investigated by a specialist who may take x-rays, inspect stools, and study the person's diet. Occasionally psychiatric observation may be necessary.

Renal colic, distress after meals and in the lower right abdomen, is usually caused by a stone in the kidney trying to descend to the bladder. The pain almost always starts in the kidney area and moves to the abdomen, leg, and genitals. Nausea and a frequent desire to urinate appear. In attempting to walk, the person will experience a pronounced tendency to tip his body to the side affected, depending on which of the kidney areas is affected. The pain may fluctuate and may even be severe enough to induce delirium. Renal colic can be

subdued by proper drugs. The pain will sometimes persist for days, but usually is limited to twelve hours or less. The stone is sometimes passed spontaneously in the urine, but frequently surgical treatment is required. *See also* CONSTIPATION; DIARRHEA; INDIGESTION; and Chapter 18, "Disorders of the Digestive System and Diet in Digestive Disorders."

COLITIS, inflammation of the colon, the part of the large intestine extending from the cecum to the rectum. Various forms of colitis can occur. Simple colitis is an acute irritation or infection of the colon, accompanied by diarrhea. Some types of colitis are caused by infection of the colon by specific organisms.

Mucous colitis is a condition in which the mucous membrane of the colon is inflamed, with symptoms of colicky pain, and constipation or diarrhea. It would seem to be primarily a psychosomatic ailment, which frequently becomes chronic.

Another form which is probably usually nervous in origin is ulcerative colitis, characterized by ulceration of the mucous membrane of the colon. The symptoms may range from only painless excretion of blood in stools to dysentery, fever, and death as a result of exhaustion, perforation of the colon and general peritonitis. Less critical cases usually recover completely, although frequently there are periods of relapse. Sometimes the disease becomes chronic, but without producing any severe disability. The entire length of the colon becomes scarred and thickened with ulcerations, and at this stage such complications as perforation, malignant disease, nutritional deficiency, and intestinal obstruction frequently occur.

Treatment of ulcerative colitis requires patient medical care, including bed rest, proper diet, sedatives, control of infection, and, if necessary, blood transfusions. Cortisone and ACTH have been used in treatment, but it is too soon to determine their value. Occasionally surgical removal of the colon is advised; and when emotional factors are thought to be involved in any way, psychotherapy is recommended. *See also* Chapter 18, "Disorders of the Digestive System and Diet in Digestive Disorders."

COLLARBONE, the common name for clavicle. *See also* CLAVICLE.

COLLODION, a coating or film used to protect and dress wounds. It is produced by dissolving gun cotton in ether and alcohol.

COLOSTOMY, a surgical operation, usually on the left side of the lower abdomen, creating a more or less permanent opening in the colon to permit evacuation after the normal rectal and anal opening is lost.

COMMON COLD, an acute inflammation of the upper respiratory tract, involving the nose and throat. It is one of the most familiar ailments which afflicts mankind yet its specific cause is little understood. Susceptibility to colds is almost universal, particularly among children. The cold is highly contagious, especially indoors, and places where groups of people congregate are excellent transmission spots for the infection.

In large urban communities where the climate is temperate, the general population averages about three colds a year. This median is higher among susceptible adults and children. The incidence is lowest in the summer, rises in the autumn, reaching its peak in midwinter and declines in the spring.

Several peak periods occur in smaller urban communities. The first is in early autumn when schools reopen and children are brought into greater proximity indoors. In addition to the winter rise in incidence of colds, a smaller rise often appears in the spring.

Colds are definitely communicable and are transmitted either by direct contact or by spread of the infected droplets of discharge. A practical method to control the spread of colds has not yet been developed. The common cold is due to one or more viruses. Scientists believe that the virus is generally present in the throat but it becomes active only when the body resistance is lowered. When the cold virus attacks the mucous membranes of the nose and throat, these tissues are weakened and become susceptible to infection by bacteria which are also generally found in the body. The bacteria are secondary invaders and the virus paves the way for their entry into the mucous membranes. Although they are not responsible for the common cold, the bacteria may initiate a secondary infection which either intensifies the local inflammation present, prolonging the cold, or causes new complications such as purulent sinusitis or otitis, an inflammation of the ear. Infants and young children appear to be more susceptible to these secondary infections than adults.

A cold usually begins abruptly, with a sense of soreness and dryness in the nose or back of the throat. Within a few hours the nasal passages feel congested, sneezing develops and a colorless watery discharge comes from the nose. After forty-eight hours the cold is usually at its peak, and is accompanied by excessive watering of the eyes, huskiness of the voice, and difficulty in breathing as the congestion spreads. The nasal discharge becomes thick and sticky and some coughing may develop. The cough does not usually bring up much discharge unless the person has a tendency to chronic bronchitis. Frequently a headache, a sense of lethargy and malaise, and vague pains in the back and limbs accompany a cold. A fever is rarely present, although in children a temperature of 102° or even higher often develops.

The uncomplicated cold generally lasts from one to two weeks and terminates without special treatment. Colds which persist or recur repeatedly, or in which there is a steady prolonged fever or chills, particularly in children or susceptible adults, may indicate complications and a physician should be consulted. As yet, a specific agent has not been developed to control the common cold and treatment is confined to relief of symptoms and control of complications. Treatment of the cold is not very different today from the treatment used by past generations. Bed rest should be enforced whenever possible and as much isolation as is practical. Plenty of liquids, hot or cold, a light diet, and keeping warm promote greater comfort. Aspirin in small re-peated doses generally gives relief as does gargling in cases of sore throat. An aspirin tablet or a teaspoon of salt dissolved in hot water is beneficial. In the latter stages of a cold, when the discharge has thickened, an atomizer or nose drops or inhaler helps clear the nasal passages. They should not be used more than once in four hours and if the person has a tendency to nasal inflammation should be employed sparingly.

Cold vaccines, which are suspensions of dead bacteria collected from the discharge of a cold, have not been found to be significantly effective either when taken by mouth or when given as an injection or nasal spray. However, continued research is being done. The routine use of sulfonamides or antibiotics for colds is definitely discouraged. These drugs should be given only in cases with a definite bacterial secondary infection —for example, in bronchopneumonia, sinusitis, or otitis media. Persons who have a consistent history of recurrent colds with accompanying complications may use antibiotics or sulfonamides, but only on the advice of a physician.

Although little is known about curing a cold, measures can be taken to ward off the infection and decrease its incidence. A well-balanced diet, sufficient rest, proper dress both indoors and out, all help to keep the body resistance high. Undue exposure to sharp changes in temperature should be avoided. Proper ventilation of rooms, with sufficient humidity in the air, helps to keep the mucous membranes in healthy condition. If humidifiers are not used, adequate moisture can be maintained by keeping a pan of water on a radiator or stove. Particular care should be taken to avoid contact with persons who have colds. Simple hygienic measures like washing the hands before eating or covering a sneeze all help to decrease the occurrence of colds. *See also* BRONCHOPNEUMONIA; CHILD CARE; OTITIS; SINUSES.

COMMUNICABLE DISEASES, those which are transmissible from one person to another. The difference, often disregarded, between infectious and communicable contagious diseases is that while infectious diseases are caused by the invasion of an infective agent like a fungus bacillus, or virus, the agents are not necessarily transmitted by a person.

COMPOUND FRACTURE. The breaking of a bone is a fracture. In a compound fracture, the point of the fracture is in contact with the outer surface of the body—for example, through a wound. If the break is covered by the skin, it is a simple fracture. *See also* BONES; FIRST AID; FRACTURES; and Chapter 28, "First Aid."

COMPRESS, a piece of folded gauze, cloth, or a soft pad which is applied firmly to a part of the body to relieve inflammations, produce pressure, or prevent hemorrhage. It may be wet or dry, hot or cold, and is sometimes perforated for drainage or observation of the underlying skin.

COMPULSION, defined in psychology as an irresistible, irrational desire to repeat certain acts. For example, a person may have the compulsion to wash his hands every few minutes, or to avoid stepping on the cracks in the sidewalk.

CONCEPTION, the union of sperm and ovum, the male and female sex cells, leading to the development of a new life. Conception is sometimes called fertilization, impregnation, or fecundation, and should be distinguished from the term copulation which refers to the act of sexual union between the male and female.

Since the egg cell of the female lives for only about twelve hours out of every month, the male seed must be deposited within the female genital tract during these few hours, or within two or three days of release of an egg. The sperm cells live about three days after ejaculation.

Conception usually takes place within the Fallopian tubes adjacent to the uterus and ovaries, and may occur within an hour of intercourse. Following union of the male and female sex cells, development is rapid, and eight to fourteen days later the product imbeds itself in the lining of the uterus where it remains until birth. *See also* REPRODUCTION SYSTEM.

CONCUSSION, a shock, severe shaking or jarring of a part of the body, usually resulting from a fall or blow. It also refers to the morbid state resulting from such a jarring. A concussion of the brain is actually a paralysis of its function, and symptoms are not due to any fracture or laceration. Signs of hemorrhage or loss of blood from the coverings around the brain may be present. Sometimes disturbances occur in the circulation of spinal fluid through the brain, and occasionally part of the soft white material of the brain is crushed or the connection cords between different portions of the brain are damaged or destroyed.

Brain concussion itself is seldom fatal. Necropsies (post-mortems) have shown that some apparent serious lesion of brain substance or vessels has occurred in fatal cases which had the characteristics of concussion but actually were contusions or lacerations. Whenever a concussion is suspected, a physician should be consulted. An x-ray examination should be made to determine whether or not fracture of the skull or other complications have occurred. While a slight crack of the skull is not critical, the pressure that may result from the bleeding inside the skull may be.

Symptoms of concussion appear immediately after the injury and vary depending on the degree of injury. Probably there will be a severe aching of the head, a weak dizzy "stunned" feeling. Disturbances in vision, cold perspiration, and shallow respiration may appear. If the jarring has been severe, more extreme symptoms may develop at once. The victim may be in partial coma or unconscious. The body will be cold and respiration exceedingly weak. Often vomiting accompanies these symptoms.

The consequences of a concussion may be of short duration or last for days or weeks or longer. Often, after regaining his senses, the person is unable to remember anything that happened during the time when consciousness was lost. Frequently symptoms of contusion and hemor-

rhage may develop and with them serious brain injuries. When the symptoms are protracted, a more serious affliction is always suggested.

During emergency treatment, the person should lie flat and be kept warm and quiet. Attempts at stimulation should not be made. No pressure should be applied or strong antiseptics given. *See also* HEAD INJURIES; SHOCK.

CONDITIONING, the development of a better physiological condition through physical exercise and training.

A great football coach once said that "a true athlete developed from the inside out, from healthy blood circulation and healthy cells to healthy muscles and nerves." Athletes are thus in "good condition," if their whole body functions as well as it can. To reach this goal, good nutrition, exercise, fresh air, rest and sleep as well as other healthful habits must prevail. Athletic coaches check carefully on the weight of their charges and keep accurate records of their physical well being. Thus they can establish whether or not an athlete works out too much or needs additional assistance to get into top form. Psychologically conditioning is the process of attaching a new stimulus to an old response, or a new response to an old stimulus. For example, in conditioning a dog to salivate at the sound of a bell, the salivation is an old response and the bell is the new stimulus which provokes the response.

CONDOM, a rubber sheath used to cover the penis during sexual intercourse to prevent the male sperm from reaching and fertilizing the female egg cell. It is a device for the prevention of infection as well as conception. *See also* CONTRACEPTION.

CONJUNCTIVITIS, inflammation of the conjunctiva, the mucous membrane covering the globe and lids of the eye. Many types of conjunctivitis exist, including allergic conjunctivitis, catarrhal conjunctivitis, the most common form which usually results from irritation or a cold, and acute contagious conjunctivitis or pinkeye. *See also* PINKEYE; EYE.

CONSTIPATION, the retention of solid waste material within the bowel for an unusually long time, or undue difficulty in its evacuation.

The excretion of undigested residue is the final step in the process of digestion. The waste material enters the colon as a loose moist mass, and there the excess water is absorbed by the body. The relatively solid mass of waste material then moves on into the rectum, where it normally prompts the desire for a movement of the bowels.

Evacuation ordinarily occurs once or twice every twenty-four hours, with a wide range of variation among individuals. With some persons greater frequency is common, while with others an interval of several days may often pass without ill effect. A fixed schedule for this function for all persons is unknown. Most doctors believe that the nature of the action, which should occur with some regularity and should produce well-formed stools, neither too moist and loose nor too dry and hard, is more desirable than the frequency.

Babies normally have three or four bowel movements a day, but the child who has less than three is not necessarily constipated. If the infant remains well and continues to gain weight, his digestion and elimination are probably normal for him. When constipation does occur, insufficient water, underfeeding, or an excessive amount of fat in the diet may be causative. Children who are weak or who have rickets may have difficulty in performing the necessary muscular actions associated with elimination.

Constipation is often the result of faulty habits and improper training. The habitual failure to respond promptly to the body's signal is often a basic cause. A lazy attitude, poorly developed habits, false modesty, or other extraneous factors often create a situation in which the signal is at first ignored and later not even felt. When such a pattern has been established by a person, he may develop chronic constipation, which, as an adult, he will usually attribute not to the bad habits which are actually basic but to nonexistent organic causes, which he will attempt to remedy by laxatives, enemas, and irrigations. These in turn may disrupt and interfere with the normal process of elimination and thus intensify his problem still further.

This type of constipation is commonly complicated even more by intricate chains of habits and misconceptions. Some constipated persons develop elaborate and mistaken notions about the shape, color, frequency, time, and consistency of the evacuation. A first step in overcoming constipation of this sort, is to correct these mistaken beliefs. Thereafter new habit patterns can be encouraged. A baby can be trained so that the simple act of placing it on the pot causes evacuation. With adults the pattern becomes much more elaborate, and can include getting up, bathing, having breakfast, even having the right magazine and a cigarette. The principle nevertheless remains the same and the development of an effective habit pattern is often the most successful treatment for chronic constipation.

Certain organic factors can, however, be involved in this digestive disturbance. The diet must contain adequate amounts of essential materials. The bulk must be sufficient to supply enough residual matter to assure an adequate mass and promote normal activity. Fruits and vegetables are best. Sufficient fluid intake is needed to prevent dehydration of the material in the colon and consequent difficulty in passing a dry mass. Profuse sweating during hot weather or as part of an acute infection can so deplete the body's supply of moisture as to react adversely on the bowel. Without adequate residue and moisture, the bowel does not function properly.

Sometimes a defect of motor activity exists. Particularly in the aged and the undernourished, the intestinal wall may lose its tone and capacity. A lack of B complex vitamins may be involved.

In some persons the nerves regulating the digestive processes are disturbed, so that the left half of the colon, its expelling section, does not function properly. Drugs are now available which overcome this condition. Other drugs which are given to combat certain conditions of disease may interfere with the action of the bowel. The physician, however, can usually deal with such contingencies as they arise.

The symptoms of constipation vary from few or none at all to a condition resembling a wasting disease. Loss of appetite comes early and halitosis is likely. The person becomes depressed and dull without apparent cause, tires easily, cannot cope with his responsibilities as usual, and may look pale and unwell. Frequent indigestion and discomfort or pain in the digestive system are common.

The doctor can establish whether bad habits and overdosing with purgatives are responsible, or whether deep-seated organic disorders may be present. In any event, only the doctor can safely outline the measures to be followed.

In most cases of dyschesia, or constipation involving largely the lower end of the digestive tract, actual re-education is necessary to start regularity and reliance on natural processes. Often, however, enemas, suppositories, or mild laxatives may be used to get new habits under way. Regular exercise is frequently advisable, especially for a sedentary person. A walk before breakfast or daily exercise of the abdominal muscles may be desirable.

Along with re-education, an adequately varied diet is probably more significant than any other factor. The major constituents of a normal diet, proteins, carbohydrates, fats, mineral salts, vitamins, and sufficient indigestible bulk, should all be assured. Fruit, especially stewed prunes and apples, are recommended for breakfast, and green vegetables and salad at both luncheon and the evening meal. Bran should be considered as a medicinal food, to be used only on the physician's advice, because it seems to accomplish little more than other bulk foods and may be irritating to the bowel.

Many drugs are available for treating various kinds of constipation. Vegetable and salt cathartics, organic and mineral medicines, substances which act mechanically, and water in various forms are among the most common. Cathartics of both the mineral and vegetable types irritate the bowel and are not advised for long use. They include the strong salts, cascara, jalap, senna, rhubarb, and aloes. Among the substances that act mechanically are mineral oil, bran, agar-agar, flax seeds, and psyllium seeds which lubricate the digestive tract or work by pushing its contents before them. Mixtures of mineral oil and such materials as agar-agar or flax seeds form a mucilaginous mass. Caution is necessary in using mineral oil because it absorbs vitamin A and may lead to a deficiency of that vitamin, and also because of a tendency of mineral oil to leak out of the bowel. Phenolphthalein is the chief ingredient of many widely used laxative combinations.

Recently attention has been given to methods of assisting the body itself to prevent overdryness of the bowel. If the amount of bile discharged by the liver is increased, making it thinner and greater in volume, the contents of the bowel remain softer and evacuation is easier and more normal when there has previously been a difficulty with overdry elimination. Bile acids have been found to accomplish this better than bile salts, which doctors formerly gave, because they thin the bile in the liver and enable it to be secreted more profusely. This is a normal body process and advantageous when constipation must be treated.

More than $50,000,000 a year is spent in the United States on constipation remedies. Cathartics, when taken habitually, end by defeating their purpose and may make elimination more difficult rather than less difficult. Some have a useful function, but they are best prescribed by a doctor. *See also* Chapter 18, "Disorders of the Digestive System and Diet in Digestive Disorders."

CONTACT DERMATITIS, an inflammation of the skin due to a sensitization to a substance with which it comes in contact. As a permanent injury to health, contact dermatitis is not a serious disturbance, but this minor allergy is persistent and often exceedingly annoying. It affects all age groups from infants to old people.

Whenever the skin is exposed to allergens, substances to which a person is sensitive, rashes, hives, cracks, burning, sores, and other irritations may develop. A good example is poison ivy in which an itchy rash is produced on the skin through contact with an oil in the poison ivy plant.

The substances to which a sensitive person may react on touch are numerous and include plants, wood, fur, silk, wool, dye, resin, plastic, rubber, metal, and many more. Some women have cosmetic contact dermatitis and cannot use ordinary beauty products such as soap, bleaches, deodorants, or powder. The active reaction of the skin to an allergenic substance makes contact dermatitis an occupational disorder too, and it frequently affects industrial workers who are exposed to certain chemicals, wood, metal, glue, or lacquer. In some instances, skin disorders spread to the nail bed and produce a condition called onycholysis. Nails may become brittle, separate into layers, or fall out completely.

When symptoms of contact dermatitis apear, the cause should be determined. A physician may discover the source through a patch test as in other allergies and then proceed with special desensitization which is possible with a number of materials. *See also* Chapter 20, "Diseases of the Skin."

CONTACT LENSES, eyeglasses that fit directly over the eyeball and fully aid the vision. A mold of the eye is made, exactly as one makes a cast of the inside of the mouth when it is necessary to have false teeth on plates. From this fragile mold a permanent one is made with dental plastic; then the glass is modeled to fit the mold. The inner surface of the contact lens must fit the eyeball so that it will not injure the sensitive tissues or interfere with the circulation of the blood. Before the mold has been prepared, it is necessary to fit the contact lenses. This means that the eye must be studied by all of the usual methods in order to determine the difficulties of vision so that the lens will meet its needs.

In fitting the contact lens to be worn, the eye is anesthetized and the contact lens shell is filled with a salt solution of the same density as the blood. The lids of the eye are then separated by the thumb and forefinger of the left hand, and the contact lens, held with a little rubber suction bulb, is inserted between the eyelids and the eyeball, first beneath the lower eyelid and then beneath the upper eyelid. This bulb must be gently released from the glass and should not be pulled in removing it. Otherwise the fluid will be lost from beneath the contact lens. If there are any bubbles under the lens they must be removed and the procedure repeated until the lens fits closely and no bubbles are in the fluid. Once the lens is fitted correctly, the person is given instructions in setting and removing the contact lens, and practices, seated by a low-cloth-covered table with a mirror before him.

Experiments have shown that the average person learns to insert the lenses in approximately nine minutes. At first, these lenses are worn only an hour or two at a time, but many who become well accustomed to them wear their lenses six to eight hours. Several months may be required, in some cases, before the person becomes sufficiently used to contact lenses to be able to wear them a long time without removing them and refilling them with fluid, and also without resting the eyes.

CONTRACEPTION, the use of a device, substance, or method to prevent conception during sexual intercourse.

Perhaps the commonest of the

various methods of contraception are the use of the sheath or condom of rubber worn by the man and, alternatively, the pessary or diaphragm worn by the woman. Chemicals, especially fixed in thick creams, which destroy or immobilize the sperm cell are also used. The American Medical Association has listed a number of such creams by name, as acceptable when prescribed by the doctor.

The physician's advice as to the proper use of such devices, materials, and methods is desirable, since not all are of equal effectiveness. The combination of pessary and cream, for instance, is probably 90 per cent or more effective; none is 100 per cent reliable. The pessary must be prescribed and fitted for the woman by the physician; otherwise, at best, its use will be haphazard protection. Creams and other chemicals are safe only on the advice of a physician. The use of douches is also common, but if they are to be effective and safe, should be employed only with medical advice. Many cleansing or sterilizing agents are dangerous to the body, or may alter normal bacterial growth undesirably in the parts where they are used.

Another method of avoiding conception is the so-called rhythm technique. The basis for this theory is the regular monthly cycle of ovulation. An egg cell or ovum passes from the ovary once every month, and consequently during the month the woman is more likely to conceive at one time than another. These intervals are commonly referred to respectively as the fertile and the safe periods. For the woman who menstruates regularly every twenty-eight days, the safe period is calculated as approximately a week before and a week after menstruation. More exactly, it lasts nine days, beginning the first day of menstruation. The fertile period, which normally is a maximum of eight days, follows, and then the next eleven days are again "safe." When the menstrual interval is shorter or longer than this, or is irregular, the physician's advice is desirable.

Another way of identifying the fertile period is to record the morning temperature, before any food is eaten or water or other fluids are drunk. Ovulation brings with it a fall in temperature, then a rise. Abstinence is practiced during the period of ovulation, and for three days before and three days after.

The latest development is a steroid called Enovid which prohibits ovulation. Five days after the cessation of menstruation a pill is taken each day for twenty days. The product is also useful in various menstrual disturbances.

CONTUSION, a superficial injury or bruise, produced by impact, in which breaking of the skin does not occur. If the skin is punctured also, the term contused wound is used. *See also* BRUISES.

CONVALESCENCE, the period of gradual restoration to health following disease, injury, or operation.

During convalescence, it is particularly important that the patient receive a well-balanced diet. To encourage strong scar tissue to form and seal over a surgical incision, a high vitamin C level is required.

Often after illness or surgery, the person may be anemic. To counteract anemia, which reduces the healing power, the diet should be rich in iron. Also important is protein, the building material of the body. The digestive tract may be sluggish at first, so food should be bland and low in residue to avoid overtaxing the digestive tract.

After diarrhea or infections of the intestines, clear fluids, such as soup, tea, juice, and plenty of water, should make up the bulk of the diet. Gradually the patient may take soft solids, such as eggs, toast, and custards.

Formerly a sick person was kept in bed for a long period of time. Physicians now tend to feel that fairly early ambulation or walking is beneficial in speeding convalescence. Getting out of bed as soon as possible prevents dangerous blood clots in the legs and also boosts the spirits. However, just that a patient feels better does not mean the body is fully healed, and the physician should be consulted before increased activity is permitted. Damage to heart, kidneys, and other vital organs can result from overactivity following infectious diseases. As soon as possible, the patient should be permitted to sit in the sun and have fresh air. Visitors, provided they are not too frequent or the visits too long, are good for the patient's morale. Of course, persons with colds or other illnesses should never be permitted to see the patient.

Some persons appear to enjoy being invalids, an attitude which is enhanced by oversolicitous and oversympathetic friends and family. The convalescent person should begin to do things for himself, to engage in intellectually stimulating activities, and to plan for return to his regular life as soon as possible.

During convalescence, the temperature is taken daily, preferably in the morning. Until the person is able to take a shower or bath, he receives a daily sponge bath in bed by a qualified person. The room should be warm during the time of the bath and only a small part of the body exposed at a time. After the bath, the bed linen should be changed, making sure that the linen fits snugly on the bed without wrinkles which can irritate the skin of the bedridden patient. Although shampooing the hair is generally permissible in most illnesses, it is best to check first with the doctor.

A person who has been in bed for a long period of time will be weak when he first gets up, so before getting out of bed for the first time it is best for him to spend a few minutes each day sitting on the edge of his bed. Next he can be assisted to a chair placed next to the bed where he may remain for a short time. Someone should always help him the first few times he attempts to walk. If dizziness occurs, he should return to bed at once and try again later.

Constipation often occurs in bedridden persons. Generally the physician will prescribe a mild cathartic. Enemas should not be given without consulting the doctor. *See also* BED SORES.

CONVULSION, an involuntary general attack of muscle contraction. In a tonic convulsion, the contractions occur without relaxation; and in a clonic convulsion, alternate contractions of opposing groups of muscles take place. The convulsion may or may not be accompanied by unconsciousness. The word fit commonly denotes an attack of convulsions.

Convulsions occur in epilepsy, asphyxia, poisoning, lockjaw, hydrophobia, apoplexy, meningitis, head injuries, nutritional deficiency, inherited tendency, and in slow-pulse diseases such as anemia of the brain. They may also appear, together with subsequent coma, as a disturbance of late pregnancy. Convulsion in infants is sometimes a reflex action connected with teething, indigestion, rickets, worms, diarrhea, breath holding, an emotional habit which some children develop, and, in particular, high fever, as in tonsillitis. When the convulsion is not brought on by high fever, it may be longer and more serious. Infant mortality rate from convulsions has dropped sharply; in 1900, 1 out of 1,000 births resulted in death from convulsions; in 1948, the figure had been reduced to 1 in 10,000, due mainly to advances in the care of infants.

Although convulsions are often frightening, especially in children, it should be remembered that a convulsion itself is not fatal. The patient should be prevented from injuring himself, but any use of force kept to an absolute minimum. A piece of wood placed between the teeth will keep the patient from biting himself. His clothes should be loosened, especially around the neck and across the chest, and he should be placed on his back, unless he vomits, in which case he is placed on his side. As the patient recovers, an effort should be made to communicate with him and to reassure him. *See also* CHILD CARE; ECLAMPSIA; EPILEPSY.

COPPER SULPHATE, bluish crystals or powder soluble in water, used in swimming pools to destroy fungi or bacteria. In medicine it is beneficial as an astringent and as an agent to induce vomiting.

COPULATION, a technical term for sexual intercourse. *See also* REPRODUCTION SYSTEM.

CORNEA, the tough transparent membrane in front of the eyeball. It occupies about one-sixth of the circumference of the globe of the eye and acts as a kind of magnifying and protective lens for the eye. Various disorders of the cornea result in serious visual defects.

Astigmatism, or blurred vision, may occur when the central part of the cornea is more curved in one spot than in another. Light rays are thus not equally refracted and bent and some of them are focused on the retina and others in front or behind it.

If the cornea is too thin or exceedingly weak, a protrusion or bulge may develop and produce a condition called keratoconus. Vision will become increasingly dim as the cornea changes, and corneal transplantation may be necessary to restore sight.

Interstitial keratitis is an inflammation in which the entire cornea becomes hazy and almost completely covers the iris. Persons with congenital syphilis are often affected.

Traumatic keratitis is a consequence of wounds or injuries of the cornea. Even slight injuries may result in an inflammation which impairs vision. During the healing process of more severe injuries, opaque scar tissue may develop instead of clear corneal tissue and a curtain is drawn over the pupil of the eye, resulting in partial or total blindness.

CORNEAL TRANSPLANTATION, an operation in which a section of clear transparent cornea is substituted in places where opaque cornea has been removed. Corneal tissue is removed from the healthy eyes of persons immediately after death and shipped by air to "eye banks," where doctors can use the tissue as needed. The tissue must be used within thirty-six hours after its removal.

Corneal transplantation has been perfected and now brings great hope of restored vision to those blinded by corneal disorders. However, the success of corneal transplantations presupposes certain conditions. For example, the operation is rarely successful when the whole expanse of the cornea has been affected, and it is not attempted in cases of opaque corneas at birth. Other components of the eye must be in good condition; certain diseases of the eye, such as glaucoma, must first be eliminated before the operation.

CORONARY THROMBOSIS, a rather loose term for a condition more accurately described as acute coronary occlusion or blocking of a coronary artery of the heart. This means that a clot of blood has formed within the heart or blood vessels, usually due to a slowing of the circulation or to alteration of the blood or vessel walls. The ability of the heart to function efficiently depends primarily on the state of the heart muscle or myocardium; thus, life itself depends largely on the state of the blood vessels which bring nourishment to the myocardium. These blood vessels are known as the coronary arteries.

Blocking or occlusion of a coronary artery may develop rapidly or slowly, and coronary disease may be mild or severe, sudden and fatal. If it develops slowly, the myocardium is gradually deprived of its blood supply and cannot function efficiently. The condition manifests itself as angina pectoris which is characterized by pain under the breastbone, produced by exertion and relieved by rest.

If the occlusion occurs rapidly as in acute coronary occlusion, one of two things may happen. Sudden death may result if the blocking involves a large artery or occurs in an already damaged myocardium. If a smaller branch of the coronary arteries is obstructed, the chances are good that the person will recover.

The primary cause of coronary artery disease, and therefore coronary thrombosis, is unknown, but is probably the same as that of arteriosclerosis, which is also not known. In a majority of cases, coronary thrombosis occurs in a coronary artery that has become thickened and hardened, or sclerosed, so that its channel is gradually narrowed. When this narrowing reaches a certain stage, the blood in that channel is liable to clot and completely block the artery, thereby depriving the heart muscle supplied by this artery of its blood supply. This hardening process, or arteriosclerosis, is similar to that which occurs in arteries in any part of the body.

Coronary thrombosis is chiefly a disease of middle life, being relatively rare under the age of forty, and is more common in men than in women. It is found more frequently among professional workers than manual workers. In many instances, the victims are active high-strung people. Mental and emotional stress may precede attacks and persons with angina pectoris, high blood pressure, arteriosclerosis, nephritis, or syphilis are particularly disposed to coronary thrombosis.

Research or prevention of coronary thrombosis has established a link between the disease and a high level of cholesterol, a fatty substance in the blood that tends to clog the arteries. Some nutrition authorities and heart specialists urge that every adult male, particularly if he is obese and has a family history of heart disease, have a periodic cholesterol test. When the cholesterol level goes above the safety point, coronary thrombosis is more likely to occur. In the usual course of coronary thrombosis, the person, even at rest, is suddenly seized with excruciating pain over the heart, which rapidly spreads all over the front of the chest and sometimes down over the abdomen. Often the person will collapse. If efficient treatment is available, this alarming condition gradually improves, but even in the mildest cases a period of at least three weeks' but preferably six weeks' rest in bed is considered essential before activities are resumed.

In the diagnosis of coronary thrombosis, electrocardiography is signif-icant. The electrocardiograph is an instrument which records the electrical activity of the heart by attaching electric wires to the limbs and chest wall of the patient and then recording the heart impulse on photographic paper. When a coronary artery is occluded, the part of the heart muscle supplied by the obstructed artery is no longer able to transmit the impulse, and therefore an abnormal record is obtained. Occlusion of either of the two main coronary arteries produces a characteristic record.

Until the true underlying cause of coronary thrombosis is known, treatment consists in resting the heart as much as possible. The area of the heart muscle, deprived of its vital blood supply by the obstruction of the coronary artery, degenerates. If this degenerative process proceeds too far, the weakened area may rupture, which means death, or the process of healing may be so unsatisfactory that the normal muscle is replaced by fibrous tissues, a poor substitute for active muscle tissue. Therefore the heart is permanently crippled.

One of the most interesting reparative processes in the human body occurs when an artery is blocked. Junctions, anastomoses, develop between the occluded artery above the site of obstruction and neighboring arteries, so that in time the area, originally supplied solely by the occluded artery, is ultimately supplied by neighboring arteries. In some cases this brings the blood supply of the affected area back to normal, while in others an adequate supply is maintained even though it is less than it was originally. This explains why rest is so essential in coronary thrombosis.

Fluid is usually restricted, and a diet of not more than 800 to 900 calories per day is prescribed. Exceedingly difficult breathing may be relieved by oxygen. Formation of blood clots may be decreased or prolonged by the drug dicumarol, or with other anticoagulants. Some surgical procedures are being tried experimentally. *See also* HEART; and Chapter 12, "Diseases of the Heart."

CORTISONE, a highly complex chemical which is a constituent of adrenal cortical extract. Its formula is known, but the chief available basic source is the gallbladder juice of cattle. ACTH, not a synthetic like cortisone, is secreted by the pituitary glands of hogs.

Hydrocortisone, a derivative, has been found more effective than cortisone for local applications, such as to the skin, or for direct injection into joint cavities. These drugs are not a cure for disease; they only relieve and suppress its manifestations.

New preparations have been developed more effective than cortisone without such side effects as disturbance of the water-salt balance. Among them are predmisolone, Meticortin, Kenacort, Aristocort, Decadron, and others.

Cortisone, quickly absorbed in the alimentary canal, is converted into hydrocortisone in the body and is thus a substitute for the natural hormone. It is used in certain acute conditions, such as the collagen diseases including rheumatic fever, rheumatoid arthritis, and polyarteritis. Corticotropin or ACTH stimulates the adrenal cortex to increase hydrocortisone production. An intact adrenal cortex must be present for ACTH to take effect. *See also* ACTH.

CORYZA, an inflammation of the mucous membranes of the nose, characterized by sneezing, discharge of watery mucus, and watering of the eyes. Translated from its original Greek, coryza means a "running at the nose." The term is used as a synonym for head cold, and hay fever is also called allergic coryza.

COSMETICS, preparations intended to beautify the skin, hair, and face. The American public spends almost a billion dollars on cosmetics each year and cosmetic manufacture is among the top twenty industries. The use of cosmetics has a long history. Four thousand years ago Egyptian women sought to beautify themselves in ways that would be familiar to the woman of today—with creams, oils, eye makeup. An Egyptian manuscript of 1200 B.C. gives treatments for gray hair, baldness, and moles. In ancient Rome, dyeing and bleaching hair was common. Honey and barley were reputed to be good skin softeners, and preparations purporting to tighten skin and remove wrinkles were available. Breasts were padded, superfluous hair removed, and skin powdered.

Women of today employ a wide range of cosmetic products and treatments. Face powder is used by most American women. Its practical purpose is to protect the skin against the weather, absorb moisture, cool, relieve irritation, and provide a faint pleasant odor. Esthetically it eliminates the shiny appearance of the skin which women regard unfavorably.

In the past face powder has been composed of various ingredients: vegetable powders of rice, wheat, and corn flour, acadia and tragacanth; mineral powders of chalk, talc, kaolin, magnesium carbonate, bismuth nitrate, or carbonate and zinc oxide, with orris root frequently used to fix them. Today most face powder on the market is a combination of finely pulverized chalky minerals, fatty acids, and soaps blended with perfume and coloring matter. Face powder is more absorbent and adheres more evenly to the skin's surface than toilet powders which contain a large proportion of inert substances such as talc, boric acid, zinc stearate, and perfume and are designed primarily to absorb moisture and perfume the body. For example, talcum powder, developed in this country in the 1890s as a protection against the weather, is magnesium silicate, slightly perfumed. Rouge is merely powder to which coloring matter and binders have been added. In the cream rouges, the coloring is in the waxes and oils.

Powder and rouge do coat the pores, but if used reasonably should not cause any particular enlargement. Pores are openings which are normally almost closed and occasionally open. With the passage of years, some elasticity is lost in these structures and they fail to close as completely as they once did, so that some enlargement of the pores is noted. The danger, although slight, in the use of face powder may be an allergic reaction to some substance in the powder. Some people are especially

sensitive to orris root, now rarely used, and the use of face powders with this ingredient may cause sneezing, eruptions, eye inflammations, asthma, or hay fever.

Creams and lotions are another part of the modern woman's toilette. Galen, one of the fathers of modern medicine who lived about 1800 years ago, developed the first formula for cold cream. It consisted of four ounces of white wax and a pound of oil of roses mixed with some water and perfumed. Today the creams do not differ radically from Galen's cream. They usually consist of mineral or vegetable oil, water in an emulsion brought about by the action of beeswax and borax, triethylamine, alkali stearates or a lanolin alcohol such as cholesterol. At one time some creams contained dangerous salts of lead or mercury.

Most dermatologists, or skin specialists, feel that creams are beneficial in cases of exceedingly dry skin and may help protect against chapping, cracking, and roughness, or soften lines and wrinkles, but not, however, prevent or eliminate them. In the application of cream, the face is usually massaged and, especially if heat is applied, a temporary swelling of the skin surface may occur with an ostensible closure of the pores; as a result, the skin may feel temporarily smoother and softer. Since the skin is a living tissue with certain automatic powers of regeneration, any improvement in its circulation will improve its condition. Proper diet and hygiene is the best way to encourage circulation and a good skin condition. Wrinkling is essentially due to a gradual loss of the elasticity of the connective tissues underlying the skin, which creams and lotions cannot correct. No method has been found for restoring elasticity to connective tissue. Face lifting does not do this; all that it accomplishes is a temporary smoothing by removal of a portion of the sagging skin, a process similar to taking a tuck in a loose dress.

Face creams can be useful as cleansing agents, but creams advertised as "skin foods" and "tissue builders" have no proven value. There is no evidence that vitamins can be absorbed into the skin to nourish it. The skin, like all other tissue in the body, must be nourished by food eaten, digested, and absorbed into the circulation.

Weight-reducing creams are also worthless for the purpose claimed, and creams promising to "rejuvenate" the skin are no better than any other cream. Hormone face creams, which contain estrogen, the female sex hormone, have been the subject of much discussion. Actually, if there is enough estrogen in the cream to restore elasticity to the skin, its use may be dangerous; if there is not enough to produce such an effect the preparation is misleading. So far it would appear that the creams available supply insignificant quantities of the hormone in comparison with medically recognized therapeutic doses. As yet there is no conclusive evidence that harm has resulted from their use although large doses of estrogen may disturb the menstrual cycle.

Vanishing creams are not entirely greaseless and usually contain potassium or sodium stearate and a little glycerin, plus some lanolin and mineral oil. The value of these creams is that in being rubbed in they serve as a slight massage which increases the blood supply to the face and produces a temporary filling-out effect.

Particularly dangerous are removers for wrinkles, freckles, moles, and warts, and bleaches and skin peels. Astringent substances produce a slight and temporary contraction of the cells around the pores but cannot remove wrinkles. Moreover, strong astringents should not be applied to the face. Egg white preparations have been made which stiffen the skin and give the impression that the skin is being straightened although actually it isn't.

Bleach creams have contained ammoniated mercury which acts as an irritant and speeds the peeling of the outer layer of the skin. They may have some bleaching effect, but cannot affect skin blemishes of internal origin. Furthermore, such bleaches can be injurious if applied excessively, too often, or to broken skin surfaces. Liver spots cannot be removed by bleach creams.

Freckles are pigmented areas of skin and freckle removers are designed to peel the skin slowly. The danger is that any preparation strong enough to remove this pigmentation may be strong enough to affect underlying tissues. Skin peels cannot remove skin blemishes of internal origin, and in addition often contain salicylic acid, resorcin, arsenic, and carbolic acid, any one of which may be dangerous to tender skin. Mole removers also generally contain a caustic which, again, if strong enough to destroy a mole can also damage surrounding tissue. The primary danger here is that every mole is a potential site of skin cancer which an irritant, such as a mole-remover preparation, can excite to malignancy. The only wise course in treating skin blemishes of any kind is to consult a physician, preferably a skin specialist or dermatologist. In the interim, harmless preparations are available which can be applied as a cover or a base for powder to diminish or conceal the defect.

Although occasionally women may be sensitive to dyes in rouges, lipsticks, or creams, more commonly a sensitivity exists to dyes for hair, eyelashes, and eyebrows. Practically all effective dyes contain ingredients that may be poisonous to some people, and may have effects ranging from serious eye injuries, skin inflammation, infection, chronic poisoning, and ulceration to baldness, fragility of hair, and loss of hair luster. Dyes which are completely harmless, the vegetable dyes such as henna or indigo, are also relatively ineffective. The metallic salts used in metallic dyes vary greatly in harmfulness. Bismuth and mercury are highly toxic. Dyes of the lead sulphur type may be poisonous and should not be used if there is a break in the scalp. Caution should also be taken against oral contact. Dyes containing a large proportion of copper salts can be poisonous, although dyes in current use contain only a minute amount of copper salts. Silver nitrate is less dangerous, but dyes containing it can produce skin irritations or blackened skin patches. Dyes containing pyrogallol, with metallic salts such as the sulphates of copper or iron, can irritate or poison. Metallic dyes act slowly, and do not penetrate the hair shaft but deposit a coating on the outside of the hair. For this reason, such preparations have sometimes been advertised as "hair-color restorers," but in general they reduce the tensile strength of the hair and tend to rub off, sometimes staining the scalp.

Aniline-derivative dyes, organic chemicals made from coal tar, act quickly and penetrate within the hair, and do not rub off or stain the scalp. Their danger is a tendency to produce dermatitis in some sensitive people and pave the way for serious infection. Some aniline-derivative dyes are safe as they are essentially nontoxic and nonsensitizing, but as a precaution a preliminary patch test is advisable before using them. This test should be repeated before each application since a person can be insensitive at one time and sensitive at another.

Dye should never be used for eyelashes and eyebrows. Mascaras or colorings with a carbon black base are harmless but preparations of aniline origin or metallic salt, particularly the former, can cause serious injury to the eyes if carelessly applied.

Chemical depilatories should be used with great caution since any substance capable of dissolving hair can also injure or irritate the skin. Even though a substance is safe for most people, there may be a few who are sensitive to it.

If reactions to cosmetics are apparent, a physician may diagnose the condition as allergic and try to discover the causative agent. Often this involves a patch test, the application of preparations to a sensitive part of the skin which is then covered with gauze. At the end of twenty-four hours, if no irritation or eruption is evident, the cosmetic can probably be used safely. Cosmetic manufacturers now produce a complete line of preparations designed for sensitive and allergic people. *See also* DEPILATORY.

COUGH, a sudden violent expulsion of air after deep inspiration and closure of the glottis, the free margins of the vocal chords. It is a symptom rather than a disease itself. The most common cause of cough is irritation or inflammation of the delicate lining of the bronchial tubes or other parts of the respiratory apparatus. A foreign substance, allergy from inhaled substances, tumors of the lungs, or nervous disease may all cause a cough. The purpose of the cough is protective. The body tries by coughing to remove the irritation or obstruction from the breathing passages. Since coughing may spread germs it is advisable to cover the mouth and nose with a tissue or handkerchief when coughing. Coughing may occur in an asthmatic attack when the passageways of the lungs are constricted or narrowed.

By listening to the chest with a stethoscope, a physician may detect signs of mucus within the chest or abnormalities of breathing which point to localization of an obstruction or infection in the chest. X-rays also detect obstructions or inflammations of the chest which produce coughing. Tuberculosis or silicosis and other diseases which cause scarring in the lungs may aggravate coughing, and a cough is especially apt to occur in certain diseases such as whooping cough. A cough may persist as a habit after the infection has been eradicated.

Any cough should be taken seriously, especially one which continues longer than two or three weeks or outlives the cold it originally accompanied. In such cases, the doctor usually examines the sputum to determine the nature of the infection causing the cough, or takes x-rays for signs of tumors. If simple infection is causing the cough, it should be thoroughly treated; an infection incompletely treated can lead to permanent lung damage. Surgery may be indicated when there is evidence of tumor growth, or special treatment in the case of tuberculosis.

Simple coughs are often relieved by medications designed to lessen phlegm within the bronchial passageways and to relieve muscle tension there. Inhalation of steam also loosens phlegm which can then be expelled by coughing. Hot drinks will relax lung tissues. Smoking and dusty atmospheres are irritating to these sensitive tissues and should be avoided. Allergic coughs can be relieved by antihistamines, but detection and treatment of the source of the cough is necessary for long-range benefit.

CRAB LICE, the body lice which attach themselves to the hair of the groin and also to underarm hair, eyelashes, and eyebrows. They are square in shape with legs well developed and adapted to clinging. This parasite feeds from the skin near the hair to which it clings, leaving pinpoint marks on the skin and causing severe itching. Phthirius pubis, the species which infests man, is ordinarily limited to the pubic region and is usually spread by direct personal contact. The female of the species, considerably larger than the male, lays eggs, ten to fifteen at a time, attaching them to hair at the site of contagion, and continues to lay eggs for fourteen days or until her death. The eggs hatch in about a week and there are three moultings in a period of about two weeks. Formerly difficult to eradicate, crab lice now succumb quickly to applications of DDT and other chemicals and ointments in a form suitable for application to the pubic area. These are obtainable by prescription. The venerable standard blue ointment is also satisfactory. *See also* LICE.

CRAMPS, sudden involuntary contraction of a muscle, or of a group of muscles.

Cramps in the calf of the leg, occurring especially during sleep, are frequent. They may be relieved by forcibly bending the knee as far as it will go, so that the muscular contraction can be released. The muscle should then be vigorously rubbed.

Nocturnal leg cramps in anemic girls sometimes occur because the leg is not receiving sufficient blood. However, the flow of blood to the legs will be increased if the person affected will get out of bed and stand up briefly until the pain departs.

Cramps of the stomach are much more painful and common than leg cramps. Application of heat is often beneficial and sometimes a drug to expel the gas from the stomach may be helpful. One teaspoon of bicarbonate of soda mixed with soda water, peppermint water, or plain water may be used for this purpose. The possibility of appendicitis should always be considered with abdominal cramps. If the cramps are not relieved within a reasonable time, a physician should be called.

When stomach cramps occur during the first day of a woman's menstrual period, the application of heat will often afford relief. Various drugs beneficial in relieving these cramps are now available. A woman who suffers persistently and severely from this type of cramp, however, should consult her doctor. *See also* ABDOMINAL PAIN; APPENDICITIS; COLIC; DYSMENORRHEA.

CRETINISM, a condition originating during fetal life or early infancy in which mental and physical development are stunted due to a severe thyroid deficiency.

The cretin may appear normal at birth, but his mental and physical deficiency usually becomes quite obvious during the first year. Characteristic symptoms of cretinism are rough dry skin, a distended abdomen, a protruding swollen tongue, apathy, and stolidity.

In many cases, regular administration of thyroid extract in early life has helped to improve the condition, but the treatment must be prolonged or even permanent.

Cretinism is more common in regions where endemic goiter is severe; otherwise it occurs sporadically.

CROSS MATCHING OF BLOOD, the technique used to determine before a transfusion whether or not the blood to be given to a patient will mix safely with his own blood. Not all human blood is the same and death can occur if cross matching is not accurately done.

Cross matching of blood deals specifically with the oxygen-carrying cells in the blood stream which are the erythrocytes or red blood cells. A deficiency of red blood cells causes anemia when hemorrhage occurs and is dangerous because the body does not have enough cells to carry oxygen to primary structures such as the brain and kidneys.

The four main groups of red blood cells, discovered by Landsteiner in 1900, are A, B, AB, and O. A person develops a certain type of cells through heredity just as he inherits blond hair or blue eyes. In addition, each cell may carry a second factor called the Rh factor, present in 85 per cent of the population. The absence of the Rh factor is called Rh negative. Therefore, blood may be grouped as A-Rh positive, A-Rh negative, B-Rh positive, B-Rh negative, AB-Rh positive, AB-Rh negative, O-Rh positive, and O-Rh negative.

During cross matching, several drops of the blood cells are mixed with blood from the donor, warmed in an incubator to simulate body conditions, and examined under the microscope to detect any tendency to form a clot or mix poorly. If this happens, the two bloods are said to be incompatible. Typing of blood cells requires only a few minutes and cross matching about an hour.

See also BLOOD TRANSFUSION; BLOOD TYPES.

CROUP, a disease scientifically known as acute obstructive laryngitis, diphtheria, or occasionally streptococcus sore throat. Croup really refers to a single symptom of throat infection since it is used to describe any condition characterized by a harsh brassy cough and difficult respiration with a spasm of the larynx and a wheezing sound. Often caused by viruses, croup may be a secondary infection in cases of lowered resistance or other bacterial infections. Although it can affect adults, croup usually occurs in small children between one and six years of age. This age group is probably affected because it cannot easily cough up the bacteria-laden mucus which drips down the throat. The shorter channel to the larynx also permits easier infection.

In croup, the laryngeal cords or the vocal cords are inflamed and swollen so that breathing has a wheezy sound. The child coughs constantly, endeavoring to get rid of the obstruction. In spasmodic croup, spasm of the cords occurs which makes them red and pulls them toward each other without the presence of any obvious infection. A form of spasmodic croup in small children is laryngismus stridulus or "false croup." The infant breathes laboriously and respiration may even stop; the face flushes and then turns blue. However, after a short time, relaxation of the spasm sets in. During a crying spell, breathing will become normal again.

The most significant step in croup is to determine exactly what is wrong.

The most serious form of the throat infection is that due to the diphtheria germ. In diphtheria, a thick adherent membrane forms in the throat. In severe forms of streptococcus of the throat, a membrane also forms, but usually is less thick and white. In the worst forms of croup, the fever is high, breathing excessively labored, and the child is exceedingly ill. In simpler cases of croup, the doctor usually advises that the child be put to bed promptly and given plenty of fluids. Steam inhalations, which may or may not be medicated with benzoin or other soothing oils, according to the doctor, usually provide noticeable relief. In cases of high fever, cool moist air may be preferred to hot steam. If coughing is severe, the doctor may prescribe sedatives which will relieve the spasms. An ice bag is sometimes used to relieve a sore throat.

The seriously dangerous cases of croup are those in which there is complete obstruction to breathing, and immediate medical attention is urgent. In these cases, the doctor may have oxygen supplied to the child through a small tube inserted into the opening remaining in the throat. A tube, known as an intubation tube, may be put into the throat which assures the passage of air through the larynx. In the most severe cases, a tracheotomy is performed; an opening is made directly into the windpipe from the outside which permits the patient to continue breathing while the inflammation is healing. Any case with severe swelling in the throat and difficulty in breathing should be regarded as serious, since stoppage of breathing for even a few minutes may be fatal.

CURETTAGE, the scraping of a body cavity with an instrument, such as a curette.

CUSHING'S SYNDROME, a group of symptoms associated with Cushing's disease, which was first described in 1932 by Dr. Harvey Williams Cushing, famous American brain surgeon.

The disease, which seems to affect women primarily, is due to a tumor in the pituitary gland. Among its symptoms are excessive obesity of the abdomen and buttocks, color changes of face and hands which make the skin look bruised and stretched, brittleness of bones, and suppression or lowering of sexual functions. Diabetes often is a complication. Women with Cushing's disease develop excessive hair growth, such as mustaches and beards.

CUTANEOUS SENSES, the four senses associated with the skin: touch, heat, cold, and pain. The sense of pain is especially well distributed over the surface of the body. The senses of heat, cold, and touch are responsive to lighter stimulation than the sense of pain. Pain develops as a sensation from stronger stimulation, and if the stimulus producing a sensation of touch, heat, or cold is increased, the sensation becomes pain.

CUTS, gashes in the skin made by a sharp-edged object such as a knife or broken glass. All cuts, even very small ones, must be carefully treated to avoid infection. They should be thoroughly cleansed with soap and water, and then covered with a clean piece of linen or sterile gauze. If the cut bleeds profusely, as it often does when blood vessels have been severed, pressure must be applied to control the flow of blood. Strong antiseptics should be avoided, but tincture of iodine, metaphen, and other mild antiseptics can be applied to destroy surface bacteria.

If the wound is deep or dirty, a doctor should be consulted, or the person taken to the nearest hospital. Suturing or sewing together a deep cut will help the healing process and avoid unsightly scars. An injection of tetanus antitoxin may be necessary to prevent lockjaw. In deep cuts, a physician must frequently determine whether or not a tendon has been severed, as tendon repairs must be made as soon as possible after the accident. A physician should always be consulted in cases of deep cuts. *See also* Chapter 28, "First Aid."

CYANOSIS, a condition which may occur during the course of certain disorders of the respiratory, nervous, brain, and circulatory systems. The face, lips, and skin may acquire a bluish tinge. Cyanosis is caused by defects in the oxidation of the blood and may also be a side effect of sulfonamides and other drugs which influence oxidation.

CYCLOPROPANE, a saturated cyclic hydrocarbon gas which has the odor of petroleum benzene. It is a potent but relatively nonirritating and nontoxic drug employed as an inhalation anesthetic—for example, to les-sen intense labor pains. Cyclopropane works rapidly and rarely leaves after-effects.

CYST, literally a bladder containing fluid. In medicine it denotes a sac which contains fluids or other semi-solid morbid substances. Cysts develop in many parts of the body and are of all sizes and degrees of severity. While their cause cannot always be determined, cysts are apt to form lumpy swellings beneath the mucous membranes or beneath the skin. A cyst is ordinarily movable, while a tumor, a new growth of cells and tissues, is firmly rooted in the tissues.

Some harmless or benign forms of cysts do not require medical attention; others do. The most frequent location of cysts which demand surgery are in the skin and glands. Whenever the opening of the glandular cell or organ is blocked, the accumulation of fluid produces a cyst. Cysts are also quite frequent in various parts of the female reproductive organs and in breasts with cracked nipples, which develop during nursing.

Among other substances, cysts may enclose foreign bodies (adventitious cysts), gas (air cysts), jelly-like substances (colloid cysts), and others.

CYSTITIS, inflammation of the bladder, acute or chronic, incited through infection by various bacilli to which the bladder is susceptible. It occurs more frequently in women than men, and pregnant women are especially vulnerable. Male inclination to cystitis is increased by the presence of stones or malignant growths. Women are often predisposed to infections of the vagina or adjacent organs which spread to the bladder.

One of the common symptoms of cystitis is a frequent urge to urinate, which is increased by standing or moving. In many cases pus is found in the urine, and painful spasms during urination radiate into the upper parts of the body. In men, pains from the lower abdomen or rectum may spread into the penis and thighs. Frequently a low fever is present and in more severe cases a rapid pulse, chills, and urinary retention.

Bed rest, hot sitz baths, consumption of large quantities of fluid, evacuation of bowels, and a soft diet without spices, condiments, alcohol, and other stimulants are the first steps in treatment. Under professional supervision, cystitis responds well to antibiotics and sulfa drugs. Among the new preparations used are furadantin and mandelamine. Irrigation of the bladder and elimination of acid in the urine are helpful, and severe pain has been relieved by prescribed suppositories. Should the symptoms of acute cystitis persist, the condition may become chronic. As the kidneys may be damaged, it is advisable to have an x-ray examination to determine the extent of the infection.

CYSTOSCOPE, an instrument used in diagnosis and treatment of lesions of the urinary bladder, ureter, and kidney. It is inserted into the opening of the male penis or the female urethra and permits the physician to look directly into the bladder. The outer sheath of a cystoscope incorporates a lighting system and room for the passage of operative devices.

DANDRUFF. *See* SEBORRHEA.

DDT, short for dichlor-diphenyl-trichloro-ethane, a potent insecticide developed during World War II. As it is especially effective as a delousing agent, after the war its use successfully lessened the spread of typhus in war-ravaged areas. DDT has also been used widely in tropical countries to control jungle yellow fever. It is most effective in and about the home against flies, mosquitoes, lice, and chiggers. The DDT may be sprayed (5 per cent DDT solution) or dusted (10 per cent DDT). This insecticide has the advantage of longer-lasting effectiveness than other chemicals. It can be purchased at most drug, hardware, or food stores. A mixture of benzyl benzoate, DDT, and sulphur used on the skin has been found effective by physicians in eradicating the mites that cause scabies.

DEADLY NIGHTSHADE POISONING. Deadly nightshade or belladonna is a plant whose roots and leaves are used medically in various forms. Atropine is a white crystalline alkaloid obtained from belladonna.

Symptoms of deadly nightshade poisoning are dryness in the throat and mouth with difficulty in swallowing, dryness of the skin, dilation of the pupils of the eyes, and blurred vision. The skin may develop a red rash, resembling scarlet fever rash. The pulse is more rapid and the person may suffer from delirium and hallucinations.

A doctor should be called immediately, and the person induced to vomit. Afterward give him strong tea (the tannic acid acts as an antidote) or hot coffee as a stimulant.

DEAF MUTISM. A person who can neither hear nor speak suffers from deaf mutism, or is "deaf and dumb." The term applies particularly if the inability to speak is due to congenital or early deafness. In other words, although he may have normal speech organs, the victim cannot form sounds because he has never heard.

Little can be done to cure such conditions. Surgical treatment of the ear and throat is of a little value. However, the victims can be taught to understand a spoken language. Ordinarily the deaf mute can learn this skill by observing and imitating the lips of others. If the mastery of this technique, lip reading, should be too difficult, the manual alphabet can be learned with relative ease by any deaf mute of normal intelligence. The education of deaf mutes must begin in the home, with the help of the family. Schools and institutions are available which specialize in the training of the deaf mute, and a child may be sent to one nearest his home. Schools for deaf mutes admit all age groups, some beginning the training of children as early as two to three years of age. In recent years, new techniques of teaching have been progressing with exceptionally fine results.

DEAFNESS, the complete or nearly complete loss of hearing due to a variety of conditions which may affect the functions of the ear. Deafness is congenital or acquired. It may be caused by an infection in one or both ears; result from another infection in the body such as meningitis, scarlet fever, measles, whooping cough, or pneumonia; or be due to damage to the eardrum from a blow or accident. It is sometimes caused by hysteria. If the ear is subjected to incessant loud noise over a long period of time, hearing may be impaired, and a sudden violent explosion can cause instantaneous deafness.

Otosclerosis, one of the most serious forms of deafness, is caused by bony growths in the inner ear which hinder the conduction of sound and thus impair the hearing. As the person grows older, these growths become increasingly worse. An ear operation called fenestration has been successfully performed by ear surgeons in cases of otosclerosis. In this operation a window is drilled into the labyrinth of the inner ear, thus permitting proper conduction of sound waves and compensating for the loss of function of the small bones of the inner ear due to the growths. Another operation mobilizes the small bones of the ear.

One of the greatest problems in medical diagnosis is to determine the exact degree of deafness. Ear specialists give the deaf person a number of highly technical scientific tests. The audiometer is one of the devices used in testing defective hearing. When loss of hearing is due to infection, steps must be taken immediately by the doctor to stop the progress of the infection. If pus or infectious material forms in the external ear, the pressure should be released promptly. The eardrum may have to be punctured before permanent damage occurs. Infections in the throat or back of the nasal passages which connect with the internal auditory system should be given attention to prevent them from spreading. Any loss of hearing, however slight and regardless of cause, should be promptly attended to by an ear specialist.

The development of the hearing aid has been a boon to the deaf and hard of hearing. Effective hearing aids at reasonable cost to fit various types of deafness have been developed. Generally the two types of hearing aids are (1) those which act by air conduction and (2) those which act by bone conduction. Tests must be made by specialists to determine the type of hearing aid best suited to the individual. In the case of children, the hearing aid should be fitted as soon as possible and the child taught to use it correctly so that he can adjust to his condition early in life.

Lip reading may also assist the deaf or partially deaf person to lead a normal active life, and schools are available where persons of all ages can learn to lip read. The person whose hearing is defective should not retreat within himself and retire from the life about him. With the help of ear specialists, hearing aids, and lip reading, plus patience and courage, he can overcome his condition and live a full life. *See also* OTOSCLEROSIS.

DECAY, DENTAL. *See* DENTAL CARIES.

DEFECATION, the act of elimination from the bowel. *See also* CONSTIPATION.

DEFICIENCY DISEASES, abnormal conditions or diseases caused by the absence in the diet of certain necessary substances, such as vitamins, proteins, amino acids, minerals, usually supplied by food. Some of the deficiency diseases are rickets, due to a lack of vitamin D; scurvy, due to a lack of vitamin C; pellagra, associated for the most part with a lack of nicotinic acid, one of the B complex vitamins; xerophthalmia and night blindness, coming from a deficiency of vitamin A; beriberi, caused by thiamine deficiency; and goiter, related to a lack of iodine.

With the increased knowledge of nutrition and of the relation between diet and health, great steps have been made toward eradicating deficiency diseases. With the exception of rickets and pellagra, the United States is relatively free of deficiency diseases. *See also* NUTRITION; VITAMINS; and Chapter 4, "Diet and Health."

DEGENERATIVE DISEASES. The deterioration or breakdown of important organs of the body, such as the heart, liver, and kidneys, leads to disorders called degenerative diseases. A group of degenerative diseases of the nervous system, such as various forms of sclerosis, both hereditary and nonhereditary, produces serious paralysis in various parts of the body.

DEHYDRATION refers to the loss of water from the body. Sometimes it occurs from perspiration due to overheating in warm weather or overexertion. The remedy is an increase in the intake of fluids such as water, fruit juices, or milk. Abnormal dehydration may result from fever, diarrhea, vomiting, or other disorders. Such conditions may be serious and the intake of fluids should be supervised by a physician or nurse. Salt deficiency may accompany both normal and abnormal dehydration. This may be remedied by adding salt tablets to the diet or by the injection of saline solution in the case of severe illness.

The dangers of dehydration lie in the development of acidosis and the accumulation of waste products in the body. If the acidosis is severe as in diabetes, injections of an alkalizing solution are often given.

Much progress has been made recently in the development of techniques for correcting dehydration, and countless lives are saved by the prompt application of such measures.

DELIRIUM TREMENS, an acute disorder of the mind and body which results from alcoholism. Visual and auditory hallucinations as well as the physical symptoms of delirium tremens may follow abstinence after prolonged addiction, or may occur at any point in a long debauch.

Ordinarily an attack of delirium tremens lasts from two to ten days. The mind wanders and sensations of pain, itching, burning, and prickling of the skin torment the victim. His hearing and vision are disturbed and he may imagine he sees animals and loathsome insects of magnified size. In short, he has "the horrors." Muttering and muscular tremors are also characteristic of this state.

The control of delirium tremens is difficult. The mental aspects are important. The lack of food during a long drinking bout brings on deficiencies of such vital elements in the diet as thiamine and nicotinic acid which are important to replace in order to eliminate some of the nervous and muscular manifestations. Therefore, concentrated feeding of vitamins is essential in the treatment. Rest, too, is essential and if drugs and sleep producers are used these should be administered under most careful medical supervision.

Proper circulation of the blood must be maintained. Until recently the victims were often placed in strait jackets or otherwise forcibly restrained and the resulting blocking of proper circulation by tight straps frequently brought on collapse of the heart and even death. In present-day treatment rest, nourishment, and a more positive approach to the total problem of the alcoholic yield better results.

DELIRIUM, a severe mental disturbance in which the sufferer is confused and disturbed by delusions and hallucinations. Extreme restlessness and excitement generally accompany delirium. The chief cause of a delirious state may be high fever, but it may result from mental disease or disorder as well as a variety of conditions stemming from structural damage of the brain.

When delirium is produced by high fever, the application of ice packs and cold compresses and other measures to lower the temperature and calm the patient are helpful. Low, muttering delirium may occur toward the end of a fever. *See also* FEVER; MENTAL DISORDERS.

DELIVERY. *See* PREGNANCY AND PRENATAL CARE; and Chapter 6, "Prenatal Care and Childbirth."

DELOUSING AGENTS. *See* DDT; LICE.

DELUSIONS, false beliefs manifested by victims of mental disturbances. A common type of delusion, occurring in melancholia, is one in which the person thinks that certain organs are missing. Frequently a delusion is the first sign of mental disorder, and calls for prompt professional attention rather than futile attempts at reasoning with the unfortunate person. *See also* Chapter 22, "Mental Illness."

DEMENTIA refers to loss or deterioration of mental faculties and is characterized by confusion, lack of contact with reality, and apathy.

DEMENTIA PRAECOX, the old word, no longer used, for schizophrenia. *See* SCHIZOPHRENIA.

DEMULCENT, any gummy or oily substance which has a soothing effect on any part of the human body, especially on mucous membranes. The white of an egg, if it acts as a mollifying agent to the stomach, is also a demulcent. Among the best-known demulcents are glycerin, acacia, flax seed, Irish and Iceland mosses, licorice, sassafras, slippery elm, and starch paste.

DENGUE (deng' ghee), an acute endemic and epidemic virus infection with severe symptoms which, however, rarely lasts longer than seven days, and from which recovery is almost always complete. The infection is transmitted by the same mosquito, the Aëdes aegypti, that spreads yellow fever. Hot weather and heavy rainfall provide ideal conditions for breeding both the mosquito and the virus, and epidemics of dengue are common in tropical areas. During World War II, outbreaks of dengue among soldiers stationed in the Pacific area were frequent. Epidemics have occurred in recent years in the southeastern and gulf sections of the United States, in Australia, Egypt, Greece, and Indo-China. In some areas, epidemics take place at five-year intervals, and sometimes affect more than half the population. An attack of dengue ordinarily produces immunity for five years or more in most people.

About four to ten days after a person has been bitten by an infected mosquito, the symptoms begin suddenly, with severe headache, extreme exhaustion, and pain behind the eyes which is aggravated by any movement of the eyelids. Within a few hours, intense pain in the back and joints makes any movement difficult. Because of this characteristic pain, dengue is also called "breakbone fever." Temperature rises rapidly, sometimes reaching 106°, the pulse is slowed, and the blood pressure drops. Often a pale pink, spotty rash appears, the face is flushed, the eyeballs congested, and some glands enlarged. After three or four days, the fever suddenly drops, there is profuse sweating, and the other symptoms disappear. This period of apparent improvement lasts about twenty-four hours, then temperature rises again and the symptoms return. A characteristic rash, resembling scarlet fever rash, appears over the knees, ankles, and elbows and sometimes spreads to the trunk, palms, and soles. The rash and symptoms continue until the fever drops again, usually within two days or on the sixth or seventh day of illness. Peeling of the skin frequently follows.

Convalescence is generally slow. Slow pulse, low blood pressure, and general loss of strength may persist for weeks. Bed rest and good nursing care are helpful. Physicians recommend large quantities of fluids, an ice cap on the head to reduce headache, and, if necessary, drugs to relieve the body aches and pains. To control the mosquitoes which spread the disease, repellents, DDT sprays, and screening should be used, and breeding places of mosquitoes detected and destroyed. Persons who are exposed to bites by the mosquito should wear protective clothing at all times and use repellents. Vaccines for immunization against dengue have been developed and may be effective in preventing the disease. *See also* AËDES AEGYPTI.

DENTAL CARIES, another name for tooth decay, a process in which bacteria form on the surface of the teeth and act upon carbohydrates to produce acids which gradually break down the enamel and dentine. Focal infection and ultimate decay and destruction of the teeth may result. To keep the teeth healthy, both preventive and corrective measures are necessary.

Prevention of tooth decay begins with proper diet. A balanced diet that includes meat, milk, eggs, fruit, and vegetables is essential for mouth health. Sweets, starches, and carbohydrates, such as candy, bread, and potatoes, which tend to cause acid formation should be limited. Regular

brushing of the teeth and use of dental floss is important. The dentist can demonstrate the correct way to brush the teeth. Teeth cleaning is most effective when it follows eating. Experiments in adding fluorine to the water supply have resulted in a significant drop in tooth decay. Another advance has been the discovery of a relationship between dental caries and Vitamin C deficiency.

Regular visits to the dentist for x-rays, checkup, cleaning, and treatment should be a routine part of dental care. Children should be taken early for their first visit to the dentist with semiannual appointments thereafter. The dentist uses fillings as the best means of stopping decay in a cavity and also of preventing new cavities from forming. Fillings may be made of amalgams, cast gold inlays, or gold foil. By removing the decayed portion of the tooth and treating the tooth to receive the filling, the decaying process is stopped. The patient should, of course, follow whatever treatment the dentist recommends. *See also* DENTIFRICE; FLUORIDATION; TEETH.

DENTIFRICE, a powder, paste, or other substance used in cleaning the teeth. The effectiveness of a dentifrice in combatting tooth decay is one of the most debated subjects in modern dentistry and medicine. Many dentists believe that despite advertising claims a dentifrice does little more than help keep the teeth clean.

Some toothpastes, for example, are supposed to kill germs in the mouth. However, the first breath taken after brushing the teeth will introduce new germs which the previous brushing will not affect. Microorganisms exist throughout nature and a variety of them may be found in the mouth at all times. Other dentifrices claim to counteract mouth acidity by their alkaline content, although the value of mouth alkalinity is not even established. A variety of other claims exist, such as sterilization of the gums and digestion of food particles in the mouth.

The significant fact regarding all these preparations is that they are only in the mouth for a very short time, and therefore any effect they may have, apart from the actual cleaning, is temporary.

Normal teeth and gums do not need any special antiseptic. A rinse with plain water is as useful as any mouthwash. However, some people like the refreshing aftertaste of mouthwash. Most mouthwashes follow a fixed formula of the National Formulary, and are known as liquor antisepticus or liquor antisepticus alkalinus. Similar preparations are sold as Listerine and Glycothymaline.

When a serious infection, such as trench mouth or Vincent's angina, canker sores or blisters, exists in the mouth, the dentist applies substances, proven by use and experiment to be germicidal, to the infected areas. These include hydrogen peroxide or sodium perborate.

Research is being done to develop a control effective against tooth decay. Products containing penicillin or chlorophyll have been produced and sold, but the claims for them have not been scientifically established.

Fluorine in the form of sodium fluoride added to supplies of drinking water has been tested and found effective in reducing tooth decay, and increasing tests further corroborate this. Similarly sodium fluoride in a diluted solution can be directly applied to the teeth by the dentist.

Although there is still no means of preventing tooth decay, certain precautionary measures can be taken by everyone. Thorough brushing of the teeth morning and evening, and preferably also after heavy consumption of sugary things such as candy, is a deterrent to decay. A good balanced diet, containing adequate amounts of proteins, carbohydrates, minerals, and vitamins, particularly A, C, and D, and calcium is an important protective measure for the health of the teeth as well as of the entire body. According to studies cited by the *Journal of the American Dental Association,* reduction of sugar intake will decrease dental caries in about 90 per cent of the people. Although some carbohydrate is essential in the diet, most people can benefit by a reduction of sugar-containing foods. *See also* FLUORIDATION; VINCENT'S ANGINA.

DENTINE, the major portion of a tooth, the chalky part, found under the enamel and under the cement of the root. Specifically it resembles bone, except that it is harder and denser and differs in structure. Dentine contains numerous tiny tubelike passages which not only branch outward toward the surface of the tooth but also contain the same pulplike material which is found in the center of the tooth.

When exposed to the air, dentine may sometimes be sensitive, and occasionally it is defective in its lime content. This deficiency, which is inherited, gives the teeth a milky brown appearance. *See also* DENTAL CARIES; TEETH.

DENTURE, an artificial restoration of several teeth. If all the teeth of one jaw are replaced, the structure is known as a full denture; and if fewer teeth are concerned, the substitute is called a partial denture.

DEPILATORY, an agent to remove hair. The hair-removing agent may be a chemical paste, a wax, razor, abrasive, or electric current. When a chemical-paste depilatory is used, the paste is placed on the skin for a short time and the hair comes off when the paste is removed. Care should be taken to leave the paste on for only the necessary time since it might be injurious to the skin if left on longer. The skin should be washed as soon as the paste has been removed, and a cold cream may be applied to soothe the skin. In the wax method, liquid wax is applied to the skin and allowed to harden. The hair comes off when the layer of wax is removed from the skin. Here the primary precaution is that the wax be applied at the proper temperature to avoid burning the skin. Electrolysis attacks the hair root, and if done by a skilled operator when the hair is still fine and thin the hair may be permanently destroyed, leaving no mark on the skin. *See also* COSMETICS; HAIR; SKIN.

DEPRESSION. *See* INVOLUTIONAL MELANCHOLIA; MANIC-DEPRESSIVE PSYCHOSIS; NEUROSIS; and Chapter 22, "Mental Illness."

DERMATITIS, the technical term for inflammation of the skin. *See also* ACNE; SKIN; and Chapter 20, "Diseases of the Skin."

DERMOID CYST, a saclike growth found, for example, in the ovary or in the chest, and containing such startling elements as hair, skin, and teeth. This type of cyst, probably prenatal in origin, grows slowly and does not spread through the body. As the person grows older, however, the dermoid cyst may irritate parts of the body. Therefore its removal, by surgery, is usually recommended. Dermoid cysts do not tend to recur. *See also* CANCER; CYST; SKIN.

DEVIL'S GRIP, also known as pleurodynia and Bornholm disease, an infection caused by the coxahackie virus which produces intense spasms of pain in the chest wall. Sometimes devil's grip occurs in epidemics throughout the United States, almost invariably during warm weather. The virus is present in discharges from the nose and throat and the infection is spread by contact. Children and young people are most often affected.

After an incubation period of from two to four days, sudden short but extremely sharp spasms of pain in the chest wall and lining of the chest, or pleura, appear. The pain may vary from day to day from a dull pressure to an excruciating seizure. Coughing, sneezing, and even deep breathing aggravate the pain. Fever is generally present.

Although the pain is agonizing during the spasms, there are usually no serious complications. A chest binder or the application of heat is often helpful.

DEXTROSE, one of the sugars produced by the digestion of starches in the body. Made chemically, dextrose is widely used in medicine to supply energy to patients who cannot be fed by mouth. It is readily absorbed into the body and is usually fed intravenously. Dextrose is also useful in prevention of circulatory failure.

DIABETES, the ordinary designation for the condition in which the body cannot utilize sugar normally, causing unusually high sugar levels in blood and urine. Properly speaking, however, the medical term is diabetes mellitus, and is entirely unrelated to a completely different disease, diabetes insipidus.

The essential factor in diabetes mellitus is insufficiency of insulin, which is secreted by specialized cells in the pancreas. This lack has a profound effect on the body. Sugar is produced by the intestinal digestion of carbohydrate foods. It is then transported in the blood to the liver where it is converted into glycogen which can be stored in the liver and muscles and be readily converted to sugar for fuel when the muscles need it. When insulin is lacking, the body is unable to transform sugar into glycogen. Then the sugar remains in the blood, is excreted in the urine, and is unavailable to the tissues and organs that require it.

Diabetes insipidus is characterized by excessive overactivity of the kidneys and overexcretion of urine. Its source is uncertain, but it is believed to be related to some disorder in the central nervous system that involves the area of the brain with which the pituitary gland is associated.

Until the early 1920's, diabetes mellitus was an extremely serious disease. All diabetics died young and a diabetic child had a short life expectancy. The discovery of insulin and its proper use in restoring order to the disrupted sugar metabolism of the diabetic has removed fear of this disease. Although diabetes requires constant attention and skillful management, even diabetic children grow up to live active lives, marry, and become parents. Dr. E. P. Joslin, an American physician who has treated diabetics for more than half a century and is one of the authorities in the field, says that in 1900 his patients averaged a life span of approximately five years. Today they can exect to live out their normal life expectancy.

Diabetes today is less menacing than a major infection. The discovery and use of insulin have made the control of diabetes possible. But insulin does not cure the condition. It can only substitute for a critical deficiency. If this outside source is discontinued, the body will be in as dangerous a condition as before.

The basic concept of diabetes is that a disorder, such as an infection or a hereditary tendency, affects the pancreas or the insulin-producing parts of it. Excessive eating over a long time or emotional stress or mental shock can incite temporary attacks of diabetes. Studies now suggest that more may be involved than pancreatic disease alone. The pituitary and adrenal glands may be implicated and the whole diabetic process more complex than was formerly believed.

Without treatment, the diabetic, although eating and drinking in an endeavor to satisfy a perpetual hunger and thirst because of the sugar circulating in his blood, loses weight, becomes weak, and is susceptible to nervous complications. He is far more prone to infection than others, especially to tuberculosis, and is disposed to gangrene and skin damage. The characteristic terminal stage of the disease, when untreated, is a typical coma. Poisoned by acidosis, which results from disturbance of body chemistry, the diabetic person loses consciousness and dies without regaining it. Coma is also a threat to those treated. Therefore, careful regulation of the condition with insulin must be properly observed.

Diabetic coma results when the blood sugar level becomes high, and acid products of the incomplete breakdown of carbohydrates accumulate in the blood. It may occur when insulin dosage is missed or is inadequate to balance food intake, or under other circumstances, upsetting the necessary balance between the sugar and the insulin in the system.

Diabetic coma is apt to be preceded by nausea and vomiting and, before these, by gradually increasing fatigue, weakness, and irritability. The physician should be consulted promptly on appearance of any of these symptoms. The patient should go to bed as a precaution against coma until the physician arrives.

Despite its slow onset, diabetic coma moves swiftly and may be critical. Once unconscious, the patient requires constant attendance by a doctor and, if possible, a nurse until he regains consciousness and during the following week or two of recuperation.

Diabetic patients need never suffer coma, according to Dr. Joslin, if they adhere to the prescribed diet, keep a check on their output of sugar, and maintain the schedule of insulin injections scrupulously. They should also know that extra insulin is needed to offset the effects of infection, which increases the severity of the condition.

During 1956, discoveries were announced of products which can be taken by mouth and which have an action like that of insulin in controlling metabolism of sugar. Extensive tests made in many countries have established the limitations of these products. They should never be used unless prescribed by a physician. In some cases, toxic side effects were observed. In the United States the two products now available are Orinase and Diabenase. The drug works best in moderate cases of diabetes and in middle-aged persons.

Untreated diabetes in young persons strikes with greater force and results in death more quickly than in older persons. In the latter, it may be quite mild and exist for years without serious effect. Diabetes does not usually appear in younger people. Two-thirds of all cases start after the person has passed the age of forty.

Overweight is one of the most significant factors associated with the development of diabetes, and modern living, with more eating and less labor of the kind necessary to burn up what is consumed, makes that condition a constantly greater problem. People become overweight, and diabetes is a price that many of them pay.

Although a hereditary tendency for diabetes does occur, it is a recessive characteristic, which means that unless reinforced by the addition of new diabetes-prone members, a family will tend to breed it out. The marriage likeliest to produce diabetic children is that in which both parents are not only diabetic but also come from demonstrably diabetic predecessors. All the children may well have the disorder. But the diabetic who marries a nondiabetic of nondiabetic stock has much less reason to fear that the children will be affected. In a marriage of two nondiabetics whose family records show a substantial number of cases, one of four children may manifest the tendency, though not inevitably.

Today control of the diet is an indispensable part of treatment. Unless it is coordinated with administration of insulin in the most rigorously careful manner, complications may occur. The phenomenon involved is not a single process and if one portion is disrupted the whole network is.

The normal quantity of sugar in the blood ranges from 80 to 120 milligrams in each 100 cubic centimeters. The diabetic has much more. Thus, one basic element of diet modification is to reduce the intake of carbohydrates, sugars, and starches. This must be done with care, since fats are not properly metabolized in the total absence of carbohydrates, and acidosis may result. Acids resulting from incomplete breakdown of fats accumulate in the blood with the excess sugar, and coma may result.

Administration of insulin must be kept constantly in balance with the intake of food and the blood sugar levels in the body. The hormone is a potent substance which can cause shock and unconsciousness when an excess gets into the blood. This reaction is the basis of its use for shock therapy in mental illness, comparable to electric shock.

Diet control for the diabetic should provide the nourishment indispensable to health and growth, without overtaxing the body's diminishing capacity to metabolize sugars. The patient should keep his weight a little lower than average for his height, sex, and age. Insulin given to excessively obese people with mild diabetes is not very effective. Nevertheless, enough food should be consumed to satisfy hunger adequately. The diabetic diet should be calculated by a physician and dietician who estimate the patient's need in calories on a basis of his weight, age, and occupation. The patient's capacity for disposing of sugar must be determined, and the doctor must decide to what extent diet may be relied on to relieve the basic condition and how much it must be supplemented by insulin.

In order to develop a diabetic's diet, his tolerance for sugar is established by beginning with an extremely simple intake and gradually increasing it until appearance of sugar in the urine begins to show that sugar capacity has been reached. At first, the patient will receive mostly vegetables with less than 5 per cent carbohydrates, such as cauliflower, celery, canned string beans, spinach, asparagus, lettuce, Brussels sprouts, artichokes, tomatoes, radishes, rhubarb, cabbage, and eggplant. The patient will receive from 150 to 200 grams of these and the bulk will relieve his hunger pangs without providing much nourishment. He should have a scale for weighing his meals. Meal plans and diet charts are available at minimum cost from the American Dietetic Association, 620 North Michigan Avenue, Chicago 11, Illinois.

In the absence of sugar in the excreted fluids, the diet is augmented on each successive day to include another five grams of carbohydrates, up to a total of twenty per day. Then the increase is slowed to the addition of five grams every other day. This is continued until either sugar appears in the urine or the patient is consuming three grams of carbohydrates for every thousand grams of body weight within each twenty-four hours.

Two or three days after the special

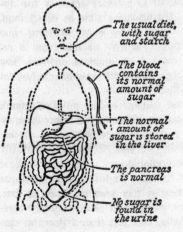

The normal sugar metabolism.

diet has been started, vegetables containing 10 per cent carbohydrates may be included in the diet to provide the added sugar intake desired. Such vegetables include canned peas, onions, beets, turnips, carrots, and squash. Later, vegetables of 15 per cent sugar content may be given, such as parsnips or canned lima beans, or even some with 20 per cent sugar content, such as succotash, beans, potatoes, and corn. Vegetables should be cooked in a double boiler, so that all juices are retained.

Bread is usually omitted from a diabetic diet because of the large proportion of starch it contains. Special breads, however, made from gluten flour are available, and the label usually indicates the amount of carbohydrates and protein present.

The appearance of sugar in the patient's urine may demand fasting for a short time until the urine is clear again, or insulin may be needed. Insulin makes it possible for diabetics to eat a greater range of foods and diminishes or eliminates the need for fasting. Health and life expectancy are increased as a result.

Since diabetics are susceptible to certain health hazards, they must observe specific hygienic precautions. Eight to ten hours' sleep at night, as well as a daily rest after lunch, if possible, are advisable, along with plenty of fresh air and an adequate amount of sunshine. Sunburn should be avoided. The diabetic's skin is low in resistance and subject to serious infection if damaged. Diabetics should not let the skin become excessively dry. Strong soaps tend to dry the skin and increase the hazard of infection and should be avoided. Cold cream or lanolin cream are good lubricants.

Proper care of the feet is essential because foot difficulties may have serious consequences. The diabetic should take care to have proper shoes, to consult a chiropodist about calluses and corns, and to secure medical attention for even a minor bruise or wound. Iodine or other harsh applications should not be used. Tight garters should not be worn because they may create disturbances of circulation and may incite gangrene.

Exercise should be taken in moderation and be gauged to the age and condition of the person, the length of time he has been diabetic and his total intake of food and insulin. Exercise should be balanced against caloric consumption.

Excessively hot baths must be avoided because of danger of injury or destruction of the tissue from burning.

Any consumption of alcoholic beverages should be accompanied by exact knowledge of the quantity of calories taken, since a single gram of alcohol contains seven calories. Soft drinks, like ginger ale and other popular beverages, are too sugar-laden to be safe for the diabetic.

Smoking is not harmful so long as moderation is observed. Excessive smoking involves definite risk, both of increasing the sugar content of the blood and of disturbing the blood circulation, particularly in the legs.

Dr. A. M. Sindoni recommends the following group of simple rules for diabetics as a safeguard against the acidosis or coma which threatens them if the sugar levels rise unduly:

1. Be careful. Never permit yourself a careless attitude toward the disease.

2. Keep all your dietary rules and, especially, never overeat.

3. Never miss a scheduled insulin injection.

4. Protect yourself from infections; even a minor one may have serious results.

5. Inform those who should know of your condition, your surgeon, dentist, chiropodist, and barber, so that proper precautions can be taken.

6. Test the sugar content of your urine at least twice a week, and, if you have failed to observe the regulations, more frequently.

7. Keep the urine free of sugar as a good assurance against acidosis or coma.

8. Whenever you feel ill, take it seriously. Go to bed, avoid chill, call the doctor, and care for yourself until he comes.

See also ACETEST; CLINITEST; DIABETES INSIPIDUS; INSULIN.

DIABETES INSIPIDUS, a disorder of the urinary system in which large amounts of urine are excreted. The urine is itself normal and sugar is not present as in diabetes mellitus. The origin of diabetes insipidus is not yet definitely established. In a specific case damage to the pituitary gland, because of hemorrhage, infection, or a tumor, may be responsible. A disorder of the pituitary is probably accountable.

As much as four to ten quarts of urine may be excreted daily, as contrasted with 1½ to two quarts normally. One report describes the case of a sixteen-year-old boy who excreted thirty-three quarts of urine every twenty-four hours, and the equivalent of his own body weight in forty hours. Intense and practically uninterrupted thirst is another symptom, and sleep is disturbed frequently because of the urge to urinate. The abnormal excretions caused by the disease result in weakness and emaciation. If a tumor or serious abscess in the pituitary region is not present, the person may get along satisfactorily; but if one of these conditions is found, fatality usually ensues. Death then is the result of the original disorder and not of the diabetes insipidus caused by it.

Both the thirst and excessive flow of liquid can be controlled for as long as six hours by injection of an extract of the posterior part of the pituitary gland. This substance when inhaled as a dry powder has the same effect but is apparently ineffective when taken by mouth. In severe cases surgical removal of a tumor or of the pituitary gland has brought control of the serious symptoms. *See also* DIABETES.

DIAPER RASH, a roughness and irritation of the skin in the area of the baby's diaper. Ordinarily infection is not involved and the rash is caused by the rubbing of the skin against a wet diaper. The irritation is aggravated if the diapers have been washed with a harsh soap, such as a soap with a high alkali content, and then carelessly rinsed. The rash is also intensified if a high degree of ammonia has been permitted to form in the diaper itself. This ammonia is produced when bacteria come in contact with urine which has soaked into the diaper.

A zinc ointment may be applied to relieve diaper rash. To prevent a recurrence of the rash, the diapers should be carefully washed with a mild soap and thoroughly rinsed. After laundering, the diapers may be soaked in a boric acid solution and hung in the sun. The presence of the boric acid will help prevent the formation of ammonia. These measures, plus careful attention to see that the baby's skin is kept dry and clean, ordinarily will bring good results. Protective lotions are available, such as silica preparations and Diaperine. *See also* INTERTRIGO.

DIAPHRAGM, a wide muscle which separates the abdominal and chest cavities of the body, contracts and expands with breathing, and is significant both to the breathing process and to the circulatory system.

A disturbance of the action of the diaphragm due to injury to the nerves may have serious effects. Inflammation or infection of the diaphragm causes shortness of breath, soreness, and a sense of pressure in the lower chest region. Spasm of the diaphragm may be either hiccups, the more common form known as clonic spasm, or a constant tension of the muscle called tonic spasm. The tonic spasm is the more severe form and results from such diseases as tetanus, rabies, or epilepsy. Tonic spasm of long duration may cause exhaustion and, ultimately, death by asphyxiation. Sometimes vigorous rubbing around the chest walls, the back, and the region over the stomach will relieve the spasm.

Hernia or rupture of the diaphragm may be caused by an injury, by a deformity before birth, or by a part of the stomach passing upward through the opening of the diaphragm at the esophagus. When a rupture occurs suddenly, symptoms of shock with severe pain in the lower part of the chest, hiccups, shortness of breath, and vomiting may be present. The most prominent symptoms of a hernia of long duration are shortness of breath and blue coloring. This is due to the possible displacement of the heart and to interference with the movement of the lungs. A child born with a large diaphragmatic hernia may also have what has been called an "upside-down stomach." Unless this condition is detected promptly and corrected surgically, the infant may not survive.

Surgery of the diaphragm for control of rupture is usually successful. Special methods of study have been developed which include the introduction into the stomach and esophagus of specific substances which are opaque to x-rays. Thus the surgeon can determine the exact point at which the displaced organ has passed through the diaphragm before the actual operation. *See also* HICCUPS.

DIARRHEA, excessively frequent and moist or liquid evacuations from the bowels of the residual wastes from digestion; a symptom and not a disease. It may result from a tremendous range of different disorders, from indigestion to an acute infection or a cancer.

Diarrhea may be transitory and pass after a brief acute episode or it may be chronic. In simple acute diarrhea the frequent evacuations gradually change in character from soft to liquid. Intestinal pain and straining to evacuate still further are characteristic; and thirst, abdominal tenderness, and sometimes fever may be present. Frequently some toxic substance or food, such as green fruit, roughage, highly spiced foods, or alcoholic drinks, may be the cause. The diarrhea usually subsides after the elimination of the causative material, although the irritation accompanying it may prolong the condition.

When diarrhea is chronic, medical attention is imperative and failure to treat such a condition can result in serious weakness. The person will lose weight, strength, and appetite, develop anemia and become prey to various infections. Chronic diarrhea has been classified under eight main headings and forty subheadings, which suggests the variety of disease conditions with which it is associated. Some of these are a stomach disorder characterized by lack of a normal amount of acid, ulcers, cancers, food deficiencies, Bright's disease, infections with different microorganisms and parasites, the taking of poisonous substances such as mercury or arsenic, or of cathartic drugs or of excessive alcohol, various internal bodily disorders, special sensitivity to a certain food, and nervous and emotional disturbance. Various major infections which involve diarrhea are amebiasis, typhoid fever, cholera, and bacillary dysentery. It can also occur with measles, pneumonia, smallpox, and influenza.

A thorough study of the person affected and of the evacuated material is essential to establish the specific cause of the diarrhea. The physician is interested not only in the patient's physical condition but also his emotional and mental state, the length of time the diarrhea has existed, the type and location of the pain, and the diet prior to the onset of the condition. The physician will try to establish the specific cause of the diarrhea and direct the treatment toward elimination of the cause rather than the symptom.

DIET. *See* DIET, REDUCING; DIET, SPECIAL; NUTRITION; VITAMINS; and Chapter 4, "Diet and Health"; Chapter 18, "Disorders of the Digestive System and Diet in Digestive Disorders."

DIET, REDUCING, a regimen of food and drink for the purpose of losing weight. In most cases of overweight or obesity, a reducing diet is the most desirable treatment. In addition to a wish to lose weight, the person should have a knowledge of the nutritional and caloric value of foods. The diet should include sufficient protein to prevent loss of body tissue protein. Carbohydrates should be limited and fat largely eliminated. To insure sufficient vitamin and mineral intake, supplementary multiple vitamin capsules should be taken daily. Losing weight involves a cutting down of regular everyday foods and does not necessitate specialized foods. Vegetables are to be cooked and eaten plain, without butter or sauces, and salads served without fatty dressings. Fruit should be fresh, or, if canned, without added sugar. Plentiful servings of low-calorie fruits and vegetables provide bulk and sat-

isfy hunger. Only lean meats should be eaten. It is important to establish regular hours for eating meals. A simple bedtime snack, such as an apple or glass of skim milk, will help prevent hunger in the early morning or the urge to eat during the night.

For an extremely obese person who is not active, a daily diet of 800 calories is possible. For moderate weight reduction, 1000 to 1200 calories can be taken daily provided the person is fairly sedentary, and 1400 to 1500 calories for persons requiring more energy for their daily activities.

To maintain health while reducing, certain foods are essential. The daily diet should include: 1 egg, 2 glasses of skim milk or buttermilk, 3 slices of bread, preferably whole wheat, 2 servings of lean meat, fish, fowl, or cottage cheese, 4 servings of raw or cooked vegetables, and 3 servings of fresh or unsweetened canned fruit. For the 800-calorie diet, the bread is omitted; for the 1200-calorie diet, an extra slice of bread and 3 teaspoons of butter are added, and the 1500-calorie diet can include 5 slices of bread, or 3 slices of bread and 2 small potatoes, and 3 teaspoons of butter. The bread in the diet can be the high-protein, low-calorie bread now sold commercially.

Following is a suggested day's menu for the 1000-calorie diet.

Breakfast

½ grapefruit
1 slice toast
1 egg
1 glass skim milk

Coffee or tea, without cream, milk, or sugar, may be taken any time.

Lunch

1 slice bread
1 cooked vegetable
3 oz. lean meat
vegetable salad
1 serving fruit

Dinner

Same as lunch; add 1 glass skim milk.

Bedtime snack: an apple or glass of skim milk.

Following are lists of fruits and vegetables which may be selected.

Fruits

Apples	Peaches
Berries	Pears
Cantaloupe	Pineapple
Grapefruit	Plums
Grapes	Watermelon
Oranges	

Vegetables

Asparagus	Mushrooms
Broccoli	Okra
Brussels sprouts	Peppers
Cabbage	Radishes
Cauliflower	Sauerkraut
Celery	Spinach
Cucumber	Squash
Eggplant	String beans
Greens	Tomatoes
Lettuce	Watercress

After the weight has been reduced to the desired level, it is essential to continue to watch carefully the diet and eating habits. The aim must be to maintain the new weight, and avoid the tendency to regain the pounds lost. *See also* OBESITY; and Chapter 4, "Diet and Health."

DIET, SPECIAL. In a number of specific diseases and bodily condi-tions, a special diet may be necessary —for example, in diabetes, heart disease, and in kidney, ulcer, and other infections. Such diets should be undertaken under the supervision of a physician. Conditions such as underweight and obesity, for safety and best results, should be properly supervised.

Some special diets may be self-ad-ministered. Among these are:

High-Caloric Diet: Add extra milk, cream, eggs, cheese, and custard to the regular diet.

High-Protein Diet: Add extra meat, eggs, cheese, and custard.

Low-Protein Diet: Omit meat and all but one egg daily; add portions of vegetables and fruits.

High-Carbohydrate Diet: Omit meat and eggs, but add extra portions of vegetables and fruits, rice, pastas, and puddings.

High-Fat Diet: Add extra butter, fats, fatty meats, oils, and cream to the regular diet.

Salt-Free Diet: Use only salt-free bread and sweet butter. Salt must not be added to food in cooking or at any other time.

See also DIET, REDUCING; OBESITY; and Chapter 4, "Diet and Health"; Chapter 18, "Disorders of the Digestive System and Diet in Digestive Disorders."

DIGESTION, the complex chemical and physiological process by which food is converted into soluble form for absorption into the tissues and cells of the body.

In digestion, the food is first ground and chewed in the mouth, which prepares it for action by the saliva. Saliva contains an enzyme which acts on starch to convert it into sugar. Then the food passes through the esophagus into the stomach, where it is further disintegrated and acted upon by the stomach juices, which contain hydrochloric acid, pepsin, and other substances such as rennin which coagulates milk. Protein is broken down by the action of pepsin and hydrochloric acid. The stomach usually requires about four hours of both mechanical and chemical action on food to complete its function. From the stomach the partly digested food

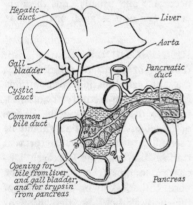

The relationships between the liver, gallbladder, pancreas and intestine.

passes into the small intestine, where both the mechanical and the chemical actions continue.

In the small intestine, bile secreted by the liver and pancreatic juice from the pancreas act on protein, starch, sugar, and fats. Intestinal juices from the lining of the intestines also act on sugars and proteins to complete the major part of the chemical process of digestion. All undigested food and debris pass, by muscular action, into the large intestine. Here water

and glucose are absorbed, and finally the remainder passes into the rectum whence it is eliminated as feces.

The process by which the tissues utilize the food substances distributed to them by the blood is the secondary phase of digestion. In this process the living cells of every tissue and organ of the body absorb various food substances that they require and synthesize them into their own structure. *See also* Chapter 18, "Disorders of the Digestive System and Diet in Digestive Disorders."

DIGESTIVE SYSTEM. All the parts of the body concerned with intake, digestion, and elimination constitute the digestive system. The digestive tract is really a continuous tube whose parts are the mouth, pharynx, esophagus, stomach, duodenum, small intestine, large intestine, and anus or rectum. The linings of this intricate, convoluted tube perform chemical and mechanical actions on the food and absorb and transmit the resulting substances to the blood and lymph.

The principal glands and organs that open into the digestive system are the salivary glands of the mouth and the liver and pancreas which open into the small intestine. Mucous glands perform a lubricating function throughout the tract, which enables food and waste material to pass through.

Numerous disorders and diseases, both temporary and chronic, affect the digestive system. *See also* Chapter 18, "Disorders of the Digestive System and Diet in Digestive Disorders."

DIGITALIS, a valuable drug derived from the dried leaves of the purple foxglove. It is a powerful stimulant for the heart, and may also be used to provoke the flow of urine in persons afflicted with dropsy or edema.

Digitalis can be dangerous and should never be used except in the dosage prescribed by the doctor. Even a slight excess over an extended period of time may cause the drug to accumulate in the system and act as a poison. The first symptom of poisoning may be palpitation of the heart, since digitalis slows the heartbeat. Often the lips tinge and at the same time the person may find it difficult to breathe. Whenever such an attack occurs, the person should be put to bed at once and a doctor called; sometimes the patient may receive a stimulant such as coffee. If his condition seems critical and the doctor is delayed, he may be given sips of tepid water to encourage vomiting. *See also* HEART.

DILANTIN, the trade name for diphenylhydantoin sodium. It is a white powder used as an anticonvulsant in the treatment of epilepsy, and is best taken with water at mealtimes, since it may be irritating if taken on an empty stomach. It should be taken only on the advice of a physician.

DISC, a plate of cartilage between the bones of the spine. When one of these discs is broken, the soft material which it contains may protrude in such a manner as to place pressure on the spinal nerves. The person so affected feels as if something has given way in his back, and will complain of a pain which seems to radiate downward along the side on which the break has occurred. This pain, constant and severe, will be intensi-fied when he coughs, bends, or stands erect for a long time. Further symptoms may include muscle spasms, a disposition to protect certain nerve areas, a diminished skin sensitivity in the affected area, and a decrease in tendon reflexes. Sometimes the break is visible under x-rays.

If the injured person is permitted to walk, he will be required to wear a girdle or cast. Ordinarily, however, he will be put in a special type of bed, in which reinforcing boards have been placed under the mattress. Removal of the ruptured disc may be necessary and usually ends the difficulty. *See also* SLIPPED DISC; SPINAL CORD.

DISINFECTION, the destruction or removal of germs or articles which may be germ-bearing from a sickroom following recovery from an infectious disease. During the course of an illness, disinfection should be carried on constantly to prevent transmission of the disease. Discharged matter from the eyes, ears, nose, throat, skin, or other parts of the body should be destroyed by burning or other sure method, after being collected in containers which can also be destroyed. Towels, bedclothes, and linens should be handled so that the infected side is turned inward, and those caring for these items should be careful to hold them by the noninfected portions.

The infectious material varies with different diseases. In chickenpox, the source of the infected discharges may be the mouth, nose, throat, or lesions of the skin; while in measles, meningitis, pneumonia, septic sore throat, and whooping cough it is usually from the mouth, nose, and throat. In typhoid, dysentery, and poliomyelitis, bowel discharge probably carries the infectious organisms. However, in poliomyelitis the mouth, nose, and throat may also be the source. In scarlet fever and diphtheria, infectious matter comes from the eyes, mouth, nose, throat, and wounded skin surfaces.

After the patient has recovered, the sickroom and everything in it should be thoroughly disinfected. During the illness, upholstered furniture, carpet, curtains, and all extraneous ornaments should have been removed. At the end of the illness, beds, chairs, tables, floors, and woodwork must be completely scrubbed with soap and hot water, and linens and other washable fabrics boiled for at least fifteen minutes. Nonwashable materials can be exposed to direct sunlight out-of-doors for at least twenty-four hours; and rubber goods, such as sheets, hot-water bottles, and ice caps, can be washed with soap and water and placed out-of-doors to air and dry for at least two hours. Books, magazines, and toys which the patient has used should be burned.

Good disinfectants are chloride of lime, creosol, or milk of lime in solution. Heat is one of the best germ destroyers. Disinfection of the sickroom with sulphur vapor is a time-honored and effective method.

DISLOCATION, the displacement of a part of the body from its usual place. The term is used ordinarily in connection with a bone, such as the elbow, shoulder, or knee, moved partially or completely out of its normal position. Dislocations usually happen suddenly as the result of a blow, fall, or other accident, and recurrent dislocations are not uncommon, especially with athletes. Because of the danger of further injury, when any type of dislocation occurs, only a physician should reset the displaced joint. Until the doctor arrives, the person should be made as comfortable as possible and kept warm. Cold compresses applied at the point of injury may relieve pain and prevent swelling. *See also* JOINTS AND JOINT DISORDERS.

DIURESIS. To release an accumulation of fluids in the blood, a physician may prescribe drugs known as diuretics. The excessive excretion of urine is diuresis. Urine contains both solids and water. Some diuretics increase the discharge of water and others increase the amount of solids released. Specific diuretics release various types of solids. Several drugs may be prescribed when a single drug to achieve the desired effect is not known. Water is a good diuretic, unless, of course, the body must get rid of an excessive amount of water. Diuretics which encourage the discharge of water are usually those which also stimulate circulation, such as digitalis, Diamox, alcohol, and coffee. Another group which includes mercury combinations may be classed as the mineral salt diuretics. For this purpose, mineral salt is effective only in small amounts, since larger doses may act instead as a stimulant to the bowels. *See also* KIDNEYS; URINE.

DIVERTICULITIS. Pouches, or diverticula, which sometimes develop on the walls of the large intestines of adults, create diverticulosis. Inflammation or infection of these pouches is diverticulitis.

The severity of diverticulitis can be determined by a test, known as the barium test, in which the patient swallows a barium mixture and is then examined by a series of x-rays of the colon. Thus, the pouches and the bowel contractions can be seen clearly, and the x-ray film will also show whether or not a narrowing or obstruction of the bowel is present.

In acute diverticulitis, ulceration with consequent perforation of the wall of the bowel may result and cause massive hemorrhage which will require prompt surgery.

In older people, one of the dangers of diverticulitis is chronic irritation with a possibility of cancer. Treatment of inflamed diverticuli includes rest and enemas to help cleanse the bowels when necessary. Sometimes mineral oil may be used to aid the passage of hardened material. Persistent obstruction or constant inflammation and pain may also necessitate surgical treatment.

Persons with diverticulitis require a soft diet, similar to that for those with ulcer. Irritating spices and sharp foods must be avoided, as well as fibrous foods and those containing seeds or skins. *See also* Chapter 18, "Disorders of the Digestive System and Diet in Digestive Disorders."

DIVERTICULUM, a small pouch which sometimes develops on the smooth wall of the intestinal tract.

Meckel's diverticulum, named for its discoverer, is a congenital deformity or abnormality occurring near the middle of the small intestine. This pouch may collect partially digested food and become inflamed or infected and cause symptoms similar to those of appendicitis; also hemorrhage requiring surgical attention may result.

Diverticula may also form in the esophagus, stomach, duodenum, or jejunum, and a single diverticulum may occur in the cecum or elsewhere in the colon. Many diverticula do not cause symptoms and will not require treatment, but when they become inflamed surgery is recommended to correct the condition. *See also* DIVERTICULITIS.

DIZZINESS, sensation of swimming in the head; one of the commonest symptoms about which people complain. Like a cough, it may be a sign of something seriously wrong that demands prompt attention.

Dizziness follows recovery from all kinds of illnesses. It may result from poisoning by drugs, or sensitivity to certain foods. It is a symptom in high blood pressure, in menopause, migraine headaches, eyestrain, brain injury, punctured eardrum, malformation of the inner ear, syphilis, alcoholism, and many other diseases or disorders.

A common form of dizziness results from inflammation in that portion of the inner ear known as the semicircular canals. Anything that interferes with the delicate mechanism of these canals will produce attacks of dizziness.

If dizziness is temporary and the condition responds to treatment such as suitable attention to diet, correction of eyestrain, or regulation of kidney action, there is no cause for alarm. However, repeated and persistent dizziness calls for most careful diagnosis. There may be insufficient blood supply to the brain or weakened heart action. Dizziness in such cases is a distinct danger signal whose warning must be promptly heeded.

Dizziness caused by seasickness or airsickness, as well as by other forms of motion, is helped by the use of drugs like Dramamine, Bonamine, or Marezine. *See also* MOTION SICKNESS; VERTIGO.

DOG BITES. Because of the possibility of hydrophobia, anyone bitten by a dog should receive the prompt attention of a physician. The wound may be carefully washed with soap and water, a weak solution of iodine applied, and the wound covered with a clean bandage. If possible, the dog should be confined and watched until it is determined whether or not it has rabies. The necessary information should be given at once to the city authorities. If the dog has rabies the person bitten is given the Pasteur inoculations against rabies. The dog is killed and its brain examined for the presence of Negri bodies which are diagnostic of rabies. *See also* RABIES.

DOUBLE VISION. *See* EYE, *Diplopia.*

DOUCHE, a jet or current of water applied for cleansing purposes to any part, organ, or cavity of the body.

The danger of germs is always greater when washing an internal portion of the body. Water used for this purpose should, therefore, be boiled, then the temperature brought as close as possible to that of the blood, about 100° F. Cold water must not be used since it is harmful when applied internally.

Certain special equipment is necessary for the administration of a vaginal douche. First is the water container which may be made of tin, glass, rubber, or plastic. A length of rubber or plastic hosing is attached to the container with a vaginal tube of vulcanite or glass at the other end. Glass is more convenient for sterilizing purposes. This equipment must be kept absolutely clean at all times.

The container should be placed two or three feet above the point where the fluid is to emerge, in order that the force of the flow of water be satisfactory. If the container is placed too high, the force might be dangerous, and the liquid could reach unintended areas.

Before the tube is inserted, the fluid should be permitted to run through the entire hose so that all of the air is expelled. Petroleum jelly, if desired, may be smeared on the end of the tube, which should be thrust inward for a distance not exceeding three inches. Afterward the fluid may be ejected into any suitable receptacle. The vaginal douche is useful as an antiseptic, as a means of removing discharge, and also for controlling disagreeable odors. The solution employed will be chosen accordingly. *See also* ENEMA; NOSE; VAGINA; and Chapter 11, "Feminine Hygiene."

DRAMAMINE, the trade name for dimenhydrinate, a compound with antihistaminic properties which has been found to be effective in the prevention and treatment of motion sickness. This drug was developed during World War II when it was successfully used in the control of seasickness among large numbers of troops.

DRESSINGS, materials used to protect such injuries as burns, abrasions, and wounds. The most significant function of dressings is to protect the injured area from germs.

Since moisture encourages the growth of germs, a dry dressing is usually preferable. When the wound is inflamed or encrusted, however, a wet dressing may be more soothing and better for cleansing purposes.

Plain white dressings of lint, gauze, cotton, or wool, sterilized with heat and wrapped in antiseptic packages, may be purchased. These are useless, however, if contaminated by unsterilized hands or brought into contact with any other unsterilized surface. Dressings may be stored in clean paper packages and kept in a suitable box, which is always tightly covered.

DROPSY. *See* NEPHROSIS.

DROWNING, suffocation in water or other liquid. A person removed from the water may be alive, even though he appears to be dead. Without delay his mouth should be cleared of any debris which he may have acquired in the struggle to breathe, and he should be placed on his stomach, the side of his head resting on his forearm. Artificial respiration should be given at once, for at least an hour, until the victim begins to breathe naturally, or the effort is found futile.

As soon as the person regains consciousness, his blood circulation should be stimulated. He should be wrapped in dry blankets, warmed with hot-water bottles, if possible, and his limbs gently massaged. Stimulants, such as tea, coffee, brandy, or whiskey in water, may be given.

Although the victim might appear to have recovered, he should not be permitted to walk alone. Instead, if at all possible, a stretcher of some type should be used. Once the person has been placed in bed, he must be carefully watched for at least an hour, since his breathing might stop again, in which case it is essential to resume artificial respiration.

In cases of drowning, every effort should be made to secure the services of a physician promptly. *See also* ARTIFICIAL RESPIRATION; ASPHYXIA; RESUSCITATION.

DRUG ADDICTION. Traffic in drugs constitutes a major problem for the federal authorities and, because of the alarming increase in youthful addicts, for parents and teachers as well.

The loss of the power of self-control through drug addiction is not only harmful to the individual concerned, but also to society. A drug addict has such an overwhelming craving for the drug that he does not count the cost of getting it; crime, violence, and murder have been the price all too often. The addict develops a tolerance to the drug so that increasing doses are necessary in order to produce the desired effect. When not under the influence of the drug the addict tends more and more to manifest typical disturbances of the nervous system. If drugs are withdrawn from the addict, characteristic withdrawal symptoms appear, with acute physical pain in addition to such symptoms as severe cramps in the abdomen and legs, muscular twitching, vomiting, and diarrhea. The addict will be irritable, restless, and unable to relax, and will break out in sweat and "goose pimples." Rest and sleep are difficult or impossible to achieve.

The chief drugs used by addicts are opium and its derivatives, morphine and heroin; cocaine; hashish; and marijuana made from hemp. The widespread use of bromides and barbiturates, sedatives and sleeping pills available to the general public, has also raised problems. The barbiturates fulfill all the requirements of habit-forming drugs. Overdose is often fatal. Therefore legal control of the sale of the drugs has been tightened.

Treatment for drug addiction is quite drastic and should be attempted only by qualified medical personnel with adequate facilities. The first step in treatment is withdrawal of the drug, abruptly, rapidly, or gradually, followed by a period of psychotherapy and rehabilitation. This final period should last at least four months, otherwise there is an even greater danger of relapse to the addiction among most patients. Information regarding treatment is available from the U. S. Public Health Service in Washington, D.C.

DT stands for delirium tremens. *See* DELIRIUM TREMENS.

DUODENAL ULCER. *See* PEPTIC ULCER.

DUODENUM, the first portion of the small intestine, leading from the stomach. It contains the openings of the pancreatic and the common bile ducts. *See also* INTESTINES; PEPTIC ULCER; and Chapter 18, "Disorders of the Digestive System and Diet in Digestive Disorders."

DUST, fine pulverized powder of dry earth or refuse, found all through the atmosphere except perhaps on mountain tops and out at sea. An atmosphere free of dust is far healthier than one which is not. Nature and industry produce dusts of various kinds, against which people cannot wholly protect themselves. In some instances, dust may be disastrously harmful to human beings.

Microscopic particles of pollen dust borne by wind come in contact with the mucous membranes of the eye and the respiratory tract and produce symptoms of allergy such as seasonal hay fever, hives, and other disorders. Industrial dusts, produced by grinding of metals and in the manufacture of wood products, flour, sugar, textiles, leather, and feathers, also affect human beings.

Most dusts contain some carbon and other organic matter. Many people are sensitive to dusts and have skin reactions when the dusts come in contact with the skin. Other dusts, when inhaled, irritate the windpipe and bronchial tubes. Coal dust may get into the lungs causing pigmentation, and may stimulate the production of fibrous tissue. Inorganic dusts containing free silica incite silicosis, a special form of change in the lungs. In silicosis the silica acts to produce nodules throughout the lungs which can be detected by x-rays. Lungs damaged in this way are prone to secondary infections, including tuberculosis.

Organic dusts, like carbon, differ from inorganic dusts in that they do not cause the changes in the lungs such as are produced by the action of silica. Organic dust particles do not penetrate lung tissue, but instead are absorbed into the tissues of the body.

Asbestosis is a special form of lung disorder in which the magnesium silicate contained in asbestos produces fibrous changes that are different from those caused by pure silica. However, asbestosis and silicosis are much alike, both being forms of the lung disorder pneumoconiosis.

To inhibit inhalation of dust, various forms of exhaust systems, air conditioning, and improved ventilation have been developed. Helmets and breathing devices worn by miners and workers employed in operations producing excessive dust have also been helpful.

Drought areas are great dust producers; but the immediate health hazard, aside from the relationship between dust storms and secondary pneumonia, is not serious. More harmful are the mental and economic hardships suffered by people living in the dust-bowl region. *See also* ASBESTOSIS; BRONCHITIS; INDUSTRIAL HEALTH; SILICOSIS; TUBERCULOSIS; and Chapter 5, "Occupational Health."

DWARFISM. *See* ACHONDROPLASIA.

DYSENTERY, inflammation of the colon. Its symptoms are pain and severe diarrhea with frequent passage of mucus and blood. *See also* AMEBIC DYSENTERY; BACILLARY DYSENTERY.

DYSMENORRHEA, pain at the time of menstruation. Discomfort in the lower abdomen or pains in the thighs and a general feeling of pressure may occur. The causes vary from anatomic malformation, such as an undeveloped womb, to disturbances of hormone balance. If pain is constant or severe enough to cause nausea, vomiting, or headache, or to interfere with normal activity, the doctor should be consulted. Mental factors also may be responsible for unusual pain. Often the young girl has been prepared inadequately for womanhood. When the pain is not severe, the use of a mild sedative is helpful.

Strenuous exercise immediately before, during, and after menstruation has been known to produce a period of pain later. Therefore, most physicians believe that violent exercise should be avoided.

While mild non-habit-forming drugs are helpful, the use of habit-forming drugs is dangerous. The relationship between the sex functions and the action of various glands studied by the physician permits him to prescribe endocrine or glandular products which are helpful in controlling dysmenorrhea. *See also* MENSTRUATION.

DYSPEPSIA. *See* INDIGESTION.

DYSPNEA, the medical term for difficult or labored breathing. This symptom occurs in attacks of asthma, acute laryngitis in children, cancer of the throat, weakness of the heart, and other conditions. *See also* ASPIRATION.

EAR, an organ which performs the function of hearing and is involved with the sense of balance. It consists of three parts: the external, middle, and internal ears. The external ear comprises the outer ear and the external auditory canal. It collects sound and transmits the waves to the eardrum, the membrane that closes off the external ear. The middle ear, or internal tympanic cavity, contains bones and nerves for further transmission of sound, and connects with the nasal passages through the Eustachian tube. The internal ear is a bony labyrinth, containing the nerves that connect with the brain, and three semicircular canals which control equilibrium. The entire inner ear structure is encased by the mastoid region of the skull. Both ears, though related, function independently, and if the capacity of one is destroyed that of the other is not necessarily impaired.

A number of disorders may affect the ear. Earache is caused by inflammation which, even though slight, should be cared for promptly by a physician, since neglect may lead to serious complications and even mastoiditis. The external ear, because of its position, is susceptible to many kinds of bruises and abrasions, as well as infection and invasion by fungi and insects. Swellings or boils on the external ear should be treated by the doctor. Bony growths on the external ear, known as extosis, are best treated by surgical removal. Congenital malformations are not infrequent and have been effectively treated by plastic surgery. Plastic surgery has also been successful on cauliflower ear, which results from repeated blows, as experienced by boxers, or from other injury.

The eardrum may also be subject to inflammation and is especially liable to puncture or rupture. A sharp instrument should never be used to remove wax or a foreign substance from the ear because of the danger of puncturing. An old saying is, "Never put anything in your ear smaller than your elbow."

Rupture of the eardrum may be caused by violent noise, such as an explosion, sharp descent from high altitude, diving into deep water, or even sneezing. Bleeding of the ear, dizziness, ringing sounds, and headache may be symptoms of ruptured or punctured eardrum. Careful diagnosis and patient treatment by an ear specialist generally corrects the condition.

The middle ear can be infected from without, through a ruptured or punctured eardrum, or from within through the Eustachian tube. Head cold, respiratory infection, diseased tonsils and adenoids, inadequate nasal hygiene, forcible blowing of the nose may all cause infection of the middle ear. These infections may be acute, chronic, or temporary, draining or nondraining. Symptoms are shooting pains in the ear, inflammation, ringing sounds, or impaired hearing. All the symptoms are danger signals and require immediate attention. Since many cases of deafness among adults are traceable to middle ear infection in childhood, the condition must be treated promptly. Children should be taught ear hygiene as a guard against ear infection.

In most cases of ear disorder, the minimum amount of manipulation is advisable, since the ear is a delicate and intricate organ through which infections can easily spread. Antibiotics and sulfonamide drugs control ear infection, thus preventing mastoiditis, once a fairly common sequel. *See also* DEAFNESS; MASTOID; OTOSCLEROSIS.

ECCHYMOSIS, the flow of blood into the surrounding tissues, after the rupture of a blood vessel. The term also applies to the discoloration of the skin caused by a hemorrhage under the skin, and to bruises which appear on the skin as the familiar black-and-blue spots after a blow and later turn brown, green, or yellow. *See also* BRUISES.

ECLAMPSIA, a serious convulsive condition occurring in pregnancy in women of any age. The cause is not definitely known. The prospective mother may suffer convulsions leading to unconsciousness. The first danger signal may be headache or failing vision. The blood pressure may rise sharply and albumin will appear in the urine. These early symptoms are pre-eclamptic. Scientific prenatal care includes constant guarding against this condition. Should any symptoms appear, precautions must be taken at once to prevent eclampsia, which is serious and in the past often resulted in stillbirth.

The woman should be hospitalized promptly. The intake of salt is restricted and a soft diet prescribed. Diuretic agents are given to induce sufficient elimination of urine, since in eclampsia the function of the kidneys is impaired and these organs must be relieved of any extra load.

Anticonvulsant drugs are administered to control the tendency to convulsions.

Fortunately the warning symptoms usually develop slowly. However, cases do occur in which serious complications closely follow the first symptoms. Most doctors believe that pregnancy itself is responsible for the development of toxic substances in the body. This toxic reaction may affect certain organs more than others, thus inducing pre-eclampsia or eclampsia itself.

Improved methods of prenatal care in recent years have done much to prevent eclampsia and reduce the mortality rate from that cause. Frequent checking of blood pressure, periodic examination of the urine, and better weight control not only tend to improve the general condition of prospective mothers but make possible recognition of the pre-eclamptic state.

Nevertheless, physicians are always on guard against any eclamptic emergency that may arise. Extreme measures, including the use of oxygen, induction of labor, and even Cesarian section may be necessary in severe eclampsia. Even after a child is born, the mother must be just as carefully watched since pre-eclampsia and eclampsia occasionally occur immediately following childbirth.

ECTOPIC PREGNANCY, an unusual form of pregnancy in which the fetus develops outside of the normal location, the uterus. It may occur, for instance, in the Fallopian tube. When ectopic gestation takes place the usual signs of pregnancy are present, though they may be overlooked. If a menstrual period is missed and slight bleedings begin to recur from the womb, a physician should be consulted. Prompt operation is the advisable treatment.

ECZEMA, a term which currently refers to a noncontagious skin rash for which a definite cause cannot be cited. Thus, a rash which is produced by a certain type of soap might be described as dermatitis, but not as eczema.

The possible causes of eczema, therefore, are always speculative. A change in the weather, in the temperature, or even in the intensity of light can be responsible. The cause may be found inside the body, perhaps in the contents of the blood, or possibly on the surface in the presence of warts or calluses, or in sensitized skin. Moreover, the area of the body may be significant. Eczema of the scalp can differ greatly from eczema of the face or groin. The skin may be sensitive to certain textiles or chemicals.

The symptoms of eczema are frequently associated with those of asthma, and often attack alternately, or they can appear at the same time. Moreover, both may start suddenly, with the swallowing of certain food or the inhalation of a particular sensitizing substance. Both diseases may involve an inherited liability.

Often the first manifestation of eczema is on the face. The skin reddens, becomes swollen and hot, and small blisters appear which may join to form larger ones. These rupture eventually and release a sticky substance. As this fluid dries it forms a yellow crust which drops off after several days, revealing a reddened and scaling area underneath. This scaling may continue for several days or weeks, after which the skin will recover its ordinary appearance. In the meantime, however, a relapse may occur and the entire sequence of blistering and healing will be repeated.

In children especially, the disease may spread and sometimes will cover the entire body. Often a high temperature is involved together with a disinclination to eat. The progress of the disease varies with the individual person; the blistering phase may predominate in one case, the dry and scaly phase in another, and the pimply stage in still another. Almost always, however, the person will suffer from severe itching. Heat may increase this itching so that it becomes almost unendurable. Eczema usually involves a thickening and breaking of the skin, and consequently the infected area is highly receptive to germs which may introduce complicating factors such as boils or impetigo.

Since the possible causes are so numerous the treatment is often broad in scope. Although it may be impossible to identify the particular food which was responsible for the attack, nevertheless general dietary routine can be of considerable value. If the attack is acute, a strictly liquid diet may even be imposed. The free consumption of water is ordinarily advised but stimulating beverages such as alcohol, tea, and coffee are seldom permitted. Medication is usually employed for special purposes only, for the relief of itching, or for the drying of open blisters. Radium, x-rays or ultraviolet rays may be used with good effect. Recently the use of cortisone ointments has permitted prompt control of this condition.

More than two-thirds of all skin diseases are classified as eczema. The symptoms and causes are so complex that successful treatment demands a qualified physician. *See also* SKIN; and Chapter 20, "Diseases of the Skin."

EDEMA. *See* NEPHROSIS.

EGGS of poultry are second only to milk in nutritive value, and many dieticians feel that every diet should include at least one egg a day. Eggs are rich in proteins, fats, phosphorus, iron, and in all the elements necessary for growth except calcium and vitamin C. They also contain cholesterol, a fatlike substance which may be involved in the growth of gallstones, cysts, and cancerous tissue. For this reason eggs in *large* amounts are not recommended for persons over forty years of age; however, anyone in this age range can safely have an egg a day unless specifically forbidden by a doctor. Ordinarily eggs are highly digestible; even a hardboiled egg, especially a minced hardboiled egg, is only slightly less digestible than a soft-boiled egg. Eggs may induce constipation, discomfort, asthma, or eczema in some persons who presumably have become sensitized to eggs, perhaps only to the albumen. *See also* ALBUMIN; NUTRITION.

ELBOW, the joint at the middle of the arm where the large bone of the upper arm, the humerus, joins

the two smaller bones of the lower arm, the radius and ulna.

This joint can suffer any of the serious conditions that affect any other joint of the body. Dislocation is the most common disorder of the elbow and one of the most serious. Any dislocation should be examined immediately by x-ray and reset accordingly. If necessary, the elbow should be put in a splint or placed in a cast until it is completely healed. Such care must be given only by a doctor. Ankylosis, or locking in place of the joint, may result from inflammation or infection. This condition requires the attention of an orthopedic surgeon who will not only treat but prescribe subsequent manipulation, massage, and application of heat to restore free movement and avoid permanent crippling. So-called "tennis elbow" results from over-

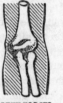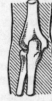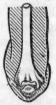

LEFT ELBOW, *front view, joint extended*   LEFT ELBOW, *back view, joint extended*   LEFT ELBOW, *back view, joint flexed*

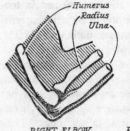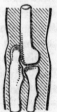

Humerus
Radius
Ulna

RIGHT ELBOW, *side view, joint flexed*   RIGHT ELBOW, *side view, joint extended*

The bone structure and articulation of the elbow.

activity in playing tennis or other sports or even nonathletic motion involving lifting, sudden pulling, or extending of the elbow joint.

Besides injury involving the muscles and ligaments of the elbow joint, breaking or detachment of the small bones may cause pain and swelling. At the end of the elbow joint is the "funny bone," which is actually not a bone but a particularly sensitive nerve; a sudden blow or pressure on it may cause considerable pain.

In growing children, cartilage which controls growth of the bone at the elbow joint can also be damaged or dislocated. If damage does occur the cartilage must be replaced; if the cartilage is not replaced, the arm will stop growing at the point where the epyphisis (cartilage) was damaged. *See also* DISLOCATION; FRACTURES; JOINTS AND JOINT DISORDERS.

ELECTRICAL INJURIES. Shock or injuries from electricity come from two major sources: accidental contact with electrical current and lightning strokes. Most of the fatal electrical accidents occur in industry, where electrical machinery and equipment are potential sources of accident to the worker. In the home, such accidents may result from faulty insulation or careless handling of lighting, heating, or refrigeration equipment.

A person suffering from electric shock must be immediately removed from contact with the source of the electric current. If a live wire must be cut, an axe with a wooden handle is the best tool to use. If the rescuer cannot cut off the current, he must be careful to handle the victim with the aid of some insulating material such as a dry rope, a wooden stick, or a leather belt. He must protect himself from receiving the shock which can be transmitted through the body of the victim. The doctor should be called immediately. If the person is unconscious or breathing has ceased, which is likely if the current has passed through the central nervous system and affected the respiratory center of the brain, artificial respiration should be given at once. Since artificial respiration may have to be continued for several hours, resuscitating equipment should be summoned if possible. The clothing of the victim should be loosened to facilitate breathing and the victim allowed to rest several hours before he is moved to a hospital.

When struck by lightning, the person falls to the ground as if he had received a stunning blow on the head. After the shock, flashes of light seem to pass before his eyes and blindness or deafness can ensue. The nervous system may be dangerously affected with resulting symptoms of paralysis, pains in the limbs, and sometimes hemorrhage.

Dry skin offers a high resistance to electricity and therefore the local burns following electric shock are greater and the general effects on the body less. Moist skin lessens resistance and permits the current to have a greater internal effect with chances of death more likely, although the surface burns may be less severe. However, the attempt to sustain the life of the victim should, of course, have precedence over any treatment of skin injuries. *See also* RESUSCITATION.

ELECTRIC SHOCK TREATMENT. When electric shock therapy is given, two or more electrodes are placed on the sides of the head and a measured electric current is passed through the brain. This type of treatment is used in mental disturbances. The application of electric shock to induce loss of consciousness has resulted in dramatic improvement for some persons, notably for those suffering severe depression, agitation, depression associated with menopause and catatonic states of schizophrenia.

ELECTROCARDIOGRAPH, an apparatus or instrument which records the electrical current created by the beating of the heart. Attached to the electrocardiograph are electrical conductors which are placed on each of the arms and the left leg. The currents of the heartbeat are conducted to the electrocardiograph where they are photographed. This resulting record of waves is the electrocardiogram. Several of these are made; one electrocardiogram is taken from the two arms, another from the left leg and right arm, and a third one from the left leg and left arm. Frequently a fourth picture is taken from the left leg and the top of the heart. The four photographs, although not identical, resemble one another.

The electrocardiograph is exceedingly useful in diagnosis. It is invaluable in the study of the heart, and in many diseases such as rheumatic fever. It aids in diagnosing suspected cases of coronary thrombosis, a disease caused by clots of blood which block blood vessels leading to the heart and damage the muscle and induce rhythm breaks and other irregu-

larities in the flow of the blood. *See also* CORONARY THROMBOSIS; HEART; RHEUMATIC FEVER.

ELECTROENCEPHALOGRAPHY, a method of recording the electrical activity of the brain, especially of the cerebral cortex. The electrical impulses are detected by means of wires attached to the scalp and are recorded graphically in waves (EEG). Valuable information is gathered by this method in case of tumor, epilepsy, infections, and hemorrhages. The apparatus used is known as an electroencephalograph. It is also useful in locating a diseased portion of the brain, if not too deeply seated.

ELEPHANTIASIS, a chronic disease characterized by inflammation of the lymphatic glands. As the condition progresses, the skin becomes thickened, the tissues under the skin swell, and, in time, the parts of the body affected enlarge incredibly. The legs, for example, may resemble the legs of an elephant, whence the name, elephantiasis. Any part of the body may be affected, but enlargement of the arms, legs, or scrotum is most common. The breasts of women are less susceptible.

The disease occurs usually as a secondary effect of filariasis. The filaria, a parasite, gets into the lymph ducts and blocks them. However, blocking of the lymphatics by other means can also produce elephantiasis.

Elephantiasis, for the most part, is a disease of the tropics and a person may have it for many years. While medical treatment of the condition itself is ineffective, tight bandaging and surgery can often reduce the deformities of the disease. Control of the mosquitoes that bear the parasite and of the worm responsible for the disease seem to be the best long-range methods of inhibiting elephantiasis. *See also* FILARIASIS.

EMACIATION, extreme thinness. Emaciation may have many causes, including a psychological basis. For example, a person suffering from depression may refuse to eat and waste away to the point of emaciation. Ordinarily the cause is basically physical, and is usually due to a degenerative disease of the muscles. Emaciation can also result from any degenerative disease of the spinal cord.

Diabetes, syphilis, or a growth in the gullet may cause emaciation. Persistent tuberculosis, in any part of the body will eventually cause extreme thinness. In addition, emaciation may also be produced by such diseases as cholera, extended diarrhea, disturbances of the thyroid glands, or even by extreme fever.

In the first six months of an infant's life, severe emaciation may seem to develop without any cause. The term "marasmus" is applied to this condition. Ordinarily the cause will be found in the baby's diet, and a change of diet will bring a cure.

Generally the treatment in cases of extreme emaciation varies greatly and depends on the source of the ailment. *See also* ATROPHY.

EMBOLISM, obstruction of a blood vessel by a blood clot or by any foreign matter floating loose in the blood stream. An embolus, as the clot or particle is known, is dangerous because it may lodge in an important arterial blood vessel or vein and block the supply of blood to an organ or tissue on which life depends, such as the brain, heart, kidney, or lungs. If an embolus reaches a vital area of the brain, paralysis and even death may follow in a few hours. Embolism in the eye may cause blindness.

An air bubble may circulate through the blood and, if large enough, block a blood vessel. A bit of fat may get loose in the blood stream following fracture of a large bone. A collection of germs from an abscess may get into a small blood vessel, plug it, interrupt circulation, and produce a secondary abscess. Any of these disturbances is called embolism.

In endocarditis, an inflammation of the lining of the heart, incrustations and growth may develop on the valves of the heart. These break off and get into the blood stream, and cause embolism. The two types of endocarditis are the acute, which arises suddenly and may cause death within a few days, and the subacute, which begins slowly and responds to early treatment.

The early symptoms of embolism are a slight rise in temperature and a rapid increase in the pulse beat. Within twenty-four hours, however, both the temperature and pulse rise rapidly, breathing becomes rapid, and the person has great mental anxiety and symptoms of shock. In postoperative embolus, the symptoms may be sudden pallor, rapid pulse, and collapse.

People past middle life are more prone to embolism than younger persons. Those who have had disturbances of the heart are affected frequently rather than those whose blood circulation has been normal.

Among the methods of treatment of embolism recently developed is an immediate surgical operation to release the blocked area, especially when the embolus occurs in the arms, legs, or in a region which can be reached. The development of such drugs as dicumarol, heparin, and others which have the power to prevent blood clotting has been invaluable. Antibiotics have been useful also in the treatment of chronic bacterial endocarditis, thus lessening the danger of embolus.

EMBRYO, a young organism in the earliest stage of development. In the human being, embryo refers to the organism during its first three months of life in the mother's womb. *See also* FETUS; and Chapter 6, "Prenatal Care and Childbirth."

EMERGENCIES IN THE HOME. At least one person in every household should know the basic rules of emergency care.

Falls. Of the millions of serious accidents which occur in the home every day, almost fifty per cent are due to falls. The first rule to observe when a person has fallen is to estimate the extent of his injuries, whether or not he has suffered a broken bone, a hemorrhage, or just a bruise.

Usually, a broken bone can be recognized immediately by failure of the limb to function. A final diagnosis, however, can only be made by a doctor with the help of an x-ray machine. While awaiting the doctor, the injured limb can be placed in a homemade splint if there is someone present able to do it. The splint may be made by wrapping the limb in a large-sized magazine or equivalent which is then tied in place by means of handkerchiefs or strips of material.

A minor hemorrhage can be controlled by placing a piece of gauze against the wound. If the hemorrhage is more severe, pressure against the gauze may be necessary to control the bleeding. A tourniquet should be used with extreme caution. However, if one is absolutely necessary, it is applied in the following manner. A large handkerchief or towel is tied around the arm or leg above the hemorrhage. A small rod of any type, a clothespin or stick for example, is then inserted under the handkerchief. On the other side of the limb the handkerchief is tied in a knot and a larger rod is inserted through this knot in such a way that the tourniquet can be easily tightened, thus closing off the flow of blood.

A bleeding tooth socket can be controlled by filling the socket with antiseptic cotton. Nosebleed may ordinarily be halted by placing the victim face down and then stuffing the nostrils with gauze, or sometimes application of hot and cold packs will bring about the same result. If placing gauze on a scalp wound fails to stop the bleeding, a tight band wound all the way around the head may be successful. A real danger is unexpected hemorrhage of the lung. A doctor should be called and the person placed in bed and kept absolutely quiet.

A bruise is an injury caused by impact in which neither laceration or external bleeding occurs. The first symptom, pain, is usually followed by redness and swelling. Since blood under the surface has entered the tissue, the skin may become black and blue, and, later, brown and yellow. Though bruises do not ordinarily require treatment, ice packs will often lessen the pain. The pain and discolor of a black eye, which is a type of bruise, will often diminish if iced compresses are applied. Later, when the blackness appears, hot compresses for half-hour intervals are more effective.

Foreign bodies. Foreign bodies accidentally penetrating any orifice of the human body ordinarily should be extracted promptly. This must be done gently, however, since violence might do more harm than good.

An infant who has swallowed a foreign object should be laid face down, or held head down, so that he can cough up the object. If anything is caught in the nostril, blowing the nose or sneezing may help to extract it. Usually, however, the best solution is to call the doctor. When a foreign object lodges in the ear, an insect, for example, it may often be removed by filling the ear with warm oil. The insect cannot live in oil and when it dies it can be floated out with warm water.

Parents are justifiably frightened when a child swallows a broken piece of glass, a pin, or some foreign substance. If small, the object may pass from the body as part of a bowel movement.

A tiny particle in the eye may often be removed with the tip of a clean handkerchief. If it is under the lid, however, the most common method of removal is to turn the eye-lid up over a small rod, such as a match.

These suggestions do not apply, however, to a speck which appears on the eyeball itself. When this happens, the wisest course is to place a pad of wet gauze over the entire eye, call a doctor promptly and keep the person quiet until he arrives. Such an accident is often extremely painful.

One should never attempt to pull a fishhook out the way it went in. Rather, it should be pushed all the way through and snipped off at the end. It may then be pulled out without damaging the flesh.

Wounds. A wound is an injury involving a break in the skin. Before caring for a wound, the person in charge should wash his hands thoroughly in soap and water, and perhaps also in alcohol. Any object applied to the wound should also be sterilized and cloth which is used as a bandage ought to be thoroughly boiled. Packages of sterilized bandages may be purchased at a drugstore or other shops.

After the wound has been washed in soap and water, or in some suitable mild solution, it should be treated with iodine or alcohol and then covered with a sterile dressing. If any pus appears in the wound, be sure to call a physician. If this is impossible, the pus should be removed before treating the wound, even if it is necessary to open the wound for this purpose.

Burns. Among the possible causes of burns are scalding water, hot irons, electricity and unexpected match blazes. Burns involving more than half the body are usually fatal. Any person who has been burned severely will suffer shock as well as physical damage and requires the immediate attention of a physician. Little can be done by the layman except to make the victim as comfortable as possible.

If a person has suffered lesser burns, however, the injured area may be covered at once with cold water or vinegar. Petroleum jelly can be used at a later stage. The wounds should never be covered with anything since these articles cannot be removed without doing serious damage to the tissues.

Burns caused by nitric or sulphuric acid should be washed at once to remove the acid. This may be done with a solution of bicarbonate of soda. If possible, the wound should then be permitted to soak in the same solution for as long as possible.

Injuries from fireworks, guns, cap pistols and similar toys are no longer as common as they were in the past. Here the greatest danger is the possibility of lockjaw, a disease in which germs, having entered a wound, are sealed in. A doctor is desirable because the wound must be cleansed, after which the victim may possibly need lockjaw antitoxin.

Resuscitation. Asphyxiation, suffocation due to deficiency of oxygen, is often caused by drowning, electric shock or by carbon monoxide gas. When a person has been under water for as long as five minutes artificial resuscitation is probably the quickest method of attempting to save his life. The most widely accepted method of artificial respiration, or resuscitation, is the direct mouth to mouth breathing, using a special tube if available. This operation may

usually be continued for at least an hour, or until the breathing has been restored. The person should be kept under close observation afterward, in case he should again cease to breathe.

If a person has suffered electric shock, the first step is always to remove the victim from the cause. Since every second counts and there is usually no time to turn off the current, the quickest solution is to throw a coat or similar article of clothing around the body of the victim and so pull him away from the current. Artificial respiration should then be administered until the doctor arrives.

Preventive action is the best method of avoiding death by carbon monoxide gas. Windows should always be kept open and an engine should never be permitted to run in a closed garage. Those who are especially sensitive to carbon monoxide gas should avoid any occupation in which such gas is prevalent.

The first symptoms of monoxide poisoning are headache, faintness, nervousness and irritability. An apparent victim of carbon monoxide poisoning should be removed at once to fresh air and kept quiet and warm. If possible, while awaiting the doctor, the patient should be covered with hot-water bottles or blankets to prevent pneumonia. At the same time, artificial respiration should be administered.

Fainting. If a person has fainted, a physician should be called. While awaiting his arrival, the victim should be placed flat on his back in the coolest location possible. If the face is pale, the head should be brought as low as possible in relation to the rest of the body. If the face is red, however, the head may be moved to a position somewhat higher than that of the rest of the body. Cold water may be applied to the face or chest, and smelling salts or a teaspoonful of aromatic spirits of ammonia in a tumbler of water may be given.

Heat Stroke. Heat stroke may occur, not only in tropical weather, but in any area, a laundry or kitchen, for example, where the heat is intense. Persons working under such conditions should take salt tablets at regular intervals throughout the day.

The signs to watch for in heat stroke are dizziness, drowsiness and fast breathing. When the attack occurs, it is essential to transfer the victim at once to a cool place and then keep him flat on his back and absolutely quiet. Sponging with cool water will help to control the temperature, and the circulation may be stimulated with coffee or other drugs.

Some authorities advise that the victim of heat stroke be placed on a bed covered with a large rubber sheet, and his entire body then rubbed with ice until the temperature drops to 101. At that point, the cold treatment is terminated and the patient is covered with blankets. If breathing stops, it is necessary to administer artificial respiration at once.

Bite Wounds. If a person has been stung by a bee or similar insect, the sting should be removed at once and a drop or two of diluted ammonia water placed on the wound. When a more serious bite has occurred, however, such as that of a centipede, spider or scorpion, bleeding should at first be encouraged as a means of removing the poison. Later, iodine may be applied, together with a cold pack to ease the pain. The sting of the black widow spider requires the additional attention of a physician who may employ a local anesthetic and also administer adrenalin to constrict the blood vessels so that the poison will not spread.

The treatment for a dog bite is the same as that which is given for any infected wound. If there is any likelihood of hydrophobia, however, the wound should be cauterized by a doctor and the dog reported to the city authorities at once.

Hiccups. A hiccup is an involuntary spasm of the diaphragm, causing an inhalation which is suddenly stopped by the closing of the glottis. A characteristic sound is involved.

Popular cures for hiccups often involve the use of a ruse which is calculated to distract the victim's attention from his affliction. If the condition persists, a doctor must be consulted. *See* HICCUPS.

Migraine or Sick Headache. Migraine may have its source in sensitivity to food, in a disease of the stomach or brain, in hardening of the arteries, in disturbances of vision, in menstruation, or in mental problems. Sometimes the cause cannot be determined.

The headache will either come suddenly or its approach may be heralded by a feeling a depression, perhaps a disinclination to work or to carry on daily activities.

When the migraine headache actually strikes, the victim is usually required to lie down in a darkened room in absolute quiet. Often the patient is so uncomfortable that he rejects any assistance or attention. Drugs provide a satisfying relief for migraine and may become habitual unless their use is carefully supervised by a physician.

Food Poisoning. When a person appears to have eaten poisoned food, an attempt should be made at once to determine the nature of the poison. Evidence may be found in an empty bottle, a cup or spoon, perhaps on the table or floor, or possibly by smelling the patient's breath or inspecting his mouth.

While awaiting the doctor, the white of eggs, milk or strong tea can be given to the patient, all of which are antagonistic to certain poisons. Vomiting can be provoked by means of tickling the back of the throat or by giving the patient a cup of warm water mixed with salt. If there is any possibility that the person has taken an acid poison, vomiting should never be induced.

See ANTIDOTE; ARTIFICIAL RESPIRATION; BURNS; DISLOCATION; EPILEPSY; ELECTRICAL INJURY; FAINTING; FRACTURE; FIRST AID; FOOD POISONING; MIGRAINE; HEMORRHAGE; POISONING; *etc.*

EMETIC, a substance used to induce vomiting for various purposes—for example, to empty the stomach of poison. An emetic should never be used for this purpose if the poison is one which might have a damaging effect on the lining of the stomach, such as an acid.

An emetic may also be used for persons suffering from bronchitis. This is indicated when the tubes which lead to the lungs are filled with a secretion which cannot be eructed except through vomiting. For old people, the emetic should be one which will not induce depression afterward. For these people, ten grains of ammonium carbonate, dissolved in water, is satisfactory.

One of the simplest emetics is a mixture of two tablespoons of salt with the minimum amount of water necessary to produce a liquid solution. Also effective is a mixture of one tablespoon of mustard in half a glass of water, or one tablespoon of alum in the same amount of water.

If an emetic is slow to act, vomiting can often be started by the old method of tickling the back of the throat with the tip of the finger, or with some object of similar shape. When regurgitation has finally begun, the process may be continued if the person drinks a large amount of lukewarm water at frequent intervals. This will also help to cleanse the stomach. *See also* VOMITING.

EMOTION, simply defined, an expression of feeling. In psychology it is a response to stimuli, involving certain physiological changes such as an increase in pulse rate, a rise in temperature, glandular activity, or a change in breathing rate. Psychosomatic medicine emphasizes the relationship of physical disorders to tension from unrelieved emotions.

In severe pain, fear, or anger, a person becomes pale because the blood vessels on the surface of the body contract. The skin feels cold and clammy, the mouth is dry because the saliva stops flowing and the tongue sticks to the roof of the mouth. Under such conditions, the heart beats rapidly and sometimes so strongly that the pulsation can be seen in the blood vessels of the neck. Other symptoms include wide opening of the eyes and dilation of the pupils. The tiny hairs of the body may actually stand on end and twitchings of the muscles may appear around the mouth and other parts of the body.

A rise in blood pressure or an increase in blood sugar may occur as a result of emotional strain due to excessive fear or to an accident involving severe emotional strain. The mere memory or association of some earlier incident later in life may provoke physiological reactions.

Continual worry is one of the significant causes of physical reactions and symptoms leading to various physical disorders. Violent emotions or prolonged minor emotional disturbances can affect the mental activity and the function of certain body processes.

EMPHYSEMA, the condition which exists when the normal air spaces in the lungs are dilated and the walls are overdistended. Various types of this disease are related to different causes. An obstruction of the breathing due to asthma or to chronic bronchitis or coughing produced by any one of a number of lung diseases may cause the walls of the small cells in the lungs to stretch and air to accumulate. The stretching occurs chiefly along the margins and upper edges of the lung where the muscular and bony framework of the lung less adequately support it. The stretching tends to destroy the elasticity of the breathing cells and causes distention of the lung.

Among the symptoms of emphysema are breathlessness on exertion and cough. The cough generally is due to chronic inflammation of the bronchial tubes. Cold air, dust, or exercise may start a coughing spell in the irritated tissues. A person with emphysema usually has a large barrel-shaped chest and prominent bones. The disease can be relieved by treatment of the asthma, bronchitis, or other chronic condition that causes it. Medical treatment of the cough which produces the distention is beneficial. Sometimes a properly fitted binder that sustains the chest walls without interfering with the movement of the ribs helps to control emphysema.

Mediastinal emphysema is caused by the introduction of air into the midchest region by a blow, strain, or coughing. It may result also from puncture wounds, or from incorrect use of machines for artificial respiration. Symptoms include swelling of the neck and occasionally of the whole face and chest. If the condition interferes with breathing, the air can be withdrawn by an operation. However, if the amount of air in the tissues becomes so great as to interfere with the circulation to the heart and lungs, death may result.

In older people, chronic emphysema may exist because of inelasticity and weakness of the lung tissues. However, the cough generally is not as severe as in the case of younger people suffering from emphysema. A really effective treatment for emphysema associated with old age has not as yet been found.

EMPYEMA, a medical term signifying pus in a cavity or organ, especially in the chest cavity, the gallbladder, or in the pericardium which envelops the heart. Usually empyema is associated with infections of the lung and is called suppurative pleurisy.

Pleural empyema affects children more often than adults. Frequently it occurs in connection with pneumonia or influenza, particularly when the influenza virus is accompanied by a secondary infection of streptococci, staphylococci, or other pus-forming germs. Occasionally the tuberculosis germ may be present and fungi of various kinds may also be found. Empyema may also follow an injury or wound to the chest and lung.

Symptoms of empyema in influenza or pneumonia may be a sudden rise of fever, pain or interference with chest movement in breathing. If examination shows an accumulation of fluid, the doctor can confirm his diagnosis by tapping the chest wall with a needle. If the amount of fluid is so large as to cause pressure on the heart and lungs, prompt removal of the fluid is absolutely necessary. Most of the infectious material can be withdrawn with the needle and a cure effected by the reinjection of antiseptics or other substances to combat the infection. In extreme cases, however, surgical operation may be necessary. The prompt use of sulfa drugs and antibiotics has made surgery unnecessary when empyema is detected early.

ENCEPHALITIS, often called "sleeping sickness," an inflammation of the brain which causes drowsiness and slowing down of mental and physical faculties. A number of distinct types of encephalitis are known, most of them caused by viruses. The condition sometimes occurs as a complication of another infectious disease, such as meningitis or measles, or may arise from poisoning or infection of a wound. Virus encephalitis should not be confused with African sleeping sickness, which is due to a parasite, trypanosoma, carried by the tsetse fly.

One of the viruses responsible for encephalitis, equine encephalomyelitis, also affects horses, birds, mice, snakes, and possibly other animals. Since 1931, when it first occurred in California, the disease has appeared spasmodically in both human beings and horses and other animals. Sometimes it has reached epidemic proportions within a two-month period, and at other times has appeared in sporadic cases in a few scattered areas.

Another form of encephalitis appeared in a major epidemic in St. Louis during the summer of 1933 and has since been called St. Louis encephalitis. Still another form, postinfection encephalitis, occurs during the course of or follows an infectious disease such as measles or influenza. Sometimes it has appeared after vaccination against rabies, smallpox, or measles. Postinfection encephalitis, which is less common than the other types, attacks persons of all ages, although children are most susceptible. There is no evidence that this type is contagious.

Symptoms of encephalitis vary greatly, depending on the severity of the infection and the area of the brain and nervous system affected. The illness may be brief and mild or severe and lengthy. Acute forms usually begin with high fever and headache, dizziness, vomiting, and pain and stiffness of the neck and back. Drowsiness, stupor, and weakness of the eye muscles are common symptoms. In severe cases, delirium, convulsions and insomnia are present.

Damage to the nervous system is the greatest danger in encephalitis. Parkinson's disease (shaking palsy or paralysis agitans) may follow an attack and sometimes a deterioration of mental faculties. Behavior disorders may develop in children who have had encephalitis.

In general, treatment consists in relieving pain and headache, reducing the fever, and making the patient as comfortable as possible. The physician may prescribe sedatives for restlessness and other drugs for insomnia or delirium. Special nursing care and regular supervision by the physician, even after the severe stage has subsided, are essential.

ENDARTERITIS, inflammation of the inner wall of an artery which occurs in certain types of endocarditis. *See also* ARTERIOSCLEROSIS; ENDO-CARDITIS.

ENDOCARDITIS, inflammation of the lining of the heart. *See also* BACTERIAL ENDOCARDITIS; EMBOLISM; HEART; RHEUMATIC FEVER.

ENDOCARDIUM, the thin layer of tissue lining the inside of the heart.

ENDOCRINE GLANDS, any of the ductless glands, such as the adrenals, the thyroid, or the pituitary, whose secretions pass directly into the blood stream. *See also* GLANDS; HORMONES; and Chapter 19, "Endocrine Glands."

ENDOMETRITIS, inflammation of the inner lining of the womb. It may follow normal birth or may occur as a result of abortion or infection. Bad-smelling discharge and fever are the two most common symptoms. This condition demands the attention of a physician. Treatment may require curettage or operation.

ENEMA, an injection of liquid into the lower bowel through the rectum. The purpose may be either to cleanse the intestines or to introduce nourishment or drugs into the body.

An ordinary ear syringe, with a rubber tip, may be used to give an enema to an infant. A single bulbful of liquid is the maximum which may be safely introduced into the intestines of a baby at one time. The injection should be performed as slowly as possible.

For enemas of larger quantity, a douche bag with a capacity of at least a pint may be employed. The bag, or can, should be hung not more than two feet above the person's head. Placing it higher gives the stream excessive force. To this bag or can a length of rubber hosing is attached. At one end of the hose is a nozzle, made of bone or vulcanite, or the end of the hose itself, rounded off may be introduced into the rectum. A soft nozzle is preferable, since it is less likely to injure the fragile inner surface of the lower intestine.

To receive the enema, the person may kneel, or he can lie on his left side with his knees pulled up to his stomach. If he lies in bed, the bed should be protected with a rubber sheet. Before the nozzle is inserted into the rectum the fluid should be sent through the entire hose so that all the air is expelled. Petroleum jelly or paraffin should be applied to the nozzle, which may then be inserted for a distance of approximately one inch. Unless the liquid is inserted slowly, it will immediately emerge. If necessary, a folded cloth or towel may be held against the rectum to aid retention.

If the purpose of the enema is to empty the lower part of the bowels rather than to cleanse the intestines, the enema may be given with the patient sitting up instead of lying down, and the liquid, once it has entered, may be permitted to emerge at once.

The type of solution used will depend on the purpose of the enema. Some enemas are nutritional, and others are intended to fill the body with fluid. As a laxative, plain water may be satisfactory or a mild soap-and-water solution, although the latter type of enema is irritating to some people. Baking soda and water, glycerin and salt or soapsuds and salt solutions are also used. An enema containing a strong medicine should not be given except with the specific prescription of a physician. A barium enema is given before an x-ray or fluoroscopic examination of the lower intestines and organs of this region of the body. *See also* CONSTIPATION; DOUCHE; SYRINGE.

ENTERIC FEVER, the technical term for typhoid and paratyphoid fevers. *See* TYPHOID FEVER.

ENTERITIS, the medical term for any acute or chronic inflammation of the intestine due to any one of a variety of causes. Pain and diarrhea are among the symptoms.

ENURESIS, the scientific name for bed wetting, urinary incontinence in the absence of demonstrable organic causes, at an age when urethral sphincter control is normally expected; a habit disturbance. *See also* BED WETTING; CHILD CARE; and Chapter 9, "Child Care and Training."

ENZYME, a complex chemical substance found largely in the digestive juices of the body which acts as a catalytic agent on other substances and causes them to split up. At least a dozen significant digestive enzymes are found in the secretions of the digestive system and aid in digesting fats, proteins, and carbohydrates. *See also* DIGESTION.

EPHEDRINE, a substance derived from a Chinese alkaloid called ma huang. When injected or taken into the body it causes smooth muscle tissue to go into spasm. In hemorrhage it constricts blood vessels throughout the body, tending to keep the blood pressure normal. As an ingredient of nose drops it shrinks the lining of the nasal passages permitting more comfortable breathing during colds. It is also useful in asthma, by relaxing the smooth muscle lining of the bronchioles, permitting easier inflow of air into the lungs.

EPIDIDYMITIS, that portion of the testicle lying like a hood over the upper end. When it becomes infected, as in gonorrhea, the condition is known as gonorrheal epididymitis. The epididymitis may also be associated with other infections. Treatment involves control of the source. The sulfa drugs and penicillin are most frequently and effectively used for these infections, but always on the advice of a physician.

EPIGLOTTIS, an elastic cartilage resembling a valve or lid, located behind and below the root of the tongue. It covers the glottis, the opening into the windpipe, during swallowing, thus preventing the entrance of food and drink into the voice box. Formerly it was assumed that the epiglottis was drawn down to cover the glottis. Actually, however, the glottis is drawn upward, to give protection.

EPILEPSY, a disorder of the central nervous system, perhaps among the most misunderstood of all human afflictions. Throughout recorded history, its victims have been, at various times, avoided, feared, scorned, ridiculed, flogged, and burned at the stake. They have been said to be possessed of the devil, and in some periods have been revered or even worshiped.

Epileptics are subject to seizures, temporary loss or alteration of consciousness, with or without convulsive movements. Five or more types of seizures are known, but only one, the *grand mal,* has the characteristics of the popular conception of a "fit" or convulsion. Even a violent *grand mal* seizure rarely lasts much longer than a minute, though it will probably seem much longer to an observer. After a seizure, the person

may sleep for a few hours or resume normal activity within a few minutes.

Contrasted with the *grand mal* is the *petit mal* seizure, a momentary blackout, with or without a twitching of the eyelids or of other facial muscles. Its manifestations, however, are so slight that it may go unnoticed even in a crowd.

Little can be done while a person is having a seizure. At the beginning of an attack he may be lowered to the floor, well away from hard objects against which he might injure himself. Any tight collars or belts should be loosened, and a folded handkerchief inserted between the back teeth to prevent biting of the tongue. The patient should be turned on his side to permit saliva to flow from his mouth.

Science has made great progress in diagnosing and treating epilepsy through the use of an instrument, the electroencephalograph, which magnifies and records the electric impulses from the brain, much as an electrocardiograph checks the heart. An electroencephalogram, the written record, is unique for each person, like a fingerprint. This record is a significant clue to the type of medication most likely to be successful.

At present, approximately 0.5 per cent of the population of the United States is afflicted with epilepsy. Seizures begin prominently in early childhood and in adolescence, but many persons are subject to them after the age of twenty-one. The number of males and females who suffer from epilepsy is almost equal. The true cause of epilepsy is not as yet known. Epilepsy is known to be related to damaged brain tissue, or to a brain tumor in some cases, but it may be present when such conditions do not exist. Tension, although it does not cause seizures, may precipitate them. A well-adjusted person who is physically and mentally active will have fewer seizures.

One of the nation's leading authorities on epilepsy, Dr. William G. Lennox, in his book, *Science and Seizures,* compares the electric impulses of the brain of a normal person to a stream with a moderate flow, controlled by an adequate dam. In the case of a person with epilepsy, the level at times rises and spills over the dam and a seizure results. The level overflows when the predisposition to epilepsy combines with minor body or emotional disturbances which most people experience without ill effects.

The hereditary cause of epilepsy is more significant than the acquired one. Among near relatives of epileptics, the illness is about three times more frequent than among the population as a whole. Certain disorders which may bring about epilepsy are thus acquired causes. Among these are (1) congenital defects of the central nervous system—as, for example, degeneration of the nervous system, congenital mental defect, and scarring of nerve tissue; (2) changes in the development of the brain after birth—as, for example, various types of meningitis, multiple sclerosis, general paresis, tumors, hemorrhages, cerebral abscess, arteriosclerosis and senile degeneration; (3) general diseases such as uremia, toxemia of pregnancy, fluid swelling of the brain, pernicious anemia, asphyxia, protein

shock, acute fever in children, hypotension, insulin or electric shock; (4) effect of convulsant drugs—for example, camphor, caffeine, ergot, epinephrine, cocaine, magnesium sulfate, and sulfathiazole.

According to the Foundation to Combat Epilepsy, the incidence of epilepsy because of acquired causes is variable. The incidence related to convulsant drugs and brain tumor is not larger than 15 per cent, abnormalities at birth around 9 per cent, infections about 5 per cent, brain tumors about 1.5 per cent, cerebral circulatory defects about 1.2 per cent, and postnatal brain trauma about 6 per cent. In approximately 77 per cent of the patients, evidence of antecedent organic diseases of the brain does not exist.

A specific cure for epilepsy is not known, but medication can reduce the frequency of seizures or eliminate them completely in about 85 per cent of those affected. Many drugs and combinations of drugs are effective when taken under the guidance of a physician. Seizures can be completely controlled—that is, prevented from occurring—in about one-half of all persons with epilepsy. An additional 35 per cent under medication have the frequency of their seizures reduced by half or more, and the remaining 15 per cent of epileptic patients are not helped by medication.

A person with epilepsy should never try to treat himself, since the drugs and dosage needed vary from person to person and only a physician, specially trained, is competent to prescribe. Mail-order remedies should never be used. For most persons with *grand mal* or psychomotor seizures, the doctor employs, among other drugs, phenytoin sodium or Dilantin; and, if this drug is not fully effective, phenobarbital may be added. Another drug, Mesantoin, can be tolerated in larger amounts by some patients than others. These drugs can be obtained only by prescription and changes and directions in dosage must be supervised properly to be effective. For convulsions, the physician may employ first phenobarbital or Mebaral. Bromides, although now replaced by newer drugs, are still useful in some circumstances. In Cases of *petit mal,* tridione, paradione, Milontin, and phenurone have been successfully used in many cases.

The person subject to epilepsy must take his medicines regularly, avoid alcohol, emotional upsets, and fatigue and live as regular a life as possible. He should not be overprotected by his family, but should be encouraged to lead a full life. Children should not be kept out of public schools and should play with their friends as usual. The epileptic must never be put into a position of feeling that he is "different."

In prevention of epilepsy as regards marriage and having children, each patient must receive individual consideration. Only the predisposition to epilepsy is inherited, not the disease itself. The chances that a child of epileptic parents will have epilepsy are about 1 to 40; and that a child will have more than one convulsion during childhood about 1 to 70. If an acquired cause is responsible for epilepsy in parents, these chances are greatly reduced.

If the number of cases of infectious diseases that involve the brain were reduced, a great step toward controlling acquired epilepsy would be made. Many of these diseases are the result of traffic accidents, occupational accidents, and war injuries. Concentrated efforts to reduce asphyxia and injuries at birth should be made.

Psychologically the illness may have a great effect. Approximately 80 per cent of all victims of epilepsy are capable of leading normal lives; those persons about them should recognize that epilepsy is not communicable and not a sign of insanity. Unfortunately, through misunderstanding of the disease, a person with epilepsy may find himself shunned by other people and discriminated against in employment. Concealment of the disease may deny many epileptics the advantages of education and marriage. Not only must the public be educated about epilepsy but the epileptic himself must learn to have self-confidence and courage.

Many people with epilepsy have achieved great heights of accomplishment—for example, Richard Wagner, Algernon Swinburne, Vincent van Gogh, and Hector Berlioz. A new organization, Epilepsy: Self-Help, sponsored and financed by the Variety Club Foundation to Combat Epilepsy, has been organized for people with epilepsy to meet for mutual association, understanding, and encouragement. The self-confidence of the epileptic can be strengthened when he has an opportunity to discuss his problems with persons who understand them. For information about epilepsy, write to the National Epilepsy

League, 130 North Wells Street, Chicago, Illinois.

EPINEPHRINE, one of the chief hormones of the inner portion of the adrenal glands. Its trade name is Adrenalin. *See* ADRENALIN.

EPISTAXIS refers to the common nosebleed. Nosebleed may be due to many factors. In children, it is usually the result of picking the nose and breaking small blood vessels. In adults with high-blood pressure, nosebleed may occur, which tends to relieve the blood pressure. Nosebleeds may result from frequent blowing of the nose, from a cold, foreign bodies in the nasal passages, or during the menstrual period. Fleshy growths in the nose, such as polyps, vitamin deficiency, food allergy, or even leukemia may all produce a nosebleed. Chronic nosebleeds can lead to general weakness.

Treatment at home should include having the victim lie down, applying ice-cold compresses about his lips and nose, and inserting small wads of cotton into the nasal passages. If this does not stop the bleeding, the doctor should be called. *See also* NOSE, DISEASES OF.

EPITHELIOMA, any benign cancer or tumor of the skin or other epithelial tissues. *See also* CANCER.

EPITHELIUM, a tissue composed of contiguous cells with little intercellular substance. It forms the epidermis, lines all the hollow organs and passages of the respiratory, digestive, and genitourinary systems of the body. The hair, nails, and enamel of the teeth are modified epithelial cells.

EPSOM SALT, a bitter white or colorless crystalline salt of magnesium sulphate heptahydrate. It acts as a cathartic and also as an antidote in lead or carbolic acid poisoning.

EQUILIBRIUM, physically the sense of balance, and mentally a well-balanced condition of mind or feeling. Physically it is controlled by information from the inner ear and elsewhere sent to the brain and transferred to the necessary muscles.

If the head is rotated rapidly and then suddenly stopped, the fluid in the semicircular canals of the inner ear continues to move. The result may be a giddiness so pronounced that the person may not be able to stand. The same sensation will be experienced if pressure is brought on the inner ear by means of a syringe, or if blood should enter the semicircular canals. Likewise the victim of locomotor ataxia may possess such a faulty sense of balance that he cannot walk without watching his feet.

Finally, if the cerebellum is itself diseased, the sense of balance is destroyed, and the victim may walk as if he were suffering from alcoholic intoxication.

ERGOT, a fungus that grows on grains and cereals. It is used to aid the uterus to contract after childbirth, to prevent blood loss. It does not affect normal pregnancy. Any form of this drug must be used only under the supervision of a doctor, since it may have adverse effects on the blood pressure as well as the blood vessels themselves.

ERGOTISM, a disease caused by overuse of ergot-containing food or drugs; it is characterized by gangrene of the fingertips and toes.

ERYSIPELAS, also known as St. Anthony's fire because the skin becomes a bright red as the inflammation spreads, a skin disease due to streptococcal infection. It manifests itself in headache, vomiting, chills, and fever, pain in the joints and prostration. The poison emitted by the streptococcus transmits the inflammation which spreads rapidly. The infection appears on the face, but may affect any part of the skin. It usually starts in a wound, fissure, or minute abrasion of the skin.

Erysipelas occurs more often in cold weather when the cracking of the skin due to exposure predisposes persons to its attack. The condition begins as an irregular round or oval patch. As it spreads, the patches become livid red, slightly swollen, hot and tender. The disease may be fatal, particularly to young children or old and infirm people, and it is essential that a doctor be called at once.

The development of sulfa compounds and antibiotics in recent years has rendered all other forms of treatment of erysipelas obsolete. These drugs reduce the fever, check the spread of inflammation, and bring the condition under control. People with erysipelas should be given plenty of fluids, at least ten glasses of water a day, and nourishing food, since the disease devastates the blood and weakens the patient. Erysipelas frequently reoccurs and therefore particular care should be taken to avoid scratching or irritating the skin.

ERYTHEMA, a redness of the skin, in uneven patches, caused externally by sunlight, ultraviolet rays, x-rays, heat, cold, friction, or by chemical irritants. Also erythema may result from the action of internal poisons, as in scarlet fever and other infectious diseases.

This condition may be caused by drugs or by poisons generated in the bowels or in other parts of the body. Sometimes it is accompanied by fever, sore throat, and pain in the joints. This type of erythema affects young people, especially girls, and may last for several weeks. Another species may occur as lesions of the skin, surrounded with red rings. The treatment includes rest in bed, a light diet, and the application of a soothing powder or lotion.

In the nodular form of erythema, round or oval nodular patches appear on the legs below the knees, and on the lower arms. The patches are tender and discolored, resembling bruises. Treatment is somewhat similar to that for the patchy type of erythema. Antihistaminic drugs, ACTH and several related drugs are sometimes effective in controlling these cases.

Another form of erythema, known as erythromelalgia, is of nervous origin and appears suddenly on the hands and feet. A more serious variety of erythema affecting the internal organs is lupus erythematosus in acute form. *See also* CHAFING; ECZEMA; INTERTRIGO; LUPUS ERYTHEMATOSUS.

ERYTHROBLASTOSIS FOETALIS. When a mother is Rh negative and the embryo is Rh positive, antibodies are developed before birth which may cause the newborn child to suffer from jaundice and anemia. This condition is known, medically, as erythroblastosis foetalis, which means destruction of red cells in the fetus. It is also called hemolytic anemia. *See also* BLOOD TYPES.

ERYTHROCYTES, the scientific term for red blood cells. For conditions affecting the red blood cells, *see also* ANEMIA; BLOOD; and Chapter 13, "Diseases of the Blood."

ESOPHAGUS, the tube, also known as the gullet, which connects the mouth with the stomach.

The modern physician possesses a special instrument by which he can actually examine the walls of the esophagus, where food will sometimes accumulate and cause irritation. Occasionally the walls will then adhere to each other, or even grow together, so that the doctor must surgically reopen the organ.

The two chief symptoms of diseases of the esophagus are pain and difficulty in swallowing. The principal disorders, besides foreign objects and irritation by food, include congenital abnormalities, inflammation, ulcers, spasm, tumors, rupture, and dilated or twisted veins. Cancer may occur in the esophagus, usually in the lower or middle portions of the tube.

Psychological problems may also be reflected in the esophagus. People have starved to death because they could not emotionally undertake the task of swallowing. However, starvation from this cause is rare, because food can be introduced into the body by means other than through the esophagus. Dilation of and operations on the walls of the esophagus are performed with a high degree of success. *See also* STOMACH; and Chapter 18, "Disorders of the Digestive System and Diet in Digestive Disorders."

ESTROGENS, the female sex hormones, are produced primarily in the ovaries. However, they also occur in the afterbirth, the adrenals and other glands. Estrogens are responsible for the development of female physical characteristics. They cause the breasts to enlarge, the deposition of fat around the hips, and development of the female reproductive glands. They make the voice high-pitched, the skin soft and delicate, and affect bone growth as well. The female sex hormones cause changes inside the uterus which lead to menstruation. Excessive levels of female hormone may lead to development of fibroid tumors of the uterus, to ovarian cysts, bone defects and possibly to aggravation of tendency to breast cancer or cancer in other areas. The female sex hormones are used medicinally for many conditions—for instance, to help regulate the menstrual periods, to lessen the severity of symptoms of the menopause, and to hasten development of female characteristics. They have been used in men with cancer of the prostate, to lessen the progress of the disease. They should never be employed without the constant supervision of the physician. Production of the female sex hormone ceases at the menopause.

ETHER, a thin, colorless, volatile, and highly inflammable liquid whose chief use is as an anesthetic in operations and as a solvent.

EUCALYPTUS OIL, an oil developed from the leaves of the eucalyptus tree, useful as a stimulant, antiseptic, and astringent.

EUNUCH, a male deprived of his testicles. *See also* CASTRATION.

EUSTACHIAN TUBE, or auditory tube, the canal connecting the nasopharynx with the middle ear. Its function is to equalize the pressure between the middle and external ears. *See also* DEAFNESS; EAR.

EXANTHEM, any eruption on the skin. Any acute disease, like measles, scarlet fever, or chickenpox, in which there is an eruption of the skin is called an acute exanthematous disease.

EXCRETION, the discharge from the body of waste products, including feces, sweat, and urine. The greater part of this function is performed by the kidneys, which are among the most significant of the excretory organs. *See also* BOWEL; CONSTIPATION; DIARRHEA; KIDNEYS; URINATION.

EXERCISE, the functional activity of the muscles. Physical exercise is a basic requirement for proper development of the body. Failure to exercise tends to produce a sluggish digestion, flabby muscles, and inadequate elimination.

Maximum benefit is derived from moderate and regular activity, rather than from violent, erratic exercise. A strenuous workout over Saturday and Sunday, for example, may be extremely harmful, unless preceded by regular training throughout the week. This warning applies to mountain climbing, sprinting, long-distance run-

ning, football, hockey, gymnastics, judo, wrestling, and boxing. Furthermore, all excessively vigorous games should be avoided after the age of thirty.

Safer exertions include walking, which is especially valuable because the distance and speed as well as the choice between level and hilly areas can be determined with relation to the physical condition of the walker. Golf and gardening can also be pursued at an individual pace. Swimming encourages deep breathing, riding develops a sense of balance, and dancing has a special asset because the sense of music and rhythm is involved. The value of dancing will be enhanced if overindulgence, late hours, and lack of sleep are avoided.

Calisthenics include such well-known exercises as the pushup and the kneebend. Activities of this type may be varied by the use of dumbbells, Indian clubs, and jumping ropes. Large muscles do not contribute to general health.

Exercises for the correction of special disorders are termed remedial. These may be active, if the patient exerts the effort, or passive, if the work is performed by someone else. A special type of passive remedial exercise is that in which a hand, arm, leg, or foot, or even the whole body is placed in a moving machine. Such exercise is helpful in the treatment of stiff joints. *See also* PHYSICAL THERAPY.

EXHAUSTION, a condition produced by loss of vital power from fatigue or protracted disease. Extreme exhaustion is known as nervous prostration or psychasthenia, sometimes referred to as neurocirculatory asthenia or weakness. The symptoms of exhaustion often include insomnia, loss of memory and appetite, listlessness, palpitations of the heart, and vitamin deficiency. Psychasthenia is rarely fatal, but it may render the person useless to himself, his family, and society. Corrective measures require a thorough examination, both mental and physical, of the person. Ordinarily a complete rest is imperative and possibly a radical revision of diet or even a change of occupation. *See also* ASTHENIA; FATIGUE; HEAT SICKNESS.

EXHIBITIONISM, a variety of sexual disturbance, seen most frequently in men, in which there is a compulsion to display the sexual organs, usually without desire for sexual union. Organized nudism is a different form of sexual disorder. The exhibitionist is typically an immature person, usually beset by feelings of inadequacy. Often he is conscientious in his daily work, and the tendency is not suspected by friends. Exhibitionists act from an uncontrollable inner tension and afterward experience depression and intense remorse. Psychiatrists believe that the disorder is the result of a subdued intense rage of some sort, a feeling of arrogance or hatred toward women and a desire to shock. Inner feelings of cruelty and sadism exist as well. The exhibitionist usually does not desire to inflict any physical harm. Treatment demands intensive psychiatric study; seldom can the person cure himself.

EXOPHTHALMIC GOITER, also known as Graves' disease, a disease caused chiefly by overproduction of the thyroid hormone with consequent enlarging of the thyroid gland. It is characterized by goiter, rapid heart action, protruding eyeballs, nervous excitability, fine involuntary tremor, loss of weight, muscular weakness, and a tendency to intense, acute exacerbations called thyroid crises. *See also* GLANDS; GOITER.

EXOPHTHALMOS, bulging or forward displacement of the eyes. Usually it is caused by an increase of pressure within the eye or by changes in the muscles of the eye. This condition is seen most often in cases of exophthalmic goiter.

EXPECTORATION, ejection of material from the mouth by coughing or spitting. Fluid or semifluid matter may be expelled from the lungs or air passages, or merely saliva. The matter expectorated, called sputum, may contain disease microbes, and spitting on floors and streets and public places is not only unattractive but also unhealthful. Expectoration should be done into a handkerchief, or in places where it cannot do harm.

EYE, the organ of sight. Constructed like a camera, the eye is intricate and efficient. All living species ordinarily have two eyes. The eyes of many other species surpass the human eye in certain respects. Many insects, for example, and some animals have eyes which are far more acute and efficient than those of human beings.

Structure and mechanism of vision. The eye is nearly a perfect sphere and occupies the anterior part of the frontal cavity of the skull. It is made of three concentric layers: the cornea, the iris, and the retina. The cornea is transparent and fits into a white membrane called the sclerotic coat. The iris connects with the choroid layer by means of the ciliary body. The iris itself is a colored, circular mem-

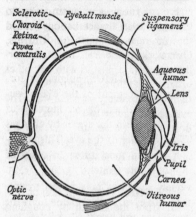

The various parts of the eye.

brane with a central perforation, the pupil. The retina, the innermost of the three layers, is a delicate transparent membrane containing the ends of the optic nerve. The vitreous body, a firm transparent jelly, constitutes about four-fifths of the eyeball. In front of the vitreous body is the crystalline lens, slightly yellow, disclike in shape, transparent, and curving out on each side. The space between the lens and cornea is divided by the iris into two parts, the anterior and posterior chambers, which contain the aqueous humor, a transparent fluid. In front the eye is covered by the conjunctiva, a mucous membrane, and posteriorly by a fibrous capsule. The entire eyeball is moved by a group of muscles attached on the outer surface. The curvature of the lens is changed by the ciliary mus-

cle, while the pupil is dilated by the action of the dilator and constrictor fibers in the iris.

To understand the mechanism of vision, some knowledge of the construction of the eye, as has been outlined above, is helpful. Actually we do not see with the eye but with the brain and nervous system. The chief factors involved in seeing are the optic nerve and the brain's center for vision. The retina, part of the nervous system, serves to convey images to the optic nerve. The lens is actually a lens, and serves to focus objects on the retina, while the muscles control the size and shape of the lens in its focusing. Accessory muscles move the eyeball. The iris controls the amount of light which enters the eye by dilating and contracting.

Ideally the lens of the eye receives light from the outside and bends it so that the image is focused on a small point of the retina. To maintain focus on the retina, the lens must change its shape when objects are viewed from different distances. This is called accommodation. When the eye is unable to accommodate properly, nearsightedness or farsightedness may result.

Nearsightedness, myopia, is the condition in which one is unable to see objects clearly at a distance. It may be hereditary and frequently is not discovered for some time.

Farsightedness, hypermetropia, is the condition in which one sees things at a distance better than things close up because the light is focused at a point beyond the retina.

The eye in its normal functioning has the ability to adapt itself to various conditions of light. Overuse will

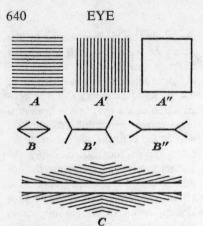

Here are some examples of figures which cause optical illusions. Figures A, A′ and A″ are all precisely the same size despite the fact that the line directions give a different impression. The horizontal lines B, B′ and B″ are all the same length although B″ certainly *looks* longer than B. The two horizontal lines in C are straight and exactly parallel despite the image they give of spreading at the center.

exhaust this ability, and proper lighting is necessary to prevent the eye from becoming strained or fatigued.

A newborn baby is farsighted and for that reason pays little attention to objects close to him. By two months, he is able to use his eye muscles to bring his eyes into range for what he wishes to see. The baby does not see small objects clearly until he is at least six months old.

As people grow older, their eyes change. The most significant changes are those in which the lens becomes clouded, resulting in cataract. The muscles connected with change of shape of the lens to accommodate seeing at various distances do not respond as well as formerly. People past forty may require glasses when previously they had not needed them. Moreover, all the tissues concerned with the nutrition of the eye change as age increases, and the eye becomes functionally a less competent organ.

Except for time spent in sleeping, the eye is used almost constantly from the moment of birth until death. Overwork of the eyes results in earlier exhaustion, just as with any other organ. Therefore, vision should be facilitated in every possible way. The eye needs regular rest periods. To reduce strain, it is essential that suitable working conditions be given the eye.

The eye may be used for measuring the general state of health. Conversely the body may reflect trouble with the eyes. If the doctor finds the eyes clear and bright he will feel less concern about any immediate danger to general health. When a severe cold, fever or weakness from any cause is present, the eye will reflect this condition by lack of luster, heavy eyelids, and sluggish movement. In jaundice, the white of the eye becomes yellowish.

The eye may also reflect general disturbances of the body, such as hardening of the arteries, anemia, and diseases of the kidney and nervous system. A tumor in the brain is sometimes discovered because of difficulty with eyesight. Frequently double vision, diplopia, is the first symptom of inflammation of the brain. The pupils of the eye may be constantly contracted, dilated, or even unequal in size because of the effects of drugs on the body.

The dominant eye. Each eye has

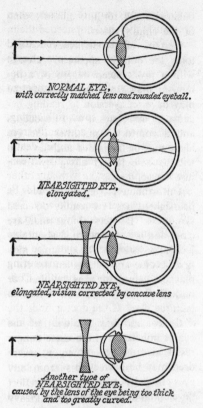

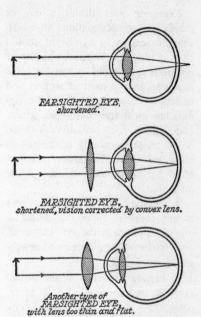

Diagrams of normal, nearsighted and farsighted eyes shown with and without corrective lenses.

an image, and these images are fused by a higher center in the brain. Eyes may differ, one from the other. When a person sees everything with one eye and depends on the image from one eye only, he is called a monocular. If he sees with both eyes and the images are properly fused, he has binocular vision. A person may be right-eyed or left-eyed, just as he may be right-handed or left-handed, and the eye on which he depends is called the dominant eye. When anything happens to the dominant eye, the other must then function. Little difficulty is encountered if the eye that has not been dominant previously worked satisfactorily. However, if that eye cannot assume dominance, a variety of symptoms may result, such as stuttering, fatigue, or various types of hysterical attacks in addition to symptoms related to vision.

Color blindness. Color blindness is more common among men than among women. Difficulty in distinguishing between red and green is the most common form of color blindness. The blue-yellow dilemma is much rarer. Color-blind persons see objects as lighter or darker, but are unable to distinguish the shades. Sometimes they may distinguish between red and green lights on roadways by their difference in brightness.

Everyone who drives a car or works in an occupation in which color detection is significant should have a test to determine whether or not he is color blind. A test for color blindness may consist of sorting and matching color samples. Traffic signals are most frequently red, green, and yellow and occasionally blue, colors most frequently concerned in color blindness. Therefore, a colorblind person should not drive a car in traffic.

A specific cure for color blindness is not feasible, since the defect is one of structure of the eye. However, color vision may be developed or substitutions found.

In certain branches of the armed services, like the navy and air force, color blindness is a bar to admission.

Vision of the child. When a child reaches one year of age, parents can, with a simple test, determine whether or not his vision is perfect. A bandage may be tied over one eye. Then a block, a ball, or any toy that the child uses may be placed near him. If the vision of the child is normal, he will pick up the object when either eye is bandaged, indicating that each eye functions properly by itself. If, however, the child is slow to detect the toy or unable to recognize it, an eye specialist should be consulted.

The next significant time for testing vision is when the child begins to read. Difficulties of vision may be present if the child holds the book too close to his eyes, too far away, or at an unusual angle. Such peculiarities call for immediate testing of the child's vision.

Certain other elementary symptoms are quickly apparent. A child with a pronounced degree of astigmatism may frown as he reads; he may have an aversion to reading because he associates it with headaches and discomfort. Sometimes one eye alone may be farsighted and the child will be able to get along by using just the good eye.

Unfortunately the child who is nearsighted has few readily detected symptoms. He sees things that are close and is not concerned about objects at a distance. The difficulty may first become apparent when the child plays a game, such as baseball or basketball, or is taken to a motion picture.

Cross-eyes. Any straining of the eye or imbalance of the muscles may result in cross-eyes or squint. Children may be born with one or both eyes crossed. A squint or walleye may develop from excessive strains placed on the external muscle of the eye by the extra effort which is required to see when there is an extreme degree of nearsightedness.

Children rarely outgrow cross-eyes. The sight of the crossed eye may never develop and, in many instances, the squint or crossed eye becomes worse. Early diagnosis and treatment are essential for the best results. As soon as one notices that a child is cross-eyed, an eye specialist should be consulted. Frequently good results are obtained merely with proper eyeglasses, which tend to hold the two eyes in position. Children have been found able to tolerate eyeglasses at the age of fifteen months. The earlier glasses are used, the more effective they will be.

The weak eye may be exercised by various training devices to correct the habit of suppressing the image of one eye. In certain disorders, when the deficiency is slight, this orthoptic training is successful. The most favorable age for such therapy is between three and six years. After the age of seven the results are rarely satisfactory.

The surgical procedure for overcoming cross-eyes is the most certain method of correction. Proper placement of the eye muscles by the surgeon tends to bring the eye back into proper relationship to the other eye and permit binocular vision. The operation is not a guarantee that vision will be improved, but it will prevent the vision from being eventually lost from failure to use the eye successfully. In addition, the correction of cross-eyes is essential in establishing a proper mental attitude in the child. Children with cross-eyes may be so sensitive to ridicule that they become shy, withdrawn, introverted personalities and their lives ruined as a consequence.

Color of the eyes. The color of the eyes is apparently largely governed by heredity. Eye color is a characteristic that comes down to people from their ancestors. When a blue-eyed person marries a brown-eyed person and there are four children, one probably will have blue eyes, one brown eyes, and two may have blue eyes with traces of brown. Brown-eyed parents may produce not only children with brown eyes but also blue-eyed children. The color of the eye is helpful in determining paternity but is hardly conclusive.

Colored rings. When one looks at bright light at night—for example, street lamps—they may seem to be surrounded by areas of color or colored rings, blue on the inside and red on the outside. This is not a disturbance of the eye, for these colors are due to the tissues and cornea of the eye. The tissues are not seen in ordinary light.

Specks before the eyes; muscae volantes. Because of the structure of the eyes, several disturbances of vision may develop which are not actual defects but merely tricks of eye function. If a person suddenly looks up at the sky or at a white ceiling after the eyes have been closed, he will probably notice a number of minute specks that move in front of the eyes. These specks are blood corpuscles moving in the smallest blood vessels at the back of the eyes. If the heart beats faster because of exercise, the blood corpuscles will move faster and the specks will also seem to move faster.

Eyestrain. Eyestrain is common. Unsuspected eyestrain may be associated with twitching of the eyelids and face. Nausea and vomiting may appear, with headache, loss of appetite, and many other similar conditions. The only conclusive way to determine whether or not eyestrain actually exists is to test the ability of the eyes to see, and then to overcome the condition by rest or with eyeglasses.

Glare or bright light places stress on the eyes. Special care should be taken to insure proper lighting in the home, schools, offices, and fac-

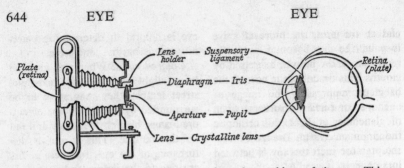

The mechanism of the camera is based on the workings of the eye. This illustration shows the parts of each that correspond.

tories. Although motion pictures and television may provoke eyestrain and fatigue, under normal conditions they do not cause serious eyestrain. However, the wrong type of lighting in the theater or home, films that are jerky, spotted, or badly lighted, and long periods of viewing may produce an uncomfortable condition.

Conjunctivitis. The tissue which lines the eyelids and runs out over the eyeball is called the conjunctiva. Inflammation of this tissue is known as conjunctivitis or pinkeye. Its symptoms are smarting and burning of the eyelids, formation of pus, and reddened eyelids. The inflamed eye becomes exceedingly sensitive to light, and tears flood it constantly. After sleep, the eyelids may be crusted together. This ordinary disorder of the eye demands care by a qualified doctor. Treatment is based on the severity of the infection and the character of the particular germ involved.

Styes. Styes involve infection of the glands of the eyelid by one of the common pus-forming germs, usually near a hair follicle, and often appear in crops. In some instances they are associated with uncorrected errors of vision. Under such circumstances the eye does not resist invasion by outside organisms as well as the normally functioning eye.

A sty behaves like a pimple or small boil. After a day or two it softens and bursts, the infectious material is discharged, and recovery usually follows. Before the sty has softened, its progress can sometimes be stopped by pulling out the hair that runs through it, and by treating the spot with an antiseptic that is not dangerous to the eye itself. Usually it is helpful to apply hot compresses to styes, to hasten the development of the inflammation. When a yellow spot appears, the infectious material should be released at once.

In the case of repeated formation of styes, physicians collect the germs causing them, make a vaccine from them, and reinject this vaccine into the patient. This may help the patient to develop specific resistance against the germs responsible for the styes.

Glaucoma. Glaucoma causes 15 per cent of all blindness in the United States, and about one-half of the blindness in adults. In this condition, pressure within the eyeball brings about loss of sight. Interference occurs with the circulation of the fluid that comes into the eye. The accumulation of this fluid causes pressure, and as the pressure increases there is pain, the eye becomes hard and reddened and the pupil gray and cloudy. This describes the acute form of glaucoma.

In a second and more serious form of glaucoma, gradual obstruction of the drainage system occurs so that the pressure increases slowly and the loss of sight is gradual.

The physician can determine the extent and effect of the pressure with the ophthalmoscope and the tonometer. Drugs have been developed which eliminate fluid and lower pressure within the eye.

As the glaucoma develops, the person finds that he can see straight ahead as well as he ever could, but not so well to the sides. Gradually the vision in front also becomes narrowed until finally there is complete loss of sight.

In the treatment of early glaucoma, drugs, such as Diamox, alone may be sufficient. In later stages, drugs prepare the tissues of the eye so that an operation to relieve the pressure, known as an iridectomy because part of the iris is cut out, may be more easily and successfully performed.

An instrument useful in measuring the width of the field of vision is the perimeter. If the field is steadily narrowing, glaucoma is present. A correct diagnosis early in the development of glaucoma is invaluable in preventing pain and pressure and in saving sight.

Older women should be particularly watchful of their eyes, as they are more likely to suffer from glaucoma than men.

Excitement is often a factor in producing glaucoma, because of the increased flow of blood to the eyes during excitement, with consequent rise in pressure. Early symptoms may include headache, blurred vision, eye pain, and nausea. Prompt attention should be paid and an eye doctor consulted.

Tumors. Tumors may arise in the lids, the eye socket, or within the eyeball, and may interfere with vision and cause irritation of the eyeball. They should be removed, even though they are generally benign tumors. Malignant tumors sometimes occur, which can spread and may require removal of the eye. The most common malignant tumor of the eye, retinoblastoma, is confined to children under ten years of age, and may even occur at birth. Malignant melanoma, perhaps the most fatal and most prevalent form of eye tumor, occurs most commonly in adults, arising inside the eye and spreading throughout the body if not checked in time and removed.

Fatigue. An eye which is fatigued and unable to work satisfactorily becomes easily irritated. Moreover, it is more apt to be invaded by foreign bodies, like cinders and dust, simply because the tissues do not react to rid the eye of such foreign material. Persons with bad eyesight frequently have red rims on the eyes, swollen eyelids and constant watering, and the eyelids may be crusted together in the morning. The appearance of any of these signs should be an indication that the eye needs medical care.

Guarding eyesight. Here are a few simple rules helpful in guarding eyesight.

1. Do not face bright windows or bright light when at work.

2. Never cleanse the eyes with a towel used by others.

3. Do not place hooks, doorstops, or other projections at the level of children's eyes. If such objects are placed near the floor or above children's eye level, there are less likely to be serious accidents involving a child's eyes.

Prevention of eye injuries in industry. Blindness or impairment of vision is one of the most serious and costly of all nonfatal accidents which workers may suffer.

Some eye disorders are known to be definitely associated with processes involving intense light and heat. For instance, a cataract occurs in the eyes of glass workers, who are exposed to the heat and glare of a furnace for many hours each week. All sorts of devices have been developed to prevent exposure of eyes of glass workers to this and other hazards. Fortunately the introduction of machinery for making glass bottles and other machinery to take the place of hand operations has minimized the dangers of furnace glare. Workers in other industries, like steel making, who are regularly exposed to glare from furnaces should wear appropriate glasses to shut out the light.

Workers in electric arc welding sometimes have inflammation of the eyes, with pain and headache. Similar symptoms affect workers in studios where photography, such as motion picture and television photography, is the chief occupation. Here again, careful attention to prevention of overlong exposure to powerful lights is imperative to overcome the hazard.

Certain industrial poisons are dangerous to the eyes, including ammonia, phosphorus, derivatives of lead, benzene, and methyl alcohol. At least fifty known poisons that can affect the eyes are used in industrial processes. Inhalation of poisonous dust or vapor and direct action of the poison on workers who have not thoroughly cleansed their hands is possible.

Adequate provision for frequent washing of hands by workers, and the use of exhaust fans for getting rid of dusts and gases are the best means of eliminating industrial eye hazards. The prevention of accidents to the eyes involves protection against flying fragments of metal, stone, and grit, and against burns from acids or strong caustics.

Properly made goggles, helmets, and shields are part of the safety program of well-managed plants.

Safety rules in eye injuries.

1. Under no circumstances should an untrained or inexperienced person attempt to remove any foreign body from the eye.

2. Immediately after an accident, the eye may be bathed with suitable mild aseptic or sterilized solutions, preferably a weak solution of boric acid made with sterilized water.

3. The eye should be covered with a sterile bandage moistened with this solution.

4. The person whose eye is involved should be sent immediately to a physician in charge of such cases.

Removing foreign bodies. Hundreds of superstitions suggest how best to remove foreign bodies from the surface of the eye. They concern sneezing or rubbing the other eye or similar notions. It is actually much safer to rub the other eye than the one in which the foreign body has lodged. Usually rubbing pushes the foreign substance farther into the eye.

Those persons who understand how to remove foreign bodies, make certain that their own hands are clean and that every instrument or other material used is clean or sterilized. The eye itself must be handled with the utmost delicacy. The person examining the eye carefully studies the eye, while the affected person first looks upward, so that the lower lid may be pulled down; then downward, while the upper lid is turned back. The upper lid cannot be turned back safely while the person is looking up or moving the eyeball constantly. With practice, skill can be developed in turning back the upper lid.

If the foreign substance is not seen, the examiner then looks at the surface of the eyeball, changing the light so as to catch the reflection of any foreign substance which may be imbedded in the cornea. Infinite care must be taken to prevent infection, as secondary infections may incite ulcers which may destroy the sight of the eye.

Viewing Television.

1. Make sure that you are getting clear reception.

2. Adjust tone setting before tuning the picture to desired brilliance. An unsteady image or too much light will produce visual discomfort.

3. Avoid intense darkness or bright light in the room in which television is viewed. Mild, indirect light is preferable.

4. Sunglasses should not be worn for viewing because they adapt vision to unnatural conditions.

5. Avoid excessively long periods of concentration on television.

6. Find the most comfortable distance for your own eyes.

7. In case of discomfort, have your vision examined. Many older persons who wear bifocal glasses may find neither segment suited to television viewing.

See also CATARACT; CORNEA; CORNEAL TRANSPLANTATION; SQUINT; and Chapter 5, "Occupational Health."

EYE BANK, a repository in which an ophthalmic surgeon may secure a cornea, to be used in an eye-grafting operation. The eye bank, in turn, secures its materials from a variety of sources, such as the eyes of a stillborn infant or on the death of an older person. Many persons now will their eyes for such transplantations. To operate such a bank is not only expensive but demands that the members of the staff possess extraordinary technical skill. However, the results are frequently so good as to justify all costs. *See also* CORNEA; CORNEAL TRANSPLANTATION; EYE.

EYE GLASSES, lenses used to correct and aid inadequate vision. They may supplement the diminishing capacity of the eye to adapt itself to distance, adjust the difficulty caused by the pull of various eye muscles, or aid in correcting poor vision caused by faulty anatomy of the eye.

Anomalies in anatomy are responsible for astigmatism, in which the image fails to focus properly on the retina, the part of the eye which receives the image. A person is far-sighted when the rays of light focus behind the retina, a condition usually corrected by a convex lens. If the person is nearsighted, so that the focus occurs in front of the retina, the adjustment can be made with a concave lens. *See also* ASTIGMATISM; BIFOCAL; CONTACT LENSES; EYE; MYOPIA; PRESBYOPIA.

FACE, the front part of the head, including the eyes, cheeks, chin, forehead, nose, and mouth. The facial skin, although not thick, contains numerous blood vessels and glands for the passage of oil, sweat, and other secretions. The tissue underneath the skin is thickened only in the vicinity of the chin; elsewhere it tends to be rather loose. Because of this looseness, space is available for swelling.

Many facial muscles, some near the surface, others far beneath, are used in facial expressions. These muscles coordinate with muscles in the forehead. In the act of eating, a muscle in the cheek poises the food between the teeth while it is being chewed and prevents food from gathering between the teeth and on the inside surface of the cheek. One of the principal nerves, the seventh or facial nerve, controls these muscles.

The main artery of the face moves upward and then forward. One of its branches is directed toward the tonsil and two other branches to the upper and lower lips respectively. Since these branch arteries to the lips are joined by two parallel arteries from the other side of the face, bleeding of the lip is difficult to control except by compressing the mouth at both ends.

The facial vein, which sometimes runs parallel with the facial artery, is connected with the cavernous sinus located inside the skull. Because of this connection, any serious infection of the face can transmit its poison to the veins in the skull. A facial infection should always be taken care of by a physician.

Complexion refers to the color and texture of the facial skin. Many ailments and conditions can affect the complexion. In chloasma, commonly known as liver spots, brown patches appear on the skin. It is often, though not necessarily, associated with pregnancy. Similar patches may occur which are not chloasma. Facial ruddiness has a variety of sources. If permanent it may be a birthmark. It may be associated with fever or with the hot flashes which sometimes accompany menopause. Redness in the vicinity of the nose often accompanies a type of acne, acne rosacea, which is produced by digestive ailments. In alcoholics, the nose may be red and the network of blood vessels chronically swollen. Prolonged exposure to weather can cause the skin to take on a red appearance. A bluish tinge to the facial skin may result from persistent bronchitis or asthma or cyanosis, a heart disease. Anemia may cause the complexion to be pallid. Any of these color tones to the complexion may be perfectly normal. In a healthy person, the gums and inside of the lower eyelid are a rosy color and, as with the skin, a deviation from this may indicate the presence of some undesirable condition. The appearance of the complexion may also be affected by such afflictions as acne, eczema, or impetigo.

A large amount of fat is packed under the facial skin. When this tends to diminish, as in old age or sickness, the skin becomes less elastic and begins to show wrinkles. *See also* ACNE ROSACEA; CHLOASMA; COSMETICS.

FAINTING, may be defined as a temporary suspension of consciousness. Originally a depression occurs in the action of the heart. This can be caused by something environmental, such as cold, heat, or hunger, or by mental shock, perhaps from pain or fright. As a consequence, the flow of blood to the brain is interrupted. Dizziness, difficulty in vision, a ringing in the ears, pallor, and an unsteady appearance may follow. The climax is a falling or sinking to the ground, possibly with a long sigh. Momentarily the victim may hardly seem alive. The breathing and pulse beat, for example, are sometimes almost imperceptible.

Treatment must encourage the flow of blood to the brain. This means that the patient's head should go down between his knees, or his entire body placed in the prone position. It is equally important that the victim should have plenty of air; the coolest place, especially in a hot and crowded room, is undoubtedly near the floor. Clothes should also be loosened, particularly those which are wound around the neck or across the chest. Alcoholic beverages, ether, ammonia, or smelling salts are often administered. Under intelligent treatment the patient will soon begin to breathe again in a normal fashion. At the same time color will come back into his face and his eyes will open. *See also* DIZZINESS; FIRST AID.

FALLEN ARCHES. *See* ARCHES, FALLEN.

FALLOPIAN TUBES, the two tubes lying close to each of the two ovaries and leading into the womb or uterus. Their function is to transport the egg cell or ovum, liberated each month by one of the ovaries, into the womb.

The potency of the Fallopian tubes is essential to pregnancy. They may, however, like other tissues, become affected by various disorders which interfere with their normal function. Painful twisting and blocking, for instance, may occur and be followed by secondary infection.

Sometimes a fertilized egg cell will begin to develop abnormally in one of the Fallopian tubes rather than in the womb. The condition, tubal or ectopic pregnancy, demands prompt surgery since unchecked growth of the developing embryo within the tube will rupture it, and serious hemorrhage within the abdominal cavity may follow, which may be fatal.

Gonorrhea is the most frequent infection of the Fallopian tubes, accounting, it is estimated, for 70 per cent of Fallopian infections. The symptoms of the acute stage resemble those of acute appendicitis. The temperature rises, the white blood cells increase, and the abdomen is tender to the touch. The infection may become chronic without acute manifestations, causing long-lasting ill health and eventually sterility.

Antibiotic and sulfa drugs are effectively used to treat gonococcal infection of the Fallopian tubes whereas formerly surgery was required. In the most serious cases, however, surgery may still be found necessary.

Tuberculosis or other infectious diseases may also attack the Fallopian tubes. Infection associated with inflammation of the tubes is known as salpingitis. *See also* ECTOPIC PREGNANCY.

FARSIGHTEDNESS. *See* EYE; PRESBYOPIA.

FASTING, abstinence from food, or limiting food, for religious, political, or medical purposes. For medical reasons, resting the stomach may aid in the relief of indigestion. Water, taken abundantly during a fast, may serve to rid the body of accumulated waste. A period of fasting is often required of diabetics, as a preparation for undertaking a diet.

Green vegetables are sometimes permitted during a partial fast. They provide necessary vitamins, help to move the bowels, and also allay the discomforts of hunger. Hunger, incidentally, does not constitute a serious problem in fasting. It is a minor inconvenience after the first day; and usually, after the second, it is hardly noticeable.

If a fast is planned for a period of more than two days, it is well to consult a physician in advance. He may suggest that the person fasting should remain in bed as much as possible, to conserve his energy and to keep warm. When the fast is broken, the consumption of food should at first be light and slow.

FATIGUE. The cells and tissues of the body have a remarkable power to recover from ordinary fatigue, but excessive, prolonged, and accumulated fatigue is dangerous. Fatigue is a warning that the person is attempting to do too much and if this warning is ignored the fatigue may develop into exhaustion, a condition in which the body is severely depleted.

A proper diet is a good preventive against fatigue. Muscles use sugar in performing their functions; numerous vitamins are essential for satisfactory functioning of the nerves; iron is required for the blood. A deficiency of these as well as other substances the body needs brings on fatigue more rapidly than when the body is receiving an adequate diet.

Fatigue can result from too little rest and sleep, from infection and disease, poor nutrition and physical and mental overwork. Some of the numerous symptoms of fatigue are a tendency to yawn, drowsiness, sweating without previous exertion, easy irritability, depression, general slowness of action or forgetfulness. Chronic fatigue induces loss of appetite and weight and increased irritability. When fatigue has progressed to this point, a doctor should determine the degree and cause of the fatigue. Rest, a change of diet, or perhaps a change of occupation may relieve the fatigue.

Four common-sense rules follow:

(1) The best treatment of fatigue is rest.

(2) Stop physical activity before exhaustion is manifest.

(3) Don't take stimulants like coffee, "pep" pills or other pick-me-ups. The feeling of relief is only temporary and induces further fatigue. Taking stimulants is like whipping a tired horse.

(4) If exhaustion is evident, medical care, including a special study of the glands, is desirable.
See also EXHAUSTION.

FATS. *See* FOOD FATS.

FEBRILE, a descriptive term meaning feverish.

FECES, the excretion from the bowels. It consists of undigested residue from food, bacteria and substances secreted from the intestinal walls and from the organs connected with the digestive tract.

FEEBLE-MINDEDNESS, mental deficiency or mental defect, a condition in which average intelligence either is not present or fails to develop. It must be clearly distinguished from mental disease, such as neurosis and psychosis, in which functions of a mind of normal capacity become disordered.

Different degrees of mental defect or feeble-mindedness are recognized. A person with an I.Q. below 20, who doesn't advance past a mental age of three, is considered an idiot. Custodial care of idiots is necessary. They usually present no special problem, since only a few live to adulthood and those who do do not pro-

create as they are infantile. Imbeciles have I.Q.'s below 50. Often they can be taught to do certain tasks, but they may require protective supervision. Morons, who have I.Q.'s below 70, generally can be trained to take care of themselves, and may even be able to support themselves. As well as doing domestic tasks, morons have held jobs in factories. Training of the feeble-minded involves sensory stimulation and development of muscular coordination. Good physical condition is important to help compensate for the mental limitation.

Symptoms of feeble-mindedness tend to manifest at an early age, although it is essential to have expert opinion regarding each individual case. A baby's failure to be as responsive to sounds and sights as normal, delay in teething and other phases of development may indicate a tendency to feeble-mindedness. However, variations in development are so great that such symptoms are certainly not inevitable indications of mental defect. The condition becomes more apparent as the child grows older and cannot adjust to other children or compete with them in studies or at play. The mentally defective person tends to remain infantile even though he grows physically.

Much can be done to prevent mental defectives from being hopeless and helpless burdens on others. Such capacity as they do have should be developed to the fullest rather than deprecated and neglected. They should be taught physical coordination to the greatest possible extent. They should be schooled as far as their capacity permits, but removed from situations in which repeated unsuccessful competition with children may give them acute feelings of inferiority and defeat. Special institutions for training the feeble-minded are available.

Individual attention is essential in caring for the mentally defective. Attempts to apply the same routine to a large group of feeble-minded persons are ineffective, because each one responds quite differently, depending on the extent of his ability.

Feeble-mindedness has a hereditary tendency. Normal people, in no sense mentally defective themselves, may be carriers of mental defect; that is, they are genetically capable of transmitting the defect to offspring. Feeble-minded persons should not marry, and those who have had a feeble-minded ancestor should recognize the potentiality of having a defective child.

Recent research has demonstrated that factors other than heredity may be responsible for feeble-mindedness. Sickness of the mother during pregnancy and injury during delivery of the infant have been suggested as possible causes, and still others may be found. Parents should not feel themselves to blame when a mentally defective child appears in the family.

FEEDING, BREAST. Conflicting ideas about breast feeding a baby— that is, feeding directly from the breast—as opposed to bottle feeding have produced some confusion in the minds of mothers, especially those who are having their first child. The weight of opinion favors feeding at the breast. A formula in the bottle, if the doctor's prescription and the

mother's preparation are correct, will provide adequate nourishment, but human milk contains valuable qualities which are not present in other forms of milk. Also, the latest investigations indicate that the breast-fed baby probably has a psychological advantage over the bottle-fed baby; even though the mother who feeds her baby by bottle holds him tenderly and affectionately, the bottle does in some way impede the direct communication between mother and child. However, breast feeding when it is done with a hurried and indifferent attitude can be emotionally unsatisfactory to the child, just as bottle feeding can give the child the feeling of security and love he needs. Above all, the attitude of the mother is important.

During the months of pregnancy much can be done to prepare the prospective mother for the task of breast feeding her baby. The doctor can recommend special care of the breasts, diet, massage, techniques for adjusting the shape of the nipples. A hospital can be selected which offers special facilities for the nursing mother.

The first days of nursing are a time in which the mother and child come to know each other. The child may at first refuse to take the breast, but if the mother is relaxed the child will probably begin to suck as soon as the nipple is introduced into his mouth. The first substance which is received is not milk but a yellowish thick liquid called colostrum. Under the stimulus of the infant's mouth the breasts quickly begin to release a thin blue milk. The nursing mother should keep in touch with her doctor during the first few weeks. The milk may not agree with the child; the child may get too much or too little milk at a feeding; he may eruct part of the intake, get colic pains, or other situations may arise which should be brought to the attention of the doctor. In general, the doctor will want to be sure that the mother is in good health and receiving the proper rest and food, exercise and recreation, and that the infant is progressing normally.

Occasionally breast and bottle feeding may be effectively combined. This may be necessary if the mother is sometimes absent from home during feeding time or if she cannot keep up the necessary supply of milk. Such a combination should be arranged with the help of the doctor. The combination of breast and bottle feeding usually will facilitate weaning.

The mother must decide which method will be used to feed the child. As stated, breast feeding is usually better for the baby, both physically and psychologically. It also eliminates the daily chore of cleaning bottle equipment and preparing the formula. Whatever method the mother decides to follow, the feeding should be administered with love and affection. *See also* CHILD CARE.

FEET. Feet are subject to a great variety of ailments. These include sprains, strains, dislocations, fractures, excessive sweating, warts, chilblains, ringworm, hammertoes, painful heels, ingrown toenails, cracked toes, blisters, bruises, circulation disturbances, fallen arches, corns, bunions and calluses, and many others.

Some of these are incurred during athletic activities, some are due to faulty footwear, and others are present at birth.

Fallen arches refers to a painful condition affecting the main bone of the foot, the astragalus. This affliction is especially common among people whose work requires many hours of standing or walking. The pain is due to the spasmodic efforts of certain muscles to overcome the strain which is placed on the tissues. Often the person can terminate the pain simply by getting off his feet.

Ordinarily, however, fallen arches require special treatment. Hot applications and massages taken at the end of the day are beneficial. Even more important is the appropriate choice of shoes. Generally shoes should be specially fitted with a medium-width rigid shank which supports the arch.

Among the most common of all foot complaints are calluses, corns, and bunions. When the skin is persistently rubbed, it tends to thicken. Such thickening, callus, develops most frequently on the bottom of the foot, usually at a point where constant pressure is exerted. For example, the golfer may develop a callus at the place on his foot where he pivots when driving the ball. A callus can be removed by the doctor. The real problem is how to prevent its return. Sometimes this can be done by padding the shoes in such a way as to shift the point of pressure on the foot.

A callus on the toes, between the toes, or—especially—on the outer part of the little toes is a corn. The soft corn, produced by a rubbing together of the little toe and the fourth toe, is a frequent point of infection, especially of ringworm. A majority of the numerous commercial cures for corns make use of salicylic acid, a drug which if given sufficient time will cause the corn to fall away. The only cure is an operation, seldom done, which removes not only the corn but also a part of the bone beneath the corn.

A bunion is a swelling produced by the inflammation of a bursa, a fluid-containing sac located between the tendon and a bone which serves to facilitate action. Bunions are found most often on the outer part of the big toe. They may also appear, however, in the middle of the top of the foot, where the person may have laced his shoes too tightly. This type of bunion can be relieved by inserting pads under the laces or by avoiding shoes which lace. Bunions resemble corns in that permanent relief may be found only in surgery. However, surgery for bunions is frequently and successfully done.

Care of the feet. The feet should be bathed once a day, then carefully dried and perhaps dusted with talcum or a germicidal powder so that moist areas will not rub together and produce infection. The general health of the feet may be improved by use of the so-called contrast bath. The person places his two feet first in one pail filled with hot water, and then in another filled with cold water. The feet should remain in each pail for about one minute, and the entire operation should continue for ten minutes. The purpose is to open and close the veins in such a manner as to encourage blood circulation. Massage of the feet is also beneficial and should be done with a circular movement of the fingers. If the skin is unusually sensitive, cold cream may be used in the massage.

For the general health of the feet, nothing is more significant than careful selection of shoes, properly fitted to the individual foot. The most crucial measurement is that from the back of the heel to the middle of the big toe. Many persons, including shoe salesmen, speak of breaking in a pair of tight shoes. This is an incorrect notion; it is the feet which are broken in. This is especially dangerous if the tightness of the shoe is longitudinal, where the tendency is to force certain toes into a right angle position, causing the hammertoe. A hammertoe may become so serious that it can only be relieved by an operation. Healthful shoes will always have round toes and shanks of only medium width. Extremes in the height and location of heels ought to be avoided. Specialists usually recommend a daily change of shoes. Shoes which are not being worn should be kept in shoe trees to retain their shape. Rubber heels possess therapeutic value because they decrease the shock effect on both feet and body. *See also* ARCHES, FALLEN; ATHLETE'S FOOT; BUNION; CALLUS; FLATFOOT.

FELON, an infection at the bottom of a fingernail which may be caused by staphylococcus or another pus-forming germ.

Home remedies like painting with iodine and other antiseptics or the application of hot wet packs soaked in boric acid solution are not always effective and the condition may get worse. If the infection penetrates muscular tissue, the bone covering, or the bone, the condition is serious and should be treated promptly by a doctor.

The doctor prevents pus and infection from penetrating deeper by soaking the finger in hot water to soften the tissue. Then by surgical procedure he releases the pus from the infected area. Hot packs soaked in boric acid are then applied and followed by painting with iodine.

If a felon is not controlled, the infection may spread along the lymphatic ducts and tissues into other parts of the body and produce a generalized infection. Indication of such diffusion is the appearance of red inflammatory lines running upward through the hand and wrist.

FERMENTATION. When a ferment, or enzyme, induces an alteration in any substance involving decomposition or effervescence, the process is known as fermentation.

Alcohol is produced by a ferment known as yeast. When yeast is added to a solution of water and grape sugar, a froth consisting of carbon dioxide is formed. In the midst of this process, the sugar content declines and alcohol begins to appear. In similar manner beverages such as wine and beer are produced. If any of these alcoholic beverages later acquire a sour or vinegary taste, it is due to another enzyme, known as mycoderma aceti, which has changed part of the alcohol into acetic acid. To further illustrate the process of fermentation, if lactic acid bacillus,

another enzyme, is added to milk sugar instead of grape sugar, lactic acid results. This occurs in the process of souring milk and also in the production of artificial buttermilk. If this enzyme produces fermentation in the stomach, the resultant carbon dioxide may lead to the formation of gas. The process of fermentation is also important in the production of bread and many other foods and industrial materials. *See also* ENZYME.

FERTILITY, the power of reproduction, has been noted in females as young as eight years and as old as sixty. Among males, the statistics are more difficult to verify.

Fertility varies greatly from one person to another. In many instances, the male may be infertile with one woman but not with another. Similarly the woman may or may not be fertile, depending on the male. Accordingly fertility must be viewed as depending on the reproductive ability of both man and woman and not on one of them alone.

The likelihood of giving birth to more than one child at a time has been estimated as: twins, once in 90 births; triplets, once in 10,000; quadruplets, once in 750,000; quintuplets, once in many million, and the recorded birth of sextuplets includes at least a few instances which are probably authentic.

By the use of x-rays, a multiple birth may be anticipated early enough so that proper preparations can be made for the arrival of the infants. Fecundity, incidentally, and this includes the tendency to multiple birth, is apparently a hereditary characteristic. *See also* BIRTH, MULTIPLE; STERILITY.

FETUS, a term designating the unborn child in the mother's womb and applied usually from the end of the third month of pregnancy until birth. *See also* PREGNANCY AND PRENATAL CARE; and Chapter 6, "Prenatal Care and Childbirth."

FEVER, the abnormal rise in temperature of the human body. Normal body temperature is 98.6° F. or 37° C. To determine whether or not a person has fever and its degree, a thermometer is used. Thermometers are generally graded from 92° to 108° F., but occasionally from 90° to 100°. Normal temperature is indicated by a tiny red arrow on the thermometer. To measure temperature, the mercury in the thermometer should always be well shaken down before the thermometer is used, and the thermometer left in the mouth at least three minutes. A thermometer placed under the arm records about one degree lower, and a thermometer placed in the rectum about one degree higher than one placed in the mouth.

Fever may arise from heat stroke, after exposure to great heat, in apoplexy, or when inflammation occurs in any part of the body. Fever may even be the sole manifestation of a mental disturbance which in turn causes tissue changes that bring about an increased temperature. By far the most common cause of fever, however, is the invasion of the body by germs, a condition known as infectious fever. Poisons produced by the invading germs affect the mechanisms which regulate the temperature of the healthy body.

Various acute specific fevers have characteristic symptoms and signs, peculiar to each, but there are symptoms associated with and common to all fevers. The person with fever does not feel comfortable or well, he may shiver severely, and in children there may be convulsions. The chills of fever are due to the spasm of the blood vessels in the skin and the exclusion of the warm blood that comes from deeper in the body. A general feeling of soreness in the muscles and bones may also accompany fever, and the pulse rate is almost always increased, except in typhoid fever. Generally the rate is increased by eight to ten beats for each degree of rise of temperature and the breathing rate also increases. The skin is dry, the urine less in quantity and high in color, the tongue is coated, the person loses his appetite and is thirsty and may be constipated. Usually the head aches and delirium may ensue. Children sometimes become delirious in slight fever attacks.

Fever in connection with microbic attack is not necessarily detrimental and may aid in combatting disease, since some microbes cannot live in temperatures above the normal body temperature.

Treatment of fever varies with type, severity, and the degree of control which the physician wishes to exercise. The diet will include plenty of water and as much food as the person can digest and enjoy. Food serves to reduce the waste of the body tissue. Many persons lose weight during fever because they feel too ill to eat. Fever also causes a definite increase in the speed of the chemical changes that go on in the body. For every rise of one degree in the temperature of the body, an increase of about 7 per cent in the speed of chemical changes occurs. The accelerated body activity indicates that a normal, and sometimes above normal, amount of food should be eaten by the person.

Drugs used to control fever, including aspirin, sodium salicylate, phenacetin, and acetanilid, should be used only when prescribed by a doctor and in the amount prescribed. Other rules for the home care of fever patients include washing the patient entirely with warm water, 85° or 90° F. or warmer, at least once a day, care being taken to avoid unnecessary exposure. If the patient's temperature rises above 102.5°, he can be sponged with tepid or cold water. If the temperature continues to rise, a wet pack, made with tepid or cold water, is often used; and for extremely high fevers, an ice pack or bath may be required, but should only by given under medical supervision. In prolonged delirium, a tepid or hot pack is sometimes beneficial. The patient should have enough sleep. In illnesses of short duration, it is not desirable to awaken the patient to give him food. In long fever cases it may be necessary, but the advice of the doctor or nurse should be sought. *See also* CONVULSION; THERMOMETER; TYPHOID FEVER.

FEVER BLISTERS. *See* HERPES SIMPLEX.

FIBRILLATION, the name of the condition in which a muscle develops a slight shivering or tremor. In certain degenerative diseases, such as amyotrophic lateral sclerosis, muscles fibrillate, but the term is applied particularly to auricular fibrillation in the heart. Instead of having a smooth powerful beat, the heart action and pulse become irregular in relationship to each other. This weakens the force of the pulsation. The condition is treated either with digitalis or with quinidine. If the fibrillation is associated with thyroid disease, surgery of the thyroid may be indicated to effect a cure.

Ventricular fibrillation, an extreme form, occurs in the ventricles of the heart in coronary thrombosis. Since little blood, if any, can be poured into the aorta from the heart, the condition is usually fatal.

FIBRINOGEN DEFICIENCY. Fibrinogen is one of the essential blood proteins manufactured by the liver. In severe liver disturbance this function may be disordered and restrict the clotting ability of the blood.

FIBROMA, a tumor of fibrous tissue. Most fibromas are benign, as opposed to cancerous tumors which are malignant. However, some tumors have both fibrous and cancerous tissue and are known as mixed tumors.

FIBROSITIS, inflammation of fibrous or connective tissue of the muscles anywhere in the body outside of the joints. Muscular rheumatism is a form of fibrositis. While rheumatic toxins may be responsible for fibrositis, other toxins, such as those from septic teeth or throat or from some other form of infection may be the underlying cause.

The condition is frequently related

to exposure to damp or cold weather, and, in the case of middle-aged or older persons, to overexertion or fatigue. Many people suffer from fibrositis after a slight draft or after an electric fan has played on a part of their body even for a short time.

Fibrositis in the lumbar region of the back may be a form of lumbago. Frequently it is involved in cases of stiff neck and sometime affects the scalp, the buttocks, and less often the muscles between the ribs. Occasionally the tendons are inflamed; and the bursas, or fluid-bearing sacs, in certain joints may also be affected.

The most common symptom is pain, increasing in intensity and lasting from a few days to a few weeks. The condition tends to become chronic, and is worse after periods of inactivity.

Temporary relief may be obtained by moderate exercise or massage. Aspirin and other salicylates may be beneficial. A combination of heat and massage as well as the application of liniment is also helpful.

If fibrositis is accompanied by fatigue or exhaustion, an attempt should be made to find the specific cause, such as infection, error in diet, or undue exposure. People with fibrositis should be protected against catching cold, chilling, dampness, or sudden changes in temperature. Wool or a wool mixture should be worn next to the skin, and drafts avoided.

Fibrositis affecting the bursa may sometimes be effectively treated by x-ray. In other instances anesthetic substances injected directly into the affected area have been successful. *See also* ARTHRITIS; RHEUMATISM; and Chapter 24, "Arthritis and Rheumatism."

FILARIASIS, an infection caused by a threadlike worm, filaria, which invades the human body. The female filaria gives birth in the human body to embryos which migrate through the body to the blood vessels and skin. From the skin, they are taken by blood-sucking flies and mosquitoes. In the insect's body they mature and migrate to the salivary glands. When the insect bites a person, the larvae get into or near the tiny wound inflicted by the insect's bite, and eventually penetrate to the interior of the person's body and travel through blood or lymph vessels until they find a permanent living site.

Perhaps the best-known form of filariasis is the tropical disease elephantiasis, or, more exactly, Bancroft's filariasis (actually elephantiasis refers only to the symptoms), in which the legs and other parts of the body become grossly swollen. The worm lives in the lymph vessels and associated tissue in the groin and in tissues associated with the external genitalia. Inflammation is followed by acute pain in these areas, then by apparent but temporary recovery. The symptoms reappear, alternating with the seeming recovery until a chronic stage is reached when lymph glands and ducts become obstructed by the worms, and the more pronounced forms of elephantiasis are observed. The larvae or microfilariae circulate in the person's blood at night when he is quiet, typically between midnight and two o'clock, and blood samples are taken by the doctor at this time. The larvae leave the blood during the active, daytime hours. The legs, groin glands, and male genitalia swell and the process sometimes extends to the interior of the body. On the surface of the skin, blood circulation is seriously impeded, cracking occurs, and finally secondary infection by bacteria and fungi sets in.

Satisfactory treatment for this infection was unknown in the past. Recent reports, however, describe favorable results with naphuride sodium and hetrazan. Sulfonamides are used against secondary infection and surgery for deformities of overgrown tissue. Prevention against filariasis consists mainly of eliminating the mosquito-breeding areas, the use of screens, and of DDT to protect persons from the infected mosquitoes.

Another filarial disease is caused by the burrowing migrations below the skin of a threadlike worm, the eye worm, which is found mostly in Africa. This, too, is transmitted by insect bite, that of the mango fly. The worm leaves an irritated, raised serpentine track as it passes on its slow way, perhaps an inch a day. It typically takes a route almost straight across both eyeballs and the bridge of the nose, down the temple and neck to the other side. Treatment consists of removing the worm with a hooked needle. The victim usually recovers.

An acute condition, onchocercosis, caused by filaria produces tumorous growths of coiled worms under the skin, sometimes as large as an orange. It is found in some parts of Central and South America as well as Africa. The microfilariae of this infection can create serious disturbances in the eye and sometimes blindness. Surgical removal of the growths and administration of the drugs used against Bancroft's filariasis are employed against this condition.

FINGER. The human hand terminates in four fingers and a thumb. The fingers are known as the fore or index, the middle, the ring, and the little finger, the first being the most mobile and sensitive. The movements of the fingers are performed by small muscles in the hand, controlled by the ulnar nerve which sometimes is paralyzed. This results in loss of function and inability to spread the fingers. The other movements of the hand are controlled by the muscles in the forearm which connect with the fingers. Sometimes an infection of the little finger will result in an abscess in the forearm, traveling along the connecting sheaths covering the tendons in the finger, palm, and wrist.

Various congenital deformities affect the fingers: too many fingers, too few fingers; adjoining fingers united by a thin or even fleshy web; contracted or bent fingers.

Various distortions of the fingers resulting from burns or accidents may be successfully treated by plastic surgery. Certain diseases, such as endocarditis or tuberculosis and other lung conditions, may induce clubbed fingers which are swollen at the ends. Arthritis may cause hard nodules to form, and deposits at the joints may result from gout.

FINGERNAILS. *See* NAILS.

FIRST AID, emergency treatment given in case of accident or sudden illness. It is necessary on innumerable occasions. Certain principles of first aid should be known to everyone, since immediate treatment before a doctor arrives may prevent more serious developments or even save lives.

Here are a few suggestions on what to do in an emergency situation:

1. Give a stricken person space—people have a tendency to crowd around the victim. Be sure he has air so that he can breathe freely.

2. Don't try to make someone who has fallen sit or stand. The effort to stand or sit may cause grave injury. Do not move the person; a bone may be broken. If the person must be moved, splints should be improvised and applied beforehand.

3. In case of bleeding, try to find the source. Merely placing a thumb on a bleeding cut and keeping it there has saved lives. Never give alcohol to a person who is bleeding externally or internally; it will only increase the bleeding.

4. When a person has fainted, keep his head below the level of the rest of the body so that the blood will flow more easily to the head. Loosen clothing about the neck and chest.

5. Since most accidents involve shock, the victim should be kept warm with extra clothing or blankets. A light massage of the limbs may be helpful.

A doctor should of course be summoned unless you are absolutely sure that the injury is slight.

Every home should have a really adequate first-aid outfit. It should include the following items kept in their original containers in a tightly shut tin box: 1 yard of 2″ gauze; ½ yard oiled silk; absorbent cotton; 2 triangular bandages; finger bandages; and clean scissors.

Also essential in the home is a properly supplied medicine chest which should include: 1 ounce bottle tincture of iodine; 1 ounce boric acid powder; aromatic spirits of ammonia; 1 ounce epsom salts; enema syringe; and clean scissors. *See also* ACCIDENTS; MEDICINE CHEST; POISONING; RESUSCITATION; SHOCK; and Chapter 28, "First Aid."

FISH. Many persons in the United States believe that a diet of fish is not as nutritious as one of meat. However, entire nations subsist largely on fish and thrive on it.

The protein content of most of the fish most commonly eaten, such as halibut, cod, whitefish, salmon, trout, pickerel, and perch, averages from 15 to 18 per cent as contrasted with approximately 21 per cent for mutton, beefsteak, and pork.

The flesh of fish generally contains, in addition to protein, fat, mineral salt, particularly iodine and phosphorus, and vitamins. It is especially valuable as a source of vitamin A and vitamin D which is significant in relation to the use of calcium and phosphorus by the body. Cod liver oil and other fish liver oils, notably halibut and salmon, are also rich in vitamins A and D. Fish roe contains vitamins B and E as well. Most of the fat in the flesh of fish is stored in the liver, except for salmon, mackerel, sardines, and herring which have about 10 to 15 per cent in the flesh. Studies of the vitamin content of various edible parts of fish indicate that oysters give the most complete vitamin value, followed closely by salmon and herring. Fish, while rich in all these things, lack calcium.

FISSURE, a division or groove between adjoining parts of similar substance. The brain contains many fissures. The term is also properly applied to certain narrow abnormal pathways, such as those which occur in the nipple or anus.

A fissure of the nipple is seen most frequently when the mother is nursing and is commonly due to lack of care, though a certain stiffness of the skin over the nipple may accentuate the breaking of the skin. To avoid this type of fissure, the mother should wash and dry the nipple with care after every feeding. Any rigidity of the skin in this area can be prevented or reduced if an appropriate ointment is applied.

The presence of an anal fissure is usually accompanied by severe pain when making a movement and often reaches down into the thighs. Blood or pus or both may also be seen in the stool. An anal fissure ordinarily occurs at the lower end of the bowel and probably near the rear. A hemorroid is often seen where it reaches the anal opening.

The pain of an anal fissure may be somewhat relieved if the person will take laxatives as needed to soften his bowel movement. The surface should then be cleansed with soft paper or cloth, and the anus and adjoining parts should be washed after every movement. After the area is dried, a soothing ointment is beneficial. Most physicians are convinced that surgery is the only successful treatment for anal fissure. *See also* ANUS; HEMORRHOIDS.

FISTULA, an abnormal narrow passage which leads from some cavity of the body to the outside skin and which may connect one cavity with another. Such an opening if not a narrow passage is not, strictly speaking, a fistula. Nevertheless, it may properly be described as fistulous.

A fistula present at birth indicates that some passageway, normal while the infant was in the womb, failed to close after birth as it should have done. Sometimes a child is born with an aperture at the navel through which urine escapes. Similarly this opening, normal in the fetus, ordinarily closes after birth.

A fistula may also stem from a wound or abscess which cannot heal because it persistently receives the contents of some body cavity. An anal fistula often originates in this manner. Two types of anal fistulae are the complete, which opens from the rectum and travels outside the bowel to the skin, usually terminating close to the anus; and the incomplete, so-called because it lacks either the surface or the rectal opening.

The incomplete anal fistula may also lead from the surface to some abscess which is created and occupied by germs which have seeped through the wall of the bowel. Early treatment of such an abscess may avoid the development of a fistula. However, if the fistula already exists it will drain persistently to the surface. The patient will not suffer pain unless the passage becomes clogged. However, at the point where the fistula reaches the skin he may experience discomfort and itching.

Another common type of fistula travels from the wall of the stomach to an abscess near the appendix, and still another is the vaginal fistula. If the lining of the vagina has been damaged in childbirth, this type of fistula may arise between the vagina and bladder or between the vagina and rectum. A fistula may also arise from either one of the parotid glands, which are under the ears, and move to a point where it enters the cheek. This is known as a salivary fistula.

If a fistula persists beyond the early stages, surgery is the only cure.

FITS. The word fit without a modifier simply means a sudden attack or seizure of any kind. The term is commonly used, however, to designate an attack of convulsions. Fits are associated not only with epilepsy but may also occur in connection with asphyxia, poisoning, lockjaw, hydrophobia, apoplexy, meningitis and in slow-pulse diseases such as anemia of the brain. They may also appear, together with subsequent coma, as a disturbance of late pregnancy. The type of fit known as infantile convulsions may sometimes be a reflex action associated with teething, worms, rickets, fever or diarrhea.

Hysterical fits are of special interest because they do not involve such symptoms as loss of consciousness or incapacity to control the bladder or bowels. Usually they occur to a person in the company of others, which seems to indicate that the victim is subconsciously trying to gain attention. Though hysterical fits are seldom physically dangerous, they do indicate a tense emotional conflict which may require the attention of a psychiatrist.

Regardless of the cause, the first step in giving relief to a convulsive patient, while awaiting the doctor, is to place him on his back. It is necessary to prevent him from doing harm to himself but use of force should be kept to a minimum. A piece of wood should be wrapped in a handkerchief and placed between the teeth so that he will not bite his tongue. His clothes should be loosened, especially around the neck and across the chest. If he vomits, he should be placed on his side. Gradually as the person recovers, every effort should be made to communicate with him and to reassure him. The patient is only half conscious at this stage, however, and must be treated with caution since he might suddenly become physically dangerous. *See* EPILEPSY; ECLAMPSIA; CONVULSIONS.

FLATFOOT, a common foot disorder which may be the result of an occupation that requires long periods of standing or walking, overweight, disease, injury, or paralysis. The condition may be based on weakness of the foot arch that is inborn, or it may be acquired through overstrain and poor position. Poorly fitting shoes may also promote the sagging of the arch. These faults which do not seem great nevertheless cause the ligaments to stretch, relax, and become incapable of returning to their original flexibility. The bones are then affected and the arch flattens, and soreness, pain, and fatigue result.

If some flexibility is retained, much may be done by proper shoes, arch supports, pads, manipulation, training, and by exercise to strengthen the muscles and other parts of the foot. All of these exercises and the course of treatment should be under the supervision of a foot specialist since slight variations of adjustment are sometimes notably effective. Even surgery may be necessary to break up the fibrous adhesions which form in rigidly flat feet. *See also* ARCHES, FALLEN; FEET.

FLATULENCE, an excess of air or gas in the stomach or intestines or in both. Often painful, this accumulation of air may adversely affect breathing, as well as the normal action of the heart.

Flatulence can be caused occasionally by fermentation in the stomach, or more often by eating of certain types of food such as beans. Most frequently it results from swallowing air while eating or drinking.

Drugs taken for relief of flatulence are carminatives. Ordinarily their active component is peppermint, ginger, dill, or anise. Any of these serve not only to expel the accumulated air but also to soothe the stomach ache associated with flatulence.

To avoid swallowing air, chew food with closed lips. This is most effective when peace and harmony are encouraged during eating. *See also* INDIGESTION.

FLU. *See* INFLUENZA.

FLUORIDATION, the addition of chemical salts, fluorides, to the water supply. It has been carried out in many communities in an effort to reduce dental decay. Fluorine is a chemical element found in the enamel of teeth, bones, and in minute quantities in other body tissues. Experiments with school children, each one receiving a regular intake of one part

per million of flourides in drinking water, have established that there is a definite reduction in dental decay when water is fluorinated.

FLUOROSCOPY, the act of using a fluoroscope; of observing, on a specially coated screen, the shadows of objects which are being x-rayed. This diagnostic technique has the advantage of offering a moving picture rather than a static photograph. The intestines may be examined in action, or the setting of a fractured bone can actually be followed with the eyes. The disadvantage of the fluoroscope is the fact that the image is less precise than that of a photograph. Great skill is therefore essential in the interpretation. *See also* X-RAYS.

FOOD ALLERGY, a disturbance affecting people who are sensitive to one or more particular foods. When eaten, such foods cause symptoms of irritation of the stomach and bowels, and often a skin rash such as hives, erythema, eczema, or perhaps asthmatic symptoms.

White of egg is a frequent cause of such allergy, as are fish, cheese, tomatoes, pork, shellfish, and other foods. The protein contained in them is most often responsible.

Food allergies in infants generally result in eczema or diarrhea and may be caused by egg white, milk, or cereals. The symptoms usually appear the first time the infant is fed these foods, and ordinarily disappear by the end of the second year. In children, sensitivity to eggs, wheat, and milk occurs less frequently as the child grows older and should disappear between the ages of four and twelve. The symptoms are dry and itchy skin eruptions. Scratching causes thickening and intensified itching, and broken skin. Because of the danger of infection, childhood eczema should be carefully watched. *See also* ALLERGY; ECZEMA; and Chapter 21, "Allergy."

FOOD FATS. Fat is a white or yellow substance, greasy to the touch, found in both animals and plants. When pure, fat has no odor, taste, or color. It exists both as a liquid and as a solid and may be dissolved in chloroform, ether, or benzene, but not in water or cold alcohol.

As a food, fat is valuable primarily as fuel, a source of energy. The most concentrated food we have, it possesses more than twice the caloric value of carbohydrates. Every ounce of fat has the same value as every other, whether it be an ounce of butter or an ounce of cottonseed oil. One type of fat, however, may be more accessible than another. In the United States, fats are consumed most frequently in the form of eggs, butter, margarine, cream, meat, olive oil, vegetable oil, and nuts. *See also* NUTRITION.

FOOD POISONING, an illness due to disease-causing organisms or harmful foreign substances, such as chemicals, in food. Misconceptions and confusion are common regarding food poisoning. For example, there is actually no such illness as "ptomaine poisoning." Ptomaines are products of putrefactive organisms which, because they were toxic to experimental animals when given by injection, were long considered responsible for the effects of food poisoning. Later studies established that

ptomaines are destroyed in the human digestive process and almost certainly do not have any connection with the symptoms of food poisoning.

Disease-causing bacteria are the commonest source of food poisoning, the most frequent probably being the staphylococcus. The same type of bacteria is responsible for many local infections of the skin involving abscesses and formation of pus. Perhaps the most severe type of food poisoning from bacteria is botulism, which occurs much less frequently than staphylococcal poisoning. As with botulism, poisoning by staphylococci is actually the effect of a toxin produced by the organisms. Probably everyone is affected by it at some time or other. Possibly what was once called ptomaine poisoning was actually caused by staphylococci. Putrefaction by itself, the process carried on by the organisms which produce ptomaines, is not harmful. Limburger cheese and other putrefied foods are safely consumed. Such foods will, of course, become poisonous just as other foods, if and when poisonous substances or organisms enter them.

Although not all staphylococci produce a substance toxic to human beings when ingested, those that are involved in boils and abscesses do, and such an infection on the hands or arms of a person preparing food can be a source of poisoning to many people. Cream and similar foods like custard and ice cream, Cheddar cheese, potato salad, many kinds of sauces and prepared meats are especially susceptible mediums for these organisms. The poison itself is heat-resistant, but whereas botulinus toxin is ineffective if boiled for a few minutes the staphylococci toxin retains its potency even after half an hour's boiling.

Staphylococci are found in the human nose and throat under ordinary conditions, although they are normally kept in check by natural balances. Another organism responsible for food poisoning is a type of bacteria called salmonella. Its effects may be more severe than those of the staphylococci, and salmonella outbreaks have occurred in which 10 per cent of those stricken died. This, however, is extreme and the usual fatality rate is about 1 per cent.

A few varieties of mushrooms may prove fatal if eaten. Mussel poisoning has been traced to a protozoan, a one-celled microscopic organism, toxic to human beings, which is sometimes eaten by the mussel. Cadmium poisoning may occur when acid food is consumed which has been left in cadmium-plated containers, such as ice trays.

Food poisoning manifests its symptoms within six hours after consumption of the poison-containing food. Symptoms are similar to those often present in intestinal disturbances, nausea, cramps, diarrhea, vomiting, and frequently headaches and sweating. Fatalities are rare. The acute symptoms tend to abate after five or six hours. Prostration may occur, generally due to loss of body fluids. The physician usually prescribes remedies directed more toward ridding the body of the poison rather than merely relieving the symptoms. Removal of the infectious or poisonous matter from the stomach is probably necessary unless it has already been evacuated by natural processes. Water and salt in the appropriate form is administered to overcome the depletion of both, and general exhaustion treated with drugs which aid circulation and heart function. *See also* BOTULISM; MUSHROOM POISONING; POISONING.

FOOT-AND-MOUTH DISEASE, an acute febrile (fever) disease, characterized by an eruption of blisters about either or both the feet and mouth. It affects chiefly cattle and other animals with cloven hoofs. The disease is contagious, involving a virus which may be spread by the infected animal, or, indirectly, through contact with the animal's straw or milk.

This affliction seldom attacks man. When it does, symptoms do not appear before three to five days after exposure. Fever and headache are followed by the appearance of characteristic blisters. In man, these appear on the hands, as well as on the feet and mouth. Treatment of human beings is primarily concerned with reducing the fever and applying antiseptics to the blisters and to the open sores which appear when the blisters break. Since foot-and-mouth disease is contagious, the patient, man or animal, should be isolated until a physician can be consulted.

FRACTURES. Breaking of a bone or cartilage is a fracture. Fractures may be classified by the type of bone or the type of break. If a broken bone penetrates the skin, the condition is a compound or open fracture. If it does not penetrate the skin, it is a simple fracture. Careless handling of an injured person may change a simple fracture to a compound one. For this reason, the patient should never be moved until a physician has advised it, unless absolutely essential.

Some fractures have descriptive names, such as a march fracture, which involves the breaking of a small bone in the foot, a type of fracture which a soldier on a long march could sustain. A greenstick or hickory stick fracture occurs when one side of the bone is broken and the other side only bent.

A broken bone will not always be evident to an untrained person. A fracture may exist even though the victim is capable of moving the injured part. Anyone who has suffered a fall or injury with ensuing discomfort should seek medical advice promptly. *See also* BONES; RIBS; SKULL; SPINAL FRACTURE; and Chapter 28, "First Aid."

FRECKLES, are harmless small brown pigmented spots or blemishes on the skin, caused by exposure to the sun's rays or to ultraviolet light from artificial sources. They are formed by the cells of the skin as a protection against further action of ultraviolet rays. People with red or blonde hair and light skin are more prone to freckles than those whose skins bronze under the sun.

Freckles appear about the seventh or eighth year and remain for life, receding in winter and reappearing in spring and summer. If the skin is shaded from the sun their appearance will be retarded.

Ointments for the skin which screen off the ultraviolet rays of the sun and prevent freckles from appearing are available, as are cosmetics that conceal freckles. Freckles may be removed with ointments containing skin-peeling properties. However, these ointments include substances that are poisonous and may cause dangerous irritation to the skin. Such preparations should not be used, especially on children. Freckles may be removed with these preparations, but they cannot be prevented from recurring.

FRIEDREICH'S ATAXIA, a rare hereditary nervous disorder which may affect several members of a family. The difficulty usually appears in childhood or early youth with a lack of muscular coordination beginning in the legs and gradually involving the whole body.

The gait becomes shambling, almost drunken, the feet deformed as in claw foot. The child will walk with the heel raised, and on the outer side of the foot. The speech is also impaired and curvature of the spine to one side is noticeable. Paralysis of the whole leg muscle may follow eventually, and the victim may never be able to walk.

The disease is caused by imperfect development of bundles of nerve fibers in the spinal cord, and so far a cure is not known. However, attempts should be made to prevent tightening of the muscles.

Although there may be a gradual hunching position, disturbance of sensation or wastage of the muscles does not occur apart from that due to the action of the disease. Death comes not from the disease itself but from pneumonia or other infections.

FROEHLICH'S SYNDROME, named after the scientist who first described it, is a disturbance of the glandular system in which sexual organs remain infantile. The disease is rare.

If the disease occurs in early childhood, it causes dwarfism, but if it appears in children before puberty, the boy or girl will be fat. The victim will be lazy mentally and have a voracious appetite for food. The sexual organs will be undeveloped. Most fat children do not suffer from this condition, and are more likely to be obese because of bad dietary habits.

The adult male becomes effeminate, his skin is soft, and the distribution of flesh around the thighs and breasts has a woman's appearance. Female patients become exceedingly fat, sometimes weighing as much as 300 pounds.

Modern hormone therapy can relieve many of the symptoms if the disease has not progressed beyond control. Treatment includes medical care and administration of hormones, such as pituitary extract. Proper therapy will reduce excessive weight, correct deformity, and restore sexual development.

FROSTBITE, a condition caused by exposure to extreme cold or cold and wind. The toes, fingers, ears, and tip of the nose are usually the first parts of the body to be affected. The frostbitten areas turn pale, the blood and moisture in the tissues freeze, and the circulation is cut off. Frostbite is dangerously deceptive since there is no feeling of pain and the victim is usually unaware of what is happening.

The old theory that a frostbitten area should be rubbed with snow or ice is completely false; such a procedure can actually cause harm. The best rules to follow in cases of frostbite are simple: warm the affected area slowly by immersing it in tepid water or bundling it up in woolen cloth. Warming too fast produces severe pain. Do not under any circumstances rub the frostbitten area as the friction can break down the cell structure of the tissue. If the skin is warmed immediately the color will usually return. However, if the frostbite is severe, the area will remain white, indicating that the cold has contracted the blood vessels to such an extent that normal blood circulation cannot immediately be resumed. A doctor should be called immediately. In time the blood will seep back into the tissues, and the affected area will appear purplish or black. In a day or two, these areas may become acutely inflamed and painful from the pressure of fluids in the skin coming through the lower layers, and blisters, characteristic of frostbite, will appear. The blisters may leave ulcers on rupturing, and the affected tissues may die. Blisters should be treated with ointments after being opened, and then covered with dry sterile dressings. In severe cases of frostbite, the tissues may be irreparably damaged and gangrene result. Amputation of a toe, finger, or entire limb has been known to be necessary in such cases.

To prevent frostbite, outdoor activity should be postponed or limited when the temperature is below 8°, particularly when there is a strong wind. If the temperature is between 8° and 15°, some danger of frostbite exists. Clothing should be warm, wind-resistant, and properly fitted. Tight shoes, socks, and gloves restrict circulation and encourage frostbite. People who must work outdoors during extremely cold weather should not stay out longer than two hours at a time without intervening rest periods of half an hour. People with diabetes or any form of heart or circulatory disease are especially susceptible to serious damage from frostbite. *See also* CHILBLAINS; GANGRENE; SKIN.

FUMIGATION. Fumigation is done with disinfectants which employ smoke or fumes. The method is used, for example, against domestic insects or as a means of cleansing the sickroom of a patient who has suffered from an infectious disease.

When a room is to be fumigated, any metallic articles present must be washed with a disinfectant and removed. Likewise cupboard doors must be opened and all drawers pulled out. The window sashes should be sealed with gummed paper, and if the room contains a fireplace, the chimney should be stuffed with newspapers. Finally, after igniting the disinfectant, the doors ought to be sealed with gummed paper from the outside.

For general purposes, the best fumigant is sulphur. This is not effective, however, unless moisture is present. Therefore, before fumigating is begun, the walls, ceiling, and floor and also the furniture should be sprinkled with water. The next step is to fill a large basin partly with water and place it on a table in the center of the room. The sulphur, in a small bowl, is then set in this larger basin. The sulphur may be either in the form of candles or roll sulphur. Roll sulphur to be inflammable must be moistened with wood alcohol.

A more recent type of fumigant, and in some ways a more effective one, is the freon bomb which was first used by the armed forces in World War II. This contains an insecticide, such as pyrethrum or DDT. Immediately upon being opened, this fumigant penetrates effectively to every corner of the room.

Approximately twenty-four hours after fumigation, the doors and windows can be opened wide and the room aired for a day or more. The wallpaper, if any, may be removed at this time and burned, and it is also advisable to limewash the ceiling and to scrub the floor, the woodwork, and the furniture with soap and water. *See also* BEDBUG; DISINFECTION; VENTILATION.

FUNGUS, a low form of plant life. Fungi, a widespread group of simple plants commonly known as mushrooms, molds, and yeasts, do not have any chlorophyll of their own and depend upon green plants or other organisms for their food sources. Fungi which invade another living organism and obtain their food at the expense of this organism are parasites. Fungi which live on dead or decaying organisms are saprophytes. They flourish in the soil and in all sorts of warm damp places where they hatch and develop prolifically.

Some fungi are many-celled and reproduce by spore formation, each spore being capable of forming a new plantlike growth similar to the parent plant. Others, like the yeasts, are unicellular and reproduce by budding. The buds break off and form new cells.

Thousands of varieties of molds have been isolated and identified. Most of them are quite harmless to man and in some cases are highly beneficial. Some varieties are used as the source of the antibiotics which have saved countless thousands of lives since the development of penicillin during World War II. Many fungi constitute a serious threat to mankind.

Disease-bearing molds are most prevalent in the soil, although they have also been found in such diverse sites as unpasteurized milk, cellars, animal excrement, cattle, and even in some community water supplies. Dangerous or undesirable fungi sometimes infest plant crops raised for food, causing potato blight and wheat rust. Some initiate and intensify certain types of asthma or hay fever; others cause the fungus or mycotic diseases which are quite common in human beings as well as in many domestic animals. These infections may be superficial, affecting only the skin, hair, and teeth, as in ringworm of the scalp, feet, and nails. More invasive fungi penetrate the tissues of internal structure and produce serious diseases of the mucous membranes, heart, lungs, and other organs. Among the more prevalent of these infections are actinomycosis, blastomycosis, histoplasmosis, coccidioido-mycosis, moniliasis, and sporotrichosis, all found throughout the south and southeastern United States and in scattered areas throughout the world. Maduromycosis, a disease affecting the feet, occurs chiefly in tropical countries. *See also* ANTIBIOTICS; and names of specific fungus diseases.

FURUNCLES. A furuncle, or boil, is a painful, pus-producing inflammation of the skin, with a central core, caused ordinarily by certain types of bacteria which enter the skin through hair follicles or sweat glands. Usually such an infection does not occur unless resistance has been weakened by diabetes, Bright's disease, or a fever. Likewise anyone suffering from undernourishment, fatigue, or constipation is vulnerable. The skin may also be weakened by local irritation, such as the persistent rubbing of a starched collar on the neck.

Boils in the vicinity of the nose or in the ear should be examined promptly by a doctor. Others, unless they get large, may be permitted to follow their own course. Larger boils may be painful and often require surgery. An appropriate antiseptic may be applied to the general area to prevent the infection from spreading and creating another set of boils.

When the entire body is afflicted with boils, a physician will sometimes administer sulfonamides, penicillin, or other antibiotics. x-rays and ultraviolet rays, as well as vaccines and similar preparations, have also been used with success against persistent boils. *See also* CARBUNCLES; and Chapter 20, "Diseases of the Skin."

GAIT, a characteristic manner of walking. Certain diseases are associated with a characteristic gait. Coordination between the two feet may be distorted—for example, by a degenerative disease of the spinal cord known as locomotor ataxia. The victim of this disease will lift each foot abruptly and higher than necessary, after which he pushes it forward and lowers it with a sudden thump. At the same time, he seems compelled to lean out and observe these movements, in order to finish them.

Another disease of the spinal cord, involving the lateral columns of the cord, produces a wooden gait in which the feet are pulled across the ground. This often involves a kind of crisscrossing of the feet, as they are dragged forward.

Several other types of paralysis have special effects on the manner of walking. When certain muscles of the leg are paralyzed, for example, a kind of drooping of the foot results. To prevent his toes from dragging on the ground, the person lifts his foot high in the air before every forward movement. Again, paralysis on one side may necessitate twisting the entire body so that the leg on the opposite side can be swung around before it advances. In paralysis agitans, the person seems to hustle and shuffle as if being shoved from behind. At the same time the body careens forward in advance of the feet, as if the person were attempting to avoid falling on his face. In muscular or pseudohypertrophic paralysis, growth occurs in the calf of the leg. Although the muscles become enlarged, they are weak. The result is a waddling gait, resembling that of a pregnant woman.

The best known of all abnormal gaits, the limp, is often caused by stiff muscles, localized pain, or a difference between the length of the two legs. *See also* ATAXIA; PARALYSIS.

GALLBLADDER, a baglike, pear-shaped sac lying usually on the underside of the liver. It stores bile which is a primary digestive substance that the liver produces almost continuously. Bile flows to the

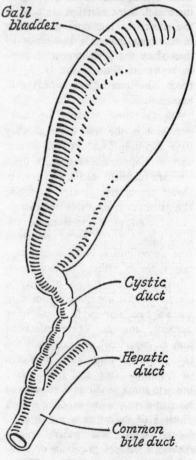

The gallbladder showing the connection to the bile duct.

gallbladder from the liver, and there is condensed by the extraction of water. When food is eaten and digestion occurs, bile enters the duodenum from the gallbladder. Bile is alkaline and neutralizes the acid semidigested food coming from the stomach.

The gallbladder is susceptible to infection and to obstructions in the tubes carrying bile, particularly by the formation of stones. The probable cause of gallstones is interruption of the bile flow by infections and digestive changes. Gallstones may range in size from that of a poppy seed to that of an egg. The stones will float in water and are soaplike to the touch. They consist largely of cholesterol, a fatlike substance found in the blood and other parts of the body, and of bile pigments. These are derived from the bile itself, but the nucleus around which they coalesce seems to be a foreign substance, such as a small cluster of bacteria or of infected discharge. Approximately 5 to 10 per cent of all adults have gallstones, and they occur in women five times oftener than in men.

Gallstones are not always troublesome, but they may block a gall duct and induce an attack of gallstone or biliary colic without warning. The pit of the stomach is seized with pain which may be agonizing and so severe that the patient collapses. Such attacks are likely to be accompanied by vomiting and fever, and usually end when the stone slips back into the gallbladder or proceeds into the intestine whence it is excreted with the solid wastes. Another attack may not occur for months or years. When the colic symptoms are repeated, the stomach feels full, pains are felt after eating fatty foods, and gas is present.

Removal of the gallbladder is advisable if the person suffers from too frequent attacks of gallbladder colic. Not only is ordinary comfort restored, but certain definite risks are thus avoided. Infection, with dangerous formation of pus, or cancer may develop if stones persist. Some persons, however, cannot undergo the surgical operation and must have continuous medical treatment and care.

Cholecystitis is the serious condition incurred by infection and inflammation when interruption of the flow of bile occurs. Acute pain in the upper right abdomen, abdomen distended by gas, and sometimes jaundice and fever accompany cholecystitis. When such attacks become a major problem, the solution is surgical removal of the gallbladder, preferably not during an acute episode. Nevertheless, if continued vomiting, rapid pulse, and indications of poisoning ensue, it may be necessary to operate immediately.

Chronic infection and inflammation of the gallbladder induce a tendency to formation of stones, and symptoms of chronic indigestion are constantly present. The patient feels too full after eating, especially if he has had fatty foods. Pain on the right side is likely, and may be intensified by stooping or bending. Heartburn often accompanies this condition and medical examination reveals hyperacidity in the stomach.

A special technique for detection of gallstones is one of the outstanding achievements of medical science. A substance, iodophthalein, when ingested or injected into the blood stream, renders the gallbladder visible on an x-ray photograph, so that the functions of the liver and gallbladder may be evaluated. The substance is carried by the blood to the liver, then in the bile to the gallbladder. If the x-ray plates do not reveal the gallbladder, further studies are made to determine whether or not the bile duct is blocked. If the gallbladder is visible in the roentgenograms, most of the stones will also be seen. Some stones are visible by x-ray without the aid of iodophthalein.

Jaundice in severe cases may be active but does not always accompany chronic gallbladder infection. Infection of the gallbladder produces a great range of internal symptoms which involve almost any organ but the one actually responsible. A tightness of the chest, palpitating heart, or shortness of breath may be quite confusing in these circumstances. Medical examination is indispensable to determine the exact cause and condition. Many persons live for years with a chronically inflamed gallbladder and without serious consequences. The risk, however, is always present. Surgical removal of the gallbladder obviates these possibilities. The operation is a major one, usually successful. Symptoms promptly disappear, but diet regulation is desirable for a number of months. *See also* CHOLECYSTITIS; GALLSTONES; and Chapter 16, "Common Disorders of the Liver and Gallbladder."

GALLSTONES, small masses of a substance composed most frequently of cholesterol, bile salts, and color-

ing matter. They often form in the gallbladder or bile ducts, and may cause symptoms varying from mild colicky pain to rupture of the gallbladder and peritonitis or even infection of the pancreas. Gallstones usually occur after the age of forty although younger women may develop them after pregnancy. In general, women are more often affected than men. Gallstones are best seen by x-ray.

Gallstones cause colicky pain as they pass into and along the bile ducts and are often followed by infection in the liver and by jaundice. They may become lodged at the entrance to the duodenem, causing intense jaundice and severe itching.

Mild attacks of gallstone colic are often treated by rest and hot packs on the stomach. However, a severe attack requires the attention of a doctor who may prescribe pain-relieving drugs. Usually the gallbladder and stones are surgically removed; the operation is performed frequently and is rarely complicated. *See also* GALLBLADDER; and Chapter 16, "Common Disorders of the Liver and Gallbladder."

GAMMA GLOBULIN, a chemical substance found in the protein globulins of the blood plasma. The blood has the power to develop antibodies to combat disease. The antibodies in gamma globulin have been found useful in developing immunity to measles in children as well as in hepatitis and other infections. Commercially available serum containing globulin has been used to advantage both in developing temporary immunity to measles and also to lighten an attack of measles in a child who has been exposed and develops the disease.

GANGRENE, the death of tissue, caused by interruption of circulation. It can result from accidental damage to the tissue, as in burns, wounds, crushing or poisoning of the flesh. Interruption of circulation with the ensuing death of the flesh can be caused by other conditions—for example, a hernia—or by a section of lung failing to receive its supply of blood. Diseases such as diabetes, hardening of the arteries, or Bright's disease may affect circulation in a similar way.

Gangrene is sometimes classified as dry or moist, depending on whether or not certain fluids flow toward or away from the area. In dry gangrene the tissue gradually shrinks and the color becomes brown and finally black. In moist gangrene the tissue is swollen, often blistered, and has the colors characteristic of a bruise. Moist gangrene is more dangerous than dry because it offers greater opportunity for infection. Since the infection can be fatal the doctor takes special precautions against bacterial invasion. The skin is thoroughly and regularly cleaned, particularly the skin around fingernails and toenails where germs might find a breeding place, and the nails themselves are usually clipped as short as possible. Antiseptic dressings are frequently applied.

Eventually a red line, the line of demarcation, will appear on the skin. This line separates the dead tissue from that which can heal. The doctor will try to save the tissue capable of healing, and stop the progress of the deteriorating tissue. Sometimes amputation is the only means of stopping rapidly deteriorating tissue. However, it may be necessary to operate without waiting for the appearance of the line of demarcation, even at the sacrifice of potentially healthy tissue.

Injury of tissue, as in wounds, encourages certain types of bacteria which cause gas gangrene. These germs behave as ferments and break up the sugars in the tissues so as to produce a gas which soon spreads through the muscles. The area becomes severely inflamed, and in later stages the color changes to yellow and then black. The progress of gas gangrene varies among patients; in some it is rapid, in others slow. As yet there is no full explanation for this difference, although the severity of the wound seems to be a primary consideration.

During World War I when gas gangrene first became a serious problem, the only medical solution was to remove all damaged tissue from the body as soon as possible. However, during World War II a serum was developed which could be injected into a person threatened with gas gangrene; and, if the infection had already started, sulfa drugs were ordinarily sufficient to bring it under control. *See also* FROSTBITE.

GARGLE, a liquid solution used to rinse the throat, pharynx, and nasopharynx, and held in this area by a stream of air from the lungs. Since some of the liquid may be accidentally swallowed, anything which might be internally harmful should never be used as a gargle. If an inflammation is so severe that gargling causes pain, the liquid may be held in the throat for a few minutes, or merely swished around, or sprayed in with an atomizer. For a slightly irritated throat, a pinch of salt or bicarbonate of soda diluted in warm water is often helpful.

GASTRIC, a term derived from the Greek word "gastro," meaning stomach. In medicine many words beginning with "gastro" are used which relate to medical conditions affecting the stomach. Accordingly gastritis is an inflammation of the stomach, gastroenteritis an inflammation of the stomach and intestines, gastrectomy the removal of all or a part of the stomach, gastroscope a device for looking inside the stomach.

GASTRIC ULCER. *See* PEPTIC ULCER.

GASTRITIS, a frequent form of "stomach upset," is inflammation of the stomach wall. When the lining of the stomach is irritated or infected, it becomes red and swollen and in a severe inflammation may even bleed.

Gastritis may be acute or chronic. Acute inflammation is often caused by food poisoning, eating spoiled food, or simply overeating. The lining of the stomach may also become seriously inflamed following the swallowing of irritating substances like lye, acid, or poison, and quick action by a physician to remove the substance is imperative. This must be followed by neutralization of the poison or the stomach wall will be perforated and acute peritonitis will set in. Surgical treatment may also be necessary.

Symptoms of acute gastritis include loss of appetite, a sense of pressure and fullness in the pit of the stomach which is unrelieved by belching, nausea, headache, and a slight rise in temperature. Vomiting then follows, producing a sense of relief. However, the person will feel extremely fatigued afterward. Examination of the material from the stomach enables the doctor to determine the nature and severity of the inflammation. Relief of acute gastritis is usually brought about in a few days by eliminating the irritating substance and being careful of food intake.

Diagnosis and treatment of constant or chronic gastritis are difficult. Many different conditions may produce these repeated irritations of the stomach lining, and treatment requires observation and control by the physician over a long period of time. Certain vitamin deficiencies in the diet produce a tendency to irritation and inflammation. Disorders of the secretion of gastric juice may also be the cause. Gastritis is generally part of the development of an ulcer in the stomach, and a chronic ulcer is likely to produce chronic gastritis. Alcohol taken in excess produces irritation, followed by inflammation.

In treatment of chronic gastritis, small meals of easily digested foods at frequent intervals are prescribed. Irritating foods must be avoided, and drugs to reduce excess stomach acidity will be administered. The physician treating chronic gastritis must carefully examine the entire system and general health of the patient. If the condition is severe, it may be desirable to begin treatment with a few days of rest in bed and a milk or light bland diet. Medication to promote regularity of the bowels may be prescribed, and later substances to promote appetite and digestion. *See also* Chapter 18, "Disorders of the Digestive System and Diet in Digestive Disorders."

GASTROENTERITIS, a general term that applies to a variety of gastrointestinal disturbances. In this inflammatory condition of the stomach and intestines nausea, vomiting, and diarrhea occur, generally accompanied by cramps.

Acute gastroenteritis of a nonspecific nature occurs in alcoholism, malaria, acute hepatitis, and as a sensitivity reaction to certain foods. Food poisoning by staphylococci is a form of gastroenteritis.

Treatment of gastroenteritis may vary from temporary change of diet in mild disorders to surgery in extreme cases. See appropriate heading for discussion of specific symptoms and treatment. *See also* AMEBIC DYSENTERY; BACILLARY DYSENTERY; DIARRHEA; FOOD POISONING; GASTRITIS.

GASTROPTOSIS, dropping of the stomach, a condition caused by downward displacement of the stomach which may be seen by x-ray.

GELATIN, an opaque substance, pale yellow, odorless, and almost tasteless, produced by boiling the skin, bones, and ligaments of animals and treating with acid. It is dry when hard and jellylike when moist. Gelatin is considered a protein, but it does not possess all of the amino acids which are necessary for growth. Gelatin is the basis for such products as glues and jellies. When used in desserts it is usually flavored and sweetened. It is medicinally used in accelerating coagulation of blood by intravenous injection, and experimental work is being done with gelatin as a blood substitute. Gelatin also stimulates healthful growth of nails.

GERIATRICS, the science of medical and hygienic care of aged people. It has broadened and expanded in recent years because of the increased number of older people. In 1890, the number of persons in the United States over sixty-five was about 3 per cent. Today sociologists estimate that in 1970 more than 20 per cent of the population will be over sixty-five. Geriatrics must therefore become more and more significant in the future. *See also* SENESCENCE; SENILITY; and Part VIII, "The Later Years."

GERMAN MEASLES, also known as three-day measles or rubella, a mild but highly infectious virus disease. German measles occurs in epidemics at three- to four-year intervals, often in early spring, together with an outbreak of measles. It affects persons of all ages, though it is uncommon in infants and children under four, and generally occurs most frequently in older children and young adults. German measles during pregnancy may be harmful to the fetus.

German measles, like measles, is transmitted most commonly by droplet infection and direct contact. The incubation period is from fourteen to seventeen days, occasionally ranging from ten to twenty-one days. The infectious period is generally a day or two before the rash appears.

The first symptoms in younger people are slight, a scant rise in temperature, perhaps a running nose and some soreness of the throat. In older persons, German measles may be accompanied by headache, weakness, slight fever, sore throat, and swelling of the glands at the back of the head and neck, with some tenderness. Usually the rash is the first symptom noted by the patient. It appears after twenty-four to forty-eight hours, first on the face, forehead, scalp, and behind the ears, then spreading over the body. The rash resembles scarlet fever rash more than measles rash. Itching may aggravate the rounded rose-red spots, which are separate at first, then tend to run together. The rash lasts about three days and fades with a fine scaling. Koplik's spots do not appear in German measles.

The general treatment is similar to that for measles. The person should remain in bed until his temperature is normal and the rash has disappeared. As in measles, he should be isolated, since he is infectious for about ten days after the appearance of the rash. German measles is not dangerous, but all efforts should be made to avoid secondary infections, since encephalitis is a rare but possible complication. One attack of German measles confers lasting immunity. The patient's bedding and linens and bedclothing should be disinfected and the sickroom thoroughly aired. Children who have been in contact with German measles should be kept out of school for at least three weeks from the date of the last contact.

If German measles occurs during the first third of pregnancy, the possibility is great that the child may have congenital defects, such as cataracts, heart malformations, deafness, or mental retardation. These serious complications have been known to occur in more than 50 per cent of such cases. Therefore, it is essential that an obstetrician be notified immediately. *See also* Chapter 7, "The Process of Infectious Diseases and Immunization of Children."

GERMICIDE, any substance that kills germs. There is a significant distinction between germicides and antiseptics; antiseptics destroy poisonous material as well as germs and also inhibit and prevent multiplication of germs.

GERMS. *See* BACTERIA.

GIANTISM. *See* ACROMEGALY.

GINGIVITIS, an inflammation of the gums. Pyorrhea is a form of gingivitis with pus, and the condition called Vincent's disease or trench mouth is also gingivitis. *See also* PYORRHEA; VINCENT'S ANGINA.

GLANDERS, a contagious disease of animals, involving swellings under the jaws and an abundant discharge of mucus from the nostrils. This disease, although found ordinarily among horses, mules, and donkeys, is occasionally communicated to human beings, primarily to persons who work with horses. This happened more frequently in the past when horses were more commonly used.

When the germ gains entrance into human tissue, it may be weeks before the first signs of the illness appear. A test exists, similar to the Wassermann test, by which the presence of the germ can be recognized. High fever, vomiting, and diarrhea accompany this disease. Where the germs localize, a swelling occurs and large ulcers and abscesses of the lymph glands appear rapidly. The latter are first seen as small knots under the skin, known as "farcy buds."

If this disease becomes chronic in a person, severe damage to the cartilage and bones is likely. In the chronic form, there is constant fever and abnormal thinness. So-called chronic glanders, as contrasted to the acute form, is sometimes curable. Antibiotics, antitoxins, and surgery are all usually necessary.

When this disease is contracted by a human being, he should be isolated at once, and all discharges from his body should be removed on materials which can be easily burned. These precautionary measures are necessary because the disease is highly contagious as well as dangerous. For the same reasons, animals infected with glanders are always destroyed.

GLANDS, organs of the body which develop a secretion, a substance which performs a specific function, as in digestion. Many of the body's most important processes are effected through the glands and their secretions.

The glands are of external and of internal secretion. The glands of external secretion include the digestive glands and the sweat glands of the skin. Those of internal secretion, also known as the endocrine glands, secrete their products, called hormones, into the blood. These are carried to other parts of the body where they exert specific effects on other glands or organs. Some glands of external secretion also produce substances which penetrate the blood as internal secretions or hormones.

Glands of external secretion include the liver, which produces bile; the stomach, which gives hydrochloric acid and pepsin for digestion; the breasts, which secrete milk; the salivary glands, which produce the saliva that moistens the mouth and contains digestive substances; the pancreas, which produce trypsin used in digestion and also insulin, an internal substance which regulates the use of sugar; and the sex glands.

The glands of internal secretion are more complex in operation and more far-reaching in effect than the glands of external secretion. For example, whereas hydrochloric acid found in the stomach acts directly on food, the products of the endocrine glands function indirectly. Together they form a system which regulates many of the body's most vital processes.

The glands control growth, the body's response to stress of all kinds, and initiate its defenses, and govern the development of sexual maturity. They induce the secondary physical characteristics which distinguish men from women, such as hair on the face and the deeper voice. They regulate the delicately balanced expenditure of energy that persists continuously in the tissues, and are intimately involved in metabolism.

The endocrine glands include the pituitary, sometimes called the "master gland" because it performs a multiplicity of functions and helps regulate other endocrine glands such as the thyroid gland involved in the consumption of oxygen; the adrenal gland, divided into two parts, the medulla and the cortex, which among other functions assist the body in emergencies; the testes and ovaries, male and female sex glands which affect both sexual processes and, even more, general body conditions; the parathyroids which control the calcium and phosphorus content of the blood; and the pineal and thymus glands which are less well understood than the others.

Endocrine disorders may have profound effects. A pituitary gland which is not functioning properly may cause giantism or dwarfism or permanent enlargement of the chin, hands, and feet. A thyroid gland deficient at birth retards the growth of the body and mind, and causes feeble-mindedness. Later thyroid disorder may greatly accelerate or abnormally retard various processes, reacting unfavorably on the heart or other organs. Lack of the hormones of the cortex, which is the outer layer of the adrenal glands, produces death in a few days if they are not replaced. Disturbances of the sex glands and their hormones may cause a woman to assume male attributes or a man to develop feminine attributes. If a duct of a gland is blocked the secretion continues. The accumulation of fluid causes the gland to dilate and form a retention cyst. An adenoma is a tumor with glandular structure.

The normal course of development of a human being comprises the initial period of growth, a plateau through the years of middle life when maturity is reached and then a gradual decline. Many unjustified or actually fraudulent claims are made that the glands promote rejuvenation. None has been substantiated and rejuvenation is as far beyond human reach as ever. *See also* ADRENAL GLANDS; ENDOCRINE GLANDS; HORMONES; and under names of separate glands; and Chapter 19, "Endocrine Glands."

GLAUCOMA, a disease of the eyes in which loss of vision is caused by a pressure inside the eyeball. This pressure occurs when optical fluid tends to accumulate there. In one form of glaucoma, this accumulation is caused by improper circulation. Pain results and soon the eyeball is hard and red, and the pupil itself becomes gray and cloudy. Another form of glaucoma, regarded as more serious, results from the accumulation of fluid caused by failure of the drainage system. The internal pressure and the loss of vision, however, develop more slowly.

In the earlier stages of glaucoma, visual difficulty occurs at both sides of the area of vision, though the person with glaucoma is able to see in front as well as ever. As the disease develops, however, the area of clear frontal vision gradually becomes narrower until finally the person is completely blind.

In diagnosis of the disease, the eye specialist employs several mechanical aids. He uses the ophthalmoscope to judge whether the internal pressure is sufficient to depress the optic nerve at the rear of the eye. With a tonometer he can estimate whether or not the pressure is increasing. The perimeter measures the breadth of vision; a progressive decrease in breadth is a sign of glaucoma. These instruments enable a prompt diagnosis which may save the sight.

In all stages of this disease, but especially at the onset, the patient should avoid excitement since the resulting rise in pressure increases the flow of blood into the arteries of the eyes, where the internal accumulation of fluid is already excessive.

In the treatment of glaucoma, eyeglasses are ineffective and in no way helpful. Drugs, however, are sometimes successfully used to contract the pupil and also to decrease pressure within the eyeball. Frequently surgery can control glaucoma and actually save the patient's sight. *See also* EYE.

GLIOMA, a tumor of the nervous tissue occurring principally in the brain, spinal cord, peripheral nerves, and the adrenals.

GLOSSITIS, an inflammation of the tip and margin of the tongue, generally caused by a vitamin B_2, Riboflavin, deficiency which occurs when the diet consists chiefly of such foods as corn, rice, or potatoes.

GLOTTIS, the opening between the vocal cords which is protected by the epiglottis. *See also* EPIGLOTTIS.

GLUCOSE, the chemical term for dextrose and for blood sugar. The glucose tolerance test is used to determine whether or not a diabetic condition exists. For this test a solution of glucose is given intravenously or by mouth and the blood and urine examined to establish the level of the blood glucose at specific intervals. The test is also used in diseases of the liver and the thyroid gland and to determine the absorptive capacity of the gastrointestinal tract.

GOITER, enlargment of the thyroid gland, located in the front of the neck. In exophthalmic goiter the gland becomes overactive and is usually but not always enlarged. Ordinary or simple goiter begins early in adolescence and is directly associated with an inadequate supply of iodine in the diet. Goiter is most common in inland and mountainous areas away from the sea where there is a deficiency of iodine in the soil and water. Simple goiter occurs infrequently in coastal areas, and is five times more common in women than men.

Within the thyroid gland are small vessels which contains a yellow substance called colloid. Colloid contains a small amount of iodine, so little that a man weighing 150 pounds has no more than 1/40,000th of a pound of iodine. Iodine is also present in thyroxin, the secretion or hormone of the thyroid gland. The thyroid absorbs the iodine from iodine-containing foods and liquids taken into the body.

As a preventive measure against goiter, small amounts of iodine are sometimes given to young people, particularly those who live in areas where the water and soil are low in iodine. Iodine is also administered to pregnant mothers to prevent undesirable changes in the thyroid gland of the developing embryo. Iodine is often added to table salt, "iodized" salt, and can be added to drinking water. Iodine-containing tablets are also available. The use of iodine should be prescribed by the doctor to assure that the proper amount is given; the actual amount of iodine taken to supplement the diet is small.

In cases in which the thyroid gland becomes so large as to be a deformity and a discomfort to the person, it is ordinarily removed by surgery. However, this condition is rare today.

Exophthalmic goiter is usually more serious than simple goiter. The processes in which the gland is involved through its secretion, thyroxin, are abnormally quickened. A typical symptom of the condition is bulging eyes, the derivation of the term "exophthalmic." The disorder occurs most frequently in young adults, especially young women, in urban areas, and is apparently associated with stresses on the nervous system. The overactivity of the thyroid gland causes the basic chemical changes throughout the body to accelerate abnormally; the basal metabolism rate rises; the heart beats faster. The person tires easily, his appetite increases, he feels warm, is more nervous than usual and inclined to excitability, he begins to lose weight, his hands may tremble, and he often engages in excessive activity. Substantially these same symptoms can be produced by ingestion of too much extract of the thyroid gland.

To establish whether or not thyroid activity is excessive, the doctor gives the patient a basal metabolism test. Normal basal metabolism ranges from plus 7 to minus 7; in exophthalmic goiter, or hyperthyroidism, this measurement may rise as high as plus 15, 30, or even higher. The heart may consequently be forced to work far beyond its capacity. Administra-

tion of extra iodine may reduce the heart action and relieve the symptoms, but this is only a partial remedy and should only be prescribed and supervised by a doctor. Physical and mental rest are beneficial to the patient.

For permanent relief part of the thyroid gland is removed surgically. Enough of the gland is left to perform its normal functions and provide the necessary thyroxin. The amount of the gland to be removed is established by the surgeon at the time of the operation. Sometimes supplemental thyroid material must be given for a time after surgery until the gland and body adjust properly to the loss of part of the thyroid gland.

Recently other means have been found for controlling excessive thyroid activity, such as radioactive iodine; thiocyanates, which lower blood pressure and depress thyroid activity; and thiouracil which controls the major symptoms. Radioactive iodine also assists in diagnosis; since the thyroid gland absorbs iodine entering the body, a test of the amount of radioactivity emanating from the thyroid can be made which guides the doctor in deciding how much radioactive iodine should be given for actual treatment. Radiation from the iodine directly affects the cells of the gland and permanently lowers its activity.

Hyperthyroidism may also result from the growth of a tumor in the gland which may in turn have developed from a simple goiter. Because of the possibility of cancer as well as hyperthyroidism, these tumors are often removed surgically. *See also* EXOPHTHALMIC GOITER.

GONORRHEA, a contagious venereal disease, characterized by inflammation of the genital mucous membranes and caused by a microorganism, Neisseria gonorrheae, more commonly known as the gonococcus germ. Gonorrhea is the most common venereal disease and occurs throughout the world. Adults are almost always infected by sexual contact with an infected person. An epidemic form occurs in young girls which is spread through nonsexual objects, such as clothing or toys.

Symptoms of infection appear in about three days, although they can take as long as three weeks, after exposure. In the male the first symptoms are usually a slight feeling of irritation or burning sensation when urinating because of the inflammation of the urethra. If the person is not treated, a large amount of pus is produced and an increased amount of discharge may be noticed. Complications can ensue which cause damage to other areas of the sex organs, such as the sex glands, and to other parts of the body, such as bones, eyes, joints, kidneys, and heart.

In women, gonorrhea affects the urinary passage and may extend to the bladder and kidneys. In the past, treatment of the infection in women was much more difficult than in men, because the organs are less accessible. Formerly a person infected with gonorrhea was incapacitated for weeks or even years, but new methods of treatment with penicillin and other antibiotics, under direction of a physician, can bring about a cure in one or two days, provided the infection is brought to the attention of a physician in time. The rapidity and effectiveness of the new drugs has brought about hopes that the disease might eventually be totally eliminated.

Gonorrheal infection of the eyes, although it does occur in adults, is more frequent in newborn infants, who become infected as they pass through the birth canal. It is estimated that gonorrheal eye infection is responsible for 10,000 cases of blindness in the United States. Doctors now administer dilute silver nitrate solution into the eyes of newborn infants to prevent this infection. Many urge the use of other drugs such as antibiotics.

In treating gonorrhea with penicillin, the physician must be particularly careful, since the patient may seem to be cured but still be able to transmit the disease, and penicillin, although it may cure the gonorrhea, may cover up, but not cure, an unsuspected case of syphilis, also present. Syphilis requires larger doses of penicillin. Therefore, if syphilis is also suspected, the physician may use a sulfonamide drug, which will not cover up a developing syphilitic condition.

GOUT, a disease in which the primary symptom is a painful inflammation of the joints of the hands or feet, and especially of the big toe. This inflammation arises when uric acid in the blood increases, is not destroyed by the body, and accumulates in the blood, where it combines with sodium to create sodium urate. The sodium urate may eventually be deposited in the cartilage and other tissues. It is not as yet known why the excess of uric acid appears in the blood, why the excess is not destroyed, or why urates are deposited in the tissue.

Gout usually begins with pain in the big toe, occasionally in the ankle, heel, or even instep, and is ordinarily accompanied by chills and fever. The pain resembles that of a violent dislocation. The affected joint becomes so sensitive that any pressure, even that of bedclothes, is unendurable. This disease attacks men, and occasionally women, in their middle thirties as well as in their sixties or later, contrary to popular belief that it is a condition resulting from a diet of rich foods in advanced years. Gout finally becomes chronic.

Among the drugs used in the treatment of gout are salicylic acid, cortisone, ACTH, Butazolidin, Benemid, anturan and colchicine, a drug used to treat gout since the fifth century. These drugs should be taken only under supervision of a physician, since they can be toxic with many side effects if improperly used. Gout is also relieved by application of heat to the painful joint and by protecting it from disturbing external contacts.

Anyone with gout should avoid excesses of diet or exercise. The diet should largely exclude foods containing white crystalline substances known as purines, which includes most meats, such as beef, veal, pork, and bacon, and most animal organ foods, such as liver, sweetbreads, kidneys, and brains. Milk, eggs, and cheese, cereals, fruits, green vege-

tables, cocoa, tea, coffee, sweets, and nuts are relatively low in purines. *See also* Chapter 24, "Arthritis and Rheumatism."

GRANULOCYTOPENIA. *See* AGRANULOCYTOSIS.

GRANULOMA INGUINALE, a disease usually regarded as venereal although no evidence exists that it is transmitted by sexual contact. It's main symptom is deep ulcerations on and around the genitals and is thought to be caused by a microorganism. There are approximately five to ten thousand cases of granuloma inguinale in the United States and it is associated with uncleanliness.

Following exposure, the disease becomes noticeable one to four weeks later. The first symptom is swelling, usually in the groin, and this swollen area then ruptures and ulcers form. As the ulcers heal, new ulcers continue to appear, and the disease may eventually cover the reproductive organs, lower abdomen and buttocks. These lesions have an unpleasant odor. A person with granuloma inguinale apparently develops little immunity and may have the condition for many years. Streptomycin and terramycin have both proved successful in treatment of the disease.

GRAVES' DISEASE, another name for exophthalmic goiter. *See* EX-OPHTHALMIC GOITER.

GRIPPE. *See* INFLUENZA.

GUMS, mucous membranes which cover the margin of the jaw and surround the roots of the teeth. Inflammation of the gum, known as gingivitis, may be general as in stomatitis of the mouth or local as in the area of an infected tooth.

Pyorrhea is the most common and serious purulent infection of the gums. Gums are sensitive and bleed easily, especially when brushed too vigorously, and in certain disorders like scurvy they become soft and spongy. The gums are also subject to tumors and alveolar abscesses which are deep-seated infections. Suppuration of the gum, or ulceration with pus, is called a gumboil. Attention by a dental surgeon will prevent permanent scars of the cheek or neck if the infection spreads. After eliminating the infection, the offending tooth or teeth must be treated. *See also* GINGIVITIS; PYORRHEA; TEETH.

GYNECOLOGY, the medical science concerned with the diseases of women, particularly those of the organs related to childbirth. A gynecologist is a specialist in these diseases.

GYNECOMASTIA, derived from two words meaning women and breasts, a condition of enlargement of the breasts which affects males only. It is usually related to some glandular disturbance. Excessive enlargement may be surgically treated.

HABIT SPASM, or tic, the habitual and involuntary contraction of a muscle. Habit spasms occur most frequently in the face, perhaps because the facial muscles are remarkably flexible, especially when stimulated by emotions. So minute and lively are some of the facial muscles that often their habit spasms are

visible only to trained observers. The tiny muscles close to the eye are particularly susceptible to these spasms.

Parents or teachers sometimes mistake a habit spasm for a symptom of St. Vitus' dance. The difference between the two, however, is easily defined. Habit spasms are predictable and always occur in the same manner; whereas the spasms seen in St. Vitus' dance are varied and therefore unpredictable.

Habit spasms can be treated effectively only after the cause has been ascertained by expert study. If the cause is physical, the cure may also be physical, via medication or surgery or perhaps merely by the adjustment of eyeglasses. Frequently, however, the cause is emotional. A habit spasm in a child might be traced, for example, to chronic fear of punishment, and the parents might find it desirable to secure psychotherapy for the child. *See* CHOREA; CONVULSION; TIC DOULOUREUX.

HAIR, slender threadlike outgrowths from follicles in the skin.

Structure. The hair root is that part of a hair beneath the surface of the skin. The sebaceous glands have their openings in the hair follicles and secrete sebum which gives the skin and scalp its oily appearance. The color of the hair is due to the presence of pigment cells. Attached to the follicles are tiny muscles which erect the follicle and incidentally the hair. These operate in excitement, when the hair "stands on end," or in chills, when "goose pimples" appear.

Growth. Hair grows at a regular rate in the average person of about an inch in six weeks. Then the follicle rests for a period varying from a few weeks to as much as ten or eleven weeks. The hair of the head, except in baldness, has an almost continuous activity of the follicles, each hair being replaced almost as soon as it reaches its full length.

Several different kinds of hair grow on the body. The hair on the scalp varies considerably, both as to the number of hairs and the length to which they grow. About 125,000 hairs grow on the scalp of the average person. Blondes have more hair on the scalp than dark people. The average length to which a hair will grow on a woman is sixty to seventy centimeters or about twenty-five inches, and it takes about four years to reach that length. Hair that is cylindrical hangs straight from the head and oval hair becomes curly.

The total number of hairs in each eyebrow is around 600 and such hair lasts about 112 days. As people become older the eyebrows tend to curl and grow longer so that they have to be trimmed. The hair of the eyelashes is practically identical with that of the eyebrows except that it is slightly more curved. The average diameter of the hair of the beard increases throughout life, so that these hairs become coarser and more bristling in advanced years. The beard is scanty among the more darkly pigmented races. Sexual differences are involved in the distribution of hair on the rest of the body.

Baldness. Alopecia or baldness involves temporary loss of hair due to various causes, or permanent loss of hair due to hereditary causes. Temporary falling out of hair may result from an infection or be related to certain diseases like typhoid, scarlet fever, pneumonia and other serious infections of the respiratory tract. In such cases, the hair may fall out suddenly, but will be replaced in time without special treatment. Falling hair may be related to excessive activity of the oil glands of the hair.

Hereditary baldness is influenced by sex-limited characteristics. Such baldness is inherited principally through the male as a dominant characteristic, and it is recessive in the female, tending to disappear if it occurs. Not only the baldness but the type of baldness is inherited. Once hereditary baldness appears, little can be done to prevent its development. Possibly the falling of hair in a hereditary case may be delayed somewhat by treatment, but even this is uncertain.

Care of the hair. The hair should be washed often enough to keep it clean; for short hair at least once in two weeks, and for long hair every three weeks will usually suffice. For most hair any good toilet soap that will lather freely is satisfactory. After the hair has been washed with soap and water it should be rinsed thoroughly and dried fairly slowly rather than with a hot blower. If the hair is too dry a small amount of oil may be rubbed into it after it has been washed and dried.

All authorites except some barbers agree that singeing the hair does not accomplish anything for hair health. When the body is in ill health, the hair is likely to react accordingly. Frequently good health and a good state of the skin and hair seem to be related.

The problem of gray or white hair cannot be readily solved. Vitamins or other substances taken internally do not substantially prevent or delay the appearance of gray hair in families in which there is a tendency to early graying. Experts can successfully dye hair. Some people, however, are particularly sensitive to paraphenyl-endiamine, which is an ingredient of many hair dyes, and a careful hairdresser will test the surface of the skin to the reaction of this chemical before using a dye containing it.

Sure methods for growing hair by artificial stimulation are unknown.

Superfluous hair. Hypertrichosis is the scientific name for excessive hairiness. Superfluous hair is not a worry to most men, but it may be a serious problem for a woman.

Expert opinion inclines to the view that the endocrine glands, or glands of internal secretion, have a definite relationship to excessive growth of hair, particularly on the upper lip and chin of women. Certain forms of overgrowth of glands may be associated with excessive growth of hair. In women excessive growth of hair is more likely to occur after they have passed the menopause. If a young girl has a fine mustache, the matter can be lightly regarded unless the mustache is too dark in color.

For removal of superfluous hair three different methods are known. The safest and the only one generally recommended is the use of the electric needle. This requires patience and endurance both on the part of the woman undergoing the treatment and the doctor. In this process a needle or wire carrying the current is inserted into the hair follicle and a weak current turned on for a brief time. Only from ten to fifteen hairs may be removed in a single session. Since there may be 1200 to 1500 hairs on the upper lip, the time involved is a major consideration. Even with the best operators, from 10 to 50 per cent of the hairs that are removed recur, depending on the efficacy of the electric current in destroying the hair follicles.

Most experts warn against removal of superfluous hair by x-ray. The results are so uncertain and the possibilities of harm so great that this method should not be used except in extreme cases. A dosage of x-ray sufficient to cause the hair to fall out is likely also to produce permanent damage to the skin.

Temporary measures for relief from excess hair are shaving, rubbing with pumice stone, application of depilatory waxes, which harden and are pulled off, taking the hair with them, and other methods. Hydrogen peroxide is sometimes used to bleach the hair so that it is not so visible. *See also* BALDNESS; CRAB LICE; DEPILATORY; SEBORRHEA.

HAIR REMOVER. *See* DEPILATORY.

HALITOSIS, the scientific name for bad breath. The cause may be tooth decay; or an infection of tissue in the mouth, tonsils, or nose; or chronic intestinal disturbances. Certain foods and seasonings, such as garlic, leave a temporary smell on the breath.

The word halitosis came into general use as a result of intensive advertising for a mouthwash. Mouthwashes cannot cure halitosis. Antiseptics like Sterisol or Listerine may destroy germs associated with decaying teeth or mouth infection. Professional medical or dental treatment of the basic cause may be required. Teeth should be examined by a dentist every six months and whatever dental work is necessary should be taken care of. Daily care of the teeth includes regular brushing every morning and evening with a good brush and whatever paste, powder, or solution the person prefers, and the use of dental floss.

When tonsils are infected or the tonsil cavities are filled with food particles, they may produce an unpleasant odor. Tonsils may be cleansed by a doctor and sometimes gargling helps, but surgical removal of tonsils is often the only effective way to combat the problem. Nose infections which may cause halitosis should also be treated by a doctor. Treatment may involve special washing.

Some foods, such as garlic, affect the odor of the breath directly from the stomach even when none remains in the mouth or teeth. In this case, flavored oils or mouthwashes may help mask the odor. Recently substances containing chlorophyll have been tried as antihalitosis agents, but evidence indicates that they do not and cannot prevent mouth odor.

HALLUCINATION, an impression, involving any of the five senses of sight, smell, taste, touch, or hearing, without actual basis in fact. Hallucinations occur frequently in alcoholic delirium, when the victim thinks he sees, for example, rats or snakes. Victims of paranoia often claim to hear voices.

HAND - SCHULLER - CHRISTIAN DISEASE, a rare disease, named for the three medical scientists who first described it, which occurs chiefly in children and young adults. Deposits of cholesterol appear in the bones and subcutaneous tissues with consequent disturbance of the metabolism. Growth and development are retarded and other symptoms usually appear, such as bulging of the eyes, a tendency to develop diabetes insipidus, and defects in the formation of the skull.

Direct application of x-ray has been the only effective form of therapy for this condition. Although complete cures have been effected, about a third of the cases terminate fatally.

HANSEN'S DISEASE. *See* LEPROSY.

HARDENING OF THE ARTERIES. *See* ARTERIOSCLEROSIS.

HARELIP, a cleft or clefts in the upper lip, so-called because of its resemblance to a hare's lip. *See also* CLEFT PALATE; LIPS.

HAY FEVER, a common allergic disorder, involving the nose and eyes. The symptoms are sneezing, watery discharge from the eyes and nose, itching, swelling, burning sensations, and general discomfort. In chronic cases, the sinuses also may become infected.

Hay fever results from sensitivity to pollen, especially to that of the giant ragweed, although many other known pollens may cause it. Seasonal hay fever is the most common form and occurs widely in the United States during the ragweed season, commencing about August 15 and continuing until the first frost. Pollen is carried by the wind and surveys have indicated that different regions vary as to the amount of pollen in the air.

Hay fever sufferers should be tested to learn the specific pollen to which they are sensitive and to make certain that the condition is hay fever and not some other chronic condition such as asthma. Scientific skin tests have been developed which are accurate and help speed the treatment.

An effective relief for hay fever sufferers is desensitization. This is accomplished by injecting gradually increased doses of pollen extracts at varying intervals, particularly at the height of the hay fever season. This treatment is continued throughout the year and the cycle of injections repeated each year. In time, improvement is such that the injections are no longer necessary.

Prevention of hay fever rather than treatment is desirable. For those who can afford to travel, a climate free of pollen during the hay fever season is helpful. For those who cannot change locale, protective glasses for the eyes, and filters and masks for the nose devised to screen out pollen are beneficial. Sleeping in an air-conditioned room is also a good preventive.

Many patent preparations and nose and eye drugs are available and can be used to relieve hay fever. Drugs like the antihistamines, ephedrine, and adrenalin, although helpful, should be used only when prescribed by a physician. *See also* ALLERGY; ASTHMA; and Chapter 21, "Allergy."

HAZARDS OF COLD. The air age has increased travel over and into the Arctic. Experience with emergency landings in which people have been exposed to the cold climate without sufficient preparation has demonstrated the need for information.

Cold and snow are the chief hazards in the Arctic. Snow blindness, which results from the glare of snow on the eyes, can and should be prevented. The Eskimo makes a crude wooden snow shield of goggles with slits, cut or burned, through which he can look. The shields, worn across the bridge of the nose and held in place by string, bar the glare of the sun. Blackening of the cheeks and bridge of the nose with soot, charcoal, or dirty engine oil is also helpful in cutting down the reflection of the sun on the snow.

Tight shoes are harmful in freezing weather and can cause damage to the feet. Therefore, shoes worn in the Arctic must be big and roomy enough to permit the wearing of at least two pairs of heavy socks. If the shoes are not large enough, they should be removed and the feet wrapped in canvas or similar materials.

The hands must also be kept warm and dry. Heavy woolen inner mitts with windproof outer mittens should be worn.

Cold metal on bare skin has been the cause of many serious accidents. Metal freezes to the skin and at the first burning sensation the tendency is to tear the part of the body involved away from the metal; this will destroy the skin. Instead, the metal should be thawed loose from the skin.

The diet of the Eskimo fits the Arctic. Since it is heat-producing, fat is the basic element of this diet. Soldiers and airmen stationed in cold regions receive special cold-weather diets. Practically all fish have enough fat to make them good Arctic food, and the liver of the cod, an especially nourishing food, can be eaten boiled.

Among the useful recommendations for health in the Arctic are those concerning frostbite. Frostbite often develops unawares. If the skin becomes stiff and grayish or whitish, frostbite has begun. Snow or ice are never to be applied under these circumstances. Heat applied to warm the affected part gradually is beneficial. Any rubbing or massage must be avoided since this may destroy the tissues. In frostbite of the feet, shoes and coverings should be removed at once, and the feet wrapped in fur or cloth until they thaw. Thawing is accompanied by a burning sensation and may be extremely painful. After frostbite the skin blisters and peels exactly as it does in sunburn. *See also* CHILBLAINS; FROSTBITE.

HEADACHE, a pain or ache across the forehead or within the head; it is not a disease but a symptom. It may be the result of profoundly complex and obscure conditions, little understood until recent years.

One theory establishes three basic types of processes underlying headaches: mechanical, such as blockage of the sinuses by infection; toxic, resulting from too much alcohol or ingestion of a poison; and functional, in which the parts and phenomena of the body involved do not manifest any detectable disease. Under these three classifications are placed alto-

gether 203 separate causes of headaches.

A common mechanical cause of headaches is dilatation of the blood vessels of the head by a temporarily excessive blood supply under too great pressure. The dilatation, in turn, may arise from different sources, such as high blood pressure or the effect of an infectious disease which evokes outpouring of fluid in the body. Thus, many infections seem to begin with a headache.

One of the most frequent sources of headache is tenseness in the muscles of the head and neck, sometimes because of local injury or a nervous disturbance, sometimes because of emotional tension. Such headaches, usually felt at the rear of the head and down into the neck, tend to respond well to heat and massage.

Brain tissue itself is not sensitive to pain, but its coverings and associated structures are capable of feeling pain. The brain rests within a membranous covering and a permanent surrounding of cerebrospinal fluid. If the supply of fluid is unduly increased so that the membrane is stretched, pain results. Any other pressure on the membrane will have the same effect. The pain may come from an abscess in the brain or from incipient tumor. Sudden movements of the head or blows upon it may similarly affect the membrane covering the brain or the other structures of the head which respond to pain.

Persons who have headaches only occasionally may find them closely related to some experience that is also only occasional, such as excessive drinking, eating, or smoking, or exposure to toxic gases or other substances. The actual source of pain is often a change in pressure within the head due to the toxic materials.

Inflammation of internal structure of the head which characterizes severe infections, such as encephalitis or meningitis, incurs acute headache, and inflammation following brain hemorrhage has the same effect.

A seemingly general headache may actually come from a disorder in a small isolated part of the head, especially from the eyes. Excessive use of the eyes, particularly in reading or working under glaring light, will induce headache. Strain and failure to correct defects of vision also bring the same discomfort. Correction of the causative factor generally eliminates the distress.

Migraine, often called sick headache, designates a particular kind of disorder marked by its intensity, its association with vomiting and nausea, and its tendency to recur. Migraine is believed to be a response by the body to some protein to which it is especially sensitive which induces fluid and swelling within the head. However, this kind of headache varies considerably from person to person and from time to time in the same person. Mental factors are closely related to the degree of acuteness experienced in a migraine attack, as are other physical conditions in the body.

In the functional headache, physical cause is not detectable, nor is tissue change discernible even to the closest examination. Frequently, however, it can be correlated to a mental or emotional disturbance. This kind of headache produces as much acute pain as if it had a clearly defined phy-

sical origin. The study and treatment of such ailments are in the field of psychosomatic medicine, which examines the interaction of the mind and body.

Frequently headache is the most acute symptom of some minor underlying condition, such as constipation, indigestion, fatigue, or menstruation.

Headache remedies are as varied as the causes, and some are dangerous for a number of reasons. The simplest and most basic remedy should be tried first: elimination of excesses in the use of alcohol and tobacco and food, adequate rest, and establishment of good hygiene relative to excretion of body wastes. A large measure of relief may thus be effected without resort to drugs.

Although the majority of commercial headache remedies are mild analgesics or pain relievers, this is not true of all. Some should be approached with great caution or not at all. Aspirin is the least injurious. Barbiturates, although they do reduce pain, may simultaneously have toxic effects. In addition, they induce drowsiness or actual sleep which can be undesirable or even dangerous, such as when driving a car. The drugs known as aminopyrine and Pyramidon have demonstrably caused serious injury to the blood. Among other analgesics are Opap, ergotamine, and others that must be prescribed by the doctor.

A physician should be consulted when recurrent headache is a new experience. Medical advice is also essential when attacks are of unusual severity or persistence. Sedatives and pain-relieving drugs merely mask symptoms. Expert diagnosis and detection of the real cause usually brings relief. *See also* MIGRAINE.

HEAD BANGING, HEAD ROLL-ING. Toward the end of the first year an otherwise normal healthy baby may roll his head from side to side at bedtime and also bang his head up and down or against his crib. Sometimes this banging will be so violent as to cause bruises on the head, or so prolonged as to rub the hair away from the scalp.

While parents are understandably disturbed by such behavior, they need not be alarmed. Head banging is not a vicious habit or a mental or emotional disturbance. Neither is it associated with any organic disease. It seems to occur at the period when the baby begins to crave some rhythmic activity; occasionally it seems to be more than enjoyment and an expression of development.

A relationship has been noted between head banging and an obstruction in breathing, such as may be caused by adenoids. Removal of adenoids is advisable and successful in many cases. Nevertheless, head banging may continue if chronic congestion of the nasal passages results from other causes.

Sedatives, which induce sleep quickly, have been found useful in correcting this condition, especially if the child has a tendency to be tense before going to sleep. Head banging, under such circumstances, is similar to thumb sucking, a means of relieving tenseness. If parents or those who attend the baby are themselves tense, this may reflect on the child. Definite or specific suggestions to cure these habits have not as yet

been developed. However, babies outgrow the tendency to head banging and rolling. Cuddling and rocking a child to relax it (and the parent) is helpful and this custom is no longer disapproved of. The bottom and sides of the crib may be lined with quilting for protection. In any case, head banging need not cause great concern.

HEAD INJURIES. A head injury can be minor, with recovery rapid, or extremely severe, requiring complicated and prolonged treatment. Cuts and lacerations of the scalp, if they are treated promptly, heal comparatively fast when infection and scarring are not present. Skull fractures may be severe, but healing, though sometimes lengthy, usually occurs without serious aftereffects. Compound fractures may sometimes involve meningitis, but the use of antibiotics has lessened this possibility. Simple fractures usually heal without complications when properly taken care of.

A head injury can be extremely serious when the brain is exposed to infection or the cranial nerves are damaged or the brain or dura has actually been injured. Injuries to the brain may be classified as (1) concussion, (2) contusion, or (3) laceration. Brain concussion—that is, a severe shake or jolt—is most common. It produces temporary unconsciousness. Victims of brain concussion generally recover rapidly and completely. Contusion, or bruise, of the brain may affect the nerve centers in a variety of ways; it can stop or diminish or accelerate their functions. In laceration, actual damage is done to the brain tissue, followed by swelling of the brain and slowing of the blood supply which further damages the tissue. After the victim has regained consciousness, amnesia in some degree may set in, depending on the degree of injury. Recovery from complete loss of consciousness comes in stages; consciousness may be regained in minutes or, in more severe cases, in hours or even days.

In serious head injuries, major brain functions may be paralyzed. If the respiratory system is paralyzed, death may occur immediately unless artificial respiration is given at once. Brain injuries may involve meningitis, hemorrhage, inflammation, and temporary or permanent personality and mental impairment. A convulsive seizure can occur immediately or months or years following the head injury and is more likely when the dura and brain have been damaged.

Treatment of head injuries ranges from first-aid measures, including treatment for shock and keeping the victim immobile, to complicated surgery entailing prolonged hospitalization. In general the older the victim of a head injury is, the slower and less certain the recovery. Children usually have fewer aftereffects than adults. Occasionally a victim of a head injury will have complications after recovery which have a psychological basis.

Repeated head injuries, as in the case of a boxer, provoke the condition commonly called "punch drunk," which is probably due to small hemorrhages throughout the brain. It involves loss or impairment of such faculties as coordination, memory, concentration, vision, and hearing. *See also* BRAIN.

HEARING, HARDNESS OF. *See* DEAFNESS; EAR; OTOSCLEROSIS.

HEART, a powerful hollow muscle which is the central pump of the circulatory system. It is pear-shaped, about the size of a fist, and weighs approximately 9 ounces. It lies in the chest, between the right and left lungs, with its narrower end pointed downward and to the left, where the heartbeat may generally be felt. The entire structure is enclosed in a tough fibrous sac, the pericardium, containing a small amount of lubricating fluid which eliminates friction in this area. The pericardium also holds the heart in position during postural changes and limits the dilation of that organ.

The thick muscular wall of the heart, the myocardium, is responsible for its contraction and expansion. The interior of the heart is completely lined with a thin smooth membrane, the endocardium, which is continu-

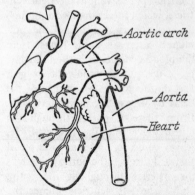

Aortic arch

Aorta

Heart

Illustration of the heart showing the aorta, the main artery which carries the blood from the heart to the rest of the blood stream.

ous with the lining of the blood vessels, where it is known as endothelium. Any inflammation of these tissues gives rise to the diseases named for them, as myocarditis, pericarditis and endocarditis.

The interior of the heart is divided into two separate cavities, similar in construction, but not communicating with each other. Each cavity contains two chambers, a thin-walled auricle above, which is the receiving depot for the blood entering the heart, and a thick muscle-walled ventricle below, which pumps the blood out of the heart. Each chamber is provided with valves, arranged so that the blood can flow in only one direction. These four chambers act in complete unison, and their ability to expand and contract without stopping keeps the blood stream in the body in perpetual motion.

The blood which has circulated throughout the body enters the right auricle by way of two large veins, the venae cavae. This muscle contracts and propels the blood through the tricuspid valve into the right ventricle, which forces the blood through the pulmonary valve into the pulmonary artery and the lungs. Here the blood deposits its carbon dioxide, picks up a fresh supply of oxygen, and returns to the left auricle of the heart by way of the pulmonary vein. From there it passes through the mitral valve into the left ventricle, which contracts and sends the blood forward through the aortic valve into the arteries throughout the entire body. The left ventricle pumps the blood through the entire systemic circulation of the body, and accordingly has the strongest muscle wall.

Both auricles contract together. This contraction, the auricular systole, is commonly known as the "heartbeat." It forces the blood into the ventricles, and the auricles then relax, or go into auricular diastole or dilation. During the latter part of the auricular diastole, and the whole period of the auricular systole, the ventricles are relaxed and fill with blood; this is the ventricular diastole. Just before the ventricular diastole is completed, the auricles begin to contract again, sending more blood into the ventricles. At this point the pressure within the ventricles increases, and when it exceeds the pressure in the large arteries that open from them, the ventricles contract, going into the ventricular systole, and the valves leading into the artery open and the blood is forced into the arteries. This regular rhythmic series of contractions and relaxations and the synchronous opening and closing of the valves is called the cardiac cycle. The period of rest for the two sets of muscles is longer than the work period, so that they may recuperate and gather fresh strength prior to each contraction. The ventricles are relaxed for a longer period than the auricles, since they have the burden of pumping.

The rhythmic action of the heart is controlled by a special structure, composed of muscle and nerve fibers. These fibers are concentrated in two centers, or nodes, but branch off into fine fibers which penetrate to every part of the heart. One node is embedded in the muscular tissue of the wall of the right auricle, and is called the sino-auricular node. This is the pacemaker of the heart; it sends out the rhythmic impulses which control contraction of the auricles. The other node, the auriculo-ventricular node, located in the lower part of the right auricular wall, controls the impulses to the ventricles. These two nodes and their common bundle of fibers, known as the bundle of His, after Wilhelm His, who first described it, with the fine network of fibers which covers the inside of each ventricle, are the only connection between the right and left hearts. The coordinated contractions and expansions of the four heart chambers results in the heartbeat.

The rate of the heartbeat is also affected by different portions of the nervous system, which exercise dual sets of controls by means of nerve cells or neurons, arising in the spinal cord and brain. Thus, heart action is increased by impulses sent over the sympathetic fibers connected to the spinal cord. Heart action is decreased by impulses sent out over the vagus, or wandering, nerve, one of the cranial nerves connected to the brain stem.

When the heartbeat is accelerated, a sensation of fluttering or throbbing of the heart known as palpitation is felt. Any normal variations in the usual rhythm may cause an awareness of the heartbeat, and persons who are acutely conscious of their cardiac output often complain of palpitation, unless their attention can be diverted. This is one of the most frequently encountered symptoms in anxiety neuroses and has no organic significance. Palpitation may also result from cardiac enlargement or changes in stroke volume or rate of the heart. Exercise or emotional stimulation

cause palpitation by increasing the stroke volume or rate of the heartbeat. Palpitation is also one of the symptoms in anemia, thyrotoxicosis, angina pectoris, and in many of the conditions in which irregular cardiac rhythm occurs.

Normally the heart beats about 70 to 80 times a minute, and continues to beat at this rate throughout life. During emotional or physical

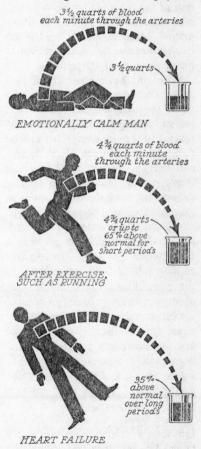

3½ quarts of blood each minute through the arteries

3½ quarts

EMOTIONALLY CALM MAN

4¾ quarts of blood each minute through the arteries

4¾ quarts or up to 65% above normal for short periods

AFTER EXERCISE, SUCH AS RUNNING

35% above normal over long periods

HEART FAILURE

Unusual work or excited emotions speed up the blood flow and increase blood pressure making the heart work harder.

strain, or in fright, the beat is increased, sometimes to over 100 beats per minute. During sleep or when the body is relaxed, the beat decreases. In a life span of seventy years, the heart beats somewhat under three billion times, and pumps more than fifty million gallons of blood.

The pressure of the blood within the arterial vessels is one of the most significant indications of the condition of the heart, and various instruments are used to obtain this information. Most commonly used is the sphygmomanometer, which measures blood pressure in the arteries.

When the heart contracts, it produces electric currents in its tissues which are just strong enough to reach the surface of the body. These currents can be measured by special electrical instruments. The electrocardiograph, for example, records them; and the recording, an electrocardiogram, notes the contraction and relaxation of the heart and reveals any abnormalities, since the recording of the normal heart presents a characteristic pattern. The electrocardiograph is used extensively in the diagnosis of heart disease. *See also* ANGINA PECTORIS; BACTERIAL ENDOCARDITIS; BLOOD; BLOOD PRESSURE; CHOLESTEROL; CIRCULATORY SYSTEM; CORONARY THROMBOSIS; ENDOCARDITIS; PERICARDITIS; RHEUMATIC FEVER; and Chapter 8, "Congenital Heart Disease in Children"; Part III, "Your Heart."

HEART BLOCK, a condition in which the muscular interconnection between the auricles and ventricles, the upper and lower chambers of the heart, is so damaged by disease that they beat independently. As a result, the pulsation of the heart is slowed, occurring in paroxysms or spasms.

HEARTBURN. *See* INDIGESTION.

HEAT CRAMPS. *See* HEAT SICKNESS.

HEAT EXHAUSTION. *See* HEAT SICKNESS.

HEAT SICKNESS. Three specific conditions commonly result from exposure to excessive heat: (1) sunstroke, called heatstroke if the cause is artificial heat; (2) heat exhaustion; and (3) heat cramps. Persons most susceptible and most likely to be severely affected are the very old or young, extremely overweight persons, alcoholics, and anyone who is ill.

Loss of salt from the body is the primary cause of heat sickness. In high temperatures, sweating is the chief way in which the temperature of the body is regulated, and profuse sweating depletes the body of large amounts of salt. For this reason, salt tablets are frequently given to men working in high temperatures.

The initial symptoms of sunstroke, or heatstroke, are ordinarily dizziness and headache, dryness of the mouth and skin, and nausea. Unconsciousness may follow rapidly and about a fourth of all serious cases end fatally. The person's face is flushed and the skin hot and dry. The pulse is rapid and the temperature may be as high as 107° or 110° or higher. Although the body is usually relaxed, convulsions sometimes occur.

The person should be placed on his back, with head slightly elevated, in a cool place, and his clothes removed. Wet cloths or ice bags should be applied to cool the head. Probably the best method of cooling the body is to wrap the person in a sheet or cloth and pour on small amounts of cold water. The body should not be cooled too rapidly. The arms and legs should be massaged, through the material, in the direction of the heart to aid circulation. Another way to cool the body is immersion in cool water for about twenty minutes. Ice bags may also be used. The cooling treatment and massage should continue until the skin no longer appears hot and flushed. No stimulants should be given, but when conscious the person may have cool drinks. A doctor should be called as soon as possible.

Symptoms of heat exhaustion differ from those of sunstroke. The face is pale, perspiration profuse, and the entire body may be clammy. The pulse is weak, breathing shallow, and weakness may be extreme. Sometimes a brief period of unconsciousness or fainting may ensue. Nausea, vomiting, dizziness, and unsteadiness are almost always present.

The person should lie down, with head level or slightly lowered, in a well-ventilated airy place. He should be lightly covered and given a half teaspoon of salt in about a third of a glass of water repeatedly until he has consumed about a tablespoon of salt. Warm coffee or tea may be drunk. If symptoms continue, a doctor should be called.

Heat cramps are extremely painful, and usually affect the muscles in the arms and legs or the abdominal muscles. Heat cramps may be accompanied by symptoms of heat exhaustion, and the treatment is the same as in heat exhaustion. A firm hand pressure on the affected area may give relief.

To prevent heat sickness, certain precautions should be taken. If possible, activity in extreme heat should be avoided or kept to a minimum. If it is necessary to remain in a high temperature, frequent rest periods should be observed and perhaps salt tablets taken. If at any time a person feels dizzy or nauseated, he should go immediately to a cool airy place. To maintain a proper sweat production, it is necessary to drink an ample amount of water, about twelve glasses a day for a person who works in a high temperature. Light loose clothing permits evaporation of sweat, and a hat will protect the head, a vulnerable area. A good summer diet includes abundant fruits, juices, and vegetables, and only limited amounts of fat food and alcoholic and iced beverages.

HEATSTROKE. *See* HEAT SICKNESS.

HEIGHT. A person's height is determined by the span of the vertebral trunk and the length of the bones of the lower limbs.

Children's growth in height is influenced by climate, including weather and sunlight, by diet, exercise, and posture, and particularly by glandular action. The growth hormone, secreted by the pituitary gland, stimulates the growth mechanism of the body for the first ten or fifteen years of life. Then the same gland begins to function is such a way as to affect the reproductive glands of both males and females. When a balance of secretion is reached, about the time of adolescence, the growth mechanism generally stops and adult growth is achieved.

Overactivity of the pituitary gland produces acromegaly or giantism. Underactivity of the same gland results in achondroplasia or dwarfism.

The injection of growth hormones in children whose rate of growth is such as to indicate that they will be abnormally short in stature has been helpful. The results have been more effective when the injections are given before adolescence, because of the relationship between the pituitary and sex glands. *See also* ACHONDROPLASIA; ACROMEGALY; GLANDS; PITUITARY; and Chapter 19, "Endocrine Glands."

HELIOTHERAPY, exposure of the body to the rays of the sun or to ultraviolet rays to treat disease. Treatment with light is generally called phototherapy. Infrared therapy, which is the use of the heat rays from the sun or from an artificial source, is a form of phototherapy.

HEMANGIOMA, a tumor composed of blood vessels. The growths appear at birth, or shortly thereafter, as reddish or purplish stains on the skin. These swellings are composed chiefly of capillaries at the surface. The blemishes may be small or large and sometimes disappear spontaneously. They are most effectively treated early in life by surgical excision or scraping. Other forms of treatment include injection of chemicals, exposure to x-ray or radium, or the application of dry ice.

Another form of hemangioma is the cavernous type. Here, spongy masses on the head and neck do not present a problem if small. However, if they are large, bruising and bleeding occur easily and are serious. Immediate medical attention for this type is advised.

HEMATURIA, blood in the urine. This condition is abnormal and requires immediate medical attention. Usually the cause can be found, but in about 2 per cent of the cases blood in the urine is of undetermined origin. In such instances, the blood appears suddenly, apparently coming from a varicose vein in the urinary tract. The loss of blood is seldom so great as to cause faintness or anemia. Usually this indeterminate type occurs in people under thirty.

A number of possible causes of hematuria, all related to the urinary system, are known. This disease may result from severe infection or inflammation of the kidneys, or when a tumor of the kidneys breaks through a blood vessel. In addition, various chemicals and drugs, such as the sulfa group, may act on the tissues of the kidney to cause bleeding. A kidney stone, rupture of the kidney, bladder, or other portion of the urinary tract may induce hematuria. Blood in the urine may also be an indication of cancer of the kidney or bladder.

A person with hematuria should be put to bed and the doctor promptly consulted. Uncontrolled or continuous bleeding may be critical if not apprehended and treated immediately and properly.

HEMOGLOBIN, the red coloring matter in blood cells, is a protein consisting of hematin and globin. It takes oxygen from the air into the lungs and transports the oxygen to the cells of the body through the arteries. Hemoglobin also combines with carbon dioxide, carrying it from the cells through the veins. Hemoglobin contains iron, which when absent from the diet causes anemia.

Various devices for measuring hemoglobin have been developed. The percentage of hemoglobin in the red blood cells and the amount in the blood is measured to determine whether or not the blood is normal as it relates to this constituent. Any deviation from the normal is an indication of some form of anemia. Excessive destruction of the red cells results in jaundice. When the pigment appears in the urine, the condition is known as hemoglobinuria. *See also* ANEMIA; BLOOD.

HEMOLYTIC ANEMIA. *See* ANEMIA; BLOOD TYPES.

HEMOPHILIA, a hereditary blood condition in which clotting is delayed or does not occur, perpetually threatening the sufferer with death from hemorrhage. In normal persons, when the surface of the body is injured and blood escapes, the blood coagulates into a solid mass within five or six minutes, and in this way seals the wound. In hemophilia, the blood does not clot properly and the person may lose quantities of blood from even a trivial wound. The inability of the blood to clot is apparently involved with a relative deficiency of specific factors in the blood. Estimates indicate that in the United States between 20,000 and 40,000 persons are affected.

Hemophilia was first recognized in the eleventh century by an Arabian physician, Albucasis, who called it "bleeder's disease." In 1803, an American, John C. Otto, accurately described it as a hereditary disease which does not affect women, but is transmitted from the mother to her children. Such women, called carriers or conductors, do not themselves have any of the symptoms of the disease. If the gene is transmitted to a son, he may suffer from hemophilia, and be able to pass on the gene to his offspring. If the gene is transmitted to a daughter, she in turn becomes a carrier, without having any symptoms of the ailment. Though it is believed that the daughter of two parents who each carry the gene of hemophilia might show the symptoms of hemophilia, a case of a woman with the symptoms of hemophilia has never been reported.

Queen Victoria, whose ancestors left no record of the disease, transmitted hemophilia to one daughter, a granddaughter, great-grandson, the czar of Russia, and to another daughter, who brought it into the royal house of Spain.

The first severe bleeding in hemophilia may be controlled, but subsequent hemorrhage may prove more serious. Persons with this tendency should always report the fact before having a tooth extracted, or undergoing the most minor surgical procedures, so that transfusions of the proper blood type can be available.

Any person who has hemophilia must avoid activity which might result in injury. When hemorrhage is not severe, it may be controlled by cold compresses, by judicious pressure, or by local application of thrombin, a basic blood factor, and Oxycel, a commercially prepared agent. Transfusions of fresh blood or preserved plasma can shorten the clotting time to nearly normal.

A recent development in this field has been the discovery of the missing factor in the blood in cases of hemophilia and its use in controlling hemorrhage. *See also* Chapter 13, "Diseases of the Blood."

HEMORRHAGE, a flow of blood, such as might result from a ruptured blood vessel. Uncontrollable bleeding indicates that the blood of the patient, because of some deficiency, will not easily clot. The supply of blood platelets may be less than adequate. Ordinarily, for every cubic millimeter of blood, at least 200,000 blood platelets are present and 50,000 are sufficient for forming strong blood clots. If the blood contains less than this number, however, the person is likely to bruise and bleed too easily, especially from the gums, from the sockets of extracted teeth, from the nose, and sometimes from internal organs. Any person who shows these or similar symptoms should have a thorough examination before treatment.

Normally a hemorrhage may be halted without excessive difficulty. A tight bandage of antiseptic gauze may be satisfactory. If a major artery is involved, as in one of the extremities, a tourniquet might be needed. Excessive bleeding after the removal of a tooth can usually be controlled by filling the socket with gauze or by the application of warm water.

In treating nosebleed, the person should lie face down, and either ice water or hot water applied, or the nostrils may be packed with gauze.

Anyone who frequently suffers from nosebleed should see a physician. *See also* WOUNDS.

HEMORRHOIDS, or piles, swellings that appear at the lower end of the bowel on the margin of the anus. These are actually varicose veins and are classified as either external or internal, depending on their location inside or outside the anal sphincter, the muscle that closes the lower end of the bowel.

Hemorrhoids result from interference with the flow of blood in the vessels of this area. A number of factors may be responsible, such as

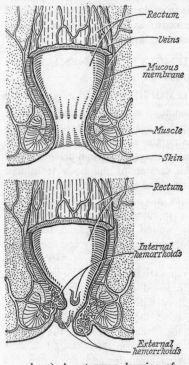

a b. a) A cut away drawing of a normal rectum and anus.
b) Internal and external hemorrhoids.

extremely sedentary habits, over-weight, constipation, or the excess use of cathartics. Pregnancy, too, may cause this condition, as may also congestion or cirrhosis of the liver.

External hemorrhoids may appear as little folds of brownish skin pro-truding from the anus, and may pro-duce little more than itching or a feeling of tightness during a bowel movement. Internal hemorrhoids sometimes become infected and in-flamed with consequent clotting or thrombosis. These may also protrude, and if scratched or broken bleed un-til the blood clots.

Treatment of hemorrhoids ranges from preventive measures to erase the cause to surgery for hemorrhoids that have become intolerable. People who lead sedentary lives must exercise. Poor circulation must be improved. Overweight must be corrected by re-ducing. Foods that may irritate and increase congestion in the blood ves-sels should be avoided or their use curtailed. Vinegar, spices, and coffee in excess are often harmful. Much can be done to regulate the movement of the bowels and a little mineral oil will help to soften the stool.

Hemorrhoids may be treated by the application of various ointments, suppositories, and hot wet packs, but such methods are only temporary and not curative. Surgery to remove piles is a radical but effective method. Electrical coagulation is effective, and injections of compounds similar to those used to treat varicose veins in other parts of the body are also means of controlling and curing hem-orrhoids. *See also* Chapter 13, "Dis-eases of the Blood."

HEPATITIS, an acute or chronic in-fectious disease of the liver, caused by a filterable virus. An acute form of the disease with similar symptoms may appear after injection of serum, as was seen during yellow fever vac-cinations given in the army, and also following transfusion of blood or plasma. In these cases, a serum was given containing a virus of which no one was aware. The disease may ap-pear after an incubation period that varies from forty to sixty days to as much as a year, and has also be-come an occupational hazard for hos-pital workers.

In ordinary hepatitis, which devel-ops without any previous injection, the spread of the virus may be traced to water or food that has been con-taminated. Here the latent period, be-fore the appearance of the disease, is much shorter.

Infectious hepatitis of the ordinary type may be mild, with jaundice as the most noticeable symptom. Other symptoms preceding the jaundice may include loss of appetite, fever with or without accompanying chills, aching of the back, joints, or eyes. Sometimes the gastrointestinal tract is affected, with heartburn, nausea, vomiting, and diarrhea as possible symptoms. The jaundice may last for weeks or months and disappear slowly or rapidly.

Treatment includes bed rest during the period of most severe jaundice, with a curtailment of activity for the duration of the disease. The diet must be controlled carefully and the invalid should be encouraged to eat since starvation is a special hazard to peo-ple with hepatitis. A high-protein, high-carbohydrate diet with few fats is a requisite.

While a few people develop chronic low-grade liver insufficiency as a result of hepatitis, the majority are completely cured in time and the liver returns to its normal functioning See also JAUNDICE; and Chapter 16, "Common Disorders of the Liver and Gallbladder."

HEREDITY, the congenital transmission of characteristics and tendencies of parents to their offspring. Genetics, the science which deals with man's origins, his mode of development and reproduction of characteristics, was given great impetus in the nineteenth century by the discoveries of Darwin, Lamarck, Mendel, and other scientists, including John Conrad Otto, the American physician who first accurately described the transmission of hemophilia from mother to son.

Certain physical traits are inherited, such as hair color and type, pigmentation of the skin, and color of the eyes. Tendencies to tallness or shortness are transmitted; tall parents generally have tall children and short parents have short children. Heredity is also accumulative; that is, many generations may contribute characteristics as well as the immediate parents.

A tendency to allergies and sensitivity to various protein substances may be hereditary. Hemophilia, the tendency to abnormal bleeding, is transmitted through the female to the male progeny, although the female does not suffer from the disease. It has occurred notably in some of the royal families of Europe. Diseases

themselves are not inherited, but possibly a tendency or susceptibility to certain diseases can be transmitted. Superstitions and popular notions about the effect of a prospective mother's thoughts and experiences on her child do not have any foundation in fact.

A child does not inherit fixed traits or characteristics. Rather, he is born with genes from both parents which interact to produce characteristics. The possibilities for interaction of genes are so numerous that several children in one family may display widely different traits.

Mental instability may be manifested through heredity by inheritance of defects in the brain structure, and many states have laws controlling propagation among insane or mentally defective people. By the same token, superior qualities in brain tissue may be transmitted. See also HEMOPHILIA.

HERMAPHRODITISM, a condition characterized by the coexistence in an individual of ovarian and testicular tissue. It is extremely rare in human beings but more common in lower forms. Hermaphroditism is sometimes confused with pseudohermaphroditism. See also ANDROGYNY.

HERNIA, or rupture, a protrusion of a part of the contents of the abdomen through a weak spot in the abdominal wall, or any protrusion of a loop or part of an organ or tissue through an abnormal opening.

Certain parts of the muscular wall of the body are less well reinforced than others. One weak point is in the groin along the lowest point of the abdomen; another is at the navel, and a third is in the area of the sex organs. When the muscle at one of these points separates sufficiently to permit part of the contents of the abdomen to bulge through, a hernia occurs. A hernia may result from any of many possible causes. A muscular weakness may be present at birth; a hernia may develop in infancy from straining—for example, in whooping cough; it may result from lifting a heavy object or other overstraining, or during childbirth, or because tissues have not healed adequately after a surgical operation.

Among several common methods of treatment are wearing a support which keeps the body material from passing through the opening in the abdominal wall; surgery in which the weak point is fastened and strengthened by surgical methods; and injection of an irritating substance which may cause the separated tissues to grow together. The doctor will decide on the basis of his examination which treatment is best suited to his patient.

In infants or young persons, support alone may occasionally, but not usually, be sufficient to permit the separated muscles to rejoin. In an older person, an inadequately controlled hernia usually tends to grow larger with time. The outward pressure of the internal organs gradually increases the size of the ruptured place in the muscle wall. Surgical repair is the most thorough and certain treatment. Permanent wearing of a truss is a possibility, especially for an elderly patient. Injection, if effective, eliminates the need for a

surgical operation, although it is usually not as reliable.

In surgery, the ruptured tissues are exposed and then sewn together, the stitches being placed to promote healing and to create an area of strength at the break. The surgical technique which has been developed is simple and the risk involved is relatively slight. The operation often does not even require a general anesthetic and is done quite satisfactorily with local anesthesia. Stitches are made of new materials which have greater strength than those formerly used. The patient must remain in bed for ten days to two weeks following the operation to assure complete healing.

The danger that an unrepaired hernia may become strangulated is always present. Furthermore, as the protrusion of the abdominal contents through the muscle break becomes greater it may be caught by a constriction of the muscles so that it will not slip back into place. Strangulation of a hernia is dangerous because the flow of blood may be partially or totally cut off in the strangulated part, threatening secondary infection, gangrene, and gradual death to this local tissue. As a consequence, the life of the patient is threatened.

An infrequent type of hernia is that occurring in the diaphragm, the muscle wall separating the chest from the abdomen. A hernia of the brain indicates a bulging of the brain through a break in the skull; and in hernia of the lung, part of the lung pushes through an opening in the chest. Hernia may affect the scrotum and other parts of the body. *See also* DIAPHRAGM.

HERPES SIMPLEX, an acute virus disorder, commonly called "cold sores" or "fever blisters," characterized by blisters or sores which appear in clusters of small painful swellings about the lips. They frequently follow severe colds, pneumonia, malaria, or other acute conditions with fever. Although usually confined to the lips, herpes simplex may occur on the conjunctivas, corneas, or on the genitals. The swellings develop into watery blisters which break, form a crust, and eventually heal.

Fever blisters are associated with digestive upsets, emotional disturbances, allergic reactions, and, in some women, with menstrual irregularities. Herpes simplex is usually mild and limited to one area, and ordinarily disappears within a week or ten days. Applications, such as zinc ointment or calamine lotion, on the affected area may relieve pain and swelling.

HERPES ZOSTER, also known as shingles, a fairly common virus disease found most frequently in adults. It usually occurs during the spring and autumn. The word zoster is derived from the Greek, meaning girdle. The condition is characterized by the appearance of clusters of large painful blisters running in a bandlike pattern on patches of reddened skin. The rash follows the course of one or more of the cutaneous nerves that transmit sensation to the skin. Generally only one side of the body is involved, though it may affect nerves leading to the eyes or other vital structures. When the eye is affected, blisters form not only on the forehead and eyelids but sometimes even on the eyeball itself. This condition requires expert attention.

Shingles (derived from *cingulum,* meaning belt) is most apt to occur when body resistance is low. It is usually preceded by severe smarting pain in the involved area and a general feeling of indisposition, with perhaps some respiratory or digestive disturbances for three to four days before the rash appears. The patches of blisters may persist for a week or two, then dry up and be covered with shingle-like scabs. The same virus that causes herpes zoster may also be responsible for chickenpox.

In treating herpes zoster, efforts are made to relieve pain and prevent any secondary infection of the blisters. Aureomycin has proved helpful and cortisone is frequently used.

HICCUPS, or hiccoughs, result from spasmodic contractions of the diaphragm caused by irritation of the phrenic nerve that controls this broad muscle which separates the chest from the abdomen. The time-honored cure is simply to hold the breath as long as possible, and if this fails to swallow cold water or gargle while holding the breath. Other popular treatments include coughing or the inducement of sneezing, swallowing ice or vinegar, or putting a pinch of salt on the back of the tongue. Breathing into a paper bag accumulates carbon dioxide and is sometimes effective in stopping hiccups. If these methods fail, a doctor should be called. The application of an ice pack to the neck, the use of ethyl chloride sprayed on the abdomen to lower the temperature, or pressure on the eyeballs or on the ribs near the place where the diaphragm connects may be effective measures. Narcotics are sometimes administered and it may even be necessary to anesthetize those with hiccups. In extreme cases, an operation may be required.

HIGH BLOOD PRESSURE. *See* BLOOD PRESSURE, HIGH.

HISTAMINE. *See* ALLERGY.

HISTOPLASMOSIS. A disease closely resembling coccidioidomycosis, histoplasmosis is probably the second most significant systemic fungus disease. The fungus histoplasma capsulatum grows chiefly in moist soil and the disease is acquired by inhaling the airborne spores of the fungus. Men are more often affected than women, and children of both sexes seem to be more susceptible to this mold than to any other mycotic infection.

At one time, histoplasmosis was considered to be rare and usually fatal. During the past two decades, however, it has become evident that the mold is also responsible for a milder form of the disease which has affected many thousands of people living in the central portions of this country, principally around the valleys of the Mississippi, Missouri, and Ohio rivers. At times the disease has reached almost epidemic proportions.

The mild phases of the infection involve the skin or lungs, beginning like a grippe or atypical pneumonia. Small localized ulcers appear in the mouth or ear and enlargment of the lymph nodes in this area may also be noted. The more advanced form reveals enlarged spleen and liver, severe anemia, and emaciation and irregular fever.

The majority of these infections heal spontaneously and drugs and antibiotics are of little help. Since the fungus has been found in the soil, in animal excreta around barns and chicken coops, persons whose work brings them in contact with these sources should be particularly careful to observe sanitary precautions, should always wash their hands before eating, and if possible wear gauze masks to prevent inhalation of spores. *See also* COCCIDIOIDOMYCOSIS; FUNGUS.

HIVES, or urticaria, a condition in which whitish elevated areas, painfully itching, appear on the surface of the skin.

These eruptions may follow the eating of certain foods, or exposure to particular atmospheric conditions. Theoretically these or other physical influences can alter the chemistry of the skin so that the absorption of certain substances will produce the rash. Psychological factors, however, may also cause the appearance of hives.

Hives often appear and disappear within the space of hours, but may persist for longer periods, become chronic, or recur persistently. Most frequently they will disappear after several days unless the person irritates or infects them—for example, by scratching.

The obvious first step in the treatment of this annoying malady is to locate the specific source. If this can be done, and if the cause, perhaps a type of food, can be eliminated, control of the disease should not be difficult. The person is advised to avoid chocolate, cocoa, nuts, peanut butter, shellfish, fish, tomatoes, fresh pork, fresh fruits, and spices.

Frequently a person may be desensitized to the food which makes him susceptible to hives. For example, the extract of shellfish can be administered in increasing amounts until the patient is able to eat this food without ill effect. Antihistamines have also been used to control the susceptibility to hives. In acute urticaria, the condition usually can be promptly controlled by injection of epinephrine hydrochloride. Severe cases also respond to treatment with ACTH, cortisone, or metacorten.

For temporary relief of the itching, certain antihistamine and hydrocortisone lotions or powders are available. Physicians often prefer the powder form, since it serves not only to relieve the itching but also to dry the affected area. Anyone susceptible to changes in temperature should select his clothes with a thought to the climate. Any garment which heats the skin or produces perspiration should be eliminated, since it will undoubtedly affect the infection and intensify the itching.

HOARSENESS, an unusual huskiness or harshness of voice, usually due to excessive strain on the vocal cords, the result, perhaps, of excessive drinking, smoking, speaking, or singing. If the person will permit himself a rest period of several days, during which he does not speak above a whisper, recovery is usually prompt.

Occasionally, if the hoarseness persists, a careful examination by a throat specialist is advisable. In singers, actors, and public speakers, certain small nodules sometimes appear on the vocal cords, the result of excessive strain.

Often a general physical checkup may be recommended, since the hoarseness may derive from a constitutional illness. Ordinarily nothing worse than a cold is encountered, or a nasal or sinus infection. Occasionally, however, hoarseness can be a valuable warning sign which points to a more serious malady, such as tuberculosis, cancer, or syphilis. Nowadays, with early diagnosis, these diseases are often curable. *See also* LARYNGITIS.

HODGKIN'S DISEASE, an ailment which involves the lymph glands. Thomas Hodgkin, an English physician, first reported it in 1832 as "multiple swellings of the lymph glands." The disease is fairly widespread throughout America and Europe and is believed to be increasing. It is most common in men between the ages of twenty and forty, although it has been reported in older people.

Hodgkin's disease is sometimes preceded by an infection of the teeth or tonsils, but a direct connection has not been established. It usually begins with an enlargement of the lymph nodes on one side of the neck, sometimes accompanied by fever. The swelling then spreads to the glands on the opposite side of the neck. The nodes are not painful or tender, vary in size, and can be felt as separate movable masses. They grow slowly and in the early stages there are no indications of other changes in the body. Sometimes a generalized itching or eruption of the skin occurs which causes great discomfort.

As the disease develops, the spleen and sometimes the liver are often enlarged, and frequently the bone marrow is affected, causing secondary anemia. When the process reaches the vertebrae and spinal cord, a paralysis of the lower part of the body results. These symptoms are accompanied by a loss of weight and the patient appears to be in extreme ill health and wasting away, a condition called cachexia. As other glands in the body become enlarged, they press in on neighboring organs. Coughing and chest pains are caused by compression in the chest, and pressure on the trachea or surrounding structures makes breathing and swallowing painful and difficult. The condition gradually becomes generalized.

Treatment consists of x-ray for the localized enlargements. When the swellings are widespread, nitrogen mustard is used in addition to the radiation of selected areas. Cortisone and ACTH have been effective in temporarily reducing the size of the spleen and lymph nodes. The periods of relief vary and are unpredictable. They may last for a week, or from two to several months, and in rare cases for as long as a year. Treatment reduces the size of the large tumor masses, and thus lessens the pressure on the surrounding nerves, giving the patient considerable relief from pain and discomfort. In view of the possible toxic effects of the treatment on the bone marrow, repeated blood counts must be made at regular intervals, and antibiotic treatment as well as blood transfusions are held

readily available. Known treatment, however, can provide temporary relief, but does not effectively halt the progress of the disease.

HOMOSEXUALITY, sexual attraction toward persons of one's own sex rather than the opposite sex. In females it is called lesbianism. In psychoanalysis the term can also include sexual interest which does not receive genital expression.

The causes of homosexuality are extremely complex and difficult to ascertain, and science or psychiatry have only partial answers to the treatment of the problem. This deviation from normal heterosexuality may develop at puberty. A lack of hormones, or such emotional factors as a father complex in the female adolescent, or a similar identification toward the mother in the male adolescent, may be the basis of homosexuality.

HOOKWORM. *See* WORMS.

HORMONES. A hormone is a substance produced by one of the internal secretion or endocrine glands which exerts a specific effect elsewhere in the body on some other gland or organ. Other glands also secrete special substances, such as the sweat of the sweat glands, the milk of the mammary glands or breasts, and the saliva of the salivary glands. The products of these glands of external secretion, however, as contrasted with those of internal secretion, do not have regulatory effects on other organs.

The pituitary gland produces several of the most important hormones. It secretes a growth hormone which produces human growth, a hormone stimulating the development of the sexual organs, hormones regulating the thyroid gland, the adrenal cortex, and other important internal secretions.

Some glandular parts of the body produce both external secretions and hormones. The pancreas, for instance, provides the body with both insulin, an internal secretion or hormone regulating the body's use of sugar, and trypsin, an external secretion involved in the digestion of protein foods.

Hormones and the glands in which they originate constitute an organized system for regulating many fundamental bodily processes in a coordinated way, including growth, reproduction, mobilization of defenses against stress and many forms of disease, and also basic aspects of metabolism, such as the use of oxygen and sugar.

In recent years, ACTH and other hormones of the cortical group have been produced from animal pituitaries and made available to the medical profession for therapeutic use in a wider variety of diseases. *See also* GLANDS; PITUITARY; and Chapter 19, "Endocrine Glands."

HOUSEMAID'S KNEE. *See* KNEE.

HYDROCEPHALUS, commonly called water on the brain, a condition in which large amounts of cerebrospinal fluid are around or within the brain. Normally this fluid flows through the ventricles of the skull and is drained off by the venous sinuses. An excess of the fluid or inefficient drainage, which may be caused by blocking of the drainage canal by in-flammation or by a tumor, will produce hydrocephalus. Obstructions may also exist at birth due to malformation of the internal portions of the skull concerned with proper drainage.

Slight cases of hydrocephalus do not present any difficulties. However, if the amount of fluid is great, the compression may impair the mental faculties and an operation may be necessary. The operation involved may be one of several kinds, depending on the nature of the obstruction. In any case, the operation is delicate and often severe, requiring special x-ray examination beforehand.

HYDROCORTISONE. *See* CORTISONE.

HYDROPHOBIA. *See* RABIES.

HYGIENE, the science that concerns itself with rules of health, both public and private, and with the methods of achieving good health by following these rules. The person who wishes to enjoy good health should observe the following general principles of hygiene.

Fresh air is important and care should be taken that rooms are well ventilated and adequate time is spent out-of-doors. *Avoid overweight* or underweight by having a well-balanced diet which includes the proper nutrients. *Eat leisurely,* chewing the food thoroughly. Be sure to drink six to eight glasses of water each day. Regular daily elimination is necessary to rid the body of waste products. Appearance and health are both improved by correct posture.

Mental attitude is an important

aspect of hygiene. As an aid to health, no drugs or medicine can fully replace a calm mature outlook on life.

Cleanliness is the first and most essential step in maintaining health. Cuts, scratches, and bruises should be given prompt attention to avoid infection and other complications. Good personal hygiene requires special attention to certain parts of the body. Hands and fingernails should be kept clean and well groomed. The teeth should be brushed with a suitable dentifrice at least twice a day. Persons who wear artificial dentures or plates may find it desirable to wash the teeth and dentures after each meal. Medicated mouthwashes and gargles are not especially recommended. The ears should be cleaned by syringing gently with warm water, being careful not to direct the force of the stream against the eardrum. Never use a hard or pointed object which could damage the eardrum. Remove excess matter from the nose with a soft handkerchief or tissue. The eye which is self-lubricating and self-adjusting seldom requires eye solutions. Beyond routine cleansing, any condition of the ears, nose, or eyes requiring special treatment should be cared for by a physician.

A yearly physical examination by a doctor and a semiannual dental checkup are recommended.

Hygienic measures relating to the community, such as sewage disposal, potable water, and insect control, are usually in the hands of public authorities and agencies. However, to be fully effective, public hygiene must be developed and carried out with the cooperation of every citizen in the community. *See also* BATHING; NUTRITION; and Chapter 4, "Diet and Health"; Chapter 11, "Feminine Hygiene."

HYMEN, or maidenhead, the membrane found at the opening of the vagina, partially blocking the entrance to the female sex organs. Although its presence is usually considered a sign of virginity, occasionally it may be entirely lacking or it may be ruptured by strain, such as occurs during horseback riding.

HYPERACIDITY, excessive secretion of gastric juice, which may appear in a temporary disturbance of the digestion or be present in chronic gastritis or in gastric or duodenal ulcers. Hyperacidity is related to the hunger pain of duodenal ulcer, as is evidenced when the pain is relieved following the neutralization of the acid with alkalies. Heartburn and belching are also caused by hyperacidity.

HYPERHYDROSIS, the scientific name for excessive sweating. *See* PERSPIRATION; and Chapter 11, "Feminine Hygiene."

HYPERTENSION. *See* BLOOD PRESSURE, HIGH.

HYPERTROPHY, disproportionate growth of any organ or tissue of the body. Vigorous exercise of the muscles can cause enlargement and bulging. Certain conditions in the heart may cause enlargement of hypertrophy, as when an improperly functioning valve impedes the outflow of blood from the chambers of the heart. Enlargement of the breasts is a common form of hypertrophy and may occur in both males and females, young or old. A compensatory hypertrophy may occur, as in the case of the loss of a kidney; then the other kidney tends to grow larger to make up for the one that is lost and even to take up some of its functions.

HYPNOSIS, a state of sleep or trance induced in a person by means of verbal suggestion by a hypnotist or by concentration on some object.

In hypnoanalysis, hypnosis is employed by the psychoanalyst to uncover the unconscious drives and mechanisms of the personality of the patient in an effort to analyze the causes of his emotional conflicts in the conscious state. The person may seem to be asleep after the hypnotist has induced the trancelike state and in this state he remains responsive to ideas suggested by the hypnotist. The unconscious mind is then exposed, repressed ideas or experiences recalled which have a bearing on the person's emotional disturbance, and a relationship later established to the conscious personality.

Narcosynthesis is a technique based on the same principle, but drugs are used rather than hypnosis. Here the hypnotic drug is introduced intravenously to induce the state which will reveal the underlying emotional conflict. This state is then followed by discussion. This form of psychoanalysis has particularly been used to treat neuroses resulting from war experiences.

Hypnosis is sometimes useful in dealing with drug addiction, dipsomania, or other injurious habits or impulses. Disorders such as insomnia, diarrhea, or constipation, due to nervous influences, have responded to this form of treatment. Certain menstrual irregularities related to a disturbed emotional state have also been treated by hypnoanalysis.

Hypnosis should be practiced only by those who are skilled and under medical supervision.

HYPOCHONDRIASIS. A person who is constantly concerned with his health or believes he is suffering from a serious disease, without factual basis, is known as a hypochondriac. The condition of morbid fear is called hypochondriasis.

In true hypochondriasis, the person's fears are related to the functioning of one particular organ of the body—the lungs, kidneys, heart, eyes, or digestive tract. Some women constantly develop imaginary symptoms concerning the organs of childbirth. A hypochondriac can mistake the slightest cough for a sign of tuberculosis. If the gastrointestinal tract is the center of anxiety, the interrelationship of the mind and the functions of the organs is such that certain symptoms can actually develop as a result. Loss of appetite, nausea, vomiting, fullness of stomach, and belching after meals are a few of such symptoms which may develop without physical cause.

The hypochondriac may be so beset with fears and symptoms that frequently the cure demands much time and patience. Persuasion that his fears are groundless is not sufficient to convince such a person. Psychotherapy is helpful, but again such treatment is slow. Persons suffering from hypochondriasis to a lesser degree have been helped sometimes by turning attention from the subject of health to new interests. Older people have most frequently responded to this type of treatment.

HYPOTENSION. *See* BLOOD PRESSURE, LOW.

HYPOTHYROIDISM, any condition characterized by deficient activity of the thyroid gland and its secretion, thyroxin.

When such a condition occurs in a child before it is born, the infant will be retarded in both physical and mental development, and will grow to be a dwarf of low mental capacity, termed a cretin. The same deficiency may arise spontaneously in later life, leading then to what is called myxedema. Abnormal tissue develops beneath the skin of the face, arms, and legs, giving a puffy appearance. The person becomes lethargic, mentally as well as physically. Sometimes this condition develops after surgical or other treatment for hyperthyroidism, when the remaining amount of thyroid tissue is insufficient for the body.

Treatment of all these conditions is by administration of thyroid substances, such as thyroid extracts, and thyroxin, which are taken daily by mouth. Only the physician should prescribe such treatment and determine the amounts to be taken, because of the dangers involved. *See also* CRETINISM; GOITER; MYXEDEMA.

HYSTERECTOMY, medical term for removal of the womb or uterus.

The presence of a tumor or any of a variety of other conditions determines the desirability of a hysterectomy. Whether or not one or both of the ovaries, the female sex glands, or the Fallopian tubes, which transport the egg cell from the ovary to the womb each month, should be removed at the same time depends on whether or not those organs are disordered in such a way as to require it.

The ovaries, especially through their internal secretions or hormones, are fundamental to a woman's health. Removal of the ovaries induces menopause or change of life, a serious development which may require administration of the missing hormones for a long time until the patient's body adjusts. Accordingly, if the ovaries are healthy, the doctor will not include them in a hysterectomy without compelling reasons. Among the most common of such reasons is the existence of cysts, encapsulated collections of fluid glandular material, which sometimes grow to unwieldy size and cause great discomfort. The ovaries may also be affected by tumors and infections in such a way as to make removal necessary. Since the ovaries supply the female body with the vital female sex gland secretions or hormones, elimination of the uterus alone will not disturb the regular onset of menopause. The womb is simply an organ to cradle the developing embryo and child until birth; it does not by itself secrete hormones. Removal of the womb does, however, permanently stop menstruation.

Hysterectomy, which is undergone by thousands of women every year in the United States, is definitely a major operation, requiring anesthesia, a stay in the hospital, and a period of careful convalescence to permit the tissues affected to mend adequately. Heavy exercise and lifting are not advisable and ample rest is necessary. The choice of the two surgical methods used will depend on the condition of the individual patient and the judgment of the gynecologist. Alternative routes, either of which may be used, are through the lower opening of the body, the vagina, or through the abdomen.

A common question of women who must undergo hysterectomy is whether or not the operation will disturb or stop regular marital relations. The answer is a definite negative. Once the postoperative repair has begun and healing is complete, marital relationship continues undisturbed.

HYSTERIA, a psychoneurotic disorder, involving intense emotionalism with various psychic and physical disturbances. It often results from repressed conflicts within the person, and occurs most frequently in young women. Irregularity of behavior is often thought to be hysteria. Most people think of a hysteric as a person alternately crying and laughing in an excited and distracted manner. The concept of hysteria was not understood, however, until the introduction of the psychoanalytic approach by Freud. There are many varieties of hysteria. In the ordinary course of experience,

the tantrum type of hysteria may be encountered, in which the person may cry, shout, walk about aimlessly, or even attack a friend. In another, more serious type, the person may not talk or move or hear what is said to him. First-aid measures, such as slapping the victim or throwing water into his face, may be effective; but if symptoms are severe, relief of hysteria requires expert medical advice.

Another dramatic manifestation of hysteria is the falling fit, which may resemble an attack of epilepsy. However, certain signs will indicate real hysteria: the person usually does not hurt himself in falling, and does not bite his tongue or have other symptoms of epilepsy; a certain degree of consciousness of action is present in the hysteric. Strange behavior may be manifested in hysteria, relating to such activities of everyday existence as eating, sleeping, working, memory, and conversation. The hysteric, being extremely impressionable, may also imitate symptoms of many diseases.

The development of hysterical paralysis may involve a single limb or perhaps half of the body, a condition known as hemiplegia. Certain signs aid the experienced observer to distinguish between paralysis due to a definite organic cause such as apoplexy and a hysterical semiparalysis.

In all types of hysteria in which real organic damage is not present, definite psychological causes are the source and are known as conversion reactions. Whatever the manifestation, the development indicates that the person to some degree has lost a sense of his own identity, and is seeking refuge in hysterical symptoms as a device to obtain attention or sympathy. Disappointment in love or some other deep frustration are examples of emotional upset which may stimulate a hysterical attack.

Shell shock or even blindness are forms of hysteria manifested in soldiers who may be seeking to escape an intolerable situation.

In the treatment of hysteria the diagnosis must be certain. Failure to detect and distinguish between a real physical cause and one of hysterical origin may be extremely serious.

Sometimes a person who for years has been blind or deaf may suddenly recover the lost sense in what is apparently a miraculous cure. Similarly people confined to bed for months because they are unable to walk or stand may unexpectedly leap from the bed if shocked by a startling alarm.

A hysterical person is unduly open to suggestion and just as he may simulate symptoms that are prompted by well-meaning but injudicious friends, so his craving for sympathy will make him respond to friendly psychotherapy, which is the most effective form of treatment. When the victim of hysteria is made to understand the basis of his disturbance, the cure of the symptoms may be as sudden as the onset. The deeper attitudes and motivations of the person must be understood to effect a real cure of hysteria.

ICE CAP, or ice bag, used when a dry cold application is required to relieve pain, affect the blood supply to a given area, or lower temperature to promote healing. A rubber hot-water bottle filled with crushed ice, a rubber or plastic bathing cap or a glove filled with ice and tied at the top may be used if an ice bag is not available.

ICHTHYOL, the proprietary name for a sulfonated coal tar derivative. Ichthyol is used in ointment or lotion form for the treatment of a number of skin disorders such as acne rosacea, erysipelas, eczema, psoriasis, etc. It may also be taken internally in the form of pills or as a mixture in the treatment of rheumatism and certain respiratory disorders. In certain inflammatory pelvic disorders it is used as a vaginal suppository. Recently it has been largely replaced by remedies having more specific action.

ICHTHYOSIS, a disorder of the skin characterized by dryness and extreme scaliness, which gives it the common name of "fish skin disease." It is a congenital disease; babies are born with scaly skin or it appears in the early months of life.

Its cause is not definitely known, although it is believed that a dietary deficiency may be responsible. Neither is there any specific treatment for its cure. The general health of the child is not affected, nor is there any itching.

Frequent warm baths to remove the scales and emollients to overcome dryness help to mitigate the condition. Complete cures have been known to occur spontaneously in connection with healing other children's diseases such as measles. In most cases, unfortunately, ichthyosis may persist throughout the lifetime.

ICTERUS. *See* JAUNDICE.

IDIOT. *See* FEEBLE-MINDEDNESS.

ILEITIS. Chronic inflammation in that portion of the small intestine known as the ileum may produce a partial obstruction which grows progressively worse. This comes from scar tissue formation such as may be caused by tuberculosis and other causes.

Crohn's disease, named for the doctor who discovered it, or regional ileitis, is a condition of unknown cause that may result in severe scarring and inflammation with chronic obstruction and often in formation of fistula.

The symptoms include cramps or colicky pain following meals. Fever and diarrhea often accompany this condition, and there is weakness and general signs of debility. Anemia may also accompany this disease.

The condition can be managed by careful attention to diet, medical treatment, and a sympathetic approach where the emotional state of the patient is a complicating factor. The disease may progress to a point where surgery is required to resolve the condition. Postoperatively patients may continue to have occasional diarrhea, but other symptoms clear up completely and in dramatic fashion. In about 15 per cent of the cases, the condition may reappear within six years and quite close to the site of the original obstruction. *See also* Chapter 18, "Disorders of the Digestive System and Diet in Digestive Disorders."

IMBECILE. *See* FEEBLE-MINDEDNESS.

IMMUNITY, the state of being temporarily or permanently able to resist an infection. Immunity to a disease exists when the antibodies, substances which combat invading microorganisms and their toxic effects, against that particular disease are present in the body. The antibodies may be present for several reasons: (1) the person has had the disease once and developed the antibodies; (2) the antibodies have been artificially provided by inducing the body to produce them; (3) the antibodies have been introduced into the body from an external source. Sometimes a natural immunity exists, such as the immunity which human beings have against many animal diseases and vice versa. Depletion of the body through deprivation may render the system susceptible to an infection to which ordinarily it would be immune.

When an infection occurs, the body's greatest defense, the anti-microbe action of the blood, especially that of the white cells, is lowered and the body becomes susceptible to further attack by the microorganisms involved. Its second defense consists of the formation of antibodies which attempt to overcome the invading organisms and bring about recovery. The continued presence of these antibodies in the blood after the person has recovered gives him immunity thereafter.

Immunization by vaccination, inoculation, or injection of an antitoxin provides such antibodies, either directly or by causing the body to produce them. Immunity may be achieved by an attack of a disease so slight as to be scarcely noticeable—for example, it is believed, in cases of infantile paralysis. Relative resistance to a disease may develop over a long period of time in a whole population which is constantly exposed to the disease. These people may still contract the disease, but are less affected by it than persons who have never been exposed to it. For instance diseases of European peoples and their descendants, such as measles and tuberculosis, often strike more primitive groups with much greater force. *See also* ANTIBODY; ANTITOXIN; IMMUNIZATION.

IMMUNIZATION, immunity, freedom from or resistance to disease, either temporarily or permanently. The body itself may produce immunity, as in the case of most infectious diseases, or it may be induced artificially. Great progress has been made in artificial immunization against disease, the Salk immunization against poliomyelitis being the outstanding recent example.

The body has the power to develop antibodies which act directly against disease-producing germs, or antitoxins which act against the toxins produced by microorganisms. In many instances, the body can develop the disease-fighting antibodies against killed bacteria or viruses as readily as against live microorganisms, with the advantage that risk of disease is eliminated. For example, the Salk vaccine is based on killed viruses, and a similar method is used against typhoid fever when killed bacilli of typhoid are injected to render the body immune to typhoid fever for a period of years.

Immunity against diphtheria is established by injecting a substance to produce antitoxin which combats the poison produced by the diphtheria germ. For smallpox, the virus of cowpox is injected which produces a mild case of the disease at the region of injection.

Schedules for active immunizations to common infectious diseases have been standardized and are followed by most physicians and clinics for diphtheria, tetanus, smallpox, whooping cough, and poliomyelitis. Whooping cough, especially dangerous to babies, and diphtheria immunization are usually given at the same time, at four to six months of age. The primary smallpox vaccination may be given at any time, generally when the child is about a year old, and should be repeated about four or five years later. The Salk vaccine schedule is usually standardized as follows: three doses of 1 c.c. each, with a two- to six-week interval between the first and second injection and the third injection seven months to a year after the second.

Immunity against plague, yellow fever, typhus, cholera, and Rocky Mountain spotted fever can be obtained by people traveling to regions where these diseases are apt to be present, and in epidemic areas. Immunization against rabies, hydrophobia, is given after a person has been bitten by an animal suspected of having rabies, or after the presence of rabies has been definitely established.

Scarlet fever immunization is available, but is not usually given except to children living in institutions or sanatoriums or in the event of an epidemic.

The value of immunization has been proved over and over again, and death rates in such diseases as diphtheria and smallpox have been reduced to relative insignificance through immunization. *See also* IMMUNITY; VACCINATION; and Chapter 7, "The Process of Infectious Diseases and Immunization of Children"; Chapter 23, "The Neuromuscular and Neurological Disabilities."

IMPETIGO, an infection, most frequently affecting children, in which the skin is covered with pus-filled eruptions. Although impetigo occurs most often on the face, other parts of the body, especially the hands, may be involved.

Impetigo is transmitted either directly from one person to another or by contact with articles used in common. If the infection is promptly treated, a cure can often be achieved in a week or two. Otherwise the problem becomes more difficult and may continue for a long time. Another complication which arises if the disease is permitted to linger is that the infected areas become susceptible to germs other than those of impetigo and thus prolong the treatment. Impetigo may occur simultaneously with infestation by lice or mites, with one condition tending to enhance the other.

Impetigo is now successfully treated not only with antiseptic ointments such as ammoniated mercury but also with preparations which contain sulfa, penicillin, and other antibiotic drugs such as bacitracin neomycin and polymixin.

Much can be done to prevent the spread of impetigo to others. Persons who resist the temptation to scratch lessen the likelihood of transmitting the disease by means of contaminated fingers. Those infected with impetigo must always use a separate washcloth and towel. Moreover, a school child with this disease should remain at home until he has recovered completely. *See also* SKIN.

IMPOTENCE, lack of power in a male to have or maintain an erection of the penis, and consequent inability to perform or complete the sexual act. Impotence must be contrasted with infertility or sterility in a male, which denotes inability to propagate offspring.

The cause of impotence may be a small or deformed penis which may be corrected by surgery, or it may be the result of some disease such as gonorrhea, diabetes, Bright's disease, or a disorder of the spinal cord. Medical treatment is necessary.

A common cause of impotence is emotional disturbance. This may occur temporarily in the early months of marriage due to self-doubts and usually disappears during the adjustment period natural to this stage of life. Impotence, unfortunately, often results from incompatibility which develops later in a marriage relationship. In such cases, psychotherapy may be the only way to resolve these marital conflicts.

Age is often a factor in impotence. Men over fifty-five sometimes begin to lose their capacity for erection and their interest in sex. Many men, however, retain their powers for years beyond this age.

INCISION. *See* WOUNDS.

INDIGESTION, or dyspepsia (a term now considered a misnomer and seldom used), denotes discomfort that accompanies or follows the intake of food. It is usually associated with difficult or painful digestion and may be related to actual failure of some phase of the digestive process.

Symptoms of indigestion are varied —a feeling of fullness or weight in the pit of the stomach; pain, either dull and steady or acute and spasmodic, which may follow immediately or occur some time after eating; nausea, or vomiting, which often relieves the pain or discomfort. Heartburn may appear, accompanied by acid, sour acrid liquid thrown into the mouth from the stomach. Flatulence and coated tongue, headache and dizziness may be present. Belching is not necessarily a sign of indigestion.

One group of gastric disturbances is caused by gastritis, dilation of the stomach, ulcers, cancer, gastroptosis, and others. Indigestion may result from disorders in organs other than the stomach, such as cirrhosis of the liver, gallbladder inflammation, appendicitis, nephritis, peritonitis, heart or lung diseases which may affect the lining of the stomach, tuberculosis, and anemia. Certain mental conditions may be the source of indigestion, such as hysteria, neurasthenia, or hypochondriasis.

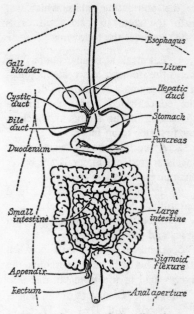

The basic parts of the digestive system.

Because indigestion may originate from such a wide variety of causes, prompt treatment should be sought. The doctor will be guided by the symptoms and treatment may vary from bicarbonate of soda to relieve stomach acidity to surgery for ulcers.

Many cases of indigestion are due to emotional disturbances rather than to organic diseases or disorder. Worry, nervousness, or frustration over a long period of time may cause constant irritation in the stomach. The person should endeavor to relieve or remove the causes of tension and to adopt a calmer, more relaxed general attitude. Plenty of sleep, relaxation, and special attention to the diet are essential for persons with nervous indigestion. In nervous indigestion, treatment includes a regimen of diet and eating habits, which will help the stomach heal itself. This often includes the following:

1. Eat meals at regular hours. This helps the stomach to secrete its juices at regular times. If meals are delayed, the concentrated acids may irritate the lining of the stomach, which is the first step to an ulcer.

2. Avoid large heavy meals. Small meals at frequent intervals are better than large meals less frequently.

3. Eat slowly and chew the food carefully.

4. Avoid irritating stimulants and spicy and greasy foods.

5. Drink a glass of milk between meals. This will help overcome the excess acid in the stomach. *See also* Chapter 18, "Disorders of the Digestive System and Diet in Digestive Disorders."

INDUSTRIAL HEALTH. Industrial absenteeism is the result, primarily, of ordinary complaints such as the common cold, indigestion, tonsillitis, nervous disorders, menstruation, rheumatism, arthritis and gout. The common cold is actually the largest single cause of absences. From 80 to 90 per cent of loss of man hours because of accident is due to psychological factors. Absenteeism costs more than ten billion dollars annually. One out of every fifty workers is a problem drinker, and alcoholism accounts for about 10 per cent of the total dollar loss from absenteeism.

Occupational Diseases. Other afflictions which contribute to loss of time at work are associated with special occupations. Silicosis, for example, is caused by breathing of silica dust, just as lead poisoning is the result of inhaling lead, and carbon dioxide poisoning by intake of carbon monoxide gas. A wide variety of chemicals, peculiar to certain industries, are also increasingly responsible for a number of inflammatory disorders of the skin as well as other diseases.

Occupational maladies also include undulant fever, which is contracted chiefly by people who work with cattle; anthrax, which results from handling of hides; caisson disease, the "bends," by those who work under conditions of great pressure or at high altitude. The newer industries which involve radiant materials, such as atomic plants, have introduced a whole new set of hazards which are being studied and for which regulations have been established in many states.

The worker should be compelled to familiarize himself with the occupational hazards involved in his particular job, so that he will be thoroughly acquainted with the nature of the diseases incurred, and alert to the first symptoms of their possible onset. Such symptoms should be reported to the medical office of the plant or to the family doctor, since the earlier the diagnosis can be made, the simpler and more certain the cure.

A working people enlightened to good health practices is the best guarantee that the advances in industrial and general medicine, safety and sanitation engineering will make their most effective contributions to the general welfare. *See also* the names of specific diseases; and Chapter 5, "Occupational Health."

INFANTILISM, a condition in which growth is retarded or inhibited because of malfunctioning of certain glands or other causes. When the pituitary gland is affected and there is a lack of growth, hormones, teeth, bones, and the sex glands will be involved and the result is an under-developed body, a dwarf, seldom over three to four feet in height. Mental retardation will take place and childish characteristics will persist into adult life. Overactivity of the same gland will produce giantism with the mental and sexual retardation characteristic of dwarfism.

Infantilism may also be the result of certain congenital defects, thyroid deficiency or other diseases. In one type, characteristics of senility such as baldness and hardening of the arteries may develop along with dwarfism. Thyroid cases respond sometimes amazingly well to injections of thyroid extract, while many of the other types have no known cure. Another form of infantilism is brought about by early kidney disease which results in death.

INFECTIONS. An infection is the condition which occurs when the body or a part of the body is invaded by disease-causing germs or organisms. One or more organs or parts sustain at least temporary damage and impairment. The body as a whole reacts protectively, in most cases, with general symptoms such as fever. An infection restricted to one fairly sharply defined area, such as a tooth or a finger, and not serious enough to provoke general symptoms, is called a local infection, as distinct from a general infection, which involves more or less the entire system.

The organisms which cause infection are practically all so small that they are invisible without a microscope, the few exceptions being largely parasites such as hookworm and pinworm. The smallest organisms, the viruses, are visible only with the ultramicroscope or electron microscope. Organisms causing disease are known scientifically as pathogenic.

Although the science of medicine is concerned for the most part with germs, which are harmful to man, many organisms are not injurious. Necessary or beneficial to human life particularly are the bacteria, present in the manufacture of milk products, alcoholic beverages, and such pharmaceuticals as penicillin and the other antibiotics.

Microorganisms are classified in a number of ways, according to their size, their shape or their mode of life. The smallest are *viruses,* which are so tiny that they pass through a porous porcelain filter. *Bacteria* are many times larger than viruses, and cannot pass through a filter, but they are nevertheless, extremely small. A third group of microorganisms are *protozoa,* one-celled animals, such as the ameba.

Fungi comprise still another group of microorganisms, and also many multicellular fungi which grow much larger. Fungi have plantlike characteristics, and those which are microorganisms are in the same general size class as the bacteria.

Parasites which attack the human body are larger, for the most part, and visible without the microscope.

In addition to the intestinal worms, they include mites, lice, and various other insects.

Midway in size between the viruses and the bacteria is a special group of microorganisms called the *rickettsiae,* after the doctor who first identified them. They cause typhus, Rocky Mountain spotted fever, and related diseases.

Bacteria are classified according to their shapes. The three main classifications are (1) the bacillus, which is rod-shaped; (2) the coccus, which is oval or spherical and (3) those shaped in one or more curves, like the *vibrio,* resembling a comma; and the spiral spirochete and spirillum. Some live singly, others together in clumps or chains.

The bacilli include the germs of many of the commonest and most severe diseases, including tuberculosis, typhoid fever, plague, whooping cough, and undulant fever. Among the cocci are the pneumococcus, pneumonia; streptococcus, familiar in "strep" respiratory infections; and staphylococcus, present in abscesses and boils. An example of the spirochete is the organism causing syphilis.

Some serious diseases caused by infecting organisms other than bacteria are poliomyelitis, smallpox, influenza, and mumps, caused by viruses; amebic dysentery, malaria, and sleeping sickness, caused by protozoa; numerous skin disorders, such as athlete's foot, caused by fungi, and other diseases which affect the whole system, such as coccidioidomycosis, a mild lung infection which is widespread in the southwestern United States; and trichinosis, elephantiasis, and hookworm, caused by worms.

An infection normally follows a regular course of development. In general, when an organ, tissue, or area of the body is invaded by an infecting organism, the body responds by taking appropriate protective measures. The nature of these responses depends upon the type of infection and its severity. For example, a boil is a localized bacterial infection of a group of skin cells. The body first walls off the area, so that the invading bacteria are prevented from entering the blood cells and other means, and the infection remains localized. In pneumonia, unless the bacteria or viruses which cause it are checked or destroyed by drugs, the whole bodily system is involved. Fever, weakness, digestive disturbances, and the other symptoms associated with the disease are all indicative of a general response by the entire body.

The body's first defense is to prevent the entrance of harmful organisms. This is the purpose of the skin, mucuous membrane, and the various devices which protect the apertures of the body. When these defenses are breached, however, the body immediately counterattacks the invading force. The white cells in the blood rapidly increase in number and attempt to envelop and destroy, actually consume, individual bacteria. A local infection, in a finger, toe or a tooth, for example, is isolated as much as possible, by a temporary protective encirclement. Blood plasma bunches up bacteria for easier disposal, and antibodies, special substances which combat specific microorganisms, are formed in the blood. The toxins, or poisons, produced by the bacteria, prompt the body to develop antitoxins to counteract them.

One of the chief reasons for complete bed rest during an acute general infection is to allow the body's energies entire freedom for these defensive activities. If these energies continue to be drawn upon for other purposes during serious illness, the body may be so weakened that it will be unable to cope with the invading organisms promptly and new and separate infections may occur. In bacteremia or septicemia, for instance, the body's system for confining an infection to a specific area becomes disorganized and bacteria escape into the blood in large numbers. In other cases, infection may leave the body so depleted than an entirely different microorganism may attack in another area before the first is overcome. This creates a condition called a secondary infection.

To supplement the body's natural defenses against infection, medical science has developed many additional protective measures. So effective have these discoveries been that many diseases that were once epidemic scourges have now been reduced to unimportance.

Probably the measure which has been most effective in combatting infections is sanitation, provisions such as those insuring pure water supplies, adequate sewage systems, and modern methods of keeping the environment and the body clean and orderly. Since microorganisms thrive in dirt, their worst enemy is cleanliness. Cholera and plague, diseases once common throughout the world, seldom occur today in industrially advanced countries. Specific disinfectants, such as chlorine in water, iodine, alcohol, and other antiseptics, are also part of the improvement in modern sanitation.

Medical science has also discovered ways by which the body itself can be stimulated to produce substances which will protect it against specific diseases. In vaccination, weakened or dead forms of microorganisms are injected into the body in such a way as to cause the formation of antibodies which render the person safe against attack by infection. By inoculation, a person can be given antitoxins which protect him against the toxins of invading organisms. Smallpox, rabies, typhoid, yellow fever, and, most recently, poliomyelitis are some of the diseases that have yielded to these methods.

In addition, research has in recent years also developed specific drugs which have disposed of many remaining major infections as serious threats. The best-known and most widely used of the newer drugs are the antibiotics, substances derived from living organisms. Penicillin was the first, and is still the most familiar. Another group includes the so-called sulfonamides, which are coal tar derivatives.

At the turn of the century, pneumonia was a serious disease, one of the most significant causes of death. Once the disease began, little could be done beyond putting the patient to bed and helping him conserve his strength for the siege. Today penicillin and other antibiotics have brought pneumonia virtually under control. Most pneumonia patients can be relieved in a matter of hours, and death, or even extreme suffering, has become infrequent. The death rate has dropped from around 60 per 100,000 population to about 7 per 100,000. Tremendous progress has also been made against the venereal diseases by use of the antibiotics. The treatment of tuberculosis has been so altered by the use of streptomycin, para-amino-salicylic acid, isoniazid, and other newer drugs that many major tuberculosis sanitoriums have been permanently closed.

Some new health problems have arisen with or because of these new remedies. The so-called "side effects" of the drugs have sometimes been disturbing. The tendency of many disease-causing microorganisms to develop strains which are resistant to one or more of the drugs has also caused concern. These difficulties are insignificant, however, when considered beside the undreamed-of protection of human life and health which these drugs have made possible.

So familiar, accessible, and sure is the shield of medicine against infectious disease today that its relative newness is often not realized. An understanding of the nature of infection did not exist before the work of Louis Pasteur, the French scientist who died in 1895. He first conceived and proved the existence of microorganisms by establishing that animal and vegetable matter do not decompose spontaneously. When he boiled such matter, it did not decompose, but the process would begin when he added unboiled matter to it.

From this simple experiment ultimately sprang all of today's knowledge of infection and medicine's power to combat it.

Before the experimental work of Lister, a British surgeon who died in 1912, virtually all surgery was accompanied by massive wound infections and suppuration. Applying Pasteur's principles, Lister showed that sterilization of operating equipment and the use of antiseptics could prevent infection. Today's improved techniques, together with drugs such as the antibiotics, have made possible the penetration and repair of the inmost parts of the body, practically without danger of infection. *See also* IMMUNIZATION; INFECTIOUS DISEASES; SANITATION; VACCINATION; and names of specific diseases, drugs, and organisms; also Chapter 7, "The Process of Infectious Disease and Immunization of Children."

INFECTIOUS DISEASES, those diseases caused by an invasion by organisms, usually microorganisms, as opposed to diseases caused by disordered functioning of parts of the body; or by foreign substances, as in allergy; or by external forces, such as heat or electricity; or by dietary deficiencies.

When a person contracts an infectious disease the offending organism multiplies within the body with harmful effects, and disrupts the function of the body by producing poisonous toxins or causing other disorders. The invading organism overcomes the body's defenses, at least until the body can rally its protective forces. Usually such an invasion comes from the exterior, the germ entering through the air, food, or some other route. Frequently, however, if the normal resistance of the body is lowered, organisms already living in the body may escape from the checks usually imposed on them by the body itself or by other organisms, and may then multiply in the same way as an external invader.

The causative organism of an infectious disease may be one of the viruses, rickettsiae, bacteria, fungi, protozoa, or minute worms. The range of infectious diseases is bewilderingly large; yet by proper attention to preventives such as sanitation, inoculation, and vaccination and by the use of the newer drugs, especially penicillin and the other antibiotics, medicine today affords effective protection against most of them.

Following are some of the principle infections caused by each type of agent.

Viruses: Smallpox, poliomyelitis, rabies, yellow fever, measles, mumps, infectious hepatitis, chickenpox, shingles, influenza, virus pneumonia, psittacosis or parrot fever.

Bacteria: Plague, tuberculosis, pneumonia, scarlet fever, syphilis, gonorrhea, whooping cough, tularemia, undulant fever, spinal meningitis, diphtheria, tetanus, erysipelas, rheumatic fever, cholera, leprosy, yaws.

Rickettsiae: Typhus, Rocky Mountain spotted fever, scrub typhus.

Fungi: Skin diseases of the "athlete's foot" type. More serious systemic diseases include coccidioidomycosis, a lung infection, and histoplasmosis, characterized by enlargement of the liver and spleen, fever, and anemia.

Protozoa, one-celled animal microorganisms: Amebic dysentery; malaria; African sleeping sickness, spread by bite of the tsetse fly; blackwater fever, a severe complication of malaria.

Worms: Hookworm; tapeworm; trichinosis.

Each disease and type of disease is spread by means intimately involved with the manner in which the organism lives. Viruses, for instance, may live within insects for a considerable time, and be passed down to later generations in insect eggs. These and the rickettsiae grow and multiply only within other living cells, whereas the other microorganisms are not so restricted.

The transmission of viral diseases is less well understood than those diseases which result from bacterial infection. Many of the latter pass from one person to another through the droplets in a cough or a sneeze, others through insects, and rabies through the bite of a rabid animal. The rickettsial infections spread only through insects, such as the louse, tick, or rat flea, the organism requiring a host. Thus, one of these diseases may be acquired by an insect bite; through a scratch which has picked up some insect excrement or remains of an insect crushed in scratching; or even, in at least one case, that of Q fever, by breathing insect excrement.

Bacterial infection may be spread in droplets from breathing or coughing, by direct contact, in food and water, in human excrement, on insects such as the ubiquitous fly, by bite of insects, and in other ways. Protozoa may be disseminated in food and water or through the bite of insects carrying the organism, as in malaria.

Infestation by worms generally occurs as a result of exposure in places where the organisms are common. Going barefooted, in parts of the United States, for instance, invites hookworm. Trichinosis is usually contracted from infected pork which has not been cooked sufficiently at high enough temperatures.

Until the advent of modern sanitation, and more especially of vaccination, inoculation, and the new pharmaceutical agents against infection, such diseases were a source of incalculable suffering and loss. Aside from the toll in human life, the economic and industrial effects of diseases such as malaria, yellow fever, smallpox, plague, and tuberculosis, before modern preventives and remedies obliterated or reduced their virulence, is beyond comprehension. These diseases were the chief deterrents in the quest for greater longevity, and by their depredations they affected the whole tempo of human development. Between 1850 and 1950, the average life span in the United States grew from approximately forty to sixty-five years, and the reduction of infectious disease was one of the primary responsible factors. Today few major types of such disorders are beyond the reach of medicine.

For further details on characteristics, mode of transmission, symptoms, and therapeutic agents *see* names of specific diseases, drugs, and organisms. *See also* IMMUNIZATION; INFECTIONS; VACCINATION; and Chapter 7, "Infectious Diseases and Immunization of Children"; Chapter 23, "The Neuromuscular and Neurological Disabilities."

INFLAMMATION, a reaction of the tissues to injury, characterized by redness, heat, swelling, and pain, regardless of the cause. (The inflammation may be a symptom of a disease or ailment, but this discussion concerns itself with the actual condition of the inflamed tissue.) The redness and heat are due to an influx of blood to the affected area; the swelling and pain are also due to blood but even more to the inflow of watery fluid or lymph which distends the tissue, compresses the nerve endings, and causes pain. The white cells of the blood accumulate at the affected area and attempt to kill the invading microorganisms. If they do not and too many white cells are destroyed, an abscess forms. Inflammation is usually due to microorganisms, but may also result from severe irritation of the skin, as from rubbing, chemical action, or heat.

When germs are involved in the inflammation the wounded area should be cleaned and antiseptics applied. Injections of serums and vaccines, and incisions to relieve the accumulation of pus are often useful measures which aid the natural process by which the tissues heal themselves. The inflamed part should be rested and if the inflammation has been caused by some irritant like a foreign object in the eye, this should be promptly removed. Hot applications to promote circulation of the blood to the affected area and ease pain may be used. Cold applications are sometimes recommended but should be applied cautiously since they can nullify the inflammation which may be part of the natural process of eradicating the effect of an irritant in the tissue.

INFLUENZA, commonly known as the flu or grippe, a highly contagious disease caused by a filterable virus, one capable of passing through a Berkefeld clay filter. It usually appears in the winter in epidemic form throughout the world and spreads with amazing rapidity during these outbreaks. Generally influenza is self-limited; that is, it runs a definite course within a specific period of time and is of short duration. While rarely serious in itself, influenza tends to predispose to secondary infections of the lungs, which may become serious.

Although influenza is believed to be a disease of antiquity—Hippocrates describes an epidemic now presumed to have been influenza—the first authentic record is a description of the European epidemic of pandemic outbreaks (epidemics 1510. Since that time at least eight which affect huge populations over the entire world) have occurred. An influenza epidemic occurred during World War I and from 1918 to 1920 spread over more than half the world with devastating results. In 1957 an epidemic broke out in the Orient; although many hundreds of thousands of persons were affected, most cases were mild and it was not serious.

The characteristic features of influenza epidemics have been the explosive aspect of the outbreaks, their rapid spread, the great numbers involved and the comparatively short duration of each wave. The spread of the disease is accelerated by the ease and rapidity with which transmission of the infection takes place from person to person by direct contact and by droplet infection in talking, sneezing, or coughing.

The symptoms of influenza appear suddenly from one to three days after exposure. Chills and fever, headache, backache, and extreme malaise are present. Usually the fever is higher and the weakness more intense than in the common cold. Discharges develop from the throat, nose, trachea, and bronchi. The infection lowers the resistance of the respiratory tract and exposes the patient to invasion by other organisms which may set up secondary infections in the sinuses, ears, or lungs.

In the absence of complications, the fever lasts from one to five days and convalescence proceeds rapidly, though accompanied by a feeling of weakness and general depression. In these cases, relapse does not take place. This type of influenza occurs in almost 95 per cent of the cases during the first phase of an epidemic.

When minor complications develop, the original symptoms are intensified and are accompanied by a more or less severe bronchitis or sinusitis or both and persistent cough which continues for weeks, bringing up pus and mucous material. This type of infection, frequently encountered in epidemic and pandemic influenza, involves the ears, the bronchial tubes, and the sinuses.

The most severe form of influenza is pneumonic influenza, which is characterized by profound weakness and exhaustion, high fever, rapid breathing, and a discoloration of the skin, which looks almost heliotrope and indicates insufficient oxygen intake of the blood as it passes through the lungs. Patients frequently cough up blood. Pneumonic influenza often results in permanent damage to the bronchial tubes and lungs, and patients require constant care until the period of convalescence is well established. During pregnancy, special precautions must be taken to prevent miscarriage or fatal results.

Since 1933, when it was first demonstrated that epidemic influenza is caused by a filterable virus, two types of viruses, designated as type A and type B, have been isolated. In 1942 a method was devised for the preparation of a concentrated vaccine which establishes immunity about seven days after injection and which is highly effective in protecting against the disease.

A specific cure for influenza is not known. Treatment includes confinement to bed as soon as the disease is suspected until convalescence is well under way and danger of complications has passed. Large quantities of liquids are recommended while the fever is present. Complete isolation avoids sources of secondary infection. Visitors should be excluded and whoever comes in contact with the patient must observe rules of sanitation. The sickroom should be kept warm, and daily baths are allowed if care is taken that the invalid does not become chilled. When the fever is high, warm sponges may be given to counteract it, or an ice cap used. When necessary, aspirin may be given, in doses of from 0.3 gm. to 1 gm., for the relief of general aches and pains. Constipation should be treated with simple enemas and the diet should be light.

The complications are treated similarly to those which appear in pneumonia, sinusitis, and other respiratory conditions. When signs of bacterial infection appear, prompt treatment with antibiotics is important.

INJECTION. Certain drugs and remedies are best introduced directly into the tissues rather than by mouth because the digestive juices react chemically upon them and nullify their effectiveness. Insulin is an outstanding example of such a substance, but it is hoped that in time a treatment will be found for diabetes which can be taken by mouth. Certain antitoxins as well as certain powerful drugs are also best introduced by injection. Injection is preferable when an instantaneous effect upon the blood stream is desirable. When a patient is unconscious, injection is the only method available for introducing most drugs.

The method of injection may vary for several reasons. Injections may be hypodermic, under the skin, introdermic, into the skin, intramuscular, into the muscles, intravenous, or intraspinal. In sudden heart failure a solution of adrenalin or atropine may be injected straight into the heart. *See also* INOCULATION; VACCINATION.

INOCULATION, the introduction of a disease agent, serum, infective material, or microorganism into the tissues through the skin or mucous membrane. The purpose may be to immunize, as in smallpox vaccination, or to increase resistance to certain diseases by introducing controlled quantities of dead germs or their poisons into the body where antibodies will develop to combat future invasion of the same microorganism. *See also* IMMUNIZATION; VACCINATION.

INSANITY, the legal term for a mental disorder. *See also* MANIC-DEPRESSIVE PSYCHOSIS; SCHIZOPHRENIA; and Chapter 22, "Mental Illness."

INSECT BITES. Bites and stings of insects produce itching, pain, and swelling. Bacterial infection may follow secondary invasion by germs.

Several serious diseases are transmitted by the bites of insects. Among these are malaria, carried by the mosquito; typhus, which is transmitted by the louse; Rocky Mountain spotted fever, which is tick-borne; and many others.

The bites of insects are rarely fatal, with the exception of that of the black widow spider. The bite of this poisonous insect causes pain and redness at the point of occurrence, weakness, dizziness, and cramps. The poison spreads fairly rapidly and should be treated in the same way as snakebite poisoning.

Most common of the insect pests that invade the body directly are lice and the itch mite. Bedbugs and spiders attack less frequently. Chiggers and biting flies also annoy human beings especially in wooded regions and in the tropical areas.

Bites from chiggers, known scientifically as *trombicula irritans,* cause intolerable itching. Thorough washing with soap and water, allowing the lather to remain on the skin for about ten minutes, followed by the application of soothing itch ointment is the best method of treatment. Dusting stockings and underclothing with sulphur powder before entering deep grass areas will help to prevent the chiggers from biting.

Lice are controlled by certain delousing techniques which remove lice and eggs from the body clothing, bedding, or wherever else they may be.

Ordinary insect bites are treated by applying baking soda and water paste, vinegar, dilute ammonia, or mentholated or phenolated calamine lotion which relieve itching and burning. Insect repellents should be applied to exposed surfaces of the skin before going into regions where biting insects that transmit disease may be encountered.

Scabies, also known as the seven-year itch, is caused by the itch mite which burrows under the skin. *See also* BEDBUG; BEE STINGS; BLACK WIDOW SPIDER; DDT; LICE; MALARIA; ROCKY MOUNTAIN SPOTTED FEVER; SCABIES; TYPHUS FEVER.

INSOMNIA, any degree of sleeplessness during the time when most people ordinarily sleep. Aside from being incidental to a number of illnesses, including fevers, heart trouble, and certain brain disorders, insomnia may be due to a variety of causes.

Occasionally insomnia may result from lack of air or overheating in the bedroom, oversupply or undersupply of bedclothing, cold feet, overloaded stomach, need of food, taking coffee or tea too near bedtime, over-excitement or worry. This type of insomnia does not present too great a problem, the remedy being obvious.

If insomnia is frequent or protracted enough to threaten health, a doctor should be consulted. He will first carefully investigate to learn whether or not the insomnia is associated with some physical disorder such as high blood pressure, hardening of the arteries, or infection. The person's emotional condition will be studied. Anxieties about family or finances, or difficulties in job or career may be the underlying disturbance. In cases in which the emotional cause is not apparent, psychotherapy may help. In any case, talking out troubles with friends or the physician may be a good idea.

When the state of health is such that a rest or change is indicated, such a change should be made. In all cases of insomnia the treatment is directed to the cause, when this is found.

Unfortunately many people are being treated with drugs for sleeplessness who could do without them, and many more are treating themselves with the widely advertised products which induce sleep quickly. These are known as hypnotics, and the strong sleep inducers are the narcotics. The habit of taking these is easy to form and dangerous.

However, one may avoid the necessity of taking drugs by certain preparations before bedtime. A fifteen- to twenty-minute walk, or a light massage before going to bed may help induce the proper state of mind and body for sleep. A snack such as hot milk or cocoa, a warm bath, or reading a relaxing book before retiring is also helpful.

With older people, who do not need as much sleep as when they were younger and more active, sleeplessness may cause frustration, irritation, or nervousness. A glass of wine or warm milk will often induce sleep. Chronic constipation may be a factor and changes in eating habits and fluid intake may be in order. Again, a study of the problem with the doctor may be helpful in finding a solution to insomnia.

INSULIN, the hormone produced in the part of the pancreas known as the Islets of Langerhans. It is significant in regulating the sugar level in the blood and in the burning of sugar to produce heat and energy. Persons who suffer from diabetes mellitus have a deficiency of insulin.

In 1921, two Canadian scientists, Frederick G. Banting and his assistant, Charles Best, isolated and produced insulin in a form that could be beneficially used to treat diabetes. Since then, insulin has been produced cheaply and is used widely by the millions of people who suffer from diabetes.

Insulin is not a cure for diabetes, but it supplements a deficiency. Care must be taken in using it. Patients who take too much insulin may have an insulin shock which involves a reduction in the blood-sugar requiring immediate attention to avoid serious consequences. Common symptoms of insulin shock are agitation, weakness, trembling, sweating, pallor, listlessness, speech difficulty, nervousness, and unconsciousness. If the victim of insulin shock is still conscious, sugar in some form, such as fruit juice or candy, is given to him. If he is unconscious, adrenalin may be injected to revive him and then the sugar given to him. In some cases of unconsciousness, glucose must be administered intravenously.

Insulin has been developed in a number of forms. Regular insulin is effective for from six to eight hours; globin, eight to sixteen hours; and protamine-zinc, twenty-four hours. The most frequently used form is NPH, a specially modified form, intermediate between unmodified and protamine insulin. *See also* DIABETES; INSULIN SHOCK THERAPY; ORINASE.

INSULIN SHOCK THERAPY. Insulin shock treatment or therapy for schizophrenia and other mental disorders was introduced by Dr. Manfred Sakel, an American psychiatrist, and is widely used in mental hospitals. By injection of insulin, the patient is put into a state of coma for a given period of time and then brought out of the coma by the administration of sugar. By this treatment, the patient during the coma period is in a condition in which psychotherapy can be more effectively used.

INTERMITTENT CLAUDICATION. *See* LIMPING, INTERMITTENT.

INTELLIGENCE QUOTIENT (I.Q.) Intelligence quotient is the rating or score obtained from certain special tests which attempt to determine the innate intelligence of a person. No test has been developed which can conclusively determine the measure of someone's natural intelligence, but many different methods have been tried, with varying degrees of success. The Stanford revision of the Binet-Stanford test is one of the most widely used at present. In this intelligence test, the rate scored on the test is divided by the age of the person and multiplied by 100. Thus an 8-year-old child whose mental level, according to the Binet-Stanford scale, is that of a 10-year-old, has an I.Q. rating of 125. A rating of 100 is considered average. Scores below this are rated as: below 70, moron; below 50, imbecile; below 20, idiot. Out of a total of 500,000 mentally deficient persons in the United States, 30,000 are classified as idiots, 100,000 as imbeciles and the rest morons.

INTERTRIGO, an irritation of the skin caused by friction between two moist adjacent skin surfaces. The most common locations for this condition are the folds of the groin the inner surface of the thighs, between the buttocks, under the arms, under the neck and behind the ears. In obese women it may occur between the breasts. In infants, intertrigo is caused by the rubbing of a diaper and is known as diaper rash.

To treat intertrigo, the opposing surfaces should be dusted thoroughly with talcum powder containing zinc oxide and then separated by a piece of lint. If the skin is macerated from the effects of perspiration, the skin should be thoroughly cleansed and dried before the powder is applied. Such care will help to avoid inflammation and infection of the skin surface. *See also* DIAPER RASH.

INTERVERTEBRAL DISC, a circular plate or pad of fibrous cartilage located between the vertebrae of the spine. The disc allows movement of the vertebrae and acts as a buffer against shocks to the spinal column. Its action is that of a cushion, the disc flattening under pressure, with the ability also to shift its position to accommodate the motions of the spinal vertebrae. Sudden strains or movements may damage the disc. "Slipped disc" is a fairly common occurrence, and refers to the vertebrae of the lumbar and sacrum. The term intervertebral disc syndrome is applied to the low back pain which results from compression or protrusion from falls, jumps, or strains in the bent-over position. A protruded disc may complicate a case of slipped vertebrae.

The intervertebral disc is also subject to degenerative changes, fracture, and calcification, or may be destroyed by tuberculosis of the spine. Rarely is it attacked by cancer. *See also* SLIPPED DISC.

INTESTINES, in human beings, the membranous tubular apparatus that extends from the stomach to the anus. The first part, or small intestine, is smaller only in diameter, being about twenty-three feet long, while the large intestine is about five feet in length. The small intestine occupies the greater portion of the abdominal cavity.

The small intestine includes the duodenum, which is about eleven inches long; the jejunum, comprising about two-fifths of the intestine; and the ileum, which makes up the remaining three-fifths. The large intestine is comprised of the cecum; ascending, descending, and transverse colons; the rectum and anal canal.

The intestines are lined with tissues which secrete digestive fluids in some portions, and with other tissues which absorb the nutrients, water, and fats at other points. The jejunum and ileum are completely covered by the peritoneum. The muscular wall of the intestine consists of outer and inner layers of fibers. The inner surface of the small intestine is covered by villi, which are tiny, fingerlike projections containing the lacteals,

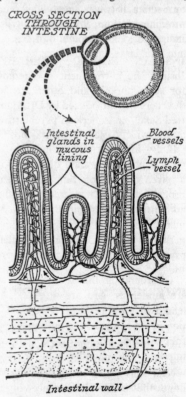

CROSS SECTION THROUGH INTESTINE

Intestinal glands in mucous lining

Blood vessels

Lymph vessel

Intestinal wall

A greatly enlarged diagram showing the structure of the intestinal wall.

which convey fats to the larger vessels of the system.

The process of digestion, which begins in the mouth and continues through the stomach, is completed chiefly in the upper part of the small intestine, after the partly digested food leaves the stomach. It usually requires about four hours for the food to pass through the small intestine.

The food is passed along by muscular contractions, in waves, which are known collectively as peristalsis. The food is also broken up by a series of contractions within the wavelike motions, by segmentation. Indigestible food remaining is passed into the large intestine through the cecum. Finally the water, and some sugar in solution, is absorbed by the large intestine, and the remainder passes out as feces through the rectum. When the contents of the bowel pass into the rectum, a mechanism responsive to fecal pressure is set up which indicates that the feces is ready to be expelled. The entire process, from consumption to ejection, takes about eighteen hours.

The large intestine is concerned only slightly with digestion and absorption of food.

Disorders of the intestinal tract are numerous, and are discussed at length in separate articles. Obstruction of the action of the intestine may follow the passing of one portion of intestine into another, known as intussusception. *See also* ABDOMINAL PAIN; APPENDICITIS; COLITIS; CONSTIPATION; DIARRHEA; DUODENUM; INDIGESTION; INTUSSUSCEPTION; RECTUM; and Chapter 18, "Disorders of the Digestive System, and Diet in Digestive Disorders."

INTUSSUSCEPTION, an obstruction in the intestine, brought about when one part of the intestine passes or is drawn into another part. It occurs most frequently at the ileocecal valve, located at the opening from the small intestine into the large intestine. It may be due to a tumor, to the presence of hardened and impacted indigestible material, or it may be caused by a rupture into which a portion of the bowel is pushed.

Acute intussusception is most common in young children, usually during the first year. It is usually caused by straining, and is characterized by severe pain and vomiting. The straining ordinarily results only in the evacuation of blood-stained mucus. Only a surgical operation will correct this condition.

Chronic intussusception occurs usually in adults and is not too serious unless the obstruction becomes acute or results in acute peritonitis, at which point an operation is also imperative.

INVOLUTIONAL MELANCHOLIA, a mental disturbance characterized by mental depression. Ordinarily this disease occurs during middle age or later. The person realizes at this time that life's long and ambitious dreams will probably never be wholly fulfilled. Moreover, as contemporaries begin to die, and as the burden of family worries and responsibilities increase, the person becomes less capable of facing and overcoming his problems. Delusions of a serious nature are sometimes experienced.

Women are more particularly the victims of this affliction, perhaps because a sense of uselessness and isolation comes to them with special abruptness.

In treating involutional melancholia, the physician stresses the importance of a nourishing diet, adequate sleep, a healthful and pleasant environment, proper exercise, and absorbing avocations. Glandular drugs have also been used with success. Another source of help is undoubtedly found in psychotherapy. *See also* Chapter 22, "Mental Illness."

IODINE, an element used in medicine in various forms. Tincture of iodine is a solution of alcohol and iodine, which can be applied to the skin in either a weak or strong mixture, depending on the purpose. The strong tincture may cause blisters on the skin. Surgeons use a weak tincture as an antiseptic paint to disinfect the skin before an operation. Tincture of iodine is a standard item in the home medicine chest, and is used as a protection against infection in cuts, bruises, or scratches. If tincture of iodine is swallowed accidentally, it may burn the mucous membranes and act as a poison. The person should be given something to cause vomiting, followed by a thin starch or arrowroot solution on bread.

An iodine deficiency in the water supply can cause goiter, and the areas in the United States which are known to have this deficiency supplement their water supplies with iodine. *See also* GOITER.

I.Q., the initials of Intelligence Quotient. *See* STANFORD-BINET TEST.

IRITIS, an inflammation of the iris, the circular disc of the eye, and sometimes also the ciliary or eyelash region of the eye. *See also* EYE.

IRON, a powder made of reduced iron or in the form of its salts, is a constituent of hemoglobin, the red coloring matter of the red blood cells, and the carrier of oxygen from the lungs to all parts of the body. Iron as a vital part of hemoglobin not only assists the hemoglobin in the disposition of waste products and carbon dioxide from the kidneys, lungs, skin, and large intestine but is essential in the manufacture of hemoglobin itself within the body. When the body is deficient in hemoglobin, and therefore iron, the body tissues fail to receive their quota of oxygen. A large number of red blood cells are destroyed each day and must be replaced.

The amount of iron needed to keep the body in good health is small, and the daily requirement of iron in nutrition is only about 20 milligrams for an adult and 10 milligrams for a child, amounts which would fit on the head of a pin. At birth, most babies are oversupplied with hemoglobin, the mothers having generously supplied them with a store of iron-rich blood from their own reservoir.

Iron in food is dissolved and absorbed into the tissues through the action of the acid in the stomach. A new baby's stomach contains little acid and the milk that is usually its main food supply is low in iron. Therefore, all babies should be fed iron-rich foods from the age of two to three months; the type and amount of food should be determined by the physician. Iron in the diet is usually found in foods which are green, yellow, or red in color, such as carrots, celery, onions, peanuts, eggs, molasses, and a number of fruits including bananas, apples, apricots, peaches, and cherries. All forms of iron, even metallic, can be assimilated. Hydrochloric acid of the stomach helps to separate the iron from the consumed food and turns it into ferrous iron, a form readily absorbed by the body. If the acid secretion of the stomach is greatly diminished, it will not dissolve the iron of the foods ingested, and the iron is wasted.

Iron deficiency and its symptoms can be due to blood loss—such as injury or bleeding peptic ulcer—diet deficiency, and defective absorption of iron in the body. The high incidence of anemia in women may generally be attributed to increased demands of menstruation and pregnancy. *See also* ANEMIA; BLOOD; HEMOGLOBIN; NUTRITION.

ITCH. *See* SCABIES.

ITCHING, or pruritis as it is scientifically known, an irritation of the fine terminations of the sensory nerves at the skin. It may be due to a variety of causes.

Itching occurs in many different diseases of the skin; it may be a result of an eruption from sensitivity to certain foods, drugs, chemicals, material, or dusts; or it may be produced by invasion of the skin by parasites, such as the louse or itch mite, or a fungus infection, such as ringworm. Abnormal states of the blood, present in diseases like diabetes, gout, jaundice, and in various

digestive disturbances, may produce itching. Nervous disorders, either of a mental or physiological type, may also cause itching. Itching often follows recovery from a case of dermatitis.

Itching may be general and nonspecific, or it may be located in one part of the body. Scratching the area may give temporary relief, but it also may lead to damage to the skin and intensify the discomfort.

Control of itching depends on locating the cause and eliminating it. For example, treatment of an allergy or sensitivity will remove the cause and cure the itching. Itching due to a lack of moisture in the skin may be helped by repeated applications of bland lubricating ointments to relieve dryness and provide flexibility.

General or nonspecific itching is soothed by bathing in a tepid bath containing oatmeal extract. Sponging with a lotion containing sodium bicarbonate may help. Rubbing on menthol dissolved in alcohol is effective in itching which also burns and witch hazel sometimes relieves general itching. Another treatment is application of cool compresses using dilute Burow's solution, which should remain on the skin 15 minutes to three hours at a time.

The doctor may prescribe various medicated ointments for specific skin disorders which cause itching, which may range from mild to antihistaminic lotions. When bacteria are present and cause a secondary itching, an antibacterial ointment may be prescribed.

In general, extremes of heat and cold should be avoided, and bathing kept to a minimum. Air-conditioning has also been helpful during the convalescent period. *See also* ECZEMA; HIVES; SCABIES.

JAPANESE RIVER FEVER. *See* SCRUB TYPHUS.

JAUNDICE, or icterus, is a symptom rather than a disease and is characterized by yellowness of the skin and of the whites of the eyes. The color of the skin may range from bright lemon yellow to dark olive green. Itching is often associated with jaundice, especially in cases of long duration.

Causes of jaundice are varied. An excess of bile from the liver or any damage to the liver which affects the normal excretion of bile pigments may be responsible. Obstruction of the bile passages through which the pigment is normally excreted into the intestinal tract from the liver may result from gallstones, tumors, or parasitic invasion of the ducts. In obstructive jaundice, the feces are clay-colored and the urine may vary in color from light yellow to brownish green. The liver enlarges and its function gradually deteriorates unless an operation is performed to remove the cause of the obstruction.

Infectious diseases such as malaria and pneumonia may damage the blood, causing excessive destruction of the blood cells and ensuing jaundice. Chemical poisoning, resulting from absorption or inhalation of toxic substances like arsenic or phosphorus which affect the liver, or other poisons or infections which affect the rate of destruction of blood cells may also cause jaundice.

Catarrhal jaundice, the most common type, is caused by an infection with a specific virus and is fairly common among young people. The acute form of jaundice is the disease hepatitis.

Jaundice is one of the chief symptoms in Weil's disease, which is caused by spirochetal infection. Chills, fever and muscle pain, are other symptoms of this tropical disease. Treatment is chiefly by chemotherapy and by transfusions of blood from patients convalescing from the disease.

The poisons of eclampsia may affect the liver and cause jaundice. Jaundice in newborn babies is usually due to excessive destruction of the red blood cells that may result from septic infection of the umbilical cord, or from other infections associated with childbirth.

Ordinarily jaundice is a symptom of damage to the liver or bile ducts. Treatment depends on the nature of the causes, but in general includes the injection of glucose to prevent further damage to the liver. Any severe case of jaundice, whatever the cause, requires bed rest and careful diagnosis by a physician who can make the necessary tests and prescribe the proper treatment. *See also* BILE; HEPATITIS; LIVER; and Chapter 16, "Common Disorders of the Liver and Gallbladder."

JAW, a facial structure composed of bones, muscles, and nerves bordering the mouth. It consists of the upper and lower jaws which meet at the back of the head. The upper jaw is two separate bones, the right and left maxilla, which meet at the middle line. The lower jaw, or mandible, is a single bone. The alveolar is the part of each jaw which carries the teeth. Except for the alveolar, the maxilla is lighter in construction than the mandible.

First-aid treatment of a fracture of the jaw is limited and the help of a physician is essential. If a fractured lower jaw can be raised to bring the lower teeth against the upper teeth without causing too much pain, the jaw may then be immobilized with a bandage under the chin and over the top of the head. The jaw should not be forced in any way. If vomiting occurs, the bandage should be removed and the injured jaw held in place with the hand until the vomiting ceases. The bandage should then be replaced.

The joint of the mandible and the temporal portion of the skull may be affected by acute inflammation of the tonsils or by inflammation of other adjoining parts of the inside region of the mouth. This may cause difficulty in opening the mouth. This joint may also be affected by chronic osteoarthritis.

In tetanus, spasmodic closing of the jaw may result. This spasmodic closing, known as trismus, may also result from irritation of the teeth and other causes. In acromegaly, the jaw is large and prominent. A condition known as parrot jaw may also affect the jaw and cause protrusion of the upper jaw. *See also* TETANUS.

JEJUNAL ULCER, an ulcer located in the jejunum, the portion of the small intestine between the duodenum and ileum. The jejunum is about eight feet long. An ulcer developing after surgery performed to create an artificial passage between the stomach and intestines is known as a secondary jejunal ulcer. *See also* PEPTIC ULCER; and Chapter 18, "Disorders of the Digestive System and Diet in Digestive Disorders."

JOINTS AND JOINT DISORDERS. The bones and cartilages of the human skeleton are held together with many joints. The joints permit movement and action, and without them the skeleton would be stiff and immovable. Some joints are fixed, as in the adult cranium; some have limited movement, as the vertebrae of the spinal column; and others have freedom of action and motion, such as the ball-and-socket joints of the shoulder and hip. The knee is another free-moving joint, but its action is limited to bending and straightening, with but slight rotation inward and outward. Its structure includes the cartilage-covered heads of the femur of the thigh and tibia of the lower leg, bound together by strong tough ligaments. Enclosing this is the joint capsule, lined with a thin membrane, the synovia, which secretes a lubricating fluid, the synovial fluid.

The joints such as the knee are moved and strengthened by muscle fibers and tendons distributed around them.

Joint disorders. A common disturbance is water in a joint such as the knee. This results from the flow of serous fluid into the joint following an injury. When the condition appears without apparent cause and disappears within a few days, it is called intermittent hydrarthrosis, accumulation of fluid in a joint.

Following an injury blood may flow into the joints of some people who bleed easily. This condition is hemarthrosis, passing of blood from its proper place into a joint.

Sprains. As a result of violence applied to a joint, the joint may become sprained. In sprains, parts of the ligaments may be torn or stretched, and the bones partially or completely displaced from contact, as in dislocations. In the knee, for example, such an injury may result in displacement, bruising, or fracture of a semilunar cartilage, which will get caught between the bones and result in locking of the knee joint. Such injury frequently occurs to football, baseball, basketball, and tennis players. The condition can be relieved by extending the leg and turning it inward. When locking occurs too frequently, a surgical operation may be indicated to relieve the condition.

Another frequent joint injury is the pulling away of the ligament which extends from the kneecap to the large bone of the lower leg. The injury can occur, for example, when kicking a soggy football. This disabling of the leg and knee is known as Schlatter's disease, after the physician who first described it.

The treatment of severe joint injuries usually requires the attention of a physician. An x-ray is ordinarily made to determine whether or not a bone is broken. If a bone has not been broken but the joint has been strained or a ligament torn, the joint should be protected and supported by a bandage. If pain is severe, a local anesthetic may be injected directly into the injured joint.

Some forms of sprains are treated by cold applications, followed by strapping or by applying an elastic bandage. Healing of a severe sprain can occasionally be hastened by bathing the affected joint in hot water or by applying heat in some other manner. Light massage, followed by more intense rubbing, helps restore circulation and motion.

In cases of chronic sprain of a joint, the constant condition of swelling, inflammation, and irritation will cause the formation of adhesions and scar tissue. In such cases the orthopedic specialist will undertake special manipulation to break up adhesions and bring about looseness in the movement of the joint. Special kinds of elastic bandages have been developed for treatment of sprains, strains, and dislocations of joints.

Inflammation of a joint. Inflammation of a joint may be limited to the synovial membrane, called synovitis, inflammation of the lining of the membrane, or it may involve the entire structure, as in arthritis. Acute synovitis may develop as a result of any of these forms of injury, or it may be due to some other disorder, such as rheumatism or gout. The symptoms are almost the same as in sprain, and the treatment too is similar to that for sprain. Pain and swelling of the joint occur; and following injury, there is discoloration from blood effusing into the joint. The best treatment is an elastic bandage and promotion of circulation by moving about until gradually the amount of fluid diminishes and finally disappears.

Acute synovitis may be followed by stiffness and adhesions, which should be overcome by movements of the affected parts as soon as possible in the course of the disorder. There is always a possibility of ankylosis, or permanent fixation, to some degree, which can be avoided by careful treatment.

Acute synovitis may become chronic, with not much pain but with weakening of the joint, thicken-ing of the membrane, and the presence of fluid. The movements of the joint are interfered with, and there may be a sense of grating or rubbing present when the joint is moved. Diathermy or hot baths may help, but in severe cases an operation may be indicated.

Dislocations. A dislocation of a joint is promptly followed by swelling to a disproportionate size and impairment of the ability to move the particular limb or part. (For first-aid measures, *see* DISLOCATION.) Once

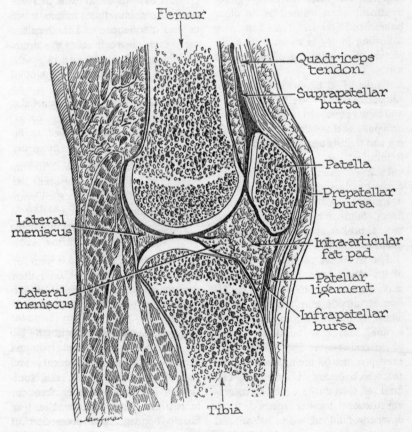

Femur

Quadriceps tendon

Suprapatellar bursa

Patella

Prepatellar bursa

Lateral meniscus

Intra-articular fat pad

Patellar ligament

Lateral meniscus

Infrapatellar bursa

Tibia

The bones and ligaments of the knee.

the doctor is called, he will make every effort to reduce the degree of dislocation in order to avoid pseudoarthrosis, the process whereby the displaced bone makes a fresh socket. Adhesions will form around the ends of the bones unless the dislocation is promptly handled.

A congenital dislocation may cause improper development, and reduction of this type of dislocation is difficult, with a tendency to recurrence.

Kneecap. The kneecap or patella requires the same sort of careful treatment when injured as do other bones and joints. The first step following injury is to have an x-ray picture. For complete discussion *see* KNEE.

Elbow. The elbow joint is often subject to breaks resulting from falls and injury sustained in sports. Certain occupations that demand sudden lifting and pulling also subject the elbow to injuries.

In most cases the injury to the elbow involves pulling of the muscles or ligaments, with the tearing of some fibers. Sometimes a portion of the bone is broken at the tip, with consequent pain and swelling.

The small sac of fluid at the end of the elbow bone, called the bursa, may become inflamed. This condition is bursitis and the pain is relieved by causing the excess fluid to escape. This may be done in any of several ways. The doctor may exert pressure on the area around the sac which causes it to break. The fluid will then flow into the surrounding tissues. Another method is to draw the fluid off with needle and syringe. Rest and application of heat

will often result in absorption of the excess fluid into the surrounding tissues. In severe injuries, it may be desirable to place the elbow in a cast and keep it immobilized for a long period. After removal from a cast or sling, exercise is needed to restore mobility to the injured elbow joint.

Ankylosis. Ankylosis, or stiffening of a joint, results from enlarging of the synovial membrane in acute forms of inflammation, as may occur in chronic rheumatoid arthritis. The joint tends to assume a position of greatest ease to avoid pain and becomes bent into this position more or less permanently. This bending may even increase if left alone. Certain optimum positions in which the various joints such as the elbow, wrist, hip, knee, and ankle may be placed have been found beneficial when there is any danger of ankylosis. These positions have proved to be the best possible ones for future use of the joint concerned. If suppuration should take place, it may be imperative to open and drain the joint. *See also* ANKLE; ARTHRITIS; BURSITIS; DISLOCATION; ELBOW; LIGAMENTS; KNEE; SPRAINS.

JUNGLE ROT, the popular term for tropical infectious diseases, used often to refer to fungus infections of the skin and more frequently to tropical ulcers.

Tropical ulcers develop usually on the feet and legs of people who go barefoot in warm moist tropical areas. Following breaks in the skin, such as may result from a bite, abrasion, or perforation by the itch mite, tiny blisters appear. These soon develop into larger, foul-smelling sores which spread rapidly and ulcerate. The ulcers become tender and painful, eating their way down into the tissues beneath the skin. Gradual disintegration of the diseased tissues occurs, followed by sloughing.

Healing is often spontaneous but recovery is slow. Scarring is common in tropical ulcers, and in severe cases skin grafting may be desirable.

Malnutrition is often seen in persons with a tendency to tropical ulcers, in whom deficiencies of vitamins, A, B, or C may be found.

In cases in which the disease is caused by the combination of bacillus and spirochete, known as Vincent's organisms, the use of penicillin and other antibiotics have been encouraging. The organisms are killed within twenty-four hours, and complete recovery takes place in a few weeks.

KAHN TEST, a procedure for detection of syphilis. It has largely superseded the Wassermann test. The test is named for Dr. Reuben L. Kahn, a bacteriologist who devised it. *See also* WASSERMANN TEST.

KALA AZAR, known also as Dumdum fever, black fever, or Mediterranean fever, a tropical disease characterized by physical wasting, progressive anemia, increase in the size of the spleen and liver, and dropsy. The bone marrow, lymph nodes, and other vital organs are also affected.

Kala azar is found chiefly in North Africa, along the Mediterranean Sea, in Asia Minor, India, and China. It is caused by a parasitic organism, the leishmania donovani, which is transmitted by the bite of the sandfly and which invades many of the vital organs. If the victim is untreated, the disease ends fatally within two years. Various antimony compounds are used to combat kala azar, but relapse is not uncommon. *See also* LEISHMANIASIS.

KELOIDS, overgrown scars which usually develop after surgery but which may occur following any break in the skin, such as a pinprick, pimple, or insect bite. Actually a keloid is a benign tumor of fibrous tissue growing in a scar. Keloids occur most frequently in young adults, and are most common among Negroes. Their exact cause is unknown.

Keloids may appear anywhere on the body, but are most frequently found on the chest and on the neck. A characteristic of keloids is their hard shiny surface, covering a mass of tissue growing out from the skin. More rare is a keloid which disappears spontaneously, leaving a depressed scar.

Keloids are usually painless but occasionally, depending on the area involved or their size, they become tender and cause pain. Sometimes a burning, itching or pricking sensation will be felt.

Surgery has been tried but found not too effective in treatment of keloids because of their tendency to recur. Electrolysis and electrical injection of drugs have also proved ineffective. More successful has been the injection of the enzyme hyaluronidase into the keloid and surrounding tissue. The use of radium and x-ray has also been found helpful in treating keloids. Special care must be taken, however, to avoid radiation of healthy tissue and to focus treatment on the keloid itself.

KIDNEYS, bean-shaped organs located high on the rear wall of the abdominal cavity. Their chief function is elimination of waste substances from the blood through the formation of urine.

The kidneys are the channels through which approximately 40 to 60 per cent of the water which is discarded passes out of the body. (The rest is eliminated largely by evaporation from the breath and in sweat.) These organs separate and incorporate into the urine the digested products of protein, substances in the blood which are formed continuously as a result of the normal constructive activity of the body. The kidneys also help to keep the fine balance between acid and alkaline conditions in the tissues by removing excess acid. The preservation of alkalinity in the tissues and blood is essential to life. They also maintain the necessary relation between salt and water in the body; a disturbance of this balance leads to overretention of moisture, as in dropsy, or to insufficiency of water, which may cause acidosis, dehydration, or reduce the necessary chemical changes.

The structure and operation of the kidneys are unique, especially for the amount of work they perform on a practically continuous basis in so small an area. Although each kidney is only about four inches, by two, by one inch, according to estimates, 600 or more quarts of blood, or 150 gallons, pass through them in twenty-four hours. Most of the blood continues on its way unaffected, but about 10 per cent of it, or sixty quarts or more, is selectively removed by the kidneys as it passes. To excrete so large a volume of liquid as urine would, however, drastically deplete the body. Therefore, most of the sixty quarts is reabsorbed by kidney cells as it passes through the kidneys. Along with it, the amino acids, building blocks of protein, sugar, and chlorides, are also reabsorbed. About 3 per cent, or 1½ to two quarts, is

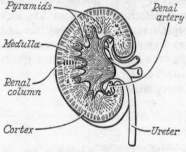

Parts of the kidney.

finally secreted as urine. Urine contains all the wastes—primarily the results of protein breakdown, urea, uric acid, and cheatinine—which the body must remove from the blood.

The apparatus which accomplishes this tremendous task is, in a sense, a bundle of tiny collecting tubes and filters. There are approximately 1,200,000 of these tubes or tubules in each kidney. Since each tubule is about two inches long, their aggregate length in the ordinary person is between 50 and 100 miles. Connected with each tubule is a minute filter, consisting of little chambers in which are packed tiny blood vessels, or glomeruli, which do the actual filtering. These blood vessels are only about 1/2500 of an inch in diameter, and total perhaps an inch in length within each filtration chamber. Yet there are so many of them that the total surface area available for filtering is about fifteen square feet.

Various disorders may involve the kidneys, and some of them may be quite serious. Fortunately, however, one kidney is sufficient to perform all the functions of both, in the event that one is incapacitated or must be removed.

One rather common kidney ailment is kidney stones. Small hard masses form in the organ and may bring a variety of consequences. Often they pass into the bladder, causing acute pain and kidney stone colic, with nausea, vomiting, and sometimes collapse. These stones may cause an obstruction of normal flow of fluid within the kidney, with various adverse effects including local infection. Frequently the stones, or occasionally the entire kidney, must be removed surgically. Internal obstruction in the kidney may also cause hydronephrosis, a condition in which urine collects and cannot escape. Here, too, surgical treatment may be required.

Other disorders of the kidney include nephritis, inflammation of the tissues; pyelitis, infection of the pelvis of the kidney; pyelonephritis, which affects both pelvis and the rest of the tissues. Such infections may result when organisms infecting some other part of the body travel to the kidney in the blood stream. High fever, tenderness in the loin, and a high white blood cell count are characteristic. Most organisms caus-

ing kidney infections are controlled by the antibiotics, such as penicillin or aureomycin, but frequently sulfonamide drugs, mandelic acid, or furacin derivatives are more effective. Tuberculosis of the kidney may arise, although the disease may not be present in any other part of the body. New drugs provide efficient means of treating this disease. If the condition is far advanced and affects only one kidney, surgical removal often results in elimination of the condition.

Bright's disease is a term commonly used to designate chronic inflammation of the kidney. The presence of albumin in the urine, albuminuria, which accompanies such inflammation, was first pointed out by a British physician, Richard Bright, in the first half of the nineteenth century. Actually albuminuria is a symptom of any of a whole group of disorders, just as fever is a symptom of infection by any of innumerable organisms.

Thus Bright's disease may designate a bacterial invasion of the kidneys, poisoning by toxins from invasive organisms or from those which originate in other infected tissues, poisoning by artificial poisons, disturbance of the kidneys caused by obstruction of the normal passage of urine, tumors or other abnormal growths, and the effects of interference with the kidneys' blood supply because of a disorder in the blood vessels themselves.

Kidney disturbances may produce symptoms ranging from those which are scarcely noticeable to those which are severe. Often the first indication is the discovery of albuminuria at the time of a life insurance examination, prompting an examination by the doctor beyond the range of the usual routine tests. A slight elevation of blood pressure, listlessness, undue fatigue, headaches, and failing appetite may also be noticed. As the disease progresses, however, regardless of the specific cause, symptoms develop such as spots in front of the eyes, dryness of the mouth and constant drinking of water, loss of weight or, conversely, gain in weight due to excessive holding of liquid within the tissues, and sometimes fever. Dizziness, nausea, vomiting, and other more acute symptoms will be noticed as the disease progresses.

Since these symptoms of kidney disorder may rise from such a variety of causes, unusual importance is attached to the exact origin in each case. Modern medicine has a number of specialized techniques for studying these conditions and, if necessary, of examining the kidney or its parts directly.

Treatment of kidney ailments is directed not only to removing the cause of the trouble but also, and of special significance, to resting the kidneys themselves. Bed rest will relieve the kidneys of much of the work they ordinarily must perform. Fewer waste products will form, and thus there will be less to be rejected. Additional strain may be taken from the kidneys by encouraging the elimination of wastes through the bowels and perspiration. Diet control also can exclude substances which require work on the part of the kidney.

Uremia occurs when both kidneys are removed or their functions totally blocked. The retention of the poisons in the body brings death in a short time. The chief characteristic of uremia is drowsiness, sometimes interrupted by convulsions. Occasionally it appears without any warning. The name of the disorder, given by Bright, was based on the assumption that urea, removed and passed off in the urine by the kidneys, is a toxic substance. Recent animal experiments, however, indicate that this may not be so, and therefore the exact cause of the poisoning that makes uremia fatal is not known.

Structural abnormalities may be present in the kidneys at birth. For example, they may be joined at one end and form a "horseshoe kidney," which does not have any notable consequences. Or the two kidneys may be fused to form one large one. Occasionally, especially in women, the kidneys change position, which is usually without significance except when twisting occurs which blocks the flow of urine. Pain and vomiting may result, but are relieved when the kidney again moves into another position. Recurrence may be prevented by wearing a suitable padded support, or by surgery.

Cysts and tumors also occur in the kidneys, blood in the urine being the most common symptom. Such symptoms should be promptly reported to a physician. *See also* ALBUMINURIA; HEMATURIA; NEPHRITIS; NEPHROSIS; URINE; URINATION; WILM'S TUMOR.

KNEE, a complicated joint with many component parts. Most significant are the capsule, the ligaments which bind the bones together and prevent untoward movements; the crescent-shaped pads of cartilage which lie on top of the shinbone and protect it from direct pressure of the thighbone; the kneecap with its powerful tendon; and the cushioning sacs or bursae that surround the main joint. The knee can tolerate much hard use, and dislocation without great violence is rare.

Inflammation of the joint can cause pain, swelling, and limited movement. The ligaments may become weakened and to some degree affect the stability of the knee in walking or even standing. In such cases, a support of some kind may be required for the knee. When inflammation of the knee is severe enough to require the person to remain in bed, proper splints are essential to prevent ultimate displacement of the tibia head.

Water on the knee. The knee, more than other joints, is liable to effusions of fluid by the synovial membrane of the capsule. This may follow any strain, twist, fall, or blow severe enough to damage a significant part of the joint. It may also be caused by infection or accompany rheumatoid arthritis. The whole joint will swell, obscuring the outline of the kneecap which is raised by the swelling and "floats." An effusion will generally subside of itself, but rest is essential.

Housemaid's knee. Housemaid's knee results from bursitis or from accumulation of fluid in the patellar bursa. This bursa is a sac in the kneecap which lies between the tendon, the anterior surface of the kneecap, and the skin. The condition occurs when a person kneels frequently. The fluid collects in front of the kneecap; whereas in water on the knee, the kneecap floats in the fluid which is behind it.

If the condition remains untreated, the fluid accumulates until a sizable swelling forms over the kneecap, and bending the knee or kneeling becomes painful. If infection reaches the fluid through a scratch or break in the skin, an abscess may form inside the bursa, and the knee becomes more painful and extremely tender. The fluid, once it forms, can be drawn out of the bursa with a syringe and hollow needle, under local anesthetic. If an abscess develops, it must be opened and drained. Often it is desirable to remove the entire bursa to avoid chronic recurrence of the condition.

To prevent housemaid's knee, always kneel on a soft pad.

Knock-knee. In knock-knee, the knee is bent inward, the foot carried outward, and the toes turned out abnormally. Both legs are usually affected. In early childhood, knock-knee usually results from rickets, but may also affect a child with weak ligaments. In the earlier stages, only the soft parts of the joint are involved and the condition may be corrected by manipulation and a correct alignment, preserved by splints or braces. When the knock-knee condition is of long standing, certain stages take place in the body structure which can be corrected only by an operation, which includes breaking through the lower part of the femur.

Broken kneecap. If the kneecap is broken, it is usually difficult to straighten the leg. X-rays which reveal the nature and extent of the injury are necessary before the doctor can prescribe treatment. If the knee-cap is broken without wide separation of the parts, the condition is frequently helped by immobilizing the leg with a cast or splint, thus permitting the parts to grow together. The surgeon usually uses a needle or syringe to withdraw the excess blood or fluid which may collect in the kneecap. The person in a cast must usually remain in bed for from four to eight weeks. When the cast is removed, manipulation of the joint will help in bending it. Application of hot wet packs or dry heat several times a day is beneficial.

In case of wide separation of the parts, surgical operation under anesthetic may be indicated. The surgeon will draw the parts together and bind them with fine steel wire or a similar material. And soft tissues that have been torn are sewed together. After the operation, a plaster cast is usually put on for four or five weeks. Upon removal, the knee is exercised and the patient permitted to bear weight with the knee straight. It may be two or three months before weight can be put on the knee in a bent position, and sometimes as long as six months before the knee returns to normal. *See also* JOINTS AND JOINT DISORDERS.

LABOR. *See* PREGNANCY AND PRE-NATAL CARE.

LACERATION, a wound made by a tear through the tissues. The damage is usually greater than when the wound is clean cut, and danger of infection is also increased.

Lacerations may be caused by a blow from a blunt instrument, from machinery, or from a fall against angular surfaces. Dirt or debris may be ground into the wounded tissues. An extensive or extremely dirty wound should be covered by sterile gauze as a first-aid measure, and then be cleansed and dressed by a doctor. A small laceration can be cleaned with soap and water, treated with mild antiseptic, and bandaged.

LARYNGITIS, inflammation of the mucous membrane of the larynx. In acute laryngitis, the usual symptoms are hoarseness and dryness of the throat, difficult and painful swallowing, coughing, discomfort and pain in speaking, and even partial or complete loss of voice. Acute laryngitis may occur in certain eruptions of the skin and mucous membranes, from swelling in certain gastrointestinal disorders, or as a secondary complication of such infectious diseases as scarlet fever, measles, and chicken-pox. It often is associated with the common cold.

Laryngitis is particularly dangerous in babies and young children. They may quickly become breathless, especially during inhaling when the breastbone may press inward and cause further complications. A doctor should be consulted at the first indication of laryngitis in a baby or child. Adults should rest in bed and refrain from using their voice. Cold moist compresses and ice packs, in other cases warmth, may be beneficial. Inhaling steam, to which aromatic oils may be added, is also helpful. In serious cases, particularly when infection is present, the doctor may prescribe drugs and soothing sprays to aid in alleviating soreness in the larynx.

Chronic laryngitis is characterized chiefly by a change in the voice, hoarseness, and often a persistent cough and need to "clear the throat." It may follow a single attack or series of recurring attacks of laryngitis, a misuse or overuse of the voice, and is also associated with chronic irritation of the nose and throat. Excessive drinking and smoking predispose to chronic laryngitis.

Any persistent hoarseness may also be symptomatic of early cancer of the larynx, of laryngeal tuberculosis, and of paralysis of the vocal cords, and medical attention should be sought as soon as possible. Treatment of chronic laryngitis always includes rest of the voice, sprays and other remedies directed toward relieving the condition. *See also* LARYNX.

LARYNX, or voice box, a cavity at the upper end of the windpipe which contains the vocal cords and serves as the organ for the voice. It consists of a number of cartilages held together by muscles and ligaments. At the upper end of the larynx is the epiglottis, an elastic cartilage which keeps food from entering the larynx and windpipe, directing it instead to the esophagus and stomach.

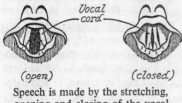

(open)   (closed)

Speech is made by the stretching, opening and closing of the vocal cords located in the larynx.

In the speech process, the vocal cords come together, leaving only a narrow passage. When air strikes the cords, they vibrate and with the supplementary aid of the tongue, teeth, palate, and lips, speech is produced. The pitch varies with the space between the cords and the degree of tension. The differences in the nature and combination of these organs determine the type of voice.

In the adult male, the voice has greater depth than that of the female, because of the greater size of the larynx and the consequent greater length of the vocal cords. A low-pitched voice is produced by slowly vibrating cords and a high-pitched voice by cords vibrating with higher frequency.

To examine the larynx the doctor uses a small mirror, mounted at an angle on a metal stem, which is put far back into the throat. By listening to the sounds made when the patient says, "Ah," and by observation, the doctor can see any modification or inflammation of the larynx.

The larynx is subject to nervous and physical disorders. Laryngitis is acute or chronic inflammation of the mucous membrane of the larynx. Paralysis of the laryngeal muscles may be due to nervous causes, to a tumor in the chest, or result from syphilis. Laryngeal crisis of locomotor ataxia is an example of a nervous condition. Laryngeal tuberculosis is generally secondary to pulmonary tuberculosis. Tumors are fairly common and are generally benign; they can be removed by surgery. Cancer of the larynx may originate in the larynx or develop from adjoining areas of the body, and surgery to remove all or part of the larynx is generally indicated.

Foreign objects drawn into the larynx may cause spasm and produce an urgent danger of suffocation. First-aid measures, such as slapping the victim on the back, may help remove the object; and if breathing has stopped, artificial respiration is necessary. If the object does not cause unusual pain and removal does not seem immediately urgent, a doctor should remove it, since unskilled efforts can cause damage. *See also* LARYNGITIS.

LATERAL SCLEROSIS, a rare disease of the brain and spinal cord, occurring primarily in men between the ages of forty and fifty years. Degeneration and scarring (sclerosis) come about gradually, leading to loss of control of muscle groups in the hands, arms, legs, and throat. As a result, the person may note tremors in the arms and legs, difficulty in swallowing and speaking, and shrinkage of the muscle of the extremities. Many factors have been attributed as a cause, such as fatigue, alcohol, lead poisoning, and syphilis, but actually the real cause is not known. Injury seems to play no part in lateral sclerosis. Treatment may include high-vitamin diet, muscle stimulants such as prostigmine, and rest.

LAXATIVE. *See* CATHARTICS.

LEAD POISONING, as the name implies, a form of poisoning due to the introduction of lead into the system.

Acute lead poisoning, which is comparatively rare, may occur when food or medicinal products are taken internally. The symptoms are severe, including sickness, colic, cramps, diarrhea, and usually constipation, leg cramps, and a feeling of drowsiness. The best treatment is an emetic, followed by plenty of milk and half an ounce of Epsom salts in half a glass of water. The victim should be kept warm.

Chronic lead poisoning occurs in workers in a number of industries, such as painting, lead mining, and refining and other industries which utilize lead compounds. The poison may be inhaled as dust, or food may have been contaminated by the hands of workers to which poisonous compounds of lead adhere. The signs of chronic lead poisoning are colic, constipation, lead palsy which affects particularly the forearm and fingers, the symptoms of arteriosclerosis and chronic nephritis, and sometimes mental depression, convulsions, and a blue line at the edge of the gums. Chronic lead poisoning is sometimes treated by the administration of magnesium or lead sulphate solution which acts as a laxative and antidote on the lead in the digestive system, followed by potassium iodide which cleanses the tract.

Persons who work in industries where lead poisoning is an occupational hazard must be careful to follow the safety regulations which have been established and to practice thorough personal hygiene.

Water which contains lead may cause slow poisoning. Symptoms may be a gradual depreciation of health, failing appetite, and signs of anemia, constipation, and colic. Formerly, when lead was the base of paints, "painter's colic" was an occupational hazard among painters, but this condition has been eliminated by the use in newer paints of a base other than lead.

LEFT-HANDEDNESS. When the left hand is stronger or more expert or used in preference to the right hand, the person is said to be left-handed. Left-handedness has been the subject of many superstitious beliefs and popular misconceptions, all of them without factual basis. Left-handedness may or may not be inherited. It presents little advantage, except to baseball pitchers, or special handicap, except to golfers. Attempts to direct a normally left-handed child to use his right hand will only confuse him and has been associated with the development of stuttering and awkwardness. True left-handed people are likely to favor using the left eye, left ear, and left foot, just as right-handed people prefer the right eye, ear, and foot. Beyond this type of preference, differences between right-handed and left-handed persons are not apparent. *See also* STUTTERING AND STAMMERING.

LEG, the part of the lower limb between the knee and the ankle; the upper part of the limb is the thigh. The bones of the leg include the tibia or shinbone on the inside, and the fibula on the outside. The two great bones are connected by a membrane. The leg contains significant muscles, nerves, and blood vessels, including the calf muscle, branches of the sciatic nerve, and the popliteal vein.

Varicose veins, which are quite common, may lead to secondary disorders such as eczema, ulceration, and discoloration. Frequent exposure to intense heat may also lead to a brownish discoloration of the legs. Eczema on the shins, apart from that caused by varicose veins, is not unusual. Dropsy or edema also affects the legs early in their development. In infantile paralysis the muscles waste away, and in another form of muscular paralysis known as pseudo-hypertrophic muscular paralysis the muscles develop unduly. *See also* ACHILLES' TENDON; ANKLE; ARTIFICIAL LIMBS; FEET; KNEE; VARICOSE VEINS.

LEISHMANIASIS, a variety of visceral and superficial infections, caused by certain parasitic protozoa known as the leishmania after the famous surgeon Dr. William B. Leishman.

This group of tropical diseases include visceral leishmaniasis or kala azar; oriental sore, an ulcerative form that attacks the skin; and a third form which attacks the mucous membrane of the nose, mouth, and pharynx. In this form the cartilage underlying these structures may also be invaded. If the larynx is affected the voice may be permanently lost.

The most effective treatment of leishmaniasis is with drugs containing antimony. *See also* KALA AZAR.

LENS, glass ground so that one or both sides are curved, giving it the power to converge or scatter rays of light. Five types of lenses are (1) spherical, in which the curved side is part of a sphere; (2) cylindrical, in which the curved part is in one direction only; (3) convex, bulging outward from its center; (4) concave, with an inward curve toward its center; (5) biconcave or biconvex, in which both sides are curved. The crystalline lens of the human eye is biconvex; that is, it bulges out to the front and back from the center. *See also* BIFOCAL; EYE; EYEGLASSES.

LEPROSY, also called Hansen's disease or Hansenosis, a chronic infectious ailment occurring almost exclusively in tropical and subtropical countries. Though generally considered, since Biblical times, to be a highly contagious disease, leprosy is actually only moderately infectious. The symptoms include ulcers, tuberculous nodules, loss of fingers and toes, abnormal coloring, either excessive or deficient, and the emergence of nerveless areas in which tissue eventually develops gangrene.

The best-known leper colony in the United States is at Carville, Louisiana. Sulphone drugs have been used to treat leprosy with some success. Streptomycin and Aureomycin are also being used in an effort to find a specific against the bacillus which is believed to cause leprosy. In addition to medical treatment, adequate diet, rest, exercise, and mental hygiene are essential in the control of this disease.

LEUCORRHEA, any whitish discharge from the vagina and uterine tract. Popularly such discharge is called "the whites." Leucorrhea may be indicative of an abnormality. The mucous glands of the vagina and cervix normally secrete small amounts of whitish material which moistens the tissues. Minor inflammation and congestion may similarly cause discharge, and premenstrual conditions sometimes stimulate ac-

tivity of the mucous glands. However, inflammation of the Fallopian tubes, which can be due to gonorrhea, tuberculosis, or some other infection, can produce an abnormal discharge. Cancer of the uterus may also be the cause. Therefore, any abnormality in quantity, color, or odor of the discharge from the vaginal tract should be referred to a physician.

LEUKEMIA, a disease of the blood in which the production of white blood cells or leukocytes increases tremendously without apparent reason. In the normal person there are about 7,500 white blood cells in every cubic millimeter of blood. In leukemia the number may increase to from 100,000 to one million white blood cells in every cubic millimeter of blood.

Although there is as yet no specific cure for leukemia, much progress has been made. Techniques of treatment are now available which help extend the life span considerably and increase the comfort of the person with leukemia.

Leukemia is generally classified as acute or chronic although several different types of leukemia are recognized. The acute form occurs most frequently in young children, the onset being sudden and the progress rapid. Chronic leukemia generally attacks persons over thirty-five years of age. Frequently the first sign of acute leukemia is prolonged bleeding after a minor operation or tooth extraction. Other early signs are anemia, fever, pain in the bones and joints, and, in some cases, a swollen mouth and thickened gums. Chronic leukemia is also characterized by anemia and bleeding. In addition, the lymph nodes and spleen are noticeably enlarged. Small lumps, composed of the infiltrating white blood cells, may appear under the skin. Chronic leukemia may also be accompanied by loss of weight, nervousness, shortness of breath, and abnormal night sweats.

Treatment of leukemia depends on careful diagnosis to determine the exact type and extent of the disease. This can be done by examining and counting the white blood cells under a microscope. The most widely used treatment involves injection of radioactive phosphorus. X-ray treatment is also widely used and now supplements the treatment by injection. X-rays affect the bone marrow and help prevent secondary anemia. Radioactive phosphorus acts on the spleen and lymph nodes to reduce them, and acts on the bone marrow to inhibit the production and multiplication of white blood cells. In certain types of acute leukemia, cortisone and ACTH have been effective in helping to produce normal white blood cells. Several new chemical substances are undergoing experiment for the treatment of leukemia. Blood transfusions may be required during the procedure to control anemia, to keep the red blood cells at a proper level, and to prevent purpura which is characteristic in some forms of leukemia. Antibiotics may also be used to prevent secondary infection. *See also* Chapter 13, "Diseases of the Blood."

LEUKOCYTES, the colorless blood cells, generally called white blood cells or corpuscles. The blood contains several varieties of leukocytes which can be differentiated and counted by straining and other techniques, including observation under the microscope.

The number of leukocytes in a person's body varies over a lifetime and during the course of a single day. More leukocytes are present in childhood and in pregnancy. After meals an increase of leukocytes occurs, due to an increase in the number of lymphocytes from the lymph glands. Any increase in the number of leukocytes is known as leukocytosis. In disease this is serious; leukemia is one of the most critical diseases affecting the blood.

In certain diseases, such as granulocytosis, leukocytes are almost totally absent from the blood. Sensitivity to certain toxic drugs may cause complete absence of leukocytes; and, since these cells are essential to resist infection, their absence may be fatal. In typhoid fever and certain other diseases, the number of leukocytes may fall below normal, a condition known as leukopenia. In cases in which it is desirable to increase the number of leukocytes, certain drugs and serums may be injected. *See also* BLOOD; LEUKEMIA; and Chapter 13, "Diseases of the Blood."

LEUKOPLAKIA, a disease affecting middle-aged or elderly persons, in which white patches develop on the tongue and on the inside of the cheeks and the gums. The exact cause of leukoplakia is unknown, but the condition has been associated with excessive smoking and was once known as "smoker's patch." Leukoplakia has also been related to drinking and, in some instances, syphilis. However, many cases do not suggest any apparent relationship to any of these alleged causes.

In time the patches become painful, especially in swallowing and talking. Continuous irritation is sometimes followed by cancer. Smoking and liquor, condiments and hot food must be avoided. Treatment by x-rays or radium and the application of antiseptics have been beneficial.

LIBIDO, sexual desire; the term also refers to the energy derived from the primitive impulses. In psychoanalysis, libido refers to the motivating drive of the sex life. In Freudian psychology, it denotes psychic energy in general.

LICE, small wingless flat insects which live on the skin of birds, mammals, and human beings. They produce irritating dermatitis and are capable of carrying disease. Three kinds of lice may infest the human body and cause discomfort and disease: the head louse, the clothes or body louse, and the crab louse. Pediculosis is the technical name for lice infestation.

The head louse is especially common among children, spreading rapidly. This insect lives only among the hairs of the head. It is small, crawling, gray in color, and visible. It lays its eggs, or nits, on the hairs to which they become attached. The eggs can be slid up or down the hair, and are best removed by sliding them off at the ends of the hairs. The eggs hatch in from six to sixteen days and the new lice mature in the next eight

to sixteen days. Head lice cause intense itching. The discomfort leads to scratching which may result in infection. Further complications, such as impetigo of the scalp and enlargement and even abscess of the neck glands, may also result. At the first sign of head lice or nits, the scalp must be disinfected to avoid the further multiplication of the lice. Treatment includes killing the lice and nits with a chemical, followed by combing the hair with a fine strong comb. A 2 per cent DDT emulsion or any of the chemicals used in scabies will kill lice. Many preparations are available in drug stores.

Body lice are comparatively rare, being found in crowded unsanitary places. During World War II, DDT was a significant factor in mass lice control. Typhus and other fevers are carried by body lice and the use of DDT on a large scale has brought these diseases under control. A thorough washing with hot water and soap, followed by the use of a disinfectant ointment, usually will rid the body of lice. It is more difficult to remove lice from clothes and bedding, and steaming or boiling the articles may be necessary.

The crab louse infests chiefly the hairy parts of the body, such as the genitals or armpits. It also lays eggs which adhere to the hair. Both lice and nits are small but visible. A 10 per cent DDT powder rubbed in thoroughly, or a 4 per cent DDT solution in liquid paraffin will destroy crab lice. As in scabies, an emulsion of benzyl benzoate is also effective. After a hot bath with plenty of soap, the emulsion should be brushed thoroughly into the affected parts. Another precaution is to clip the hair short. Soiled pajamas, undergarments, and other clothing should be soaked in an antiseptic solution and laundered. *See also* BODY LICE; CRAB LICE; DDT; TYPHUS.

LIGAMENTS, tough fibrous bands of tissue connecting bones at the joints and holding them in place. They do not stretch, but are placed in an interlacing arrangement so that they permit the movements required at these poinits. Another type of ligament, which is really modified peritoneal tissue, holds the major organs in place. An elastic form of ligament is found at the vertebrae, where considerable range of movement is required, as in bending the back. Here the ligaments stretch and then become taut, keeping the parts steady.

Ligaments can be torn from the bones at the points where they are attached, or otherwise damaged. They may heal of themselves if the part that has been injured is immobilized. In some cases surgery may be imperative to bring together torn ends of ligaments. Plastic surgery is also employed to restore motion in cases of paralysis by transferring ligaments from one part of the body to another. *See also* JOINTS AND JOINT DISORDERS; SPRAINS.

LIGATION, tying off of a blood vessel to constrict it, or the application of any type of ligature, either cord or thread. Ligation is often indicated in surgery and may be required in cases of accidental bleeding. Sometimes warts, piles, or small tumors are constricted by a ligature at the point of attachment to the body. Catgut, usually used as a ligature in sur-gery, is readily absorbed into the tissue. Sterile linen or silk are also used as ligatures in various types of operations.

LIMPING, INTERMITTENT, or intermittent claudication, a symptom of disturbance in the circulation of the blood vessels of the legs; it may result from disease or inflammation or hardening of the blood vessels. The first symptoms may be numbness, tingling and burning sensations in the toes, and in some cases a heavy painful feeling, cramps and weakness in the legs and feet. When the condition is severe, cramping pains are felt in the muscle of the calf, causing a lump when walking.

Intermittent claudication results from narrowing of the blood vessels and failure of the circulatory system to function properly in supplying blood to the leg. Rest will alleviate the pain.

Intermittent limping is a particular symptom of Buerger's disease. Other disorders associated with limping are dislocation of the hip, breakdown of the arch, various nervous and muscular disorders, and even ill-fitting shoes. All require diagnosis and treatment by a specialist in orthopedics. To treat limping, a thorough study of the circulation is made. Color of the skin is associated with circulation, and a test is made by raising the leg and flexing the foot toward the knee; if circulation is adequate, the color will return when the leg is lowered to a normal position.

LINIMENT, an oily preparation which is rubbed into the skin to help circulation, relieve pain, and promote the cure of stiffness and inflammation. There are many different types of liniments, including the anodyne or pain-relieving liniments which contain aconite, belladonna, and opium; liniments mixed with irritants that cause redness of the skin and stimulate circulation, including those containing ammonia, camphor, mustard, soap, and turpentine; chloroform liniments which are both pain-relieving and stimulating to the circulation; calcium oxide or lime liniments which soothe inflamed areas; and liniments compounded with mercury and potassium iodide which both stimulate the circulation and help reduce swelling and inflammation.

All these types of liniments are liquid except the last which is a soft solid and may be applied with a fine cloth. Liniments are helpful primarily because of the vigor with which they are applied, and are not specifically curative of any condition.

LIPOMA, a fatty tumor or a tumor made of fatty cells. Although lipomas are painless and not malignant, they are unsightly and may become the seat of gangrene or fat necrosis. If infected or annoying, they should be removed by surgery.

LIPS, the two fleshy folds surrounding the cavity of the mouth. They are composed of the skin covering the outer surface, mucous membrane covering the inner portion, connective tissue, and a ring of muscular tissue and the artery that supplies blood. The functions of the lips include feeding and speech.

Harelip, a congenital condition, results from failure of the lips to grow together properly and is a serious and often unsightly handicap. Plastic surgery performed in early infancy is most effective in correcting it. Another condition of the lips which is successfully treated by surgery is overgrowth of the glandular tissue, which ordinarily results in enlargement of the upper lip.

Chapping or inflammation of the lips is often due to exposure to sun, wind and cold. Sensitivity to chemical ingredients of lipstick may also produce similar conditions. Cracking of the lips may follow. A protective ointment helps give relief.

A deficiency of riboflavin provokes cracking and blistering in the corners of the mouth. Supplementary vitamins together with careful hygiene and protective ointments usually cure the condition.

More serious are carbuncles and abscess of the upper lip. Because of the presence of large blood vessels in this area, care must be taken to prevent spread of infection to vital parts of the body. Use of sulfa drugs and antibiotics has greatly reduced the danger of this condition, which was formerly fatal in some cases.

Also serious is cancer of the lip which may be induced by chronic irritation, as in pipe smoking. Early detection and treatment by surgery is imperative; treatment by irradiation or electric coagulation or a combination of both has proved effective.

In the common cold and in fever, blisters known as herpes frequently form on the margins of the lips. Nervousness in menstruation and sensitivity to certain foods may also induce blisters. *See also* HARELIP; HERPES SIMPLEX; HERPES ZOSTER.

LIVER, the largest gland, and one of the largest organs in the human body; it is located in the upper right abdomen, immediately under the diaphragm and attached to it by ligaments.

The liver is involved in many significant body processes, such as affording protection from disease, supplying sugar to meet the needs of muscle tissues, and regulating clotting of the blood. It weighs three to four pounds in the adult male, and is estimated to be approximately seven times larger than requisite, thus assuring the body of a substantial safety factor when liver functions are concerned. In addition, the liver possesses special power of regeneration. After being damaged, it can regenerate its own tissue almost immediately.

The digestive process is especially closely related to the liver. Every vein from every part of the digestive tract empties into the liver through the portal vein. The proteins, sugars, and starches absorbed by the blood vessels of the stomach, by the small and large intestines and the pancreas are brought to the liver in the blood. These products result from the digestion of meats, starches, and sugars consumed as food.

Among its other activities, the liver produces and distributes a pint or more of bile every twenty-four hours. Bile is a bitter-tasting, yellowish golden or brown fluid which is strongly alkaline and thus neutralizes the acid which enters the duodenum from the stomach. The bile is composed largely of bile salts and bile pigments. Bile salts assist in breaking down food fats in the intestine and

in the absorption of fat through the intestinal wall. The fats are not excreted, but are absorbed in the intestinal wall and reused.

Bile pigments are derived from hemoglobin of discarded red blood cells, excreted with the solid waste of the body. The term "jaundice" arises from the yellowish cast which bile pigments give the mucous membranes and the conjunctiva of the eye when they circulate in abnormal amounts in the blood. Bile is continually produced by the liver. Among other functions it serves as the medium for excreting various harmful substances which the liver removes from the blood.

A bile duct, formed by the joining of two lesser ducts, carries bile from the liver to the duodenum. On the way, part of the bile is deposited as a reserve in the gallbladder, where it is concentrated by the absorption of moisture into the walls of the gallbladder. This organ supplies bile to the intestine after the passage of food into the small intestine from the stomach. When solid substances in the bile precipitate and settle they form gallstones, which may vary considerably in color, size, and consistency, depending on their exact composition.

The liver takes sugar from the blood and stores it as glycogen, which is quickly converted back to sugar when it is needed by the body, especially the muscles. The liver produces urea, which is taken by the blood to the kidneys for excretion. The liver also forms fibrinogen and antithrombin, two substances essential to normal conditions in the blood and in its clotting. Fibrinogen forms a clot. Antithrombin prevents the constant disintegration of the white blood cells and prevents coagulation of the circulating blood, which is extremely dangerous.

Another vital biochemical activity of the liver is the formation of many antibodies, the substances developed by the body to counteract invasive organisms and their toxins. The liver synthesizes proteins, stores copper and iron, and produces both vitamin A and one of the ingredients essential to the creation of the red blood cells.

Since it is so crucial in the functioning of the body, a serious condition results when the liver becomes infected, inflamed, or otherwise disordered. One significant factor is the effect of the liver on the body's sugar supply. Liver cells respond to major damage by discharging their glycogen. Injection of glucose may then be indicated to supply the required sugar. This in turn may demand the injection of insulin to assist the body in taking care of the replenishment of sugar. Unusual fatigue, listlessness, drowsiness, and confusion are symptoms of a relative lack of sugar or, often, a relative excess of insulin. The same circumstance may arise from sources other than liver damage, and the cause can be established when the quantity of sugar in the blood is checked.

Among the serious diseases of the liver are cirrhosis, or hardening; atrophy, or wasting; overgrowth; and bacterial or parasitic infection, which cause abscesses. Recent research indicates that the liver is vulnerable to dietary deficiencies, especially those of vitamins. Vitamin deficiencies may be associated with hardening of the liver.

Acute hepatitis is a form of liver disease caused by a viral infection, and the proper diagnosis is urgent, since the symptoms often resemble other disorders. Fatal complications may ensue with little or no warning.

Abscesses in the liver may originate from infection by amebae, as in amebiasis, or from a general infection of the blood, as in pyemia. Abscesses caused by amebae are more serious, since they tend to be single rather than multiple, and thus to concentrate their virulence in one spot in the liver. Frequently, though not invariably, the history of the patient reveals previous dysenteric infection. Usually a liver abscess must be treated surgically. It must be exposed and cleansed or it is likely to rupture and empty its contents into the abdominal cavity and result in peritonitis which might be fatal. Sometimes an operation is advisable to establish the actual existence of an abscess. Operative treatment is accompanied by injection of amebicidal drugs.

The proportion of fat in the liver is increased by its reaction to various poisons, to a high-fat diet, sometimes to general obesity or chronic alcoholism. In reacting to poisons, the liver replaces functioning cells with fat. Storage of fat in the liver occurs with an overfatty diet. Carbon tetrachloride, a common drycleaning substance, phosphorus, arsenic, and chloroform are all particularly damaging to the liver. *See also* ALCOHOLISM; BILE; CIRRHOSIS; HEPATITIS; JAUNDICE; and Chapter 16, "Common

Disorders of the Liver and Gall-bladder."

LIVER EXTRACTS, pharmaceutical preparations containing soluble fractions of mammalian livers or solution of liver and purified solution of liver. The liver contains a substance which stimulates the formation of red blood corpuscles. Persons with pernicious anemia are successfully treated with intramuscular injections of highly concentrated liver extracts, which increase the number of red blood corpuscles in their blood. *See also* ANEMIA.

LIVER SPOTS, or chloasma, yellow and brownish spots and discolorations in patches on the skin. They may occur in pregnancy, tuberculosis, and digestive disturbances. They may also follow exposure to sun or heat and may appear in areas where pressure from a pad or belt has been exerted on the skin.

Pigmentation has been successfully treated with an ointment containing benoquin, a drug derived from an Egyptian plant, ammi majus. In certain instances, peeling techniques have also been used successfully.

LOA LOA WORM DISEASE. *See* FILARIASIS.

LOCKJAW. *See* TETANUS.

LOCOMOTOR ATAXIA. When the spinal column is infected by syphilis, serious progressive damage occurs in the nervous system. The resulting condition, which may appear anywhere from five to fifteen years after the initial infection, is known as locomotor ataxia.

Many symptoms accompany this disorder, all coming from the destruction wrought by the infection in the spinal nervous tissues. One of the most serious symptoms is the loss of ability to coordinate body movements. In walking, the feet seem to flip up and down, and the legs have a jerky motion. Walking in the dark is difficult, and touching the tip of the nose with the forefinger may be impossible.

Some essential reflexes are disorganized or lost. Normally the pupil of the eye opens wider in the dark to admit any light, and narrows when exposed to light. The eyes and the pupils of a person with locomotor ataxia react in a disorganized way.

Acute pains, resembling the symptoms of an inflamed appendix or a severe intestinal infection, are sometimes felt in the organs of the abdomen. Similar pains attack other parts of the body, such as the face and legs. Strange sensations, like sharp changes of temperature, are experienced on the skin, without any apparent cause. A common symptom is an illusion that insects are crawling on the body.

Since the discovery of blood tests that enable prompt diagnosis of syphilis, and the use of antibiotic drugs like penicillin to control it, syphilis of the nervous system and general paresis are becoming exceedingly rare.

LOEFFLER'S SYNDROME, a group of respiratory symptoms without specific causes. These may include mild fever, coughing, asthmatic breathing, and fatigue. In such cases, the doctor makes careful tests to make sure that pneumonia, asthma, or another respiratory disorder are not present. Bed rest, which is the best treatment, is usually prescribed.

LONGEVITY, long life or the condition or quality of being long-lived. It is an inherited tendency, but a higher standard of living, better nutrition, and advances in medicine have in recent years increased the life span. Today the average life expectancy in the United States is more than sixty-five years of age; the prospect for succeeding generations is an increase of sixty-eight or seventy years.

Statistics indicate that women in the United States generally live longer than men. Certain occupations are also associated with longer life than others. Increased longevity has created certain basic problems concerning the aged which are as yet far from a satisfactory solution. These include economic independence for the aged, emotional security and recognition of their status in the community, and proper standard of living and adequate medical care. *See also* SENESCENCE; and Chapter 26, "Geriatrics."

LORDOSIS, or sway back, a condition caused by an increase in the forward curvature of the lower spinal column or small of the back. It comes from an effort to improve the body's balance, as in the later stages of pregnancy.

Lordosis is also associated with hip-joint diseases and other disorders. In a person with a large heavy abdomen, a strain is placed on the muscles and ligaments which can produce pain and an increase in curvature of the lower spine. *See also* SPINAL CORD; SPINAL CURVATURE; SPINE.

LOW BACK PAIN, one of the commonest complaints brought to the attention of doctors. A symptom rather than a disease, low back pain may be caused by a great variety of conditions which are classed as congenital, mechanical, produced by disease, or the result of injury or strain.

Some of the mechanical causes are poor posture, overweight, or occupational strain. Injuries to or strains of the vertebrae, their ligaments, muscles, or nerves can cause low back pain. Such diseases as lumbago, rheumatoid arthritis, tuberculosis, syphilis, osteomyelitis, and degenerative arthritis of the sacroiliac joint produce low back pain.

Low back pain can originate in a number of areas of the spinal cord and may result from disorder of the sciatic nerve, which passes through the thighs, legs, and feet from the back. The sacroiliac joint may also be the seat of low back pain, as the result of strain, injury, or disease.

Early treatment is essential in order to avoid development of chronic conditions or complications such as arthritis. A physician should be consulted at the first sign of pain in the lower back. In most cases treatment is nonsurgical, and, if the diagnosis is correct, largely effective in at least 90 per cent of the cases. Treatment includes rest, physical therapy such as heat, baths, and radiant light; strapping; drugs; and mechanical aids such as splints, belts, and braces.

Most therapy can be carried out at home, although more prompt and efficient treatment can be administered in a hospital. *See also* BACKACHE; LUMBAGO; NEURITIS; SACRO-

ILIAC; SCIATIC NEURITIS; SLIPPED DISC.

LOW BLOOD PRESSURE. *See* BLOOD PRESSURE, LOW.

LUMBAGO, an acute attack of pain and stiffness in the lower back region which may appear without warning and without a sign or symptom of general illness. It may occur after ordinary housework or gardening, exposure to cold or wet weather, or sitting for a period of time in a draught of cold air blowing on the lower back region. It is usually characterized by a twinge of pain on moving.

Lumbago can generally be cured by heat from a hot-water bottle, heating pad, infrared ray, or with diathermy. Drugs such as aspirin may be taken or the doctor may inject a local anesthetic to be followed by limited movement and rest periods. Repeated attacks of lumbago may be due to an infection elsewhere in the body which the doctor will try to locate. *See also* LOW BACK PAIN.

"LUMPY JAW." *See* ACTINOMYCOSIS.

LUNGS, the respiratory organs. The lungs lie on either side of the chest and occupy a large part of the chest cavity. The right lung is larger than the left and contains three parts or lobes, whereas the left lung has only two lobes.

Structure and function. The general structure of the lung resembles that of an inverted tree. The main stem is represented by the bronchus, which leads into the lung from the windpipe and subdivides into smaller and smaller branches or tubes, end-

ing in the minute ones called the bronchioles. These lead to the alveoli or air sacs on the surface of which are the capillaries.

Blood is supplied to the capillaries by the pulmonary artery, and carried off by the pulmonary veins. Lymphatic vessels also pass through the lungs, which are covered by the pleura, a membrane.

Primarily the function of the lungs is to provide oxygen to the red blood cells and to eliminate carbon dioxide. In the rest of the body the capillaries expend oxygen and take up carbon dioxide, whereas in the lungs the capillaries take up oxygen and throw off carbon dioxide.

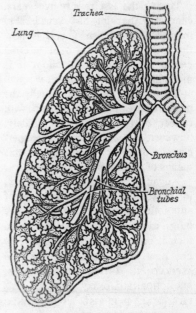

A cross section view of the lung.

In the course of twenty-four hours' breathing, an active man absorbs more than twenty cubic feet of oxygen, and his blood emits more than twenty cubic feet of carbon dioxide. The lungs normally take in air and expel waste products seventeen times a minute, and can speed up to seventy or eighty times a minute during extreme muscular effort or in pneumonia.

Diseases of the Lungs. Tuberculosis and pneumonia are among the most serious diseases infecting the lungs. Other infections may cause bronchitis and bronchiectasis. The lungs may be affected by various viruses, by parasites and fungi, and by different poisons and dusts found in industry. Certain other disorders like abscess and emphysema or dilation of the air cells may invade one or both lungs.

During the last twenty-five years, cancer of the lung has considerably increased in incidence, and is now the most common form of internal cancer among men, in whom it is more likely to occur than in women.

Removal of the lung is usually the preferred treatment for patients with cancer of the lung. Unfortunately, however, detection in a large percentage of cases is too late for this means of control of lung cancer.

Advances in surgical techniques, in anesthetics, and in the use of antibiotics have made surgery on the lungs more possible and successful than it once was, and the death rate has now been decreased. *See also* ASPIRATION; ASTHMA; BRONCHITIS; BRONCHOPNEUMONIA; CHEST; EMPHYSEMA; PLEURISY; PNEUMONIA; TUBERCULOSIS; and Chapter 15, "Respiratory Diseases."

LUPUS ERYTHEMATOSUS, usually a chronic, but sometimes severe acute disease, marked by the appearance of red scaly patches of various sizes on the skin.

The disease may seriously affect the internal organs. Infusion into the joints may occur, and the toxic effects may be extreme, sometimes fatal. This acute form of erythema requires drastic treatment. The use of ACTH and cortisone, and the injection of gold salts have been found effective in many cases. *See also* ERYTHEMA.

LYMPHATIC SYSTEM, an interconnected series of spaces, ducts, and glands within the body which carry lymph, a fluid which is constantly being circulated throughout the body. Lymph is similar in composition to a clear dilute blood plasma without red blood cells. It is formed in the blood capillaries and fills all spaces between the cells of the body. From the intercellular spaces the lymph is emptied into the lymph capillaries, from which it passes into larger lymphatic vessels. These vessels join together to form larger and larger vessels, finally forming the thoracic and right lymphatic ducts which lie immediately under the collarbone.

Lymph nodes are found along the ducts, occurring in groups imbedded in connective tissue. These nodes are small bean-shaped aggregations of lymph nodules and cords between which lymph flows from one lymph vessel to another. The lymph itself contains white blood cells which combat bacteria. The lymph glands filter out infectious material and other debris from the tissues and act as the body's defense against the spread of infection. Lymphatic tissue is also found in the digestive tract; and the lacteals, which absorb fat from digested food, of the small intestines are the smallest form. The circulation of lymph does not depend on the action of the heart, but is accomplished by the movement of body muscles, such as in breathing and walking.

Certain disorders may affect the lymphatic system—for example, infectious mononucleosis and glandular fever in which the lymph nodes become swollen and tender. In agranulocytosis, the production of white blood cells stops. The lymph vessels and glands may become inflamed. Septic sores on toes and fingers may result in acute inflammation of glands in other parts of the body through spread of the infection. Tuberculosis frequently causes inflammation of the lymph glands. Malignant and benign tumors may occur in the lymph glands or the glands may enlarge as a result of malignant growths carried to them from other parts of the body. Cysts often form in the glands when the lymphatic vessels are dilated.

Any disturbance of the lymphatic system must be taken care of by a physician. Proper treatment of the causes of the infection will usually relieve the symptoms affecting the lymph glands. *See also* ELEPHANTIASIS; HODGKIN'S DISEASE; LEUKEMIA.

LYMPHOGRANULOMA VENEREUM, known popularly as bubo, a world-wide virus-produced disease usually spread by sexual contact.

The chief symptom is swelling of the lymph glands following infection. Five to fourteen days after the disease is contracted, a small ulcer, or papule, appears on the sex organs. This may heal within a few days, but frequently a secondary infection results in a larger sore. The infection spreads along the lymphatic ducts and in a short time reaches one of the large lymph glands.

In the early stages, fever, inflammation of the joints, skin rashes, and infection of the brain and dura may be present. Other symptoms are stiffness and aching in the groin, followed by swelling. These swellings, hard and about the size of a walnut, are known as buboes. They may break down and leave a draining abscess but this is rare. Elephantiasis in which the whole vulva may swell sometimes occurs in women, and in more severe cases the whole body may be affected.

After healing, men are generally considered incapable of transmitting the disease, but women may be carriers for years. Although rarely, the disease may be transmitted other than through sexual contact, by way of the mouth, nose, and eyes.

The Frei test may be used to confirm the diagnosis of lymphogranuloma venereum. Injection of a tiny amount of the causative virus, followed by formation of a crusted inflamed area on the skin, is positive proof of the ailment.

The duration of the disease can be controlled successfully by vaccines, made from material taken from infected glands. Sulfa drugs, penicillin, and other antibiotics including terramycin and aureomycin are used; lymphogranuloma is one of the few virus diseases that yields to such treatment. *See also* BUBO.

LYSOL, a proprietary product of the cresol compounds, dark brown in color, oily with a characteristic tarry smell, widely used as an antiseptic. Caustic and poisonous in high concentration, lysol is most effective and safe to use when only a teaspoonful is added to a pint of water.

MADURA FOOT, a chronic fungus infection usually limited to the feet although occasionally it attacks the hands or other parts of the body. This disease was first described by Henry Vandyke Carter while he was working in Madura, India. Madura foot, or mycetoma, is most prevalent in India, China, and Africa, but sporadic cases have been reported in Italy and Greece and the United States.

Madura foot is caused by a number of different fungi which enter the foot through a minor cut or abrasion in the skin. The skin grows discolored and boggy as the fungus eats its way into the deep tissues, forming open sores, and the foot becomes swollen and deformed. The disease progresses slowly, gradually invading the bony structure of the foot and causing crippling deformities. The graphic term, jungle rot, denotes a condition in which deep open sores break down skin tissue, regardless of the cause. The infection is usually confined to the foot.

When treatment is begun early, the ailment is greatly benefited by huge doses of the sulfonamides. Deeper abscesses are removed by curettage.

MAGNESIUM CITRATE. Magnesium is a bluish white, hard but malleable metal, widely present in organic and inorganic nature. As a component of muscles, bones, body fluids, and tissues, it is vital to life. Its salts, magnesium citrate, are used in medicine. Magnesium citrate is a popular mild laxative, which should be taken upon arising in doses prescribed by the doctor.

MALARIA includes a group of diseases which are manifested by periodic attacks of chills, fever, and sweating. The disease is transmitted by the anopheles mosquito in a rather complex manner. A female mosquito must bite a person whose blood already contains both the male and female malaria parasites. These parasites enter the body of the mosquito where they undergo fertilization, the male parasite ejecting small filaments which break loose and come into contact with the female parasite. The fertilized forms then leave the stomach cells and gradually enlarge until finally they rupture into the body cavity of the mosquito and make their way to the salivary glands. When the mosquito bites another person, these parasites pass with the mosquito's saliva and start the development of the parasite in the person who has been bitten. About ten days later, parasites can be observed in the red blood cells of the infected person. This parasite devours the red pigment and iron-containing material; the red cell ruptures and parasites are released which attach themselves to new red cells. There are various other types of the parasite which produce different forms of malaria.

On about the fourteenth day after infection, the person will have backache, muscle soreness, and fever with paroxysms and chills. Paroxysms occur on alternate days when there are two types of the same parasite developing in the blood, which gives the condition a cold, a hot, and a sweating stage. The cold stage is characterized by chills with chattering teeth, uncontrollable shaking, and cold bluish skin. Then comes a high fever followed by sweating, when the temperature drops to normal.

In quartan malaria there is a four-day interval between the sets of symptoms. In falciparum malaria, which has an incubation period of about twelve days, the fever is high and irregular, and bleeding, including blood in the urine, frequently occurs.

The physician determines the type of malaria from a study of the blood and from the symptoms and the order in which they occur. Quinine and camoquin and totaquine are drugs used to prevent malaria. These plus atabrine, quinacrine, chloraquine, and primaquine are used in the treatment of malaria. Prevention of malaria depends ultimately on the control of the anopheles mosquito. In areas where the anopheles is present, swamps must be cleaned out, breeding places sprayed with insecticide, and water not allowed to accumulate. In tropical regions, people who are constantly exposed to malaria should take quinine every day one hour before sunset, screen their beds at night and keep the air moving, and wear suitable protective clothing. Very powerful and effective insect repellents are available today which help in the fight against the spread of the anopheles.

MANIC-DEPRESSIVE PSYCHO-SIS. A psychosis is a serious mental illness and manic-depressive psychosis is a form of such mental disturbance. It is almost as common as schizophrenia, the most frequent mental disorder, and about one-third of all the patients in mental institutions belong to this group. Manic-depressive psychosis may attack at any age, but is more prevalent in the age group between twenty and sixty. Women are more subject than men, comprising about two-thirds of all cases.

Manic-depressive psychosis has been called cyclical insanity, because it is characterized by periodic and alternating cycles of mania and depression. In the manic phase, the person may manifest overabundant energy, incessant activity, and exaggerated well-being. Impulsiveness and motor excitement will be pronounced, and his ideas lofty and unmistakably pleasurable, expressed in incessant talk. His judgment will seem disordered and his ability to make decisions weak. The mood may suddenly change to extreme irritability, temper, and anger, and then he may give advice and criticism to others in an attempt to show his superiority.

As in other psychoses, the afflicted person is apt to have lofty goals. The manic-depressive psychotic imagines that he is an exalted and powerful personality, perhaps a great scientist, actor, king, or savior of mankind. He will aggressively demand attention to his claims, which he may express without cessation. During the manic phase, he may completely change his former moral and ethical standards. In most instances, pronounced eroticism and sometimes alcoholism and drug addiction occur.

Hypomania or lesser mania is a milder form of mania. Here, too, an overabundant energy and quest for incessant activity appear. The person's humor and talk will be boisterous or childish and giggling. While delusions of grandeur are absent, the hypomaniac still manifests an irritating and overdone self-esteem. Outbreaks of anger and irritability are frequent.

The manic phase alternates in manic-depressive psychosis with a painful emotional condition in which the person is dangerously depressed and miserable. In this state he will be self-derogatory, driven to deep despondency by some sense of guilt about often illusory misdeeds and sins. He may contemplate suicide, considering himself unworthy to live. Delusions and hallucinations are habitual, and symptoms such as sluggishness, inability to make decisions, and lack of power of concentration are pronounced. This depressive stage of manic-depressive psychosis may be accompanied by physical symptoms such as constipation, coated tongue, sleeplessness, loss of weight, and many others. Intellectual activity is suppressed while the person is deeply involved in his harrowing delusions, and stupor is not uncommon. Women become antagonistic to sex and men.

Manic-depressive attacks, which may occur originally from great emotional tension, may be short or last for many months. If they are isolated and infrequent, chance for recovery is possible; however, full and complete recovery is rare. *See also* Chapter 22, "Mental Illness."

MARASMUS, a word derived from the Greek *marasmos* or decay, is a disease characterized by progressive wasting of body tissue of infants. It also denotes severe malnutrition due to poor diet or protracted intestinal disorders that prevent proper utilization of food. Only rarely is the underlying cause of marasmus a constitutional disease, such as syphilis or tuberculosis.

The symptoms of marasmus are similar to those of gradual starvation. The infant has a low temperature, loose skin in folds, wasted limbs, large sunken eyes, and a general appearance of old age. Marasmus occurs most frequently in bottle-fed babies, in slum and unsanitary conditions, and in institutions.

Treatment, if in time, may restore the health of some infants, especially those older than six months. Large quantities of mother's milk must be given; if necessary it can be procured from a mother's milk bank. If human milk is not available, powder or evaporated milk may be substituted. Vitamins A and B complex, massages, and an abundance of fresh air have been found helpful.

MARIHUANA, also known as hashish in the Orient, a habit-forming drug. It is the dried leaves and flowers of the Indian hemp plant, usually smoked in cigarettes. Addiction to marihuana is as widespread in the United States as in other countries. Every country in Asia has a centuries-long history of marihuana drug addiction.

The effects of marihuana have been

recognized since the beginning of recorded history—an Assyrian medical tablet in the British Museum refers to hashish as "an intoxicant which cheers the spirits and sharpens the erotic impulse." Vivid descriptions of hashish debauches abound in ancient Arabian literature. Marco Polo in his discription of his travels tells of the desperate band of Persian highwaymen, the Assassins, who initiated new members into their order by a licentious hashish carnival. It has even been suggested that the words assassin and hashish are derived from the same root.

Marihuana or hashish affects its users in many ways, since it stimulates the nervous, respiratory, circulatory, digestive, excretory, and genital systems. The drug clouds the mind and reduces self-control; the person becomes restless and talkative, relaxed and exhilarated with a sense of well-being, followed by drowsiness. Generally difficulty in focusing and sustaining mental attention is noted.

Marihuana has long been a major problem for government narcotic squads, for the Indian hemp plant grows wild in many areas. Smoking the drug in the form of "reefers" has become increasingly prevalent. In 1934, the United States Congress enacted legislation which prescribed almost as severe penalties for the use and sale of marihuana as for narcotics. *See also* DRUG ADDICTION.

MARRIAGE, the physical, personal, and legal union between a man and woman for the establishment of a family. The beginning of marriage is a new experience for both partners. Sexual adjustment must be made and techniques adapted to the needs and preferences of the husband and wife. Although sex is the biological foundation of marriage, many adults are misinformed or confused about it; the family physician can be helpful to the person who feels he needs guidance.

Differences exist between men and women which affect the degree of sexual gratification, and for women especially the success of the sexual life depends in large measure upon the degree of emotional accord enjoyed with her husband. Sex is of course not all of a marriage; but if this area is a source of satisfaction to the husband and wife, success in the other areas will be more easily assured. *See also* CONCEPTION; CONTRACEPTION; IMPOTENCE; ORGASM; STERILITY.

MASSAGE, treating the body by rubbing and kneading. Ordinarily the purpose is to stimulate circulation or to increase suppleness of the muscles. The hands are most often used to massage, though mechanical devices are available.

The type of massage employed depends on the purpose. The simplest massage is a rhythmic stroking motion, applied superficially to relieve pain or induce sleep. To encourage the flow of blood and lymph, the stroking motion is deeper and directed toward the center of the body. This technique is also effective to relax the muscles and reduce swelling, or, when applied in the area of the stomach, to provide a substitute for the normal contraction and relaxation of the stomach muscles and thus stimulate motion in the intestines.

In the squeezing type of massage, the tissue is pulled up and then pressed between the fingers or hands. Alternatively the tissue may be pressed, not between the hands, but between a hand and the bones or muscles. This method is often employed to aid in preventing adhesions, to stimulate circulation, or to induce heat. Circulation may be further encouraged if this deep massage is performed with a vibrating motion. Likewise the induction of heat is enhanced if massage is forceful enough to cause friction between the hands and the tissues.

Another style of massage is percussion. This involves using a hammering action with the fingers, the side of the hands, or with certain instruments.

If massage does not bring about the desired results, medical advice is recommended. Massage is best applied under proper supervision. *See also* OSTEOPATHY; PHYSICAL THERAPY.

MASTITIS, inflammation of the breast; it occurs in various forms and degrees of severity. An injury to the mammary glands can produce an infection by staphylococci or streptococci. The breast becomes swollen, reddened, knotty, and tender to the touch. Pain may be severe and fever high.

The acute form, puerperal (pertaining to childbirth) mastitis, is frequent among nursing mothers, occurring a few days or weeks after delivery. A so-called "caked breast," the result of excessive milk secretion with retention, may precede it. In some instances, chronic mastitis follows the acute form. However, it may be the outgrowth of an injury to the tissues of the breast or due to menstrual disorders, miscarriage, or abortion. Women during menopause are frequently affected. Young girls may suffer a painful swelling and hardening of the breast during puberty. Mastitis at puberty is rarely a serious inflammation and in most cases quickly subsides.

Mastitis must always be diagnosed and treated by a physician. Treatment may involve surgical emptying of abscesses and extraction of milk with a pump. Drugs, such as the sulfonamides and antibiotics, are prescribed to act specifically against the germs. *See also* BREAST.

MASTOID. The mastoid (breast-shaped) bone is a part of the skull just behind the ear. This spongy network of bone connects with the middle ear. Disorders of the middle ear, nose, throat, or upper part of the breathing system may cause infection to spread into the mastoid. When this occurs with inflammation of the bone, the condition, mastoiditis, is dangerous, not only because it may cause permanent damage to the inner ear but because the close proximity of the mastoid tissues to the brain may lead to meningitis, the spread of infection into the membranes around the brain.

Symptoms of mastoid infection include high temperature, pain, and redness behind the ear, and occasionally a stiff neck. Often earache, sore throat, or a cold have preceded the symptoms. Infection of the mastoid may follow measles, scarlet fever, or diphtheria.

Prompt treatment of infections of

the nose, throat, tonsils, and ear with antibiotics has made mastoid infections rare; twenty years ago the condition was common. Treatment of severe mastoid infection may include surgery in which the diseased inner contents of the mastoid bone are removed.

MEASLES, an acute, highly communicable disease, common throughout the world. The characteristic symptoms resemble those of the common cold with fever and the early appearance of a rash on the mucous membranes of the cheeks and lips and later over the entire body. The disease is found everywhere, regardless of climate, race, social or economic status. Epidemics usually occur in late winter, at two-year intervals in large communities and four- to five-year intervals in smaller communities. Everyone is susceptible to measles and the transmission of the disease takes only an infinitesimal dose of the virus. Most of the cases occur among children, adults usually having had it in childhood. However, older people have been known to contract measles in areas where an epidemic appears after a long absence. Measles during pregnancy is apt to cause miscarriage; it has been observed in newborn infants when the mother has had it simultaneously.

Measles is transmitted through secretions from the eyes, nose, and throat by direct contact or droplet infection and is spread through the air by coughing, sneezing, or talking. It may be transmitted from seven to eleven days after a person has contracted it. Transmission is at its highest peak just before the rash appears. Complications that may follow measles do not spread the disease, though they may transmit the secondary infection.

The first symptoms generally resemble a cold, with running nose, sneezing, an irregular fever and chills, pains in the head and back, and watering eyes. There may also be inflammation of the upper respiratory passages and congestion of the mucous membranes of the nose and mouth. A day or two later, bluish white specks, called Koplik's spots, appear opposite the first molar teeth and inside the lower lip. They are pinpoint in size and surrounded by a bright red area. At first there are only a few, but soon the spots increase and run together. Koplik's spots may be seen two or three days before the rash appears. As soon as these spots appear, the person should be isolated, not only to avoid spreading the disease but also to aid his own recovery. Fever will be fairly steady, gradually rising to its height when the rash appears.

The rash, which usually appears over the body about fourteen days after exposure and about three or four days after the fever begins, seldom lasts longer than four or five days. It first appears in the hairline, behind the ears, on the neck and over the forehead, then extends downward, gradually covering the entire body. These tiny red pimples become larger and redder and tend to increase and group together, giving the skin a blotchy appearance. Temperature often ranges between 104° to 105°, the skin itches and burns, the face is puffy, the eyes red and swollen and sensitive to strong light.

A discharge from the nose ensues, as well as a hoarse cough without discharge, and the patient generally feels miserable. When the rash has reached its peak, the fever drops rapidly, the symptoms disappear, the cough lessens, and the patient begins to improve rapidly. As the rash fades and dries, the skin sheds gritty brownish scales.

Uncomplicated measles is not a particularly severe disease, but, like many of the virus infections, it tends to reduce the normal resistance of the body so that the patient becomes susceptible to secondary infections, which may involve the upper respiratory tract, the ears, nose, sinuses, larynx, and lungs. The most serious complication is bronchopneumonia or conjunctivitis which may damage the eyes. At one time tuberculosis was a frequent aftermath of measles, particularly in cases in which prolonged signs of lung involvement and persistent low-grade fever were present. In addition to these secondary invasions by bacteria, another serious complication due to the virus of measles itself is inflammation of the brain or encephalitis. Fortunately this is rare.

In recent years, use of convalescent serum in prevention and treatment of measles has modified the severity of the disease and in some cases averted it successfully. Immune globulin, extracted from normal human placental tissue, and gamma globulin, a substance taken from pooled blood collected by blood banks, have all proved effective in weakening the virulence of the disease.

Of utmost consideration are all measures which will prevent develop-

ment or spread of measles. Children who have been exposed to it should be isolated for fourteen days after their first known contact. If globulin has been given to modify the disease, the child should be isolated for a minimum of eighteen days following the last exposure. Unnecessary exposure should always be avoided, particularly of older infants, preschool-age children, and pregnant women. This is important not only as a preventive of transmitting the disease but also to minimize the incidence of secondary infection.

While a specific drug for treatment of measles is not yet known, the improved methods and drugs used to treat the complications have materially reduced the already low death rate as well as the effects of secondary complications.

If a person has been in contact with measles or in the presence of an epidemic, a physician should be consulted promptly for preventive treatment. When the symptoms appear, the person should be put to bed immediately in a warm, well-ventilated room. He should be fed a light diet, given plenty of fluids, his bowels kept normal, and his eyes protected against strong glaring lights. Drugs or sedation may be prescribed by the doctor to sooth nasal irritations or cough. Warm alcohol or sponge baths are preferable to alleviate fever and aspirin may be given. All activity must be restricted and the period of convalescence prolonged until full strength is regained. As an added precaution, persons caring for the patient should wear an outer garment which can be removed before contact with other people, and hands should be scrubbed on leaving the sickroom. When the disease has subsided, the patient's dishes, linens, bedding, and the entire room should be disinfected. *See also* INFECTIOUS DISEASES; and Chapter 7, "The Process of Infectious Diseases and Immunization of Children."

MEAT, ANIMAL, the flesh of domestic animals, such as cattle, sheep, and pigs, used as food. The flesh of wild animals is usually called game, and of domestic fowl, poultry. In addition, the "fleshy" edible part of other foods, such as fruits and nuts, is known as the meat. Usually meat for human consumption consists of lean or muscular tissue, and gristle or connective tissue. Varying quantities of fat are either plainly visible or present in small particles throughout the meat and between tendons and membranes.

Digestibility of meat does not significantly depend on cuts or on different methods of cooking, and while meat contains less roughage than grain foods, 98 per cent of its proteins and fats are digested.

Meat should be a part of every well-balanced diet. Besides being a good source of carbohydrate, meat supplies the body with minerals and vitamins, such as riboflavin (B_2), thiamine (B_1), and also vitamin (B_{12}). Its high iron content makes it a valuable adjunct in overcoming nutritional anemia. Particularly significant is the protein which meat supplies. Meat, composed almost entirely of animal protein, is one of the best and most complete sources of protein, which is essential to maintain body tissue and to promote growth. High-protein

diets are often prescribed after burns, surgical operations, and infectious diseases.

Most meat to be sold commercially is inspected by the federal government and stamped U.S. Insp'd. The meat packer usually grades the meat, with the rating enclosed in a shield. The grades commonly purchased are prime, choice, good, standard, and commercial, in order of the quality of the grade, prime being the most select, and commercial the lowest grade. Following is a list of calories per pound of meat.

BEEF—all edible portions

Chuck	1005
Loin, Porterhouse steak	1270
Loin, Sirloin steak	1130
Round steak	835
Rump	1325

VEAL

Breast	840
Chuck	610
Legs, cutlets	705

LAMB

Breast or chuck	1350
Loin	1540

PORK

Ribs and Shoulder, chuck	1635
Flank	1280
Ham, fresh	1700
Loin, chops	1655

POULTRY

Chicken, broilers	205
Fowl, as purchased	775
Goose, young, as purchased	1505
Turkey, as purchased	1505
Chicken, gizzard	1075

APPROXIMATE PROTEINS PER POUND

BEEF, Fresh

Chuck, edible portion	19.2%
Loin, Porterhouse steak, edible portion	21.9%
Loin, Sirloin steak, edible portion	18.9%
Round steak, edible portion	20.9%

VEAL, Fresh

Breast, edible portion	20.3%
Cutlets, " "	20.3%
Chuck, " "	19.7%

LAMB, Fresh

Breast, edible portion	19.1%
Loin, " "	18.7%

PORK

Ribs and Shoulder, edible portion	17.3%
Ham, fresh, edible portion	19.5%
Loin chops, edible portion	16.4%
Flank, edible portion	18.3%

POULTRY AND GAME

Chicken broilers, edible portion	25.1%
Fowl, as purchased	13.7%
Turkey, as purchased	16.1%
Chicken, gizzards	24.7%

MEATUS, an opening or passage. The term is applied to various orifices or openings of the body, such as the auditory or external ear, the meatus of the nose which connects the pharynx and the nasal passage, and the urethral meatus through which urine is discharged.

MEDICINE CHEST. Every household should have an orderly, adequately stocked medicine chest—that is, a cabinet or container in which medicines, drugs, bandages, and other related supplies are kept. Too often the family medicine chest is a catchall, and the medicines and drugs it does contain are old or unlabeled or their original purpose forgotten. Drugs wrongly used can do infinite harm, and all old medicines for illnesses since cured should be thrown out. Not only can random taking of medicine be harmful, but many drugs deteriorate and are not safe after a certain time. Every item in the medicine chest should be labeled and, if necessary, dated. It may be a wise idea to keep the cabinet or container locked if there are children in the household, since even a seemingly mild medicine can have fatal results. The key should be kept in a safe place where it can be found promptly. Following are items which most families will want to keep in their medicine cabinets.

Laxatives and cathartics. A wide variety of substances are used as laxatives. Castor oil and epsom salts are not generally advisable, since they are irritants and may drastically disrupt the normal pattern of bowel movement. Mineral oil, a mechanical lubricant, is somewhat less potent; however, if used over a period of time, it may interfere with the absorption of vitamins A and D. Perhaps the safest laxatives are the so-called bulk laxatives. Some persons, however, are sensitive to the natural type, and synthetic bulk producers are more consistent in their action, nonallergenic, and do not swell until they reach the intestine. Other common popular preparations include phenolphthalein, Seidlitz powder, sodium phosphate, milk of magnesia, aromatic cascara, and mineral oils mixed with sugars. A laxative or cathartic should never be taken when the abdomen is painful, since it may cause serious harm—for example, in the case of appendicitis. Persistent use of laxatives will eventually chronically interfere with the normal bowel movements, and is a habit to be avoided.

Pain relievers. Most pain relievers are used for headache, although they are sometimes taken for neuritis, neuralgia, toothache, colds, and pains of unknown origin. Most headache powders purchased commercially contain phenacetin or acetanilid in varying doses. The most common general pain reliever is acetylsalicylic acid, commonly called aspirin, which is usually sold in 5-grain tablets. If kept in a tightly-capped bottle, aspirin will keep indefinitely, except in the tropics. Aspirin does not cure, but will relieve certain types of pain. It acts as both an antipyretic (antifever) drug, and an analgesic (antipain) drug. Various combinations of aspirin are available—for example, with phenacetin and caffein. Although it is one of the safest drugs, serious and even fatal effects from aspirin poisoning point up that no drug is always safe.

Aspirin is available for children in smaller tablets, which are sometimes flavored. This has proved to be a mixed blessing, since children may confuse the aspirin with candy and consume large quantities of it. An editorial in the *Journal of the American Medical Association* has advised against the use of sweetened aspirin and aspirin chewing gum. Hundreds of cases of aspirin poisoning occur each year and usually because through negligence the bottle of aspirin has been left in a place accessible to children.

Most cases of aspirin sensitivity are not serious, but two or three persons out of a hundred have reactions, usually nausea or stomach upset. This is especially likely in those who have allergies or asthmatic conditions, and such persons should be especially cautious in using aspirin.

Sleep-producing drugs. Most of the sleep-producing drugs are chiefly derivatives of barbituric acid—for example, Seconal, Amytal, veronal, Trional, and combinations of barbituric acid with other drugs. These drugs should be used only under medical care, and then extreme caution should be taken to keep them out of the reach of children, and to have the bottle clearly identified.

Narcotics. Among the strongest of medicinal preparations are the narcotics and anesthetics, which should never be used by anyone without a doctor's prescription. A drug that must be administered with a hypodermic syringe should not be kept in the family medicine cabinet. Some persons with diabetes have been taught by their doctor to inject themselves with insulin, and they usually keep the syringe outfit in a special separate place.

Antibiotics. Formerly antibiotics could be obtained only by prescription, but now, in some states and in certain dosages, they can be purchased at a drug store without a prescription. Antibiotic lozenges for mouth infections or sore throats, and bandages medicated with antibiotics are now available.

Any antibiotic preparation should be used with discretion. Locally they can produce definite sensitizing effects and result in irritations far more serious than the one the drug was purchased to cure. Also, taken orally, antibiotics, such as Aureomycin, Terramycin, penicillin, are known at times to produce serious side effects. Any antibiotics that are left over from a prescription should be destroyed; and if, for any reason, old antibiotic preparations are taken and signs of nausea, vomiting, or other unusual symptoms appear, the doctor should be contacted at once.

Antiseptics. Many different antiseptics are available for use on the skin, for cleansing parts of the body, or as a gargle. Iodine, Metaphen, Mercurochrome, Zephiran, and similar preparations are often used.

First aid. Among the materials needed for first aid are adhesive tape of various widths, sterile cotton, sterile gauze bandages, sterile gauze pads, petroleum jelly, zinc oxide ointment, and scissors, which should be kept in the medicine chest exclusively for such purposes. Other first-aid items which may be included are ready-made sterilized bandages to cover small wounds, which can be purchased in a waterproof type and premedicated, and milk of magnesia and sodium bicarbonate (baking soda) which are frequently recommended by doctors as alkalies.

Poisons should never be kept in the family medicine chest, or any chemicals used around the household for bleaching, killing insects and rodents, drycleaning, and similar purposes. Even when children have been cautioned again and again to stay away from such chemicals, accidental poisonings do occur; the rate of accidental poisoning in children under five is 2.6 per 100,000 children. Too often the labels on, for example, cleaning fluid bottles, do not tell of potential dangers or the precautions which should be taken when the solution is used. Many such solutions contain carbon tetrachloride, a toxic chemical. Inhalation of a small amount can poison a child, and be dangerous for an adult.

In addition to first-aid materials, most families will find it desirable and convenient to have a bedpan, glass drinking tube, syringe for giving an enema, atomizer, hot-water bottle, electric pad, ice bag, and sometimes a special device for creating steam, to be medicated with small amounts of tincture of benzoin or other drugs for relief in various types of throat conditions.

The family medicine cabinet should be checked at least four times a year, and all unnecessary items thrown away, such as old razor blades, which should be kept in a special container and then discarded.

Following are several rules to be observed.

1. Do not save poisonous preparations of any kind, unless absolutely necessary. Keep them separate from medicines, and label plainly.

2. Every drug should be clearly labeled, and the correct dose plainly marked.

3. Keep bottles tightly closed;

drugs may concentrate and become dangerous, or evaporate and become useless.

4. Do not keep samples of any patent medicine whose composition is not known.

5. Never keep any opium or morphine preparations in the family medicine chest.

6. Discard all prepared prescriptions when the special purpose for which they were prescribed is past.

7. Read labels carefully, especially again before giving any drug or medicine.

MELANCHOLIA. *See* INVOLUTIONAL MELANCHOLIA.

MELANOSIS, the condition which exists when abnormal deposits of melanin are formed in the blood or placed in organs or surfaces. Melanins are metabolic, dark brownish, granular pigments which are produced by the activity of cells. As a normal pigmentary matter, melanins occur in hair, skin, or muscles. Pigmentation of the skin or some internal organs is not always associated with a medical disorder. Tanning or freckling result from exposure of the skin to the ultraviolet rays of the sun, or from radium therapy. Prolonged treatment with certain chemicals—such as arsenic, for example—will also result in skin pigmentation. The nipples of the breast and other parts of the body may be pigmented during pregnancy.

Melanosis, however, is sometimes related to serious ailments. In Addison's disease, some skin disorders, and ochronosis, a discoloration of cartilage and allied tissues, melanosis is a symptom. It also occurs in pellagra and other disorders resulting from vitamin deficiencies.

Tumors containing melanins, the so-called malignant melanomas or melanocancers are especially serious. They originate in discolored flattened moles and spread, adding pigmentation to other parts of the body. In such cases, melanuria is pronounced. Since pigments may be involved in all sorts of tissues, the prefix "melano" may also refer to the pigment in sweat (melanidrosis), to the pigment in the menstrual flow (melanorrhagia), to the pigments in the mucous membranes of the mouth (melanoplakia), and to the black fungus growths (melanomyces). *See also* FRECKLES; SUNBURN.

MELANURIA, the condition in which urine takes on a brownish black color because large quantities of pigments are present.

MEMORY, the capacity to retain and revive impressions, to recall or recognize previous experience. Some recollections seem to appear without any exertion on the part of the person, whereas sometimes a recollection will entail a certain amount of mental activity. It is probably true that every experience and impression is permanently recorded in some way on the brain; however, intervening happenings and thoughts "block" or cover the great majority of impressions, which, from a practical point of view, are "forgotten." Forgotten impressions are sometimes recalled in specialized circumstances, such as under hypnosis.

Very little is known about the way in which memory operates. Some information has come from experiments on the brain. For instance, persons who have tumors of the frontal lobes of the brain suffer some loss of memory, particularly of recent events. Hardening of the arteries and diminished circulation of the blood associated with old age also have an influence on memory.

Memory is sometimes spoken of as "good" or "bad." The amount and accuracy with which a person can remember is usually a matter of his degree of concentration. A person preoccupied with his own introspective thoughts rather than with what is happening around him will often have a "bad" memory. *See also* AMNESIA.

MENIERE'S DISEASE, a chronic ailment in which the major symptoms are dizziness, deafness, and noises in one or both ears. It is usually due to an interference with the function of the inner ear or labyrinth, and is frequently accompanied by nausea and vomiting. It begins in late life and affects both sexes. This group of symptoms is often called aural vertigo or Ménière's syndrome, since it was first noted in 1861 by the French physician, Prosper Ménière.

The disease begins with mild deafness and head noises, called tinnitus, which are high-pitched and hissing, roaring, or ringing. The noises are generally heard on one side of the head only, and vary in intensity from day to day. The vertigo, which is a strong feeling of swaying, rocking, or turning, begins abruptly, and may last from a few minutes to several hours, and is generally associated with nausea and vomiting. It recurs at long, irregular intervals. Complete rest helps to lessen the severity of the attacks. Impairment of hearing is progressive, and on rare occasions, during an acute attack of dizziness, there may be a rolling of the eyes from side to side, known as nystagmus.

Treatment of this condition is still experimental. It includes a low-salt diet and daily doses of ammonium chloride. Antihistaminic drugs, Dramamine, Marezine, and Bonamine, are now being used with fairly good results. The course of the disease varies with each patient. There have been long periods of relief in many cases.

As in many disorders which recur periodically, emphasis in treatment is placed upon giving the patient a feeling of complete reassurance and confidence; and this, together with well-regulated living, sufficient rest, and moderate sedatives such as phenobarbital, frequently bring about noticeable improvement. Psychotherapy is recommended when extreme emotional tension is present.

When the attacks are persistent and do not yield to treatment, surgery is employed. The eighth cranial nerve, which supplies the branches to the ear, is cut. In those instances where hearing is present on only one side, especially if deafness has already begun in the opposite ear, the nerve is not completely cut, so that as much hearing as possible may remain. This operation has helped relieve the patient of vertigo in almost all cases, except, of course, those in which it originally started on both sides.

MENINGES, the three membranes which cover the brain and spinal cord. They include the pia mater, which contacts the cord and the brain substance; the dura mater, which lines the spinal canal and the cranial cavity; and the arachnoid, a substance resembling a fine web which is between the pia mater and the dura mater.

Meningitis is an inflammation of these meninges. The prefix "mening" generally denotes disorders that affect the membranes, such as meningioma, a tumor in the meninges, or meningism, an irritation of the meninges. *See also* MENINGITIS.

MENINGITIS, an inflammation of the meninges, the membranes covering the brain and spinal cord, caused by infection of the cerebrospinal fluid by various microorganisms. The term is, however, usually applied to an epidemic form, caused by the meningococcus.

The doctor diagnoses meningitis not only from the history of the patient, which may indicate that he has been in contact with the infection, and from the symptoms, but also by obtaining specimens of the spinal fluid which are studied for the presence of germs and for other changes which indicate infection and inflammation. Occasionally examinations are made of the blood to find out whether or not there is a meningococcemia, which means germs of meningitis in the blood.

The symptoms of meningitis arise from the changes that the germs and their poisons produce in the tissues of the nervous system. During the period of invasion, sore throat, dull-ness, fever, chills, rapid pulse, and a general soreness of the body indicate that an infection is present. Then a rash of pinpoint-sized red spots or even large spots appears over the body. In the stage when the infection has spread to the nervous system, severe pain is felt, with intolerable headaches, vomiting, and even delirium and convulsions.

The conquest of meningitis is one of the great triumphs of medicine. Before the discovery of a serum which could be used against meningitis, the death rate used to be 80 or 90 out of every 100 cases. Sulfa drugs, antibiotics, and other advances in treatment have reversed the situation so that today recovery is the rule and death the exception, even in the most stubborn form of the disease, tuberculous meningitis, a variety caused by the tuberculosis germ. Medicine may well be within sight of a meningitis recovery rate of 100 per cent. Because of the many possible complications, hospital care is necessary for persons with meningitis. *See also* CEREBRAL MENINGITIS.

MENOPAUSE, or, more popularly, change of life, the characteristic physical changes which most women undergo between the ages of forty-five and fifty, though sometimes earlier or later. Early onset of menstruation is usually associated with late appearance of the change of life.

The basis of the retrogression is the gradual cessation of the secretion of certain major endocrine glands. The most noticeable aspect is the gradual or abrupt disappearance of menstruation. Loss of sexual desire and sexual activity are rarely involved. Not only do the ovaries, the female sex glands, become relatively inactive, but other changes take place in the body. The spleen, the lymphatic system, and the intestines are affected, at least slightly.

The manner in which the changes of menopause take place is subject to tremendous variation among women. With some it occurs quickly and with only minor disturbances. With others, however, the change of life lasts three or four years, accompanied by much difficulty. The most troublesome factors sometimes associated with the menopause are mental depression, heightened irritability, and excitability. Unless these are extreme, however, little medical treatment is necessary. Nevertheless, mental difficulties may develop at this time and then medical advice is desirable.

The most common physical symptom is the hot flush, which sweeps the entire body with sudden warmth and perspiration, then leaves it chilly. Flushes occur without perceptible reason or often in association with excitement. Itching skin and constipation of the bowels may be noticed but are readily controlled, and heart palpitations, headache, dizziness, and insomnia are not unusual.

Most of the unpleasant developments of menopause are of minor consequence, and these, and others of a more serious nature, can usually be controlled with hormones. Because of the complications which may be involved and the long duration of change, medical supervision is helpful. The same symptoms may characterize other developments within the body and demand prompt medical attention when they occur.

Men often experience many of the unpleasant symptoms of menopause, related to retrogression of the sex glands. *See also* MENSTRUATION.

MENORRHAGIA, the loss of an exceptional amount of blood at the monthly menstrual periods, in contrast to metrorrhagia in which an excessive flow of blood occurs between menstrual periods. Several possible causes have been found for this uterine bleeding, including poor functioning of hormones involved in the menstrual cycle, poor blood clotting, an unusual condition of the blood, or some emotional or psychological factor.

A physician must be consulted to diagnose the cause. Among successful therapeutic measures employed are complete bed rest and drugs to relieve anxiety and to bring about contractions of the womb. Hormones, such as estrogen, progesterone, and androgen, have also been used successfully.

MENSTRUATION, the periodic flow of blood experienced by women in the years of sexual maturity and the associated changes that occur in the body at this time.

When the discharge ceases, the lining of the uterus or womb begins to thicken and continues the process for a week or longer. In the next stage, lasting about two weeks, the lining of the womb becomes engorged, in readiness to receive a fertilized egg. Approximately two weeks before the regular menstrual flow begins the ovary releases an egg. If the egg is not fertilized and pregnancy has not taken place, by the end of the cycle the womb lining, called the endometrium, breaks down, alterations in the blood vessels occur, and the menstrual flow washes away the residue.

Characteristics peculiar to this cycle vary greatly in different women. Although the average period is exactly four weeks or 28 days, some women complete the cycle in three weeks and some take as long as five. In others, irregularity may be usual. Although the age of sexual maturity is usually between the twelfth and the sixteenth years, development earlier or later is not abnormal.

Slight variations in the individual cycle are not significant, but sudden major changes, such as complete cessation of menstruation in the absence of pregnancy, should receive prompt medical attention. Suspension of the menstrual period may be caused by a variety of factors. Undernourishment and associated disturbances such as anemia, or severe infections like tuberculosis, rheumatic or typhoid fever may be responsible. Disorders of the pituitary gland or thyroid gland or the ovaries themselves may be involved. Two ovarian secretions or hormones, estradiol and progesterone, are the chief regulators of the menstrual cycle, and the ovaries in turn are controlled to some extent by the pituitary.

Conspicuous delay in the onset of menstruation in a young woman should be investigated by a physician. Although nothing more serious than personal variation may be involved, other difficulties may be responsible. Delayed development, if it persists, may eventually lead to psychological changes, rendering normal childbirth impossible.

Menstrual pain may be caused by such factors as a narrow cervix, the passageway from the womb, by fibroid tumors in the uterus, by cysts, or by variations in the position of the uterus. Most of these conditions can be remedied by a physician. Pain and discomfort which sometimes accompany menstruation may often be relieved by simple measures such as mild sedatives, application of heat, and plenty of rest and sleep. Nevertheless, a physician should be consulted if these remedies are not effective. Glandular substances, to modify the behavior of the mechanisms involved, or the use of more potent pain-relieving drugs may be necessary. Some drugs are harmful if not employed under medical supervision and milder ones may become habit-forming if care is not exercised.

Menstruation is a normal physiological function, and is not concerned, as some suppose, with ridding the body of "poisons." Unless special factors are involved that prompt medical advice to the contrary, young women need vary only slightly their ordinary routines. Violent and competitive athletics are not advisable or should be closely controlled because of the general stress they impose on the body, and bathing need not be interrupted. Swimming may cause extra blood to be lost, but there is rarely any risk of infection from the water itself. *See also* DYSMENORRHEA; MENORRHAGIA; MENOPAUSE; METRORRHAGIA; and Chapter 11, "Feminine Hygiene."

MENTAL DISEASES AND DISORDERS. *See* Chapter 22, "Mental Illness."

METABOLISM. *See* BASAL METABOLISM.

METASTASIS, a process in which primary agents or cells, through blood vessels or lymph channels, transfer the seat of a disease from one part of the body to another. For example, tumors of one organ may spread to the brain, especially from a focus in the lungs and breasts. Cancer in any part of the body may metastasize—that is, transfer—from the kidney, uterus, prostate, or breast and become secondary cancer in another part of the body. The condition is dangerous since it can become widespread before any symptoms are apparent.

Another example of metastasis is the wandering course of acute rheumatism, which has the tendency to involve the lining of the heart and the pericardium, the membranous sac which it envelops. In mumps, the testicles of males or ovaries of females may be involved, as a result of metastasis.

METICORTEN. *See* CORTISONE.

METRITIS. In medicine, diseases of the uterus are referred to by the prefix "metro," denoting relation to the womb. Metritis is an infection of the uterus by gonococci or other organisms. A metroscope is an instrument used for examination of the uterus.

METRORRHAGIA, a hemorrhage from the uterus between menstrual periods; it may be a sign of a serious disorder. Full examination and treatment by a physician is desirable. The excessive flow of blood between menstrual periods is often related to disorders in the womb and pelvis, and sometimes to acute fevers and glandular conditions. *See also* MENSTRUATION.

MIGRAINE, commonly called "sick headache," has an age-old history dating back to the ancient Greeks. The name is believed to be derived from the Greek word *emikrania,* meaning half head, which became *mikrania* and eventually migraine. The complaint is widespread, usually beginning some time around puberty and lessening in late middle age. Migraine is more common in women, and often more than one member of a family suffers from it.

Certain features distinguish migraine from other types of headache. It is limited to one side of the head, recurs periodically, and for each person follows a rather consistent pattern, so that it can often be predicted where the headache will begin, how severe it will be, and how long it will last. The headache is described as a throbbing, aching pain, limited to the forehead, temple, or back of the head. In some cases it seems to arise from the back of the upper teeth and strikes the face and the area below the eye, or it may spread behind the angle of the jaw, reaching down the neck and into the shoulders. This pattern of pain is often accompanied by an unusual throbbing in the neck. In some instances the first symptoms are not confined to the head, but instead the person will suffer pain in the abdomen, chest, or arm, or an attack of vomiting or diarrhea, or a passing fever. A frequent accompaniment to the migraine headache is a disturbance in vision, which may take the form of temporary blindness, blinding flashes of light, or a general blurring of vision. These symptoms disappear as the headache abates.

Migraine, primarily a tension headache, is believed to result from continued muscle contraction which causes distention of the blood vessels in the brain. The general tightening of the body associated with anxiety and emotional tension contributes in most cases to the preliminary symptoms—the tingling sensations in the hands and feet, the impairment of vision, and noises in the ears or mental depression.

In the treatment of migraine, much emphasis is now placed on prevention of the attack. At the first indication of its approach, steps are taken to avert the headache or reduce its severity. Complete quiet, a dark room, hot or cold applications to the head and a hot-water bottle at the feet are often helpful. Aspirin and ordinary analgesics give little or no relief once the headache has begun. Histamine and intramuscular injections of ergotamine tartrate, administered by a physician, have been effective.

The psychological factor is of primary significance in treatment of migraine. The patient must feel that he is receiving the best possible care and that his physician has a thorough understanding of those emotional factors in his background and environment which may be at the root of his condition. Patients with migraine headaches almost invariably fit into a common pattern. They are tense, driving, rigid in their standards, conscientious, and constantly striving for perfection. The treatment of migraine must include and evaluate all the factors that may give rise to the disorder. The patient must be made to understand the nature of his drives and how these create frustration and anxiety. Psychotherapy, a long-term project in these cases, has yielded fruitful results and promises to be even more successful in the future.

MILK, the whitish liquid secreted from the mammary glands of all mammals; it is the only natural food, intended for the very young, which comes straight from the living body. Nature provides it in abundance, and more than eighty different animal sources have been classified.

Milk has always been highly esteemed and from time immemorial many nourishing, healing, and spiritual qualities were attributed to it. Mother's milk was long considered the only suitable food for an infant, and children were breast fed for three years or longer before animals were domesticated and the milk of cows, goats, camels, and sheep able to be substituted for that of the mother. The ancients believed that without the milk of the mother a child could not possibly survive. In the seventeenth century, the famous Dutch chemist, Jean Baptiste van Helmont, proved that mother's milk was not essential for the child, and today many substitutes are available.

Milk is often called a food of near perfection. It furnishes proteins to replace and repair body tissues, it supplies minerals such as calcium to build sound bones and teeth and to perform other functions, it is a good source of natural sugar and of vitamins A, C, D, B₁, and B₂, and it is abundant in fats which are more easily digested than any other edible fat.

Chemically milk is a watery compound of milk sugar, casein, albumin, and ash, with suspended fat globules. When the water is removed, the dry matter is milk solids. Richness of milk is related to the proportion of these solids. About four ounces of nutritional value are found in a quart of milk. Standards for marketed milk, adopted in different states, vary somewhat, but on the average are 12.5 per cent of solids and at least 3 per cent of fat. Most milk on the market has been pasteurized. Some nutritional experts feel that pasteurization affects the nutritional qualities of milk only slightly, while others feel that some of the vitamins C and B complex are lost and minerals precipitated and rendered less soluble. Today much of the milk supply is sold in homogenized form, involving a special process in which cream is distributed evenly throughout the milk.

Dried milk is one of the forms now widely used, particularly since it is now available in a form which is instantly soluble in water. By the method of preparation, dried milk is free from danger of bacterial contamination. In dried milk, less than 2 per cent of moisture remains. The fat, sugar, and protein of the milk are not chemically changed, and the food value is just about the same as that of fresh milk, except for vitamin C, much of which may be lost in the drying process. In addition to dried milk, dried skim milk, in which the butterfat content is much less, is available.

Evaporated milk is fresh milk from which the water has been evaporated to a point where it contains not less than 7.9 per cent of milk fat and not less than 25.9 per cent of total milk solids. Condensed milk is a liquid made by evaporating a mixture of sweet milk and refined sugar or corn sugar so that the sweetened condensed milk contains not less than 28 per cent of the total milk solids and not less than 8.5 per cent of milk fat. Sugar is used to prevent spoilage.

Canned whole milk which does not need to be refrigerated either in transit or storage is the latest milk product to be marketed. Bacteria-free, the sealed milk will keep at least six months. When served chilled, it tastes much like regular milk and has the same food value.

When fresh milk is not available, or in places where the available fresh milk does not meet proper sanitary standards, canned or dried milk is certainly preferable to doing without milk. While medical authorities recommend that the adult diet include milk, it does not necessarily have to be consumed plain, but can be used in combination with other foods. Some persons cannot digest milk easily and in some cases milk may act as an outright toxin. In spite of its stronger taste, some people prefer goat's milk. It is considered to be more easily digested, because its fat globules are smaller so that finer curds are formed in the first stages of digestion. *See also* CHILD CARE; FEEDING, BREAST.

MINERALS. *See* CALCIUM; GOITER; IRON; NUTRITION.

MISCARRIAGE. *See* ABORTION.

MONGOLISM, a type of idiocy, with some similarities to myxedema and cretinism. The name apparently derives from the slightly oriental look, due to the obliquity of the eye slit, mongoloids have. However, mongoloids occur throughout the world. Three mongoloids are born in every thousand births, all resembling one another. They are small, rarely reaching the height of a normal twelve-year-old child. They have broad faces with flat or stubby noses, and an open, apparently undeveloped mouth with large protruding lips. Their legs and arms are abnormally short, the hands thick and the muscles flabby. In most instances the senses are deficient, with weak eyesight, impaired hearing, and an undeveloped sense of smell. Mongoloids have speech difficulties and very limited vocabularies and usually are only able to utter unintelligible sounds. They reach puberty exceedingly late and may learn to walk as late as the age of eleven or twelve. Frequently mongoloids show little or no interest in their environment, live in a stupor, and seem unable to perform even simple tasks or to take care of themselves. Thus their retardation is pronounced enough for them to be considered true idiots.

Often organic defects are present. Mongoloids may have a faulty circulatory system, or underdeveloped brain, liver, and kidney. Physical weakness and a susceptibility to lung and intestinal infections have always been high contributing factors to the high death rate among mongoloids before the age of maturity. However, antibiotics and other drugs have increased their life span considerably.

The cause of mongolism is not known, but some medical authorities believe that it is an interaction and interrelation of various factors rather than a single cause. Hereditary factors have not been established as related to mongolism. Since mongoloids are prenatal casualties, they can be considered as part of the broader problem of congenital anomalies.

A specific cure for mongolism is not known. Even under the most ideal circumstances, mongoloids will only become about 30 per cent normal. Yet the attitude that nothing can be done and that efforts are useless is rather severe. Glandular remedies and calcium phosphate are used; but the greatest help is patience, compassion, and love. Dr. Thomas Benda, an authority on this subject and author of *Mongolism and Cretinism,* reports that mongoloids can learn to do simple manual chores such as household or farm work. He points out that they learn by imitating others. *See also* CRETINISM; FEEBLE-MINDEDNESS; MYXEDEMA.

MONILIASIS, a disease caused by a yeastlike fungus, Candida albicans, and occurring throughout the world, among all races and ages, and in both sexes.

The fungus causes a wide range of infections, from mild disorders of the skin and mucous membranes of the mouth or vagina, to invasion of the deeper tissues, particularly the bronchi, lungs, or meninges. The fungus is widespread in nature, and has been found in the normal mouth, throat, and gastrointestinal tract, as well as in patients with long-standing diseases, in which the wasted tissues offer a good medium for the growth of this organism.

The most common infection, oral thrush, is an acute inflammation of the mouth, tongue, gums, or pharynx, often found in undernourished children and during the first few weeks in infant life. It is highly contagious. Another variety is vaginal moniliasis, which often occurs during pregnancy and in diabetics. Monilia infection of the skin of the hands often develops in bakers, waiters, bartenders, housewives, and others whose hands are softened from continual soaking in water.

The symptoms vary with the location and the intensity of the infection, from creamy whitish patches in the mucous membranes to fever, cough, abscess formation, and meningitis.

The infection generally responds to treatment. Alkaline mouthwashes or irrigations with dilute solutions of gentian violet clear up infections of the mouth. Skin infections have been controlled by potassium permanganate soaking, and daily application of an ammoniated mercury ointment. Nystatin (Mycostatin), a new antibiotic which is the first of these drugs to be effective against this fungus infection without causing undesirable reactions, has brought encouraging results.

MONONUCLEOSIS, INFECTIOUS, a virus infection which causes a swelling of the lymph glands and changes in the white blood cells. The condition occurs in epidemic form as well as in scattered cases, most commonly in people between the ages of ten and thirty-five. Recent research has demonstrated passage of the virus in saliva during kissing.

Some five to fifteen days after exposure to the disease, there may be a flulike feeling of malaise, fatigue, and headache. Fever develops and the lymph glands, especially those of the neck, become enlarged, giving the condition its common name, glandular fever. Sore throat is generally present.

The condition develops in many different ways. Sometimes skin eruptions with discolored rashes are perceptible; the liver may be affected, causing a jaundiced appearance of the skin; and occasionally the heart, lungs, and central nervous system are involved. The spleen is also frequently enlarged. In still other cases, all the symptoms may pass unnoticed. Infectious mononucleosis is manifested by characteristic changes in the blood, an increase in the white blood cells and some changes in their structure.

Infectious mononucleosis usually runs its course within three to six weeks, and recovery is generally uncomplicated and complete. Occasionally the spleen and the lumph nodes may remain enlarged for some time after the other symptoms have disappeared.

Bed rest and limitation of activities are considered essential and in severe cases may have to be prolonged, even after all fever or acute symptoms have subsided. Hot salt gargles or throat irrigations are often given to relieve sore throat. Special diets are usually prescribed when jaundice develops. Aureomycin and chloramphenicol have recently been used, and may be effective in controlling the condition.

MORON. *See* FEEBLE-MINDEDNESS.

MORPHINE. Of the approximately twenty alkaloids in opium, morphine, a glossy colorless crystalline narcotic base, is the chief one and largely responsible for the effects of opium. As morphine acts reliably and quickly and is especially suited for hypodermic use, medicine employs it widely as a pain reliever. Morphine can be habit-forming. *See also* DRUG ADDICTION.

MOSQUITO, an insect, the female of which has a long proboscis with which it can puncture the skin of man and animals to draw blood. Some species transmit certain diseases, such as malaria, yellow fever, dengue, and some forms of filariasis.

The anopheles, which carry malaria, usually lay their eggs in fresh water which has surface vegetation, although some also breed in polluted water or marshes. The aëdes, which carry yellow fever, are usually found breeding about dwellings, as are the culex, which carry the filaria worm.

The primary protective measure against mosquitoes is to prevent their breeding. This involves getting rid of stagnant water, draining and filling pools and marshes, covering wells, open cisterns, water-filled barrels or tubs. Chemicals are used in large-scale mosquito control, and DDT is effective against the larvae of all mosquitoes but must be carefully employed since it is toxic to wildlife.

DDT sprays are also effective around and in the house. Every home should have drains and windows effectively screened. People living in regions where mosquitoes are prevalent should wear protective clothing and use repellents such as dimethyl phtholate, which is available as a cream. *See also* DENGUE; MALARIA; YELLOW FEVER.

MOTION SICKNESS, a condition produced in some persons when they are in a moving boat, car, bus, airplane, elevator, swing, or other conveyance. The exact cause of motion sickness has not been established, but it is thought that the semicircular canals in the internal ear which are associated with balance are involved, and the senses of sight, smell, taste, and hearing also seem to be factors. Characteristic symptoms are nausea, headache, dizziness, and vomiting.

Certain conditions aggravate the tendency to motion sickness—for example, a stuffy unventilated enclosure, unpleasant odors, or irritating or loud noises. More people become sick during the day than the night, some persons are sick when they ride backwards but not when they ride forwards, and reading or other close use of the eyes will sometimes be contributory. Persons with chronic infections of the sinuses and of the ears are more likely to suffer from airsickness than others.

The best and most effective drugs now available for prevention or treatment of motion sickness are Marezine, Bonamine, and Dramamine. Marezine does not bring on as much drowsiness as the other drugs and its effect is almost immediate. It lasts about four hours and should be taken fifteen minutes before departure. Bonamine lasts an entire day, but, like Dramamine, is apt to cause drowsiness. Dramamine is excellent for quieting the nerves and therefore of benefit to nervous travelers and persons with organic conditions in whom vomiting might be injurious. For severe cases of vomiting, the doctor may prescribe a combination of Dramamine and Marezine, which is administered in the form of rectal suppositories.

Several measures can be taken to help prevent motion sickness. When riding in smaller vehicles, sitting low near the center of gravity subjects the person to as little motion as possible. Children may sit on the floor of a car. In an airplane, a left-hand window should be avoided, since most turns and banks are made to the left. Rich, heavy, and gas-forming foods should not be eaten before beginning a trip. It is a good idea to eat moderately and not overload the stomach, and keep alcoholic beverages at a minimum. If symptoms of motion sickness appear during flight, the person should slide down the seat as far as possible with his head and neck supported. In severe cases of motion sickness, ample bed rest is advisable, and a plentiful intake of fluids, intravenously if necessary. The person susceptible to motion sickness should be kept warm, but make sure he gets plenty of fresh air at all times. Adequate sleep before and during the trip will also help stave off motion sickness.

MOUNTAIN SICKNESS, an illness of discomfort suffered by those who climb high mountains. Most people are accustomed to living at altitudes of less than 5,000 feet above sea level, and at altitudes of 12,000 feet or more they are likely to undergo radical physical changes. For example, as the oxygen pressure goes down, an increase is likely in the depth and rhythm of breathing, and also in the number of red blood cells. At the same time, the hemoglobin, the red coloring matter in the blood, will probably take up more and more of the oxygen for its use.

A lack of sufficient oxygen is the cause of mountain sickness. The symptoms include dizziness, headache, vomiting, and difficulty in thinking, reading, writing, hearing, and seeing. Nosebleed may also occur in advanced cases, and the temperature is likely to rise. The person may suffer a weakness in the limbs so pronounced that he will find it difficult to continue walking or climbing. The need to keep the tissues supplied with oxygen may also increase the pulse rate.

Treatment of mountain sickness is primarily a matter of slowing down the entire body function until the person has learned the technique of accommodating his body to the higher altitudes.

MOUTH. The mouth is the opening through which animal or man takes in food, or the cavity containing or the parts including the masticating apparatus. The mouth consists of the vestibule, which is the space between the cheeks and teeth and the cavity of the mouth proper behind the teeth. The roof of the mouth is formed by the hard palate and the floor of the mouth is occupied by the tongue. The large salivary glands, known as the parotids, open into the vestibule and are on each side, and there are also numerous small salivary glands. The whole cavity of the mouth is lined with mucous membrane. Saliva moistens the mouth, enables the food to be rolled into a plastic mass, and lubricates the food. Saliva also cleanses the mouth of bacteria and food particles.

The mouth is one of the most vulnerable areas of the body as regards disease-producing organisms. It is also affected by disturbances of nutrition, endocrine and metabolism balance of the body.

MULTIPLE SCLEROSIS, one of the commonest disorders of the nervous system. This disease is marked by interference with muscular movements which are finally lost. Degeneration and scarring of the nervous tissue develop very slowly, and outward symptoms of multiple sclerosis appear only gradually over the years. Symptoms depend on how and where the nervous system is damaged. Frequently the first symptom is a gradual failure of the leg muscles. Leg movements become jerky and spastic and eventually paralysis occurs. Another common symptom is the slowing down of speech. The person talks in a monotone, and each syllable is uttered with great effort and difficulty. The hands tremble, especially when a purposeful movement is attempted. Sometimes, too, the head tends to shake. Those suffering with multiple sclerosis generally maintain a good frame of mind, even when the disease reaches an advanced state. Occasion-

ally they become depressed and emotionally and mentally disturbed, but this is not characteristic.

The rate of development varies in all cases. However, eventually the basic functions, such as sight, hearing, and digestion, are involved, and constant nursing becomes a necessity. Sometimes this point is not reached for many years.

As yet, nothing is known that will arrest or cure the disease. Nevertheless, the adequacy of the care given can make a real difference. General and medical care must be properly given in order to secure any relief. Also, the patient can be protected from those conditions which are especially threatening to his condition. Only with such meager methods can the effects of the basic disorder be held to the minimum at this time.

Medical researchers are still working to determine whether or not a virus infection or inflammation coming from some toxin is responsible for multiple sclerosis. No organism has yet been found to which it can be attributed. There are instances in which the disease makes its appearance after childbirth or a major operation, but apparently this is a matter of coincidence. No special hereditary factor seems to be involved. It generally appears before the age of forty. *See also* Chapter 23, "The Neuromuscular and Neurological Disabilities."

MUMPS, an acute contagious disease of early winter and spring. It is more dangerous to adults than to children. Mumps usually attacks children between five and fifteen years of age and is rare among infants of less than ten months of age. While complications are serious, they occur in only about one out of a hundred cases. The commonest complications, according to a report of the U. S. Public Health Service, are "inflammation of the sex glands, sometimes causing sterility in men, and inflammation of the brain. Mumps may also lead to deafness, inflammation of other glands or kidney disease." However, mumps is usually such a mild disease that approximately a third of those who contract it recover without having definitely known that they have had it.

Mumps is caused by a tiny virus, the smallest form of infective organism. The mumps virus, which was only definitely isolated in 1937, is larger than those causing poliomyelitis, influenza, and yellow fever and smaller than those causing rabies, cowpox, and typhus.

Mumps is a communicable disease, though not as contagious as measles and chickenpox. The mumps virus is found in discharges of the nose and mouth, most frequently in the saliva, and is spread to others by personal contact or contaminated objects. Usually a person has mumps only once in a lifetime, since the first attack gives the body protective substances against subsequent attacks. Cases are known, however, in which the disease has occurred two or even three times.

The first symptoms of mumps appear from twelve to twenty-six, but usually eighteen, days after exposure. Usually pain under the ear is preceded by chills, fever, headache, and loss of appetite. Vomiting and nosebleeding may occur, with gradual swelling of the gland in front of and below the ear and along the angle of the jaw. The parotid gland of the cheek is the most commonly affected, and the technical term for mumps is parotitis. The face of the patient becomes puffy, and usually the swelling is confined to first one side of the face for a few days and later both sides. The pain increases when food is swallowed. The temperature may reach 101° to 104° during the second or third day. Fever and swelling will subside within a week or ten days.

While treatment of mumps is not specific, it is simple. The patient should be kept in bed. His mouth must be kept clean, and an antiseptic mouthwash and gargle is of great value, especially when tonsils and throat congestion tend to aggravate the symptoms. Elimination of the bowels can be regulated with mild laxatives. A soft diet including broths, gruel, soft-boiled eggs, and custards, but especially liquid foods, is given while the temperature is about normal. Hot compresses, more soothing than cold, applied locally will make the patient more comfortable, as will sponging with hot water and keeping the face warm and protected from chills.

Isolation of all mumps patients is now recommended. Those persons who nurse them should keep away from their faces, since most infections come from the nose and mouth, and it is also advisable to wear a mask in the sickroom.

Fortunately few persons die of mumps. The rare but dreaded complications usually develop as the swollen glands in the face subside. Pain and swelling may evolve in the testes of the male and, on rare occasions, in the ovaries and breasts of the female. A form of meningitis may result and middle-ear congestion may lead to deafness. Other exceptional complications which may occur in both sexes are pancreatitis, optic neuritis, facial paralysis, and permanent enlargement and dysfunction of the parotid gland.

In 1945, researchers, adapting the mumps virus to eggs, developed a mumps vaccine which has been available since 1950. It is not particularly significant for children who have not reached puberty, since mumps in children is usually mild, and therefore routine immunization is not recommended. The vaccine is sometimes indicated for children and young adults who live in close quarters with persons having or likely to have mumps. For adults, however, in whom mumps can be a serious illness, the vaccine may be paramount. *See also* Chapter 7, "The Process of Infectious Diseases and Immunization of Children."

MUSCLE, an organ composed of muscle tissue, which causes movement of some part of the body because of its ability to contract. Muscle is also the muscle tissue, which is made up of individual muscle fibers or cells. It can be classified as nonstriated (smooth) or striated, according to its appearance under a microscope; as body, skeletal, or cardiac muscle, according to its location in the body; and as either voluntary or involuntary. For example, the intestinal muscles are unstriated involuntary muscles.

Muscle tissue enjoys an ample blood supply, since in doing its work it requires much energy and causes a rapid turnover of food materials, more than other body tissue. Muscles also are well supplied with nerves, both motor, for movement, and sensory, for feeling. Besides controlling the movements of muscle, the nerve cells in the spinal cord also control nutrition; and if the cells become diseased, or the fibers are cut or fail to function in any way, the muscle atrophies from disuse.

Contraction of muscles calls for energy and consequent production of waste in the form of lactic acid. This causes the tiredness following strenuous work or exercise. If the muscles are forced beyond the limits of endurance, muscle fatigue ensues, which calls for a period of rest. During rest, waste products are eliminated from the tissues and normal muscle activity is restored.

Skeletal muscles are attached to their respective bones by tendons, which are a specialized form of muscle. Some tendons, such as the hamstring tendons at the back of the knee, and the Achilles' tendon above the heel, are near the surface. *See also* MUSCLE DISEASES AND DISORDERS; and Chapter 23, "The Neuromuscular and Neurological Disabilities."

MUSCLE CRAMPS. *See* CRAMP.

MUSCLE DISEASES AND DISORDERS. In most cases, diseases affecting the muscles result from damage to nerves which control the feeling and motion of the muscles. Muscles are sometimes damaged by physical activity; for example, a muscle fiber may be torn by a sudden jerk or sharp blow or overstretching.

The biceps muscle in the arm may be torn, or occasionally the large muscles which manipulate the thumb are pulled away. Frequently tendons, the fibrous structures by which muscles are attached to the bones, are torn. Tearing of muscles in the thigh and back of the foot occurs in running and athletic sports in which there are sudden turns of the foot and leg.

Sudden severe pain at the point where the break of the tendon or muscles has occurred is usually the first sign of such an injury. This is followed by weakness, and frequently there is a flow of blood between the fibers of the muscles. Clotted blood produces pain or irritation.

In treatment of such injuries, the nature and severity of the injury, the age of the patient and his general condition are significant factors. In some cases surgery, to repair serious tears of muscles and tendons, may be essential as soon as the doctor has diagnosed the injury. Skillful surgery combined with immobilization by cast until healing takes place bring good results in most cases. After the injury has healed, it is advisable to use heat, massage, and controlled movement to promote complete recovery of the function of the muscle. Specialists in the branch of medicine known as kinesiology are trained to carry out this treatment.

Muscles may become infected and inflamed due to invasion by microorganisms. Inflammation of a muscle, or myositis, may produce pus and abscess, with serious danger to life. Trichinosis is an inflammation which is localized in the muscles; the parasite causing the disease grows in the muscle tissue of the body after having entered the body through the digestive tract.

In poliomyelitis, inflammation causes the destruction of nerve cells affecting the action of the muscles, and wasting away of these muscles is characteristic. Wasting away of muscles and loss of strength is also typical of a group of diseases known as muscular dystrophies. The sources of these conditions vary and in many instances the cause is not known. In a typical case, a child, seemingly normal at birth, will begin at about the age of four or five to be unable to use his legs properly. The back muscles become weak, so that the child cannot sit erect and he soon has difficulty getting up from a prone position. In some cases, complete wasting of the muscles occurs, whereas in others, continued progressive weakness follows without as much destruction of tissues. As the affected muscles become weaker, the stronger or opposing muscles pull, so that the body may become twisted and distorted.

Muscular rheumatism, or fibrositis, is inflammation in the connective tissue which is mingled throughout a muscle.

A tumor in a muscle is called a myoma. Cancer of the muscle is curable, provided an early diagnosis is made. Therefore, any lump in a muscle should not be neglected or disregarded, but thoroughly examined by a doctor. *See also* ATROPHY; BACKACHE; CRAMP; FIBROSITIS; LUMBAGO; POLIOMYELITIS; RHEUMATISM; SPRAINS; TRICHINOSIS; and Chapter 23, "The Neuromuscular and Neurological Disabilities."

MUSHROOM POISONING. Mushrooms are fleshy fungi of the basidiomycetous variety. Mushroom poisoning occurs from eating the poisonous type. Sporadic causes of mushroom poisoning appear, usually due to inexperienced mushroom gatherers who have not learned the simple directions for distinguishing the poisonous from the edible mushroom.

The amanita phalloides, which yield the toxic phallin, and the amanita muscaria, which yield the toxic muscarin, are mushrooms most commonly responsible for poisoning. From time to time other specimens, some of them previously undescribed, are reported to have had poisonous effects. For example, medical authorities in Oregon have warned of eating the mushroom galerina venenata, which has brought about many deaths.

In most cases, symptoms of mushroom poisoning are apparent within six to fourteen hours after the fungi have been ingested. The victims have severe abdominal pains, watery diarrhea, unquenchable thirst, and the skin quickly becomes blue. Muscular convulsions are followed by collapse and frequently death. The galerina venenata causes severe damage to the gastrointestinal, renal, cardiovascular, liver, and central nervous systems. Treatment must be given as promptly as possible in all cases of mushroom poisoning. Purgatives are used to empty the intestines and a stomach pump to evacuate the stomach. Atropine has proved a good antidote for muscarine poisoning. *See also* FOOD POISONING; POISONING.

MUSTARD, a yellow powder made of the ground seed of a yellow-flowered genus of plants, Brassica.

Medically mustard is used as an emetic in digestive disorders and as an agent to cause redness of the skin. In first aid for poisoning, it induces vomiting. A footbath of one tablespoon of mustard to a gallon of hot water is a time-honored comfort in the common cold and stimulates the circulation in the feet and legs.

A mustard plaster, made of a mixture of mustard, flour, and water, acts as a counterirritant to draw blood to the area where the mustard plaster is applied. In bronchitis, for example, a mustard plaster applied to the chest relieves the feeling of congestion. Since a mustard plaster can be so strong as to blister the skin, it should be milder for women and children than men, and should not be left on for more than fifteen to twenty minutes at a time.

MYASTHENIA GRAVIS, a chronic disease of the nervous system, affecting the voluntary muscles and rendering them exceedingly weak and exhausted when they are used. The muscles of the eyes, face, neck, throat, tongue, and lips are especially involved, but others, like arm and leg muscles, may be affected later. In many cases, the person with myasthenia is so fatigued that he cannot hold anything in his hands, keep his eyes open, or even feed himself.

More often than not the development of the disease is gradual, but its onset may also be sudden. Early symptoms are general debility, weakness of one or the other voluntary muscles, double vision, difficulty in swallowing and chewing and talking.

Remission of the disease may occur for longer or shorter periods—as, for example, during pregnancy. In some cases, however, myasthenia gravis may prove rapidly fatal, and before the new treatments were developed was almost always fatal.

Myasthenia gravis usually begins in adulthood, but cases of affected babies have been known. Women are generally attacked in the early thirties and before the age of forty, much more often than men, whereas the incidence is higher in men in the later periods of life.

Medical science is still not certain of the cause of myasthenia. It may be stimulated by a deficiency in the transmissive connection between nerves and muscles. Enlarged thymus glands have been found in some sufferers and thus the disease has been associated with overactivity of the lymphatic tissues of the thymus gland. In young patients removal of the thymus gland has brought encouraging results. Some physicians have used x-ray treatment for the thymus gland, with some success. Most cases of myasthenia are helped by a drug, Neostigmine, which is administered first intravenously and later by mouth. The physician must strengthen the muscles of a patient and in most cases this drug acts rapidly. Sometimes Neostigmine is combined with potassium chloride, ephedrine sulfate, and other drugs.

MYOCARDIAL INFARCTION. *See* CORONARY THROMBOSIS.

MYOPIA, nearsightedness, an optical defect. The vision of distant objects is blurred, and in some cases close objects as well. In myopia the eyeballs are longer than normal. Parallel rays of light do not focus on the retina, the lens of the eye, but are brought to a focus before reaching it. When a myopic person brings an object closer to his eyes, he helps the image to be formed farther back in the eyeball and thus the lens gets a clearer picture. While temporary nearsightedness may result from infections or injuries of the eye, myopia is usually a result of heredity or excessive use of the eyes, especially in close work, and the condition should be corrected by glasses with concave lenses. *See also* EYE.

MYXEDEMA, a constitutional disorder, usually due to degeneration or absence of the thyroid gland, because of disease or surgical removal. The incidence of myxedema is much higher among adults between thirty-five and forty-five, principally women, than other age groups. The condition, therefore, has been called "acquired cretinism." Cretinism is a condition due to thyroid deficiency which is characterized by stunting of physical and mental development.

Juvenile myxedema, which usually afflicts children around puberty, is treated as a form of cretinism. Generally it is not as serious in its mental and physical consequences if treatment is instituted early enough.

Symptoms of myxedema, manifold as they are, develop slowly and many months may pass before they are distinct enough to be easily diagnosed. Some of the more significant symptoms are absence of perspiration, loss of hair, decay of teeth, general weakness, thickening of the skin of the nose and its mucous membranes, swelling of the lips, abnormal sensitivity to cold, a stiff walk, pronounced hoarseness, and often mental abnormalities.

Before treatment with thyroid was introduced, the chance of survival was usually very low. The milder form of the disease can now be cured by administration of sufficient and graduated doses of thyroid gland extract. In severe cases the symptoms can be controlled by similar treatment, which must be carefully adjusted by the physician, sometimes by trial and error.

Strict surveillance and hospitalization may be essential in the early period of treatment because of possible pronounced changes in the general condition of the patient during prolonged treatment with thyroid. Symptoms may disappear, one after another, after a short time, and the physical change in the patient's appearance will be remarkable. Continued administration of small doses of thyroid gland during the lifetime of the patient has been found essential to sustain the improvement. *See also* CRETINISM; THYROID GLAND.

NAIL BITING, a behavior problem common among children and not unusual among adults. Children often put their fingers in their mouths unconsciously—for example, while reading a book or watching a motion picture when they are apparently calm. High-strung children will usually succumb to biting their nails more easily than calm ones. The reasons for a person to bite his nails are varied, including tenseness, lack of manual activity, or emotional disturbance. Scolding, nagging, threatening, shaming, or applying bad-tasting ointment or mechanical restraints to the fingers will aggravate rather then help overcome nail biting. More successful is an appeal to the pride or vanity or maturity of the child. Sometimes a change in the parents' general attitude toward the child will make him feel more secure and subsequently stop biting his nails.

NAILS. The nails, located at the end of the fingers and toes, are elastic horny plates, composed of cells with abundant quantities of keratin, the basis of all horny tissue. They are thin, flattened, and slightly rounded at the edge. Concealed in the skin are the roots of the nails and the producer of the nails, the matrix. The thin and therefore white "half-moon" or lunula extends into the visible part or body of the nail. Average healthy fingernails grow about 1/30th of an inch a week and toenails about a fourth this speed. A healthy nail is pinkish, smooth, and naturally shiny. Temporary ridges or spots may be evident even in healthy persons.

Abnormal conditions in the strength, texture, color, brittleness, and growth of nails are indicative of the state of health of the body. Dark brown or blue spots may result from some undesirable condition, possibly an infection or inorganic poisoning. Pale and soft nails may occur from a deficiency of calcium, and nails with a bluish tinge sometimes indicate poor circulation. White spots are usually due to minor injuries or pressure, and repair, as in most nail conditions, is rapid if the matrix is not destroyed.

The matrix of the nail may be injured by burns or frostbite so that growth is impeded. Nutritional deficiencies and circulatory disorders may result in unduly fragile, brittle, or split nails. Similar symptoms, together with irregular development, can be observed as an indication of digestive changes and in some skin diseases. In many cases, nails stop growing during infantile spinal paralysis and hemiplegia paralysis.

Paronychia, a pus-producing inflammation characterized by swelling, shininess, and extreme tenderness of the skin around the nail, is a fairly frequent condition. It heals quickly if measures are taken to prevent its spread under the nail.

A nail that has been struck or pinched may turn purple or black, due to blood that forms beneath the nail, and the nail may detach from the bed. If pain is severe, the doctor can relieve it by releasing the blood from under the nail. Splinters or thorns are sometimes pushed under the nail. If they do not work out naturally, they may have to be removed by a doctor, who splits the nail.

Among workers who are exposed to certain chemicals, contact dermatitis may develop. This skin inflammation sometimes results in a complete separation of the nail, called onycholosis. If the matrix is injured, the nail will not grow again. In some nervous and vascular diseases or some vitamin deficiencies, the nails become inflamed and fall out.

Hangnails, as annoying and painful as they may be, have little medical significance other than that they serve as an entry for bacteria, and trimming and use of an antiseptic is the only treatment required. Ingrowing nails are a more serious problem. Most often due to constant pressure against a toe by tight shoes, ingrown nails may result in swollen and inflamed feet, and the nail may be embedded in an exceedingly sensitive inflamed area. At times, a portion of the nail must be removed by operation, which is not painful under local anesthesia. Toenails should not be trimmed down at the corners, since this will aggravate ingrown toenails. Other care of the nails includes keeping the cuticle soft, so that it will not tear and cause hangnails, and clipping or filing off rough edges of the nail.

Peeling of the nails can result from injury, but more often is due to their long length, or occurs among persons who constantly use their hands, such as typists or pianists. Housewives, whose hands are frequently in water and soap and harsh cleaning fluids, often have dry brittle nails. Wearing protective rubber gloves will greatly help to keep the hands and nails in good condition.

NARCOLEPSY, recurring sudden attacks of irresistible sleep. In some cases it may be accompanied by a cataplexy, or tonelessness of the muscles. Here the person has spells of muscular weakness, often following anger, laughter, fright, or a startling noise. The knees may give way and the person fall to the ground, but without loss of consciousness.

Narcolepsy occurs in persons suffering from certain brain diseases, and has also been known to develop after serious injury to the head. Some cases have been associated with tumors involving certain portions of the brain. In other instances, excessive sleepiness or ease of falling asleep has been part of a mental condition.

Narcolepsy usually occurs in people who are rather undynamic and lethargic. The person with narcolepsy generally manages to stay awake while working at something that interests him, but when left alone or when lying down he quickly falls asleep. Persons with narcolepsy have even been known to sleep while standing in a bus. Narcolepsy is sometimes also associated with a condition of hunger called bulimia. Few people die of narcolepsy, unless as a result of an accident.

In treatment of narcolepsy, amphetamine, or Benzedrine, has been found useful in preventing the attack of sleep. People who are subject to certain forms of heart symptoms, such as palpitations, tremulousness, and internal tension, as a result of taking Benzedrine may take Dexedrine. In especially severe cases of cataplexy, potassium chloride is given. These drugs are powerful and should never be used unless prescribed by a doctor.

NEARSIGHTEDNESS. *See* MYOPIA; EYE.

NECROSIS. *See* GANGRENE.

NEPHRITIS, inflammation of the kidneys. Like Bright's disease, with which it is often considered synonymous, this term actually covers not one but a group of disorders with similar symptoms. Albumin is almost always present in the urine. Dropsy is another condition in which a breakdown in the excretory system of the kidneys causes the retention of liquid and swelling in various parts of the body.

The intimate connection between albumin in the urine, dropsy, and disordered kidneys was first pointed out by a British doctor, Richard Bright, in 1827, and his name became a designation for any condition in which these symptoms appeared. Several different kidney disturbances are distinguished, each with a special technical name, a few of which are acute and chronic glomerulonephritis, chronic pyelonephritis, and arteriolar nephrosclerosis.

Nephritis is a major health problem. More than 100,000 people annually die of nephritis in the United States. This is 7 per cent of all deaths, making it the fourth greatest cause of death.

The discovery of albuminuria, or albumin in the urine, is a symptom which must not be regarded lightly, because nephritis is detected most easily and quickly by the discovery of albumin in the urine, which may have grave consequences. Albuminuria, which may be found during a general medical examination, must always be followed immediately by further study. Albuminuria by itself does not necessarily or inevitably point to nephritis. It may be found in persons who do not have other symptoms and in many whose kidneys are affected but not sufficiently to justify a diagnosis of nephritis. In one test, 5.3 per cent of 20,000 men had albuminuria when first examined. However, in a followup, two-thirds of this 5.3 per cent proved to have shown it only temporarily, and in only 6.5 of those who did show it was there real evidence of kidney disease.

Wastes are extracted from the blood which passes through more than two million tiny filters in the kidneys. From each of these tubules the blood emerges through a channel that is only a seventh as large as that by which it entered. The result is a squeezing effect. Blood flows back into the general blood stream by being forced under pressure through the walls of the channel. The wall filters out waste products which ultimately are collected in the urinary bladder and excreted as urine. Albuminuria is a signal that there has been interference with this process.

The first symptom of nephritis may be detection of albumin in the urine or a vague feeling of illness or minor disturbances of other functions, such as a slight elevation in blood pressure. Unusual fatigue and listlessness, diminished appetite and headaches may be manifest. As the disorder progresses, a typical train of events usually ensues. The sight is slightly disturbed. The need to urinate at night may interrupt sleep. Weight may be either lost or, with waterlogging of tissues, gained. Gradually more serious symptoms appear, including nausea, sometimes diarrhea, vomiting, and enlargement of the abdomen due to fluid associated with lung and liver congestion. As the condition becomes more se-

vere, unconsciousness and convulsions may supervene.

Acute nephritis or glomerulonephritis ordinarily has a rapid course, but if treatment is sufficiently early and adequate, fatality is rare. Typically a disease of young adults and of children, this is the form of kidney disorder most frequently called Bright's disease; the exact cause is unknown. Secondary effects of infection elsewhere in the body caused particularly by streptococci are frequently suspected to be the primary source. The kidneys themselves, however, are not infected nor can the specific organisms be found in them. Toxic substances such as certain metals can incite acute nephritis.

When kidney inflammation is suspected, the urine should be examined without delay. If albumin is present it will collect and coagulate when tested with heat or strong acid. In nephritis, examination of the urine will also show red blood cells and tiny molds of the minute tubes in the kidneys, which may be composed of any of numerous substances; these are called hyaline, granular or blood casts, or some other name. Urine tests are essential not only as an initial diagnostic aid but also to trace the progress of the disease. Acute nephritis may persist for a few weeks or some months, but usually terminates in eight to ten weeks.

Acute nephritis was formerly considered a fatal disease. Actually, however, about 90 per cent of those who have nephritic symptoms get well, with prompt diagnosis and adequate treatment. The other 10 per cent tend to become eventually chronically nephritic.

Rather than a specific remedy, treatment of nephritis demands adherence to certain basic procedures which assist the body to overcome the disease. The primary objective is elimination of the condition before it becomes chronic. Usually the acute disease is amenable to treatment, whereas a full return to normal from the chronic type is infrequent.

Probably the prime and most basic single item of therapy for acute kidney inflammation is immediate and complete bed rest as long as the kidneys function improperly. Protein intake may be limited, but since it is needed to repair tissue depleted by fever or inflammation, the doctor must consider each case separately. If dropsy or edema is present, salt and liquids may be kept to a minimum. Retention of liquid in the tissues can be so pronounced that the eyes are closed with swelling and the legs can be moved only with difficulty. The condition may be deceptive so that a moisture-swollen person will appear stout and robust when actually he is emaciated. Sweating and frequent bowel movements are often encouraged in order to eliminate as much waste as possible and thus take work off the kidneys.

When acute nephritis eventually becomes chronic a transitional stage, called nephrosis, may intervene. The manifestations include reduced amount of urine, high urine albumin, general edema, and fluid in the abdominal and chest cavities. This may persist for weeks or years, and is best treated in a hospital where the complicated tests of internal conditions on which prescription of treatment depends can be made most easily and satisfactorily.

Chronic glomerulonephritis occurs both as a sequel to the acute form and without any positively definite precursor. Sometimes such a nephritic stage will persist for years, then become latent, punctuated by acute attacks. The latent condition may also endure for years and permit the person to live a reasonably normal life. Repeated flare-ups in acute form, however, occasionally reinforced by rising blood pressure which generally is a part of this condition, cause increased damage to the kidneys, lower their capacity, and eventually induce uremia. This is the toxic state resulting from retention of poisons and wastes in the blood and tissues when the kidneys cannot perform their normal function. When the toxicity is complete, death results almost immediately because of removal or total blockage of both kidneys.

This chronic form, first described by Richard Bright, gave rise to the incorrect assumption that any type of nephritis is extremely serious. It is often only one aspect of a general condition of disordered blood vessels. In such instances death may come not only from uremia but from a stroke or failure of the heart. Some patients become invalids and live only a few years, while others are active, under certain restraints, for much longer periods.

Treatment is focused on the prevention of further infection, regulation of the intake of fluids and other substances, and constant observation by the physician of the progress of the disease. Nephritis is so variable from patient to patient that standard rules for diagnosis or treatment cannot be set forth.

Any person whose urine has revealed albumin should have a general medical checkup at least once a year. The kidneys possess great reserve power. Even when substantial parts of them no longer function the remaining healthy portions maintain a necessary minimum activity. *See also* KIDNEYS.

NEPHROSIS, any degeneration of the kidney without signs of inflammation, one of the commonest chronic diseases of children and one of the least understood. It produces serious disturbances of other bodily functions as well as that of the kidney. The fluid that should be passed on through the kidneys to the bladder for disposal is instead distributed throughout the body, causing swellings called edema. The face is so badly swollen that the eyes are almost closed. The stomach may be distended to about twice its normal size and the swelling extend down to the feet.

Frequently a few days or weeks or months after the illness is first observed, the child will pass a large quantity of urine and his swelling will disappear within a few days. This is known as diuresis and it may occur spontaneously and frequently throughout the course of the disease, although there is no consistent pattern. The edema-free period following diuresis may last only a few days, several weeks, or even months, or it may be permanent. Complete recovery rarely occurs in less than two years after the onset of the disease

and sometimes much longer. Why nephrosis disappears has not yet been explained. A low-salt diet and ACTH or cortisone seem to have been the prime factors in helping some patients. Formerly approximately 50 per cent of all nephrotic children died. New methods of treatment have reduced this rate to some degree. Many of the deaths have not occurred as a direct result of the disease, but from peritonitis or other infections to which these children are highly susceptible. Today these infections are usually controlled by antibiotics.

After the child has returned from the hospital, every possible precaution should continue to be taken against infections, since even tonsillitis may lead to fatal complications. The psychological well-being of the patient is also significant, and his life should be as normal as possible. *See also* KIDNEYS.

NERVE. *See* NERVOUS SYSTEM.

NERVOUS BREAKDOWN, a popular, inexact term which covers a wide variety of mental disorders. Any form of mental or emotional difficulty, from the mildest anxiety state to the most severe form of insanity, can be called "nervous breakdown" by the layman. Since the term is so broad as to elude definition, it is never really applicable to any condition. *See also* Chapter 22, "Mental Illness."

NERVOUS SYSTEM, the entire nervous apparatus of the body. It controls all muscular movements, both voluntary and involuntary; is responsible for thought processes; regulates such body functions as circulation, respiration, digestion, and elimination; and conducts pain and other sensations to the brain.

The nervous system includes the central nervous system, comprising the brain and spinal cord; and the peripheral nervous system which consists of the twelve pairs of cranial nerves arising from the brain, three pairs of nerves coming from the spinal cord, and the nerves of the sympathetic or autonomic nervous system which supply the internal organs and blood vessels.

Nerve cells with their fibers are the units of the nervous system. The operation of the central nervous system depends on these nerve cells (gray matter) and their nerve fibers (white matter). The function of the gray matter is to generate and dispatch nerve impulses. The function of the white matter is to conduct these impulses to and from the cells in the gray matter.

Nerve tissue itself consists of cells with nuclei and threadlike axons which conduct impulses from the nerve cells. Most nerve cells also have relatively short processes called dendrons which conduct impulses into the cell. Impulses normally flow in one direction only. In the afferent nerve they flow toward the nerve centers and in the efferent nerve they flow away from the cell. A nerve cell with its axon and dendron is called a neuron and the entire structure of the nervous system is made up of relays of neurons.

A nerve consists of bundles of nerve fibers and is supplied with blood vessels, lymphatics, and nerves. Some nerves are afferent, some are efferent, and others are mixed.

Impulses of many sorts travel down the paths in the spinal cord, while others enter it and travel upward to the brain.

Injuries and diseases of the nerves. When nerves are divided, the part separated from the nerve cells undergoes degeneration. Regeneration may take place in time, depending on the extent of the injury. However, when the fibers within the brain and spinal cord are divided, regeneration does not follow.

Certain drugs, like bromides and the new tranquilizers, may diminish the activity of the nerve cells. Other drugs can increase activity. Similar effects are produced by the toxins of various disease germs. In some cases nerve cells may be killed. Physical injury can also damage nerve tissue.

Nerve cells weakened by inflammation may recover if the damaging cause is removed, but nerve cells that are destroyed, as in poliomyelitis, cannot be replaced.

Sclerosis is the name given to a fibrous change of the supporting tissue in the brain or spinal cord. Nervous tissue may be converted into a fibrous mass, and may also be damaged by pressure from tumors from within or from tumors or other swellings in adjoining tissue.

Poor nutrition may weaken nerve tissue. Degenerative softening of nervous tissue is caused by deprivation of the blood supply. Disorders of the endocrine glands may also upset nerve cell metabolism. If a nerve is blocked, loss of sensation and paralysis and wasting of muscles ensues. Diseases affecting the brain are dangerous to the nerve centers. These include centers for the heart, respiration, blood pressure, and others. *See also* ATAXIA; BRAIN; MULTIPLE SCLEROSIS; NEURALGIA; NEURITIS; PARALYSIS; POLIOMYELITIS; SCIATIC NEURITIS; SPINAL CORD; SYMPATHETIC NERVOUS SYSTEM; and Chapter 23, "The Neuromuscular and Neurological Disabilities."

NEURALGIA means pain in a nerve, and the term implies that the pain is felt along the nerve or the part of the body supplied by it without any corresponding physical changes.

There are many different types of neuralgia, depending on the nerve involved. Nerves especially apt to become irritable and produce severe pain are the brachial nerve in the arm, the intercostal nerves running between the ribs, the nerves of the scalp, and the sciatic nerve. The fifth cranial nerve, also known as the trigeminal nerve, which supplies the forehead, face, and jaw, is most often affected with neuralgia. The nerve may be so sensitive that even a cold current blowing on the face or a light touch of a finger to the face causes stabbing pain.

In severe cases of neuralgia, or when medical treatment fails, a surgical operation which destroys the nerve roots usually gives permanent relief and involves little risk, even for elderly persons. In neuralgia affecting any nerve, the doctor first determines the nerve area involved and then takes steps to prevent the sensation of pain from traveling along that nerve. To do this, he may use sedative drugs, inject local anesthetics or alcohol, or treat the nerves with x-rays. Diagnosis is more difficult in

those cases in which the sensations of pain are mental rather than physical in origin. *See also* TIC DOULOUREUX.

NEURITIS, inflammation of a nerve or of a nerve sheath. It is distinguished from neuralgia, in which there is pain but not inflammation. In neuritis, pain and tenderness are felt over an area supplied by the particular nerve affected. It may be limited to one nerve or affect several, as in multiple neuritis or polyneuritis. Neuritis of the optic nerve can cause temporary or even permanent blindness.

Other symptoms of neuritis include loss of feeling or disturbance of sensation and sometimes paralysis, so that it is impossible to move the affected area. Many different causes of neuritis are recognized. Some types result from frostbite, dislocation, poor posture in sleep, drugs or injections, cold or radiation treatment. Neuritis occurs in cases of chronic alcoholism, arsenic or lead poisoning, with or following diabetes, in infectious diseases like diphtheria or malaria, in rheumatism and occasionally in influenza. It can also be present in cases of nutritional deficiencies, especially when vitamin B is deficient, as in beriberi.

Treatment of neuritis depends on the doctor's diagnosis of the underlying cause, and the treatment is directed toward removing that cause. For relief of pain, analgesic drugs and barbiturate sedatives are given. Limiting movement of limbs and providing rest, followed by moderate movement, is helpful. During the acute phase, heat also helps to alleviate pain. Other specific measures, such as diet adjustment, which may include vitamin B supplements, may be prescribed by the doctor as the individual case demands. *See also* SCIATIC NEURITIS.

NEUROSIS, an emotional disorder, but without a severe accompanying personality change. It refers to the type of adjustment a person has made to situations which he unconsciously feels may cause him anxiety. The type of adjustment constitutes the nature of the neurosis. The cause is usually attributed to the existence within the person of an emotional conflict, contradictory desires, usually of a highly complex nature.

Several types of neurotic reaction can be identified, all of which are an attempt by the person to shield himself from his inner conflict. In the depressive reaction, the person experiences a general sense of physical and mental inertia, marked by an attitude of general pessimism, self-deprecation, and self-absorption. The neurotic depression is provoked by seemingly nothing, or if it is a response to a particular event—for example, the death of a friend—it becomes exaggerated and lengthy and eventually seems to exist for itself.

Amnesia is an extreme type of dissociative reaction. Here the person loses awareness of who he is for a time, in order to protect himself from some unpleasant situation. He literally refuses to be himself. Unlike delirium states, a person who has suffered from amnesia can recall under hypnosis events which occurred during the time, although consciously he cannot.

In conversion reaction, the person, rather than face a painful situation, imagines that he has some physical disorder, such as blindness or inability to move one arm. Since he usually has no knowledge of body function, the symptoms he describes are often inaccurate.

In phobic reaction, the person develops an intense fear of some particular thing, such as water or cats. This object becomes a substitute or symbol for his inner anxiety and since he can usually avoid the object, he can thus avoid his anxiety.

These and other neurotic reactions constitute an elaborate defense which the person sets up to protect himself from acknowledging some inner emotional trouble. They operate as safety mechanisms which allow the person to cope with and adjust to his environment. Thus he stays in contact with reality, as opposed to a psychotic person, who undergoes severe personality disorder and loss of contact with reality. *See also* AMNESIA; INVOLUTIONAL MELANCHOLIA; MANIC DEPRESSIVE PSYCHOSIS; PARANOIA; PSYCHOANALYSIS; SCHIZOPHRENIA; and Chapter 22, "Mental Illness."

NIEMANN-PICK'S DISEASE, an acute systemic disorder affecting young children in whom there is an enlargement of the liver and spleen. This rare disease occurs most often among infants of Jewish parentage. Malnutrition and retardation of mental and physical development are common symptoms. Treatment is seldom effective and a child with the disease often dies early from secondary infections.

NIGHT TERRORS. Children sometimes experience nightmares which are intensely disturbing to them. Physical factors, such as indigestion, intestinal worms, adenoids, or febrile disorders, may be the cause; but more often night terrors occur in emotionally disturbed children, and if they recur, the child should probably receive psychiatric help.

NOCARDIOSIS, a rare fungus disease which may be acquired through a superficial skin wound, especially on the feet. The infection tends to be chronic and spreads through the system, affecting the lungs. The symptoms resemble those of tuberculosis. Afternoon fever, night sweats, cough, loss of weight, and general malaise are present.

Nocardiosis is commonly treated with sulfadiazine, supplemented by bed rest and a nourishing diet for several months.

NOISE. Noise raises the blood pressure; and hardness of hearing, dizziness, and headache may develop in persons whose occupation exposes them to excess noise. Repeated exposure to irritating sounds may cause echeosis, which is a nervous reaction to excessive noise.

Tinnitus is a ringing, roaring, or hissing sound in one or both ears. It may be due to many causes, such as disease, brain disorder, or as a result of certain drugs. When associated with deafness, tinnitus can be caused by wax in the ear; when it occurs in connection with acne, infection or growth in the ear is sometimes the origin. The treatment depends on the cause. *See also* DEAFNESS; EAR; MENIERE'S DISEASE.

NOSEBLEED. *See* EPISTAXIS.

NOSE. The nose is primarily composed of bone, cartilage, and tissue. The adjoining sinuses are cavities in the bones of the head which are connected with the inside of the nose by narrow passages. The mucous membrane which lines the internal surface of the nasal cavities is extremely sensitive and easily damaged, and susceptible to invasion by germs and infections. These internal cavities also contain hairs which help to protect the inside of the nose from foreign substances, such as germs or dust, which might otherwise find too easy access. The hair follicles constitute another source of infection.

Care of the nose. The nose should be cleaned with a handkerchief or a piece of tissue. Any substances which cannot be removed in this manner may be loosened with a spray or lubricating ointment. A number of mild sprays are available, but should not be used with force. When a person picks his nose, pulls out internal hairs, or attempts to pinch internal pimples, he risks damaging the mucous membrane and consequent danger of certain pus-forming germs entering and spreading throughout the body.

A nasal infection can usually be recognized by its characteristics of redness, swelling, and pain. If the condition appears to be severe, a physician should be promptly consulted. Furthermore, when disease or accident produces a condition which is likely to lead to deformity, the necessary plastic surgery should be done as soon as possible since better results can be obtained if the operation takes place before the organ has improperly healed.

Foreign bodies in the nose. Worms, such as maggots and screw worms, sometimes infest the inside of the nose. This rarely happens, however, unless some abnormal situation already exists in the nose. For example, if a disease with some characteristic odor has localized in the nose, worms may be attracted to the area and infestation begins. The membrane will become irritated and the person will sneeze more often or have a more abundant discharge, perhaps with blood. The correction of such an infestation is seldom difficult. Often it can be cured by simply washing the interior of the nose several times with a suitable antiseptic solution.

Polyps. The mucous membrane of the nose contains cells which sometimes grow too large, with the result that little bodies or polyps protrude into the cavity and obstruct normal breathing. Their presence may also heighten asthmatic symptoms or certain chronic infections. The polyps should be removed. If there is a nasal discharge present which comes from only one side of the nose, it is probable that a foreign substance has accidentally lodged in the nose. A doctor should be consulted. He will examine the nose thoroughly to decide whether or not polyps are present.

Polyps are usually easily removed; if they recur, they should again be removed. As yet little is known concerning the growth and regrowth of polyps. Some scientists believe that they are the result of some previous infection, but others feel that the infection is the result of polyps rather than the cause. The use of radium after the removal of polyps will often prevent their reappearance, and surgery is frequently followed by mild radium treatment, usually after the postsurgical inflammation has disappeared which may be several days. The presence of polyps in the sinuses is more difficult to diagnose. Usually a substance opaque to x-ray is introduced into the sinuses before the x-ray picture is taken, and the polyps can then be seen in the x-ray picture.

Nosebleed. Since the nose is well supplied with blood, its internal tissues are highly sensitive and nosebleed occurs frequently. Nosebleed is usually present in diseases like hemophilia or purpura in which bleeding is common and coagulation defective. Scurvy, severe anemia, and hardening of the arteries may also include nosebleed. In arterial hardening involving high blood pressure the nosebleed has the effect of lowering the blood pressure. Nosebleed can also result from breaking the blood vessels of the nose by blows, bruises, or internal tumors.

In treatment of nosebleed, the victim should be placed on his back in order to lower the blood pressure. The bleeding will probably stop in a few minutes. The person should be cautioned against blowing his nose since this might start the bleeding again. If the nosebleed persists, a physician should be called. He may pack the nasal cavities with sterilized gauze which will be allowed to remain in the cavities for only a short time because of the danger of blocking the tubes leading from the ears to the nose. Other measures to halt bleeding include closing off a blood vessel by pinching, cauterizing, or use of drugs which aid in coagulation of the blood. Drugs may be used to prevent the loss of too much blood, but the loss of blood from nosebleed is seldom serious. Nosebleed is a symptom, not a disease, and is an indication that a nasal disturbance or other undesirable condition exists. *See also* SNEEZING; OZENA.

NURSING, care of the sick, wounded, or infirm. Good nursing in sickness can hasten recovery, prevent complications and perhaps even save a life. Often just keeping the patient as comfortable as possible and in good spirits is of great significance. During the doctor's absence, a good nurse carefully observes the patient and accurately reports to the doctor what she has noted.

The nurse may help select and prepare the room where the patient will be, seeing that it is clean and properly ventilated, with all excess furniture and decorations removed. She will make the bed each day, and in between keep it smooth and tidy. In most cases she will wash the patient once a day with warm water and soap, washing and drying only one part of the body at a time, with the rest covered. If the patient cannot be completely washed each day, his face and arms should be kept clean. The teeth and mouth should be cleansed several times a day. As in a hospital, the usual time for full toilet is in the morning, about an hour before breakfast.

The temperature of the sickroom should be moderate, and kept as even as possible. Good ventilation is essential; if windows are opened, a screen should be used to prevent air from blowing directly on the patient. *See* *also* BED AND BEDDING; BED SORES; CONVALESCENCE; FEVER.

NUTRITION, the sum of the processes involved in the growth, repair, and maintenance of the entire body. Persons who work in the field of nutrition are concerned with food and feeding and its relation to the state of the body. Nutritional substances supply the energy and are the raw material with which the body performs its myriad functions and produces the various internal chemical substances necessary to life.

The concept of feeding is rapidly being revised from a standard of "adequacy," or one that will prevent deficiency diseases, such as scurvy, rickets, beriberi, to "optimum," that which will produce the highest condition of well-being in the body.

States hitherto not recognized as related to nutritional inadequacy are now attributed to it—for example, capillary fragility. Deficiencies so slight that they do not produce reliably observable symptoms are now evaluated by laboratory methods as nutritional deficiency states and corrected as such. Nutritional substances are being investigated and applied as curative agents in conditions not directly but often indirectly attributable to nutritional deficiency, such as cirrhosis of the liver and atherosclerosis, in which the ratio of fats to other substances in the blood stream may be imbalanced. Disease, injury, and other conditions of stress may affect the nutritional status of the body. Negative nitrogen balance, the result of protein depletion, calorie deficiency, and certain vitamin disturbances are known to occur in injury, shock, and in a number of infectious ailments. Several pharmaceutical companies are preparing antibiotics and other medications fortified with vitamins, notably vitamin C, significant in antibody formation and wound healing.

The nutritional elements needed by the body may be classified in five essential groups: proteins, carbohydrates, fats, vitamins, and minerals. Protein foods contain the element nitrogen, an adequate amount of which is required to keep the body in nitrogen balance. Unlike other food elements, proteins are not stored in the body, and a constant replenishment is necessary to sustain health; if the body does not receive them, it will consume its own substances. Proteins are digested in the stomach by the action of the gastro juices, which contain hydrochloric acid, are changed to peptones, and reduced by pancreatic enzymes to amino acids in the small intestines. Twenty-eight amino acids are known, only ten of which are thought to be vital to health. Specific amino acids, however, are essential to specific processes, and a deficiency in any may upset normal functions. Protein foods are used by the body to rebuild proteins for growth, repair, and maintenance of tissues; for production of hormones, enzymes, and antibodies in the blood; and for removing toxins.

The metabolism of carbohydrates supplies energy. When large amounts of carbohydrates are consumed, however, the body stores the part it does not need as fat.

Fats provide a longer, more sustained supply of energy than do carbohydrates, and have a unique initial lymphatic circulation. Fats, whose role is not completely understood, are thought to be indispensable to many chemical processes. Since the body can manufacture fat from carbohydrates and, if necessary, even from protein, they are not considered as essential as other elements. Two to three ounces of fat in the diet each day is sufficient.

Fourteen minerals are known to be essential to an adequate diet, and they are found in varying amounts in all varieties of food. Calcium and phosphorus are significant to the bony structure of the body, including the teeth. Insufficient calcium may cause painful tonic spasms of the muscles. Iodine is used by the thyroid gland to produce a hormone called thyroxin, essential for the cellular use of oxygen. Iron combines with oxygen breathed in through the lungs, in a way not dissimilar to the combining of an iron object with oxygen in the air to form rust. Copper, cobalt, manganese, potassium, magnesium, cadmium, and other minerals are involved in various biochemical actions, such as enzymes, and some are used for body structure.

Vitamins, like the other elements, are organic compounds, substances which contain carbon. Unlike protein and the others, however, they do not furnish energy, but are essential for the transformation of energy and regulation of metabolism in the body. Without vitamins, normal growth and maintenance of life of men and animals could not occur. Vitamins are sometimes called "exogenous" hormones, hormones from outside the body, and certain vitamins bear a strong chemical resemblance to certain hormones produced by the body. A deficiency of specific vitamins might cause a deficiency of specific hormones. In animal experiments, for example, a diet deficient in pantothenic acid, a B vitamin, causes the adrenal glands to shrivel. Vitamin D bears a strong chemical resemblance to the sex hormones. The body must obtain an adequate supply of vitamins through food consumed, since it can produce little of the essential vitamins. Vitamin D can be synthesized by action of sunshine on tissues; vitamin A from carotene; and vitamin K and some of the B vitamins from bacteria in the intestines. *See also* MEAT; PROTEIN; VITAMINS; and Chapter 4, "Diet and Health."

NYMPHOMANIA. The excessive desire of a woman for sexual gratification sometimes results in a pathological condition known as nymphomania, which manifests itself in an insatiate urge for sexual intercourse. Since the causes of the condition are emotional, psychotherapy is necessary.

NYSTAGMUS, an involuntary rapid movement of the eyeball. The movements may be from side to side, up and down, or the eye may roll on its front-to-back axis. Nystagmus generally affects both eyes. It is especially associated with disturbances of the nervous and brain tissues which control eye movements. In miner's nystagmus and in nystagmus due to disorders of the ear, giddiness occurs and objects may appear to move. It sometimes affects persons who work in poorly lighted, cramped quarters.

Often the person is unaware of the movement of his eyes. In all cases of nystagmus an eye specialist should be consulted.

OBESITY, a condition in which excessive fat is stored in the body, due to a positive energy balance. Usually obesity comes from overeating. Far less common is obesity resulting from an organic disease or deficiency which occurs because of disturbance of the pituitary or thyroid glands. Obesity also results from changes in the secretions of the sex organs, as occurs in pregnancy and in menopause.

A tendency to obesity seems inherent in certain races and in families, but for the most part it is individual and directly related to the rate of intake of food and the use of that food to supply energy to the body. The unused food is stored as fat and deposited in parts of the body which usually are first to show excessive fatness, such as hips, stomach, breasts, and buttocks. Fat may also be stored around important internal organs— for example, the heart and liver—and interfere with the proper functioning of the organs.

As well as being unattractive and uncomfortable, obesity is dangerous to health, especially in middle age and thereafter, when it is increasingly difficult to correct. An obese person tends to fatigue and shortness of breath; there is a strain on the joints of the feet and legs, with a consequent predisposition to flat feet and to osteoarthritis of the knees and lower back. Heart disturbances, diseases of the pancreas and kidneys, gallbladder and certain cancers are more common in the fat person, as well as diabetes, which presents special problems among obese persons. The mortality rate in surgery is higher and the general life span is shorter.

In the great number of cases, the body weight can be reduced by modification of the diet. Foods containing starches and sugar are limited and fats virtually eliminated. Emphasis is placed on fruits and vegetables, which may be eaten in large quantities to give a feeling of satiety and supply vital mineral salts and vitamins without adding large numbers of calories. Drastic reducing diets, or "fad" reducing diets are seldom satisfactory for any length of time and a diet which can be sustained over a long period should be selected. Gradual reduction of weight is better than rapid reduction and usually not more than two pounds a week should be lost.

A reducing program that includes drugs or reducing salts should never be undertaken without the advice of a doctor, since drugs, such as amphetamine, which discourage appetite have a stimulating effect which may cause insomnia, and thyroid extract, unless obesity is directly related to thyroid deficiency, may produce serious effects on the heart and nervous system.

In some cases when it is desirable to reduce weight quickly, such as in preparation for an operation, the person may require hospitalization. Here the doctor can exercise strict control and calorie intake can be reduced to as low as 500 calories a day. However, for the average person, a diet of 800, 1000, 1200, or 1500 calories a day may be prescribed, with vitamin and mineral-salt supplements in the lower brackets.

The biggest problem in weight reduction is sustaining the weight loss. In many cases the person gradually gains back the pounds lost. To be able to maintain the correct weight often requires a whole new attitude toward food, a re-education of taste. The emotional factors relating to obesity have received special study and it has been discovered that many fat people eat as a compensation for some dissatisfaction in their lives. For example, a person may consume large amounts of food, much beyond the amount necessary to satisfy a normal appetite, because he is upset, bored, or unhappy. However, usually the person is unaware of the relation between his attitudes and the amount and type of food he eats. Realizing why he has, for example, a compulsion to consume several pieces of chocolate cake in the evening may help him control his eating. In a sense, each obese person is a special case, and for lasting results in weight reduction the unique aspects relating to his overweight must be dealt with. *See also* DIET, REDUCING; and Chapter 4, "Diet and Health."

ODORS. *See* ANOSMIA; BODY ODOR; OLFACTORY SENSE; SMELL.

OLFACTORY SENSE, the sense of smell, which depends on the system of nerves and specialized tissue known as the olfactory nervous system. The olfactory nervous system begins as specialized cells in the lining of the upper part of the nose. These nerves pass up into the olfactory bulbs at the base of the skull. Nerve cells in the cortex of the brain complete the system, which includes the olfactory tracts connecting the cortex with the olfactory bulbs. *See also* ANOSMIA.

OMENTUM, a large membrane covering the lower part of the stomach and hanging down in apron fashion over the coils of the intestine. It is part of the peritoneum, the membrane lining the interior of the abdominal cavity and surrounding the contained soft organs, and is a storage place for fat. The omentum may be involved in hernia and require surgery. Certain infections, inflammations, and tumors may affect the omentum which also may require surgery. *See also* PERITONITIS.

ONYCHIA, inflammation of the matrix of the nail, resulting in the loss of the nail. *See also* NAILS.

OPHTHALMIA, severe inflammation of the eye, especially the conjunctiva, the mucous membrane covering the anterior part of the globe of the eye. *See also* CONJUNCTIVITIS; EYE; PINKEYE.

OPHTHALMOSCOPE, an instrument for examining the interior of the eye, invented in Berlin in 1851 by the famous German physicist, Hermann von Helmholtz. It consists of a mirror mounted on a handle. By means of an electric bulb light is thrown into the eye and the ophthalmologist is able to examine the eye through an opening in the center of the mirror. *See also* EYE.

OPTIC NERVE, the second cranial nerve connecting the retina of the eye with the brain. It conducts the sensory impulses of sight. *See also* EYE.

ORCHITIS, inflammation of the testicles, the sex glands of the male (the prefix "orchi-" refers to the testicle). The condition is characterized by swelling, pain, and a sensation of heaviness in these organs. Various infectious organisms, including those of gonorrhea, syphilis, or tuberculosis, may cause orchitis. In many cases of mumps, in young men from fifteen to twenty-five years of age, the infection spreads to the testicles. The incidence may be reduced by intramuscular administration of mumps serum, if it is given within thirty-six hours. When orchitis is a complication of gonorrhea, treatment is determined in each case by the specific cause. Drugs relieve the pain, and sometimes cortisone and antibiotics are also recommended. Surgery may be imperative.

ORGASM, the climax of sexual excitement, during which the sense of pleasure is at its height. It is followed by a period of relaxation and a feeling of fulfillment. In the normal male, ejaculation of semen accompanies an orgasm. In the female, orgasm, and ejaculation of fluid may or may not take place in intercourse during the early period of marriage. However, with experience this inability to come to climax may be overcome, being largely due, in many cases, to mental causes rather than physical. *See also* IMPOTENCE.

ORINASE, a new drug to be taken by mouth by persons with diabetes mellitus. This product has been tested in many thousands of cases, and has been effective in reducing blood sugar and the presence of sugar in the urine. Furthermore, Orinase has been found helpful in curbing the passage of excessive amounts of urine, and excessive appetite, and it also eradicates itching.

This drug cannot be used as a substitute for insulin in every case of diabetes mellitus, and is most likely to aid those in whom the diabetes is relatively mild and stable, and in whom onset took place some time after the age of thirty. Care must be used in determining which diabetics can be transferred from insulin to Orinase. The drug should not be given to children with diabetes, or to those who have diabetes complicated by acidosis, coma, infection, fever, or gangrene, to diabetics whose nerve or thyroid function is impaired, or when surgical procedures are contemplated.

Special care should be taken in the management of persons who are being transferred from insulin to Orinase to make sure that the urine is tested for sugar at least three times daily during the period in which Orinase is being substituted for insulin. Symptoms which may appear in the transition period include hunger, nervousness, sweating, paleness alternating with flushing of the face and dizziness.

Other reactions, none of them too serious, may be gastrointestinal upset, headache, skin allergy, and intolerance to alcohol. In such cases, the dosage must be reduced in size and made more frequent. *See also* DIABETES; INSULIN.

ORTHODONTIA, the branch of dentistry concerned with malocclusion, or deviation from normal alignment of the teeth. The purpose of orthodontia is not only to improve the appearance of the person; by properly adjusting the placement of the teeth the general efficiency and health of teeth and gums is improved and future trouble caused by misaligned teeth is avoided.

The orthodontist first makes a complete x-ray examination of the mouth, takes measurements and makes a cast of the teeth and gums. He then places braces, or frames, made of wire and gold on the teeth and the often lengthy process of redirecting the growth of the teeth has begun. After this, the braces are frequently manipulated, moved and changed by the orthodontist. The whole process sometimes takes several years.

OSTEITIS, or ostitis, inflammation of the bone. In common practice, osteitis refers to inflammation of the dense shafts of long bones, the spongy portion of the ends of the long bones, or the tissue of the short or flat bones.

Tuberculosis is a common cause of osteitis, but it may also be produced by various organisms, such as the staphylococci. Some degree of osteitis will also be found in such bone disorders as osteomyelitis.

Paget's disease, also known as osteitis deformans, begins in the bone marrow, spreads to other portions of the long bones, and also affects the skull. The sacrum, pelvis, and lower extremities are also involved. The long bones lengthen and thicken, often becoming twice their normal size. At the same time, they soften and become bowed where weight is placed on them. The skull grows progressively larger.

Outside of neuralgic pains and headache, the health of the person is unaffected. The disease generally occurs between the ages of forty and sixty, and is rarely fatal. However, other complications such as spontaneous fracture, secondary anemia, and bone sarcoma may cause death. Paget's disease is of unknown origin, and no positive treatment for it has as yet been found.

OSTEOMYELITIS. Certain pus-forming germs, and sometimes those of tuberculosis, pneumonia, or typhoid fever, produce infection in the bones which is known as osteomyelitis. Though the germs may enter from infected tissues close to the bone, usually they are carried by the blood stream.

Osteomyelitis may appear in any bone of the body, but is more common in the leg and arm bones. The greatest danger arises when this infection attacks the jawbone.

Osteomyelitis in its early stages often gives an inflamed and swollen appearance at the point of infection, and a blood test will reveal an increase in the number of white blood cells. Fever and rapid pulse are also present, pain is felt in the bone, and sensitivity in the diseased area is likely to be great.

Since the blood stream is involved, this infection can be carried throughout the body and may travel from bone to bone. Fortunately prompt

diagnosis is now possible with x-ray so that treatment can be started before multiple osteomyelitis, infection of several bones, develops. Moreover, the modern sulfa and penicillin drugs will actually penetrate to a deep infection of the bone. The dramatic success of penicillin in treating osteomyelitis of the jawbone helped to bring this drug to immediate general attention. Surgery of the bone is still required so that the infected material can be removed. Only then can the doctor apply the drugs to the infection within the bone.

OSTEOPATHY, a system of treatment of disease by manipulation of bones, joints, and other body tissues. It is based on the theory that the body is a mechanical organism whose structures and functions are coordinate and interdependent and that a disturbance of either constitutes disease. The theory also holds that when the structure of the body mechanism is normal, environmental conditions favorable, and nutrition adequate, the body is capable of making its own remedies against disease and other toxic states.

Osteopathy places chief emphasis on body manipulation, although it sometimes also includes generally accepted medical and surgical methods of diagnosis and treatment. In many states osteopaths are limited by law to treating patients only by manipulative methods, but in some states they may also undertake surgical procedures and prescribe medicine.

OTITIS, inflammation of the ear which can involve the outer ear, the passage to the drum and the outer surface of the eardrum itself, and the middle ear. Rarely is the innermost ear affected in this type of inflammation. Otitis can be acute or chronic.

In otitis of the external ear, the skin is inflamed and may produce a discharge that apparently comes from inside the eardrum. However, the drum is not perforated, and only the skin of the outer ear is involved. Application of antiseptics and systematic and thorough cleansing is the usual treatment, and most cases respond fairly rapidly after treatment is begun.

In otitis media, or inflammation of the middle ear, suppuration usually occurs and the condition is commonly referred to as running ear. It develops from acute infection of the upper respiratory tract and enters the ear passages by way of the Eustachian tube. Generally it follows a head cold or sore throat, especially if neglected. In children, adenoids are often a factor in recurrent cases of running ear; and measles, diptheria, and scarlet fever also frequently cause otitis in the middle ear. In adults, sinus trouble may sometimes be involved as well.

The usual symptoms of acute otitis media are earache, fever, headache, pain, and deafness. Upon examination the eardrum is red and it loses its normal shape and luster.

In the early stages of treatment the patient should be put to bed. If the pain does not subside within a few hours, the doctor will probably prescribe aspirin or codeine to relieve the distress. The application of heat is also helpful.

In treatment of otitis in its acute form, the use of antibiotics has suc-cessfully replaced many other forms of treatment. However, surgical incision of the eardrum and drainage of the ear is still the most effective method of relieving pressure. In many cases a combination of surgery and drainage, followed by the use of antibiotics, is most effective. However, sensitivity tests must be made for each patient's reaction to antibiotic treatment. In numerous instances it may be found best to drain the ear and keep it clean, allowing nature to take its course without the use of drugs.

Even without treatment, a mild attack will subside. But in other cases, especially if treatment has been neglected or the ear improperly cleansed, a state of chronic otitis media may be established. There is danger of acute mastoiditis, and constant or recurrent discharge may provoke a gradual impairment of the hearing.

Chronic otitis is classified as serous or suppurative, depending on whether or not there is pus formation. The source of the infection must be located by the doctor, and treatment is essential since there is always a serious threat of acute inflammation as well as gradual destruction of the hearing. It is therefore advisable to seek treatment promptly in case of earache or running ear. *See also* DEAFNESS; EAR; MASTOID.

OTOSCLEROSIS, a chronic disorder of the ear in which spongy bone forms in the capsule of the labyrinth of the ear and the small bones lose their power to conduct sound. The exact cause of otosclerosis is unknown. Tests have been made to determine whether or not it is hereditary, due to vitamin deficiency or to failure of glandular function, but none of these has been conclusive enough to establish the underlying cause.

Otosclerosis affects women more often than men. Frequently the first sign is an annoying ringing in the ears, and a gradual and progressive loss of hearing. It may affect only one ear at first, but eventually both ears become involved. Sometimes enough hearing is retained for the person to follow ordinary conversation, but in other cases it is necessary for him to use a hearing aid or learn to lip read.

Gradual loss of hearing is an almost certain indication of otosclerosis, but tests have been developed by ear specialists to confirm the diagnosis and to make sure that other factors that may affect hearing are not involved.

Various types of treatments are used in otosclerosis, including careful control of diet, vitamin supplements, drugs to allay the ringing sensation, glandular extracts to correct glandular failure, and surgical procedures. The most positive treatment is the Lempert operation in which a window is drilled from the outer healthy bony structure into the inner ear. Fenestration, as this method of surgery is called, has been successful wholly or partially in a great number of cases, but is usually only possible when the nerves are unimpaired. Another operation restores movement to the stapes, one of the three small bones which make contact with the eardrum. *See also* DEAFNESS; EAR.

OVARIES, the two sex glands of women. They lie in the lower part of the abdomen and perform two essential functions: they germinate the female reproductive or egg cells, one of which passes through the Fallopian tube to the uterus every month; and they provide internal secretions or hormones which influence most feminine physical characteristics and which are related to the reproductive process.

The hormone estradiol determines the familiar feminine attributes; it causes both external and internal sex organs to grow to adult size and the development of the typical figure with lines softened by a layer of fat under the skin. Estradiol also appears significant to the development of more mature attitudes and concerns in the young girl.

The other hormone secreted by the ovaries, progesterone, cause changes in the uterus and prepares it to receive the fertilized egg cell. Progesterone is secreted approximately for only a week, or a little more, each month after the egg cell has been released by the ovary.

The female phenomenon, menopause or change of life, is bound intimately with the discontinuance of these hormones. When ova are no longer released each month progesterone is no longer developed. Gradually the estradiol diminishes and finally ceases. Estradiol normally is produced from the second until approximately the fifth decade. Endocrine disorders can cause changes in younger women similar to those of menopause.

Removal of the ovaries because of infection or for some other reason results in the termination of the hormones and causes definite bodily changes regardless of age. One of the great advances in medicine has been the discovery of the exact chemical character of the hormones and the method of extracting them from natural substances or of manufacturing them artificially. Now these are substituted for those hormones lost. The removal of one, or part of one ovary has no such effects.

One of the principal disorders of the ovary is the formation of cysts, sacs which contain liquid material of glandular origin of various kinds which may grow to considerable size. If the cyst remains small, difficulty may not ensue, but if it enlarges it must be removed surgically.

The ovaries may be affected by growth other than cysts, such as tumors and cancers. Since the physician cannot ascertain the exact nature of such a growth by external examination, an operation is usually necessary in order to determine the type of growth involved and the proper course to be pursued.

Infection may reach the ovaries through the Fallopian tubes, the passages which each month ordinarily carry the egg cell into the uterus. Gonorrhea, streptococcal and tubercular infections are common. Fever and pain as well as swelling may be relieved quickly by application of heat or cold, with a hot-water bottle, heating pad, or ice pack. Sulfa and antibiotic drugs used under the doctor's direction usually are effective. However, the infection may not respond to treatment and the removal of the ovary or the Fallopian tube by surgery may be necessary.

Another ovarian disorder is caused by strain, stretching, and twisting of the tissues which fasten the ovary to the abdominal wall. The affected ovary may stop functioning temporarily and as a result its blood supply may be interrupted or the ovarian ligaments themselves, as they are called, may be involved. Surgery is sometimes required to correct this condition.

OVULATION, the process in which the egg or ovum is released from the Graafian follicle of the ovary. In the sexually mature female, ovulation occurs every twenty-eight days. This cycle ordinarily produces only one egg at a time; infrequently it produces two or more eggs which can result in multiple birth. Following ovulation the egg enters the Fallopian tube where fertilization by the male sperm takes place following intercourse. If fertilization does not occur, the egg undergoes degeneration and a new cycle begins. Failure to ovulate results in sterility. *See also* CONTRACEPTION; MENSTRUATION; OVARIES; STERILITY.

OXYGEN, a colorless, odorless, gaseous element which constitutes about one-fifth of the volume of the atmosphere. Formerly used by physicians only in life-and-death emergencies, today oxygen is used frequently in the treatment of many diseases.

Among modern mechanisms employed are the incubators for premature infants as well as oxygen rooms and oxygen tents. Many of these devices involve the danger of fire and explosions unless they are supervised by experts.

Generally speaking, oxygen is prescribed for all patients who either cannot breathe easily, or who, for some reason, are suffering from a limited supply of air. Such a need arises, for example, in pneumonia or carbon monoxide poisoning.

Oxygen is not often administered for diseases of the heart because the shortage of air which occurs in connection with these afflictions is usually due to a diminished circulation of the blood. An exception, however, is angina pectoris in which an oxygen deficiency occurs in the heart muscle. If attacks occur often, unexpectedly and with slight provocation, oxygen can be of great value.

OZENA, or atrophic rhinitis, a disease affecting the mucous membrane of the nose and characterized by an extremely offensive odor. A gradual degeneration of the nasal membrane is followed by discharge of matter and formation of large foul-smelling crusts. The sense of smell is affected so that the person himself is unaware of the odor coming from the nose. The interior of the nose is dry and the internal structure so affected as to make the airway through the nose unusually wide. Continuous coughing and hacking to clear the passages of the crusts which get into the throat also occur.

Treatment formerly included frequent syringing of the nasal passages with alkaline and antiseptic solutions. Now attention to diet and tests to determine the glandular condition and general health are part of the treatment. Surgical procedures which were helpful in the past are now usually replaced by more effective hygienic measures.

Ozena, which was once quite common, especially among young girls, has largely disappeared. However, ozena may affect children in whom an early nasal infection has gone untreated and atrophy of the nasal membrane followed by symptoms of ozena may result from negligence.

PAGET'S DISEASE. Two separate and distinct disorders are named Paget's disease. Sir James Paget, a famous British surgeon, first described them in 1871. One of the disorders is osteitis deformans, a disease of the bones, which is discussed under osteitis, and the other is Paget's disease of the nipple.

Paget's disease of the nipple is a cancer of the breast. It generally affects only one breast and is manifested by redness and dryness of the nipple, cracks and ulceration. The nipple is usually tender and frequently there is an abnormal discharge. Cancer of the breast is ordinarily detected a year or two after the nipple is affected, which in most cases is considered an early warning sign. *See also* BREAST; CANCER; OSTEITIS.

PAIN, a disturbed sensation, causing suffering or distress. Pain is produced by irritation of the trunk, root, or terminal of a sensory nerve. Nerve endings in the skin are also sensitive to touch, heat, and cold as well as pain. Pain may be considered a protective mechanism in that it directs attention to some disturbance in the body.

Pain varies with the cause and

among different people, some persons being more sensitive to it than others. Pain may be described as boring, gnawing, cutting, burning, throbbing, and in other ways. The description of the type of pain often helps to determine its cause—for example, a throbbing pain is associated with suppuration. The situation or point of origin is an even better indication of its cause. However, the area of the pain may be misleading, as in the case of a referred pain in the temple resulting from a bad tooth, or

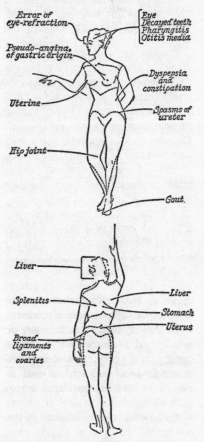

Error of
eye-refraction

Eye
Decayed teeth
Pharyngitis
Otitis media

Pseudo-angina,
of gastric origin

Dyspepsia
and
constipation

Uterine

Spasms of
ureter

Hip joint

Gout.

Liver

Liver

Splenitis

Stomach

Uterus

Broad
ligaments
and
ovaries

Examples of referred pain.

a pain in the back of the shoulder caused by irritation of the liver. The system whereby pain originates in the nerve endings and is channeled into the spinal cord and up into the brain may also cause pain to be felt in tissue that has been removed—as, for example, a pain in a leg which has been amputated.

Pain which is entirely mental in origin is called psychogenic pain. Frequently it is vague and irregular and the person often exaggerates in describing it. The pain usually disappears when the mental cause has been erased.

Much study and research has been devoted to pain and the effects of various drugs and techniques in relieving it. For example, in surgical operation pain is relieved by blocking or cutting various nerves. It is diminished or blocked chemically by the use of pain-killing drugs. *See also* ACUTE ILLNESS, ACUTE PAIN.

PALATE, the roof of the mouth. It is composed of the hard palate and a soft palate. *See also* CLEFT PALATE.

PALSY. *See* PARALYSIS AGITANS.

PANCREAS, one of the vital organs of the body, ranking in importance with the liver. It is situated in the abdominal region, behind the stomach, close to the liver and gallbladder with which it shares a common duct leading into the duodenum, the first part of the small intestine. The pancreas is about six inches long, yellowish in color, soft, with a head, body, and tail.

The pancreas performs two distinct functions. The first is to secrete the pancreatic juice into the intestinal tract. This fluid is one of the chief chemical aids in digestion, containing certain enzymes essential in the digestion of starch, proteins, and fats. The pancreas also acts as an endocrine gland, secreting insulin directly into the blood stream. Insulin is valuable in the regulation of blood sugar levels and in the conversion of sugar into heat and energy.

Insulin is produced by the part of the pancreas known as the Islets of Langerhans, groups of specialized cells found scattered throughout the organ. A disorder of the pancreas which cuts down the production of insulin results in the disease known as diabetes mellitus. Tumors may also develop in the Islets of Langerhans and cause an overproduction of insulin. This combined with an insufficiency of blood sugar gives the symptoms of an overdose of insulin and may include coma, convulsions, or periodic attacks of fatigue and shortness of breath. Surgery to remove these tumors is the most effective method of controlling the condition.

The pancreas may be affected by infection of the gallbladder, the bile duct, or stomach, and jaundice may result from such inflammation. If cancer is involved, it may also produce jaundice.

Acute damage of the pancreas may occur from direct invasion of the organ by bacteria, or by blockage of the pancreatic duct resulting in the retention of powerful digestive ferments. Violent symptoms may develop suddenly in the abdomen, including severe pain, vomiting, hemorrhage, paleness, and shock.

While surgery was once the first step in treating acute pancreatic infection, current management resembles that practiced in other hemorrhagic acute gastrointestinal disorders. The patient is put to bed and blood transfusions are given. Intravenous feeding is begun and continued until the acute stage is passed. Surgery is avoided in this stage, and pancreatic secretions are inhibited by nasal suction from the stomach. Drugs to relieve pain are given, and in some cases blockage of the nerves is effected. When the condition warrants, the patient is placed on a bland diet, as in cases of duodenal ulcer.

In most instances careful treatment results in complete recovery, but patients should be examined within six weeks thereafter to make certain that complications, such as biliary disease or pancreatic cysts, are not present. In some cases, however, there may be recurrence of the acute symptoms, or development of chronic pancreatitis. In the chronic form, the pancreas is so affected as to cause permanent damage to the insulin-producing cells, and there may be a development of fibrous tissue which gradually blocks off the production of pancreatic juice. Treatment may include administering pancreatic extracts to make up the deficiency of digestive fluid and insulin to control diabetes. Occasionally surgery is desirable to remove cysts which develop. When great pain is present and does not respond to direct surgery, the splanchnic nerves leading to the pancreas may be cut.

Cancer of the pancreas usually affects middle-aged or elderly men, and is only one-third as frequent in women. It is generally accompanied by severe deep pain in the back between the shoulder blades. Whether or not it begins in the head, body, or tail of the pancreas, surgery of the entire organ is indicated when cancer is detected. Such an operation is now possible, with the means developed for controlling shock and the availability of substitutes for the secretions of the pancreas. *See also* DIABETES; INSULIN; JAUNDICE; and Chapter 18, "Disorders of the Digestive System and Diet in Digestive Disorders."

PARALYSIS, temporary or permanent loss of muscle function, sensation, or voluntary motion, usually caused by injury to nerves or destruction of nerve cells which control the function of the affected muscles or muscle tissue. An example of paralysis is the cutting of a motor nerve, as may happen in injury to the wrist or forearm. The muscles supplied by the nerve cease to function and begin to degenerate. Unless the cut ends are successfully joined together by surgery and unless nerve fibers grow into the old nerve trunk, these muscles will be permanently inactive.

Damage to nerve cells or fibers may be caused by disease, pressure, or destructive injury to the brain or spinal cord, any of which may produce partial or total paralysis of several muscles. Paralysis due to brain damage is most likely to be a stiff or spastic type, and paralysis due to damage to the cells in the spinal cord is generally a limp flaccid kind.

Specific terms are used to describe various types of paralysis. Paralysis of both arms and both legs is called quadriplegia. Paralysis of one side of the body is hemiplegia. Diplegia is paralysis of similar parts on each side of the body. Monoplegia is paralysis of a single arm or leg or a single muscle or group of muscles, such as those on one side of the face. Paralysis of both legs is paraplegia.

As well as being caused by injury to the brain, spinal cord, or nerves, paralysis can be brought about by embolism, thrombosis, or brain hemorrhage, known as apoplexy or stroke. Tumors and various progressive diseases and degenerations can affect the spinal cord and produce various types of "creeping paralysis." Various forms of neuritis affect the muscle through the nerves and cause a temporary paralysis. Paralysis which is mental in origin occasionally occurs, as in hysteria.

To treat paralysis, both nerves and muscles must be considered. In paralysis from strokes, poliomyelitis, and neuritis, the tendency for recovery or improvement is strong once the underlying disease or condition has run its course. Paralysis due to pressure on a nerve tends to disappear if pressure is removed before the nerve cells or fibers are completely destroyed. Treatment involves treating the nerve or tissue causing pressure on the nerve as well as treating the muscles that have been affected.

Muscles that have been paralyzed are protected until nerve impulses once again reach them. Of utmost importance is preventing the paralyzed muscles from being stretched by the pull of healthy opposing muscles. This is most frequently done by immobilization in splints or braces. Paralyzed muscles must also be kept warm and tone maintained by gentle massage, increasing in vigor as the muscle improves. Rehabilitation of paralyzed patients requires much special training and long hours of tedious work. *See also* APOPLEXY; CEREBRAL PALSY; PARAPLEGIA; POLIOMYELITIS; STROKE.

PARALYSIS AGITANS, a disease distinguished by muscular weakness and trembling of parts of the body at rest. Dr. James Parkinson of London described it in 1817. Scientifically the condition is known as paralysis agitans, and it is also called Parkinson's disease or shaking palsy. The disorder is typically one of elderly people, striking mostly persons in their sixties and seventies. On rare occasions brain inflammation, such as encephalitis, may cause a similar disturbance.

Paralysis agitans ordinarily affects first a single arm or leg, then the second limb on the same side, and finally those on the other side. Often an arm first betrays symptoms by losing the typical swing that accompanies walking, and the face begins to lack its customary expressiveness and changes slowly or not at all with passing moods. Involvement of the limbs is followed by that of the trunk muscles, which gives the body a stooping posture. Steps become shorter and more rapid and develop into a combination of a shuffle and run. The rate at which the disease advances varies in different persons. Often it progresses slowly, leaving the health good in other respects. Intervals as long as a year may occur between the phases of development from one limb to another.

Changes in the brain, in other nerve tissue, and in blood vessels of the brain have been observed in association with paralysis agitans. Although exact knowledge as to its cause is not known, special or direct relationship to either brain hemorrhage or high blood pressure is doubtful.

Treatment of paralysis agitans is usually limited to relief of symptoms, to efforts to keep the patient comfortable, to maintaining his general health and thus to endeavoring to retard the progress of the disease.

Drugs of the belladonna type reduce rigidity; they may be administered in various ways to give relief. Baths and massage relieve the tensions in the muscles and are soothing to the skin.

Operative procedures have been developed which diminish the circulation of blood to the areas in the brain concerned with the tremors. Success has been reported in many cases of paralysis agitans. *See also* Chapter 23, "The Neuromuscular and Neurological Disabilities."

PARANOIA, a rare psychosis characterized by delusions of persecution and often hallucinations, usually of an auditory type. Contact with reality is still maintained, but it is distorted. The paranoid person feels that a person or group is persecuting him, perhaps trying to kill him. Often this intense fear and suspicion is combined with excessive but unrealized ambitions and delusions of grandeur. The paranoid person blames the "persecutor" for his failure. In the true type of paranoia, one thing becomes the "persecutor," rather than the person being suspicious of everything, and this thing dominates the person's life. *See also* Chapter 22, "Mental Illness."

PARAPLEGIA, paralysis of the lower limbs, due to severe injury to the spine or spinal cord. It may result from a severe blow to the spinal cord, fracture or dislocation of the spinal column, or from bullet or knife wounds.

Surgery may be required to correct damage to the injured area or to remove bone or metallic fragments. In some cases an operation may not be indicated or practical at the time of injury.

Whether or not an operation is performed, a long period of hospital care is essential following injury to the spine resulting in paraplegia. Experience in World War II, which produced thousands of disabled veterans, proved the significance of supervision and patient nursing in the ultimate rehabilitation of a great number of paraplegics.

In the early phase of treatment meticulous attention is given to maintenance of healthy bone structure, care of the skin, proper drainage of the urinary tract, bowel activity, and diet. Once partial recovery is attained long-term care of the patient is paramount. The patient must be helped through the trying period of adjustment to his disability. Skillful physiotherapy and occupational therapy and sometimes psychotherapy play a considerable part in rehabilitation. Much has been accomplished in preparing paraplegics for useful occupations. They have been taught to walk with braces and to drive specially equipped automobiles. Many have married, established homes, obtained employment, and taken their places as useful, self-sufficient citizens. *See also* PARALYSIS.

PARATHYROID GLANDS, the four small glandular bodies attached to the back of the thyroid gland in the neck, two lying on each side. Together they are about the size of a small bean and are the smallest glands of internal secretion.

The function of their secretion or hormone is to regulate the use of calcium and phosphorus in the body. When the glands are underactive and the quantity of the secretion deficient, the amount of calcium in the blood drops and the amount of phosphorus increases, eventually producing tetany, a spontaneous muscle spasm. Overactivity of the glands results in withdrawal of too much calcium and phosphorus from the bones, rendering them soft and fragile.

When tetany occurs as a result of underaction of the parathyroids, the muscles have a tendency to go into painful prolonged spasms; tingling, numbness, and sometimes twitching may accompany the spasm. The forearms and hands are most often affected; the throat is the most troublesome part. The muscles eventually become abnormally sensitive to stimuli. People with tetany frequently are subject to nervousness and emotional depression. Tetany often results from inadvertent removal of the parathyroid glands, which are so small that they can be unknowingly removed or destroyed during a surgical operation on the thyroid gland.

The symptoms of tetany may arise from causes other than parathyroid deficiency, but are all characterized by inadequacy of the supply of calcium received from food. Similar symptoms may come from too much alkali.

In the past, treatment of tetany was difficult, but today the calcium deficiency can be remedied in various ways—for example, by regulating the diet to keep the phosphorus intake low which requires a reduction of meat, egg yolk, and dairy products. Before treatment can successfully be planned, the condition of the blood must be determined and the specific factors producing the symptoms isolated. Diet control alone is sometimes sufficient to restore normal function. Glandular extracts of parathyroid may be prescribed.

Excessive parathyroid secretion stimulates the kidney to remove from the blood and excrete in the urine too much phosphorus. The bones, functioning as a reserve supply of phosphorus, release the phosphorus to compensate for what the blood lacks and in doing this also release calcium, thus depriving the bones of an essential constituent and giving the blood an excess. The result is a bone condition, called osteitis fibrosa or osteoporosis, in which the bones are so fragile that they can be cut with a knife. They are easily broken by a mild shock. Such accidents may occur repeatedly and healing may be accompanied by permanent deformity in the bones unless great care is taken to prevent it. The deformities caused by twisting and other abnormalities are called osteomalacia. The excessive calcium in the blood tends to form stones or calculi at various points in the body.

Excessive parathyroid activity may be the result of a tumor of one or more of the glands; and when this occurs, surgical removal is the only effective measure.

Another serious effect of parathyroid overactivity is damage to and gradual inflammation of the kidneys from the excretion of too much calcium and phosphorus through them. This condition is not necessarily fatal since the underlying cause can usually be treated effectively, after which the kidneys resume their normal state. *See also* Chapter 19, "Endocrine Glands."

PARESIS. Persons who have had syphilis over a period of time sometimes develop in later years a condition known as paresis. It is also called general paralysis, general paresis, general paralysis of the insane or dementia paralytica, or paretic neurosyphilis. The syphilis has infected the brain and coverings of the brain, resulting in a tissue damage sufficient to cause paralysis and mental disturbance. Paresis is three to five times more frequent in men than women.

Among the first symptoms are slight changes in behavior, such as irritability, carelessness in dress and hygiene, lack of judgment, forgetfulness, inability to concentrate, and slowness of comprehension. Besides these symptoms of nervous disorder, certain signs of motor disturbance are manifested, including disturbances in dexterity, lack of coordination, and tremor of the hands. Changes in facial expression may develop, and often there is difficulty in pronunciation and speech defects with sibilants. In the pupil of the eye, dilation or reaction to light is lost, but adjustment to objects at different distances, accommodation, is retained.

As paresis develops, new symptoms of mental disorder are manifested. In some cases the person feels euphoric and has grandiose ideas of wealth and power, sometimes expressed in eccentric behavior. Or he may feel depressed, persecuted, and be self-deprecatory. Still another case may display a pronounced loss of memory and difficulty in calculation and writing.

Eventually the damage to the brain becomes so great as to cause general paralysis and require hospitalization with bed rest. The use of penicillin has largely replaced all earlier forms of treatment and has been effective in a high percentage of cases where damage has not progressed to a hopeless state. When the patient cannot tolerate penicillin, other antibiotics, especially the group known as the tetracyclines, have been found effective. *See also* SYPHILIS.

PARKINSON'S DISEASE. *See* PARALYSIS AGITANS.

PARRY'S DISEASE, a name given to toxic goiter. It is named after Caleb Hillier Parry (1755–1822), the English physician who described it. It is also called Graves' disease and Basedow's disease. *See also* GOITER.

PARTURITION, the act of giving birth to a child. *See also* PREGNANCY AND PRENATAL CARE; and Chapter 6, "Prenatal Care and Childbirth."

PATCH TEST, an allergy test in which a small patch of adhesive containing a substance to which a person may be sensitive is applied to the skin. The appearance of redness and inflammation is considered to be positive proof of such sensitivity. *See also* ALLERGY; and Chapter 21, "Allergy."

PEDIATRICIAN, or pediatrist, a specialist in children's diseases. His special field is called pediatrics.

PEDICULOSIS. *See* LICE.

PELLAGRA, a dietary deficiency disease, once prevalent in the United States, especially in the South. It is due to malnutrition and is caused by a diet deficient in, among other essential vitamins and minerals, nicotinic acid or niacin, which is absolutely vital for growth and health of the human body. Symptoms of pellagra are chiefly inflammation of the mouth, redness and soreness of the tongue, secondary cracking of the skin and ulceration around the mouth. The skin of the back of the hands and the forearms may become red and thickened, and the neck and chest are sometimes similarly involved. The alimentary tract is affected and diarrhea, vomiting, and loss of appetite appear. Other symptoms may be headache, irritability, anxiety, muscular weakness, and—in extreme cases—melancholia and dementia.

In the South, persons with pellagra had often existed on a diet of pork fat, corn bread, and corn syrup. The United States Public Health Service has attempted to reduce the frequency of pellagra by educating these people to the need to supplement their diet with tomatoes, green peas, other green and yellow vegetables and foods.

To treat pellagra, usually an improvement in diet is all that is required. Nicotinic acid deficiency is corrected by large doses of nicotinamide.

If pellagra has existed for a long time and much weight has been lost, a high-calorie diet is given the patient, and sometimes bed rest is required. In a severe case, the person may have been so weakened by his condition that he must be urged to eat and rest.

Antibiotics are used to treat the skin until it has healed through proper diet and rest.

PELVIS, a basin-shaped ring of bones at the base of the trunk, joining the spine and the legs. The gaps in the skeletal structure are filled with muscles and membranes, actually forming a closed basin.

The female pelvis may be deformed from birth or as a result of disease, presenting special problems in childbirth. The obstetrician measures the dimensions and capacity of the pelvis of a pregnant woman to determine whether or not difficulties will be encountered in parturition, the act of giving birth. This is known as pelvimetry, or measurement of the pelvis.

The pelvis of either men or women may be fractured as the result of accident.

PEMPHIGUS, an acute or chronic disease of the skin, characterized by the appearance of large blisters which develop in crops or in continuous succession.

The chronic form of pemphigus,

pemphigus vulgaris, was formerly fatal in a large number of cases, but is now successfully treated with ACTH and cortisone, and fatality almost never occurs. The disfiguring and annoying skin lesions which the disease produces are now also successfully treated.

Acute febrile or fever pemphigus most frequently attacks butchers and persons who handle animal carcasses. The symptoms are usually fever and headache. Provided treatment begins early enough, the different types of pemphigus respond well to cortisone and ACTH.

PENICILLIN, an antibacterial drug. In 1929 an English bacteriologist, Sir Alexander Fleming, observed that the mold known as penicillium notatum interfered with growth of cultures of staphylococci and that germs did not grow for some distance around the penicillin mold. This observation later led to the extraction of penicillin by other scientists into a form which could be used in treatment of disease.

Penicillin is used against germs which cause pneumonia, meningitis, gonorrhea, boils, common throat infection, and various staphylococcal diseases. It is also extremely effective in treatment of syphilis, replacing most of the earlier remedies. Subacute bacterial endocarditis, formerly fatal in a great number of cases, has been found to be controllable by penicillin. Penicillin is also used for trench mouth, rat-bite fever, and other infectious diseases.

The discovery of penicillin led to the development of streptomycin, Aureomycin, and many other antibiotics which have helped enormously to combat a great number of infectious diseases. *See also* ANTIBIOTICS.

PENIS, the male organ of copulation, which also contains the urethra which carries urine from the bladder to the outside of the body.

The penis and urethra are subject to various disorders, infections, and structural irregularities. Hypospadias is a structural malformation of the urethra, in which a splitting of parts of the penis occurs so that the opening of the urethra is at the lower side of the penis instead of the front. Epispadias is a condition in which the floor of the urethra transverses the top of the penis instead of the underside. An operation is required in both cases to correct the condition. Tumors, either benign or malignant, may also occur in the urethra or penis. *See also* TESTICLES.

PEPTIC ULCER. An ulcer is any sore or break in the surface usually of the skin or mucous membrane, resulting from destruction of the underlying tissues or from loss of the covering layer of tissue. Peptic ulcer, commonly known as "ulcers," is a chronic condition in which the lining of the stomach or duodenum, the first part of the small intestine, is inflamed as a result of the action of digestive juices on the mucous membrane.

Peptic ulcers are found four times as often in men as in women, and ten to twelve times as often in the duodenum as in the stomach. They usually occur in definite locations which are bathed freely or regularly in gastric juices. Thus the upper part of the

duodenum, which receives partially digested food along with a certain amount of gastric juice as it is sent to the intestines, is a place where peptic ulcers are particularly apt to develop.

Pain, the outstanding symptom of peptic ulcer, usually occurs at certain regular times and is relieved by eating. Constipation is another common symptom. Nausea, vomiting, loss of appetite, and even anemia may occasionally be symptoms. Unfortunately most persons suffer symptoms over a period of five to eight years before seeking medical advice.

The doctor diagnoses peptic ulcer with x-rays, which will reveal the presence of an ulcer in the stomach in a great majority of cases but an ulcer in the duodenum with less accuracy. The gastroscope and fluoroscope with the aid of barium often can indicate the presence of ulcers when the x-ray has failed to do so.

Continued neutralization of the gastric juice relieves the pain, and this may be accomplished by use of antacids, which combine aluminum hydroxide and magnesia products. They are taken every two hours, alternating with food of some kind or milk so that the person takes milk, food, or antacid every waking hour.

Besides antacid powders and pastes to insure neutralization of the acid present in the gastric juices, drugs are prescribed which block the nerve impulses to the stomach and have an antispasmodic and sedative effect.

In addition, the doctor will prepare a diet which is suited to the condition. The diet will avoid seeds, skins, and foods with coarse fibers, as well as being nutritionally balanced to promote general health and healing of the ulcer.

One of the most serious complications of peptic ulcer is acute perforation of the wall of either the stomach or the duodenum, which often occurs without warning. In most cases, surgical treatment is required to repair the damage. A more frequent complication is destruction of a large blood vessel in the wall of the stomach or duodenum, causing massive hemorrhage with vomiting of blood and appearance of black tarry stools. Treatment of hemorrhage includes complete bed rest, blood transfusions if needed, and intravenous feeding until the patient can be fed orally. Then small but frequent meals of milk and cream are given and soft foods gradually added until a fairly strict ulcer diet is effected. Surgical treatment is usually not required. Under such management the bleeding stops and the ulcer is brought under control. Antacids, antispasmodic and sedative drugs are also part of the treatment.

Smoking, use of alcohol, and overexertion may aggravate ulcer formation and delay healing, and therefore doctors recommend abstinence from tobacco and alcohol and only moderate exercise.

Since psychological factors seem to be involved in the development of peptic ulcers, and since tense hard-driving persons appear to be more likely to develop them, treatment often emphasizes the need for reduced anxiety and tension. This can sometimes be effected by a change in occupation, a long restful vacation, or by psychotherapy. *See also* Chapter 18, "Disorders of the Digestive System and Diet in Digestive Disorders."

PERICARDITIS, an acute or chronic inflammation of the pericardium which covers and encloses the heart; it is caused by infection in the heart, or from infections in other parts of the body, from rheumatism, or wounds or tumors in the heart.

Some of the usual symptoms are pain over the heart, a rise in the pulse rate and temperature. In the dry or fibrinous form of pericarditis, the doctor can hear the sound of friction in the heart region made by the roughening of the wall of the pericardium and the formation of fibrinous material. In more extreme cases, so much fibrinous material may develop that the heart becomes encased and constricted in its movement. Surgery is sometimes successful in removing such calcified material. Occasionally fluid forms in such quantity that it becomes imperative to tap the pericardium and drain the fluid. This occurs mostly in cases of pericarditis which result from rheumatism. In another form of pericarditis, adhesions form which anchor the heart to surrounding tissue; these also require surgery.

In most cases of pericarditis, the infection which is the cause is treated. The use of antibiotics has been effective. When pericarditis is associated with tuberculosis, a long period of bed rest must accompany the antibacterial treatment.

PERINEUM, the part of the female body between the external genitals and the anus. In childbirth, these tissues are subject to great pressure and often tear and must be sewn up by the obstetrician. To prevent tearing during delivery, the doctor often makes an incision of the appropriate length in the perineum, which is later sewn and permitted to heal. After the delivery, the application of analgesic ointments and other preparations, as well as sitz baths, are helpful measures in healing the torn or incised perineum.

PERITONITIS, inflammation of the peritoneum, the membrane which lines the abdominal cavity. The peritoneum can be affected by many disturbances and inflammation is the most serious. Occasionally peritonitis is the result of direct injury to the abdomen, but usually it is a by-product of infection of one of the organs lying within the peritoneum, or of infection of the blood.

Acute peritonitis develops rapidly and a physician should be consulted as soon as possible. Death can result within a few hours or days following the onset of peritonitis.

The basic treatment is usually surgery and antibiotics. The peritoneal cavity must be opened and the infectious material removed. The microorganisms ordinarily involved in peritonitis are usually susceptible to effective control by penicillin and the sulfa drugs, and these drugs have been largely responsible for decreasing the once high fatality rate. However, successful treatment depends on early diagnosis and treatment.

Peritonitis is the most serious complication of appendicitis and may also follow the rupture of an ulcer of the stomach or intestine. Infection and pain begin almost simultaneously, the pain being most intense at the point of infection. A generalized feeling of acute illness follows as the body absorbs the poisons from the infection. The temperature rises, the abdomen is sensitive to touch, the abdominal wall is rigid, and vomiting begins. *See also* APPENDICITIS.

PERNICIOUS ANEMIA. *See* ANEMIA.

PERSPIRATION, or sweat, the fluid, largely water, excreted by the sweat or sudoriferous glands, situated beneath the outer surface of the skin with ducts opening into them. The chief function of sweating is to regulate body temperature. As moisture evaporates, heat energy is absorbed and in the process the surface on which evaporation takes place is cooled. Sweating is one of the main methods by which the body maintains the constant temperature vital to health and life.

The sweat glands are situated in the deepest of the several skin layers and communicate with the skin surface by corkscrew-shaped tubes. More of these glands are found per square inch in the palms of the hands and soles of the feet than elsewhere in the body. Those in the armpits and groin are the largest. The fluid exuded is 98 to 99 per cent water, plus a slight amount of salts and urea. Perspiration is normally acid, but when sweating is profuse, it becomes alkaline. About a pint to a pint and a half of water is exuded as sweat daily.

The body releases water in other ways than by sweating. About two quarts of water a day are exhaled in the breath; another quart and a half to two quarts passes in the urine.

Sweat passes through the skin to

the surface constantly. When it evaporates immediately without dampness, it is called insensible perspiration. When the sweating is more profuse and noticeable, it is called sensible perspiration. The amount of sweating varies according to the external temperature and the amount of exertion, part of the body, individual differences, and emotional factors. During an exciting motion picture, a person may sweat 50 per cent more than usual. One investigation indicated that sweating from the bottoms of the hands and feet was five to ten times greater than from other areas of the body.

The odor of sweat depends on the part of the body from which it comes. In winter, when persons perspire less, the urine will be lighter colored than during warmer weather.

Disorders of the sweat glands range from simple excessive perspiration to a serious underlying condition. Usually the annoyance of excessive perspiration can be alleviated by proper clothing, dusting powders, and an effective deodorant or antiperspirant. Some drugs limit sweating, but should not be applied to large areas of the body without a doctor's prescription. Profuse sweating occurs in malaria, tuberculosis, and rickets, which, of course, require medical attention. Light sweating is not uncommon; however, total failure of the body to sweat is rare. Drugs to encourage perspiration are available. Other conditions are bromidrosis, in which the perspiration has an offensive odor, and chromidrosis, in which the sweat turns black, blue, green, red, and yellow, believed to be due to in-

fection by specific microorganisms. *See also* BODY ODOR.

PERTUSSIS. *See* WHOOPING COUGH.

PHARYNGITIS. *See* PHARYNX.

PHARYNX, the area in the throat between the mouth and the opening of the esophagus or gullet. It functions as a resonating organ in speech. A group of semicircular muscles in the pharynx also help in the swallowing of food. The pharynx is generally divided into the nasal pharynx, extending to the nose, and the laryngeal pharynx, leading to the larynx and trachea.

The mucous lining of the pharynx may be affected by acute or chronic inflammation as the secondary effect of a severe cold, sore throat, or acute tonsillitis. It may also be infected by streptococci, as in septic sore throat. In most forms of acute pharyngitis the infection attacks suddenly, and the mucous lining becomes swollen, purple, and glazed, and covered by thick mucus. The uvula may swell and the tonsils also be seriously affected. Sometimes the swelling is severe enough to interfere with breathing; and fever, coughing, and a feeling of fatigue may develop.

The most effective treatment includes complete bed rest, hot drinks, drugs to control the fever, and gargling with warm salt water to allay the soreness. The doctor will employ intramuscular injections of penicillin in streptococcal sore throat and in other forms in which the organisms are responsive to penicillin. When penicillin is not tolerated by the patient, other antibiotics are used. Antibiotics are also effective in treating Vincent's angina, another form of throat infection which affects the pharynx.

Chronic pharyngitis of various types may result from repeated attacks of acute pharyngitis, and it is frequently associated with chronic colds, sinusitis, and nasal infections. Simple persistent inflammation of the pharynx is characterized by symptoms similar to the acute form, but is much less severe and without complications. It may be caused by smoking or inhalation of dust. The doctor usually applies medication while he searches for the underlying cause which he endeavors to eliminate.

In hypertrophic pharyngitis, another chronic form, the lymph nodes are also involved. A small amount of thick mucus in the throat may cause difficulty in expectorating and the patient will have a cough.

In atrophic pharyngitis, or dry sore throat, thick crusts form in the throat which produce a foul odor and are difficult to remove. Dry sore throat is often induced by diabetes, but may also result from decreased secretion of mucus in the throat during old age, or it may follow a similar condition affecting the nose. If it spreads from the throat to the larynx, hoarseness and coughing will result and the surface of the pharynx have a shellacked appearance. The doctor can apply proper medication and take steps to eliminate the causative condition.

PHENOLPHTHALEIN, a drug used as a laxative in constipation. In general it is less toxic than most other laxatives and is a constituent of many commercial laxatives. Although

rarely, certain persons are sensitive to it.

PHLEBITIS, inflammation of a vein, accompanied by swelling and pain. When infection and clotting occur, the condition is thrombophlebitis. Blood vessels that are swollen and knotted are often described as varicose.

Any illness which slows the blood circulation and which entails a long period of lying down may induce formation of clots in the blood vessels of the legs. After such an illness, when the person walks, clots may form, the legs swell and become blue, and even lameness result. To relieve this type of phlebitis, the foot of the bed is elevated and the legs kept free of pressure with a bed cradle. The legs may also be wrapped in soft cotton and placed on a pillow when the patient is sleeping, or a semielastic bandage worn. Moderate exercise is sometimes helpful. Recovery usually occurs in about ten days.

The greatest danger in phlebitis is that a clot may break off and form an embolism and lodge in a vital blood vessel leading to the heart, lungs, or brain. Fortunately this rarely happens. More frequently the clotting divides into small infected clots which travel to other parts of the body where secondary infections or abscesses may form.

Acute phlebitis is often painful. However, with modern treatment, the pain usually disappears as soon as the condition is brought under control. Treatment may include injection of drugs which both bring relief from pain and prevent clotting or coagulation. Dicumarol, which prevents blood coagulation, is widely used to treat acute phlebitis and other thromboses. Treatment may continue for weeks and sometimes months, and care must be taken to prevent pressure on veins.

PHTHISIS, an old term used for tuberculosis or any disease characterized by emaciation and loss of strength, especially diseases of the lungs. *See also* TUBERCULOSIS.

PHYSICAL THERAPY, the treatment of disease and disability by physical means, often by use of water, air, heat, massage, electricity, and exercise. This branch of medicine has undergone extensive and specialized development in recent years and enormously benefited innumerable paralyzed and disabled persons. Physiotherapy, as it is often called, has restored function to limbs or organs stricken by poliomyelitis, arthritis, muscular dystrophy, effects of tumors in the brain or nervous system and accidental injury. Even parts of the body totally disabled are sometimes restored to partial or complete use.

A variety of equipment and methods are utilized in physical therapy. High-frequency electrical current can be directed deep into the tissue of the body with a diathermy machine or infrared lamp, and is frequently used in treating inflamed joints, bursitis, infections of the sinus, and other conditions difficult to penetrate. Hydrotherapy, treatment by water in tanks, pools, or large baths, makes use of the buoyancy of water to treat paralyzed arms and

legs. The whirlpool, a special water device in which water circulates in a whirling motion at any desired temperature, produces a mild massaging movement and is used, for example, on a leg in which circulation of the blood has been retarded. In the constant-flow bath, the disturbed patient is placed in a canvas-type cradle with only his head above the surface and gently circulating tepid water soothes the nerves and induces relaxation and sleep.

Treatment to restore weakened muscles usually begins by subjecting them to a gentle motion, as in hydrotherapy. The patient performs simple exercises which increase in complexity as the muscles strengthen and become better coordinated. The treatment may include special devices such as stationary bicycles, weight lifts, and walkers. In the case of a paralyzed diaphragm, a machine which alternates air pressure and partial vacuum, such as the iron lung, enables the lung to move.

Occupational therapy is in a sense a variation of physical therapy and often is an essential part of rehabilitation of disabilities. The patient engages in activities which not only require him to use his disabled parts but which also help him develop new skills and crafts.

The development of new equipment has aided in the advancement of the entire field of physical therapy and today highly trained and specialized technicians are required to administer treatment under the supervision of the doctor. Physical therapy has come a long way from the hot-water bottle and heating pad.

PIGMENTATION, coloration of the skin; it is determined not only by the amount and nature of the pigment in the epidermis, but also by the color of the blood and the size of the blood vessels, especially those which are close to the surface.

The skin of a light-haired person contains little pigmentation, so that the blood shows through rather clearly. In a brunette, the pigmentation is heavier and the blood less visible. When the skin is almost black, the blood underneath is virtually invisible.

Flushing of the skin, a special aspect of skin pigmentation, is due to a temporary enlarging of the blood vessels close to the surface of the body, set off by certain nerves, and is provoked physiologically—by direct exposure to the sun, for example—or psychologically by emotional experiences such as embarrassment or confusion. *See also* FRECKLES; LIVER SPOTS; MELANOSIS; SUNBURN.

PILES. *See* HEMORRHOIDS.

PILONIDAL CYST, a term which goes back to ancient times and comes from two Latin words, *pilus* and *nidus,* meaning nest and hair or nest of hair. A pilonidal cyst develops from an improperly formed glandular organ, found under the skin at the end of the spine, which contains hair follicles and which secretes sebaceous and other fluids that have no outlet. This causes formation of a cyst, which may become infected and cause pain. The cysts seem to occur most frequently in men between the ages of twenty and forty-five. During World War II, men who sat for long periods in bumpy jeeps, trucks, and planes sometimes developed pilonidal cysts due to the irritation at the base of the spine. In some cases the cyst became as large as an egg.

The cysts are sometimes treated with temporary measures, including sitz baths and a minor incision to draw off fluid under pressure. However, when the opening of the cyst is blocked with hair, dirt, and body secretions, surgery is required. Considerable abnormal tissue must be excised and sufficient time spent in the hospital to allow complete healing. In some cases the excision is so extensive that plastic surgery and other reparative measures are required.

PINEAL GLAND, an organ, about the size of a pea, located in the head near the lower part of the brain. Its function, although considered vital in the human system, is not clearly understood. Recently researchers at Yale University discovered a hormone which is secreted from the pineal gland, but thus far its function is not completely known. One hormone is melanotonin concerned with pigmentation.

Enlargement of the pineal gland may crowd the passage through which the cerebrospinal fluid flows out of the brain into the spinal cord. When the canal is closed entirely, the brain fluid, seeking escape, creates such pressure that death may result.

Attempts to learn the function of the pineal gland in experimental work with animals have included both destruction of the gland and administration of excess amounts of a pineal extract. When the gland is eliminated in guinea pigs, their sex organs grow to greater size and more rapidly than normal. Results with pineal extract are less certain, because a pineal extract has not yet been made which has demonstrable and unquestioned activity. Animals fed such an extract seem to grow larger and become stronger than others; however, they also manifest retarded development of the sex organs. The supposition is that pineal extract slows down excessively rapid growth and retards overactivity of the sex glands.

Tumors of the pineal gland are rare, and in young boys cause development of sexual organs to adult size and function. They do not have the same effect on young girls. A pineal tumor in an adult woman may cause menstruation to cease, and in an adult man may provoke the sex glands and testes to degenerate.

Although surgical removal of the pineal gland is not often advisable, because of the high mortality rate, in some cases permanent cure has been achieved by this means. Radiation therapy may bring a temporary cure.

PINKEYE, an inflammation of the conjunctiva, the tissue which covers the inner surface of the eyelid. It may be caused by a germ often carried on towels or on soiled hands. The eyes become red and the eyelids swollen and puffy. Often the eyelids are stuck together with pus when the person awakens from sleep. Medical treatment varies, depending on the type of germ involved. A similar appearance, called vernal conjunctivitis, may develop as the result of allergy. *See also* CONJUNCTIVITIS.

PINWORM. *See* WORMS.

PITUITARY, the most important gland of the endocrine system, or glands of internal secretion. This gland secretes substances into the blood which are carried to organs in other parts of the body where they exert significant effects. Thus, the endocrine system regulates many of the most important of the bodily functions. These include growth, sexual development, defenses against emergencies and disease, and many metabolic processes. The pituitary performs an unusual number of these and, in addition, controls other endocrine glands. Endocrine secretions are called hormones.

The pituitary is divided into two distinct portions: the anterior and the posterior. The anterior is much more important, having a profound role in bodily growth, the development and activity of the adrenal cortex, the sex glands, the thyroid, and the pancreas. The posterior is related especially to water retention by the kidneys.

The mechanisms involved in control of growth are not fully understood, but the significance of the pituitary in the process is well established. The growth hormone, if excessive during childhood and adolescence, will produce giants, and if insufficient, dwarfs. If pituitary overactivity occurs later in life when the principal bones have lost capacity to grow further, those of the extremities —the head, hands, and feet—may enlarge, resulting in a condition called acromegaly. The face may assume a coarse look and the tongue grow. Usually due to a pituitary tumor, acromegaly can be treated by surgery or x-ray.

When the pituitary is removed from an immature animal, its long bones soon cease to expand and its total size and weight remain smaller than normal.

Another function of the pituitary is the stimulation of the sex glands to maturity. This occurs at puberty, until which time the pituitary growth hormone controls growth. When the sex glands, under the pituitary stimulus, develop to a point of secreting the full amount of their own hormones, the growth hormone ceases to affect increase in height. The pituitary continues throughout life, however, to secrete growth substance, but its function after the attainment of physical maturity is not yet fully understood.

When pregnancy occurs, a hormone related to the female periodic cycle becomes superfluous for the time being and is excreted in the urine. The Aschheim-Zondek test for pregnancy is based on this fact. In this test, immature rabbits or mice are injected with urine from the patient. If the hormone is being excreted and is present in the urine, the animals mature in a few days which signifies that the person is pregnant. This test achieves 98 to 99 per cent accuracy.

Slow sexual development in young people and reduction of fertility because of underactive testes or ovaries in adults can be treated by extracts of pituitary gland containing the sex-stimulating pituitary hormones.

One of the most significant pituitary secretions is ACTH, the initials of the term adreno-cortico-trophic hormone, which means that the substance has a special affinity for the cortex or outer part of the adrenal gland. Since the adrenal cortex is greatly involved with meeting stresses of practically all kinds which the body bears, the function of the pituitary substance which stimulates it is particularly significant. ACTH is now used, with much the same effect as cortisone, an adrenal-cortical hormone, to relieve several diseases, including arthritis, asthma, hives, and exceptionally high fever.

When the pituitary is removed, the adrenal glands degenerate. Degeneration of the adrenals also causes Addison's disease, which was formerly fatal. Now the lives of patients with such disorders may be extended by use of hormones derived from the adrenal cortex.

Other pituitary substances are associated with the secretion of milk and the activity of the thyroid gland.

The posterior pituitary is connected with retention of water by the kidneys. Many nerve fibers connect it to the section of the brain involved in regulating weight, sleep, muscular coordination, and emotional activity. It affects the system of involuntary muscles when these are inactive and so is sometimes used in aiding childbirth and stimulating the bowels. The posterior pituitary also is involved in controlling blood sugar.

General pituitary inactivity renders a person dull and slow, in mind as well as body. Sleep occurs easily and fat accumulates. In young children this inactivity retards both mental and sexual development. Overactivity of the pituitary induces a variety of symptoms.

Other pituitary functions include a relationship with the parts of the pancreas producing insulin, which regulates body utilization of sugar, and another relationship with the thyroid gland. When the pancreas is removed from an animal, sugar appears in its blood and urine, since sugar cannot be used properly without insulin. If the pituitary is also removed, these symptoms are relieved. Removal of the pituitary with the pancreas left intact causes a diminution of sugar.

A pituitary secretion partially controls the thyroid, and deficient thyroid activity leads to pituitary enlargement. The thyroid is enlarged, in turn, by administration of the pituitary hormone related to it. Pituitary deficiency tends to lower the basal metabolism which functions closely with the thyroid. The pituitary also influences the parathyroid glands which are involved with the body's use of calcium.

A possible relationship between the pituitary and growth, and the processes which lead to cancer is being investigated. Cases have been recorded in which a cancer of the prostate gland and of the breast have been controlled by removal of the pituitary.

Among the most serious disorders which involve the pituitary is Cushing's disease, in which a tumor in the anterior lobe causes, among other symptoms, obesity of the abdomen, face, and buttocks. Atrophy, or degeneration, of the anterior lobe in adults results in Simmond's disease, characterized by extreme emaciation. In rare cases of Froehlich's syndrome, the anterior lobe is so affected as to produce extreme obesity and infantile sexual organs. *See also* CUSH-

ING'S DISEASE; and Chapter 19, "Endocrine Glands."

PLACENTA. *See* AFTERBIRTH; REPRODUCTION SYSTEM.

PLAGUE, a contagious disease, endemic in eastern Asia and in former times occurring epidemically in Europe and Asia Minor. In the Middle Ages, epidemics of various kinds used to devastate populations. Called the Black Death, the plague spread throughout Europe, often wiping out entire sections of population. For example, Florence, between 1345 and 1350, lost almost half of its inhabitants from the bubonic plague. The plague is thought to have been introduced into Europe from China, via the trade routes. Medieval physicians believed that the air was filled with the contagion of the plague.

Today it has been learned that such plagues are due to the spread of small, rod-shaped germs, pasteurella pestis, which are transmitted to man by the rat flea.

The two most common forms of plague are bubonic and pneumonic plague. In bubonic plague, swollen abscesses appear in the groin, commonly called the bubo, accompanied by swelling and hypertrophy of one or more lymph nodes. The disease also affects the blood, spleen, and liver. In pneumonic plague, the germs infect the lungs.

Modern science has developed methods of vaccination against plague and techniques of control to prevent its spread, so that it is exceedingly rare in civilized countries. Only a few cases of pneumonic or bubonic plague have been reported in the United States in the past fifty years.

PLATELETS, also called thrombocytes. *See* BLOOD.

PLEURISY, a group of symptoms produced by inflammation or infection of the pleura, the lining of the chest cavity covering the inside of the chest wall, the top of the diaphragm, and the outer side of the lungs.

The most common sources of pleurisy are pneumonia, tuberculosis, and influenza. The first signs are usually pain, which may become severe on taking a deep breath, a cough, fever, and rapid shallow breathing. In some cases, a quantity of fluid is effused. This accumulation is known as pleurisy with effusion or "wet" pleurisy. Sometimes a large amount of pus is formed by secondary infection, producing a condition known as empyema which is extremely serious and requires immediate care.

In the form called "dry" pleurisy, which almost always follows an acute case of pneumonia, pain appears over the site of the infection and with a stethoscope the doctor can hear a sound of rubbing inside the chest cavity. When the underlying infection is cured, the pleurisy disappears.

In management of pleurisy, the patient should remain in bed, as bed rest is almost as significant as medication in relieving the condition. In mild cases, application of heat may be helpful. When breathing causes severe pain, the doctor will sometimes strap the chest to limit its movement. Tapping, to drain off pleural fluid, and use of solutions containing anti-

biotics is often effective, and acute cases of pleurisy respond rapidly to this treatment, and the incidence of chronic pleurisy has been greatly reduced. An operation may be imperative in cases of severe empyema.

PNEUMONIA, an inflammation of one or both lungs. Many types of pneumonia have been distinguished, but usually when the word pneumonia is used without qualification, lobar pneumonia, in which one or more entire lobes are infected, is implied, and the causative organism is the pneumococcus. Other organisms may also produce pneumonia, such as the streptococcus and staphylococcus, which may cause bronchopneumonia.

The symptoms of a typical case of pneumonia may follow a slight cold or infectious disease or may appear suddenly without warning. A shaking chill may be followed by a sharp stabbing pain on the side of or in the chest, with coughing and expectoration of brown or bloody sputum. The pulse is rapid, the cheeks flushed, temperature rises sharply, and weakness and even prostration, headache, nausea, vomiting, and diarrhea sometimes ensue.

The person with pneumonia must be put to bed immediately, and carefully watched, since restlessness, sleeplessness, and even delirium may provoke the patient, despite his weakness, to try to get out of bed.

As the infection progresses, changes may take place in the lung itself. It may become filled with inflammatory material and solidify, causing shortness of breath and shallow noisy breathing. The blood cannot obtain sufficient oxygen and so the skin and mucous membranes may become bluish, a condition known as cyanosis. The patient must be placed in an oxygen tent to assist his breathing as well as correct the cyanosis.

During the acute stages of pneumonia, care must be taken to prevent complications, such as heart failure, empyema, distention of the abdomen, and abscess. The development of other diseases, including pericarditis, endocarditis, meningitis, and arthritis, must also be carefully prevented.

For a long time pneumonia was a dreaded disease with a high mortality rate. Treatment depended on the use of serums, which were developed to combat specific infections, and the condition usually led to an acute stage with a definite "crisis," in which the patient appeared near collapse. After the crisis, a sharp drop in temperature followed and the patient fell into a deep sleep, with subsequent recovery in some cases.

Today the use of sulfonamides and antibiotics, such as penicillin, terramycin, aureomycin, and streptomycin, have decreased the development of lung abscess and empyema, and the death rate has fallen sharply. Good nursing care in pneumonia still continues to play a considerable part. The recovery period is especially significant. The patient should not get up from bed or engage in activity too early. A complete physical checkup, including a chest x-ray examination, is strongly advised following pneumonia.

The number of cases of virus pneumonia has sharply increased, at the same time that bacterial pneumonia has yielded to treatment with sulfa drugs and antibiotics. Although the nature of viruses is not completely understood, and few specific measures have been developed to combat them, it is known that virus pneumonia is produced by a number of specific types of virus. Virus pneumonia may vary from a mild or "walking" state to a serious condition requiring hospitalization. In a mild case the patient may not suspect that he has anything more severe than a slight cough and fever, which he may ascribe to a cold. In the more severe form, fever, sweating, malaise, headache, sore throat, weakness, and a dry hacking cough are involved.

Treatment of virus pneumonia includes bed rest, even in a mild case. Antibiotics are frequently effective in preventing complications. It is essential to treat the fever and cough; and in severe cases in which cyanosis is present, an oxygen tent may also be required. In general, virus pneumonia does not persist more than a few days to a week. However, convalescence, usually characterized by weakness, is often long and slow, and x-ray examination of the chest may reveal shadows for several weeks.

POISONING. Any substance which is capable of producing a harmful or deadly effect can be considered a poison. For most such substances there is both a safe dose and a poisonous dose, the severity of the effect depending on the amount taken and on the age and physical condition of the person involved.

Poisoning is an emergency situation; *the doctor should be called immediately,* and first aid given at once.

Symptoms, although there may be no early ones, include nausea, vomiting, cramps, and stomach pains. If a corrosive poison has been taken, burns and stains may appear on and around the mouth and tongue. Headache remedies and sleep-producing drugs produce drowsiness, sleep, and sometimes unconsciousness.

In first-aid treatment for poisoning, two points are important. The first is that a poison diluted with a large amount of liquid is absorbed less quickly than in concentrate and vomiting can be induced more easily when the stomach is filled. Second, once the poison is removed from the body it can do no further harm and so in some types of poisoning it is imperative to induce vomiting repeatedly until the fluid ejected is as clear as when it was swallowed.

To dilute the poison and induce vomiting various liquids may be used: warm soapsuds, soda water made with common baking soda, or salt water. The liquid should preferably be lukewarm. It may be necessary to give six or seven or more glasses of liquid.

After the stomach is thoroughly cleaned out, an antidote may be given. A good universal antidote which can be given for all cases of poisoning and which every household should keep on hand consists of the following: two parts powdered burnt toast, one part milk of magnesia, one part strong tea. The carbon in the toast absorbs poisons; the magnesium has a soothing effect on the mucous membranes of the stomach and a laxative action which also neutralizes acid poisons; and the tannic acid in the tea tends to neutralize caustic alkaline materials. A heaping tablespoon of Epsom salts also can be given.

Two important exceptions are alkali and acid poisoning. In these cases, vomiting *should not be induced,* to avoid danger of perforation. In first-aid treatment for *acid poisoning,* neutralize the poison with an alkali, such as baking soda, lime water, milk of magnesia, or chalk. Then give a demulcent, such as milk, olive oil, or egg white. The victim should be kept warm.

For *alkali poisoning,* neutralize the alkali with a weak acid such as dilute lemon juice or vinegar. Then give milk. The victim should be kept warm.

Shock is frequently present in all types of poisoning and must be controlled. The victim should be kept warm and if breathing stops, artificial respiration applied.

In poisoning from a sleep-producing drug, it is especially important that the stomach be washed out by whatever means possible, and a cup of strong coffee every half hour or so is also recommended. The danger that breathing may stop is particularly imminent and artificial respiration may be necessary.

There are a vast number of substances which when swallowed or inhaled can be poisonous, such as insecticides, polishes, sprays, cleaners. When poisoning is suspected, it is sometimes difficult to determine what the poisonous substance has been. If the victim is unable to give the information, perhaps an open bottle or his physical symptoms can help decide. In the case of some substance taken from a container, the container often but not always gives the remedy for poisoning. Some cities maintain special bureaus which give information about poisoning and its antidotes, including all the new products on the market which might conceivably be poisonous.

Following is a list of some of the more common causes of poisoning, with symptoms and treatment.

ACETANILID POISONING. Acetanilid, phenacetin, and Pyramidon are frequently constituents of headache remedies which, in sufficiently large doses, can cause death, especially in children. The person will have disturbed hearing or deafness, rapid breathing, blue lips and nails, nausea, vomiting, and sometimes convulsions, stupor, or coma. Vomiting should be induced unless the person is unconscious or has already vomited excessively. Then the universal antidote is given. Since respiratory failure is a dangerous possibility, artificial respiration may have to be given. When the doctor arrives, he may have the victim placed in an oxygen tent.

ARSENIC POISONING. Arsenic is present in many insecticides, rodent killers, paints, dyes, and cosmetics. Small doses of arsenic taken into the body over a long period produce irritation of nerve endings. The person who has swallowed an arsenic product will have burning pains in the throat and stomach, and the odor of garlic on his breath. Other symptoms may be vomiting and diarrhea and extreme thirst with a choking sensation. Vomiting should be induced, followed by an antidote of egg whites in water or milk, and the vomiting-antidote procedure repeated. Afterward strong coffee or tea is given,

and then Epsom salts in water or castor oil.

BARBITURATE POISONING. The barbiturates include such well-known drugs as Luminal, Seconal, phenobarbital, pentobarbital, Amytal, Dial, Ipral, neonal, and Evipal. Either intentionally or unintentionally people sometimes take overdoses of "sleeping pills," which in many cases leads to death, and most states have laws governing purchase of these potentially harmful drugs. Symptoms of barbiturate poisoning include headache and confusion, bluish color of nails and lips, uneven breathing, drowsiness, stupor and coma. Vomiting should be induced. The chief problem is to maintain proper breathing and to control shock. Strong coffee or tea is given and artificial respiration if necessary. The doctor will make certain that the throat is free of mucus and that the victim is receiving enough air.

BENZENE POISONING. Benzene, a widely used solvent, is frequently a constituent of floor waxes, floor cleaners, varnish removers, and numerous other products. Benzene vapor is heavier than air, but when warmed it rises and spreads easily. A person who has inhaled benzene fumes will act, at first, as though intoxicated, appearing flushed, dazed, and staggering. He will become drowsy and gradually unconscious. He should immediately receive fresh air and be given artificial respiration if necessary. In case the benzene has been swallowed, the person will breathe with difficulty and have a slow pulse. Nausea and vomiting will probably occur and maybe convulsions. Vomiting is *not* to be induced, but strong coffee or tea given. The victim must receive fresh air and artificial respiration if necessary. The doctor will support the action of the heart with drugs. A victim of benzene poisoning must be particularly careful to receive adequate nutriments in order to build up the blood.

BORIC ACID POISONING. Infants have been seriously poisoned by mistakenly being given boric acid solutions instead of water, although boric acid in ordinary quantities is not a dangerous poison. Vomiting should be induced, coffee given as a stimulant, and large amounts of alkaline drinks to protect the kidneys.

COAL OIL OR KEROSENE POISONING. The first symptom of ingestion of kerosene is a burning sensation in the stomach, mouth, and throat, followed by nausea and vomiting with slow breathing and feeble pulse, and convulsions and coma. Strong coffee or tea should be given and artificial respiration if necessary. Vomiting should *not* be induced. If kerosene fumes have been inhaled, the person's face is flushed or his lips blue, and he has difficulty breathing. He should be removed from the area of the fumes into fresh air, and artificial respiration given if necessary. Persons who work in an atmosphere where they inhale great amounts of coal, oil, kerosene, or naphtha fumes develop symptoms of "naphtha jag," characterized by a sense of excitement and lack of self-control, followed by depression, headache, nausea, a roaring sound in the ears, irritation in the throat, and a trembling of the hands and arms. If sufficient fumes have been inhaled, shallow breathing, weak heart, convulsions, and death may

ensue. The doctor may give antibiotics to prevent pneumonia, and blood transfusions may be required.

CYANIDE POISONING. Cyanide, used in the silver industry and in certain insecticides, is lethal in small quantities and acts with extreme rapidity. Hundreds of deaths occur each year from cyanide poisoning and in most cases it is difficult for the doctor to determine just how much cyanide has been taken. Treatment has been unsatisfactory because the poison is so rapidly fatal. Antidotes used are methylene blue, glucose injections, amyl nitrate inhalation, and sodium thiosulphate and sodium nitrite injections. Lavage with potassium permanganate is also part of current treatment.

The person who has swallowed cyanide has the odor of bitter almonds on his breath, is confused, and has a headache. Vomiting and diarrhea are present, followed by convulsions, unconsciousness, stoppage of breath. First-aid treatment includes inducement of vomiting and drinking large amounts of hydrogen peroxide in water.

LYE POISONING. Lye is a caustic alkali used as a cleansing agent in washing powder, drainpipe cleaner, and paint remover, and is a household menace, especially to children. The person who has swallowed lye has burns and stains on the mouth and a burning pain in the mouth, throat, and stomach. Vomiting occurs. Vomiting should *never* be induced. The alkali should be neutralized with a weak acid such as diluted vinegar or citrus fruit juice—as much as the person can drink. The doctor may reopen the throat passage so that the person can breathe and swallow by using a rubber eyeless catheter which is gradually increased in size. Treatment to dilate the passage with this device may in some cases continue for as long as a year. The doctor may also give sedatives to relieve pain and treat the local burns.

MERCURY POISONING. Bichloride of mercury acts rapidly on the tissues of the body. In severe cases, the victim suffers pains in the abdomen, vomiting. Egg whites and milk help to inactivate the mercury. The doctor may give BAL for several days. It forms an easily excretable combination with the excess mercury.

NARCOTIC POISONING. The victim of narcotic poisoning is drowsy and may fall asleep, pass into a coma, and die. Vomiting should be induced and strong coffee given as a stimulant. It may even be imperative to move the person about forcibly to keep him awake and avoid respiratory failure. Artificial respiration may be required.

NICOTINE POISONING. Nicotine is a constituent of a group of insecticides. Ingestion of nicotine causes a hot burning sensation of the stomach; it is rapidly absorbed and may cause heart failure, convulsions, and respiratory failure. Initially the person is nervous and excited, then depressed. He may suffer vomiting and diarrhea, breathe deeply and rapidly, and have pale clammy skin. Vomiting should be induced, followed by hot tea and burnt toast, or the universal antidote. Artificial respiration may be necessary and the doctor may give oxygen inhalations.

STRYCHNINE POISONING. Some cathartics and tonics contain strychnine. Symptoms of strychnine poisoning

are nervousness and excitement, stiff neck, and twitching muscles and convulsions. Vomiting should *not* be induced except immediately after the poison has been taken. Burnt toast is given and the victim kept in a quiet dark room. The doctor may control the convulsions with barbiturates and wash the stomach with potassium permanganate solution or tannic acid. Artificial respiration or oxygen may be necessary.

THALLIUM POISONING. Thallium sulfate is an ingredient of some depilatories. The symptoms are nausea, pain in the stomach, diarrhea, delirium, and convulsions. Vomiting should be induced and strong coffee or tea given.

TURPENTINE. Turpentine comes in straight form, and floor polishes may contain this potential poison. Symptoms are abdominal pain, nausea, vomiting, and diarrhea, and later excitement, stupor, and coma. Sometimes the urine contains whole blood. Treatment includes inducement of vomiting, followed by Epsom salts in water and large amounts of water to promote urination.

See also CARBON MONOXIDE; DEADLY NIGHTSHADE POISONING; FOOD POISONING; MUSHROOM POISONING; LEAD POISONING.

POLIOMYELITIS, an inflammation of the anterior horn cells in the gray matter of the spinal cord. It is caused by a virus, the smallest living material. Viruses differ from bacteria mainly in that they cannot move by themselves and cannot live outside a living body. The virus of infantile paralysis, or poliomyelitis, as it is more properly called, is one of the smallest known. Man is affected almost exclusively, although monkeys may be infected.

Poliomyelitis can exist in one of three forms. Many people have had poliomyelitis without realizing it, having contracted a mild case which rendered them immune to further attacks. Poliomyelitis may cause only a little diarrhea, stomach upset, cold, or muscle aches, which last for a few days. This is known as abortive poliomyelitis. If temporary paralysis of arms or legs occurs, the condition is known as nonparalytic poliomyelitis. The third type, paralytic poliomyelitis, may cause lasting damage or death if respiratory muscles are involved.

Epidemics of poliomyelitis usually occur during the warm months, July to October in the United States, and February through April in Australia. The virus is present in the nasopharynx and bowel movements and may be spread by sneezing, coughing, or by contamination of water or food with sewage. The poliomyelitis virus affects the cells of the spinal cord, brain, and other nervous tissue, leading to the familiar paralyses. Adults as well as children may be affected. Symptoms may be vague at first and include fever, headache, spasms of the arms, neck, thighs, and weakness. Treatment, which is not yet wholly satisfactory, consists of exercising the affected muscle groups to prevent withering and shrinking from lack of use; employment of the iron lung to carry on respiration when the respiratory or breathing muscles are damaged, and other such supportive measures.

Innumerable numbers of children have become permanent cripples as a result of polio, and many adults and children have died from it.

The development of the Salk poliomyelitis vaccine has been a particular blessing to all parents and children. The vaccine can produce immunity to the poliomyelitis virus, and this may last for many years. The vaccine is produced by growing virus on the tissue of the kidneys of monkeys. The virus is then denatured, or killed, making it safe for injection into human beings. Even though denatured, the vaccine can cause the human body to produce resistant substances, or antibodies, to poliomyelitis. All human beings should be vaccinated. For a more detailed discussion of the Salk vaccine, *See* Chapter 23, "The Neuromuscular and Neurological Disabilities."

POLYCYTHEMIA, a disease of unknown origin in which the production of red blood cells in the bone marrow is greatly increased. The average number of red blood cells is about five to six million per cubic millimeter of blood. In polycythemia, the number may reach as many as fifteen million red blood cells per cubic millimeter of blood. Usually white blood cells and platelets increase also, adding to the viscosity of the blood and affecting its flow to the brain and other parts of the body.

The symptoms in polycythemia may include dizziness, severe headache, and a feeling of fullness in the head. In some cases, fainting occurs and numbness and tingling in the hands and feet. The person may feel irritable and sluggish and have occasional spells of amnesia. Sometimes the vision is disturbed and there is a constant ringing in the ears. The spleen becomes greatly enlarged in order to act as a storage reservoir for the increased production of blood cells. The person's skin often has a bluish cast because of the prominence of small veins.

Treatment for overproduction of blood cells with the consequent enlarged spleen may be done by x-ray of the entire body. Radioactive phosphorus seems to be the most effective treatment, bringing relief for long periods.

When great overproduction of white blood cells and platelets also occurs, other drugs are effective. Blood-letting to relieve severe attacks of polycythemia is sometimes practiced, and has been found effective when thromboembolism is a complicating factor. In mild cases of polycythemia, periodic blood-letting may be the only treatment. However, there is danger of loss of iron and consequent anemia, in terms of hemoglobin content and oxygen-carrying capacity of the blood. Besides thromboembolism, hemorrhage and gout can also be complications of polycythemia.

POLYP, a nonmalignant tumor which hangs by a pedicle or stalk from the surface of a body cavity. Polyps vary widely in structure and nature, depending on their location. In the ear, a polyp consists of granular tissue caused by chronic irritation. A nasal polyp contains a soft overgrowth of mucous membrane and generally indicates disease of the underlying bone tissue. A rectal polyp is usually a glandular tumor. Polyps are frequently found inside the sinuses as inflammatory growth on mucous lining. A gastric polyp is a nonmalignant tumor in the stomach.

Surgery is generally employed to remove polyps. In the nose, the base must also be excised after the polyp has been removed. Sometimes polyps occur in groups in the large intestine and must be removed and the entire area excised because of the danger that one may have become malignant. Electric current is often used to remove polyps in the urethra. Polyps on the walls of the uterus may not require treatment unless they endanger health. Rectal and gastric polyps also may become malignant and should therefore be removed.

POSTURE, position or bearing of the body. Good posture means that the body is held in the correct position when standing, sitting, lying down, or in motion.

In standing, the ideal posture is one in which the person stands tall and erect, the abdomen drawn in, the shoulders square and high, the chin straight back and held in, the weight properly distributed on the feet, and the curve of the back well within normal limitations.

In a correct sitting position, the body is erect and the head poised to bring the center of gravity in the line joining the bones of the hips. A constant bent posture or droopy position while at work or at rest results in stretching and relaxing of ligaments, with a tendency toward permanent sagging. As a result, the back becomes rounded and the chin pushed forward.

Good posture through life is desirable because it will prevent many disorders and help cure others. Both the home and school can cooperate effectively in training children to observe the rules of correct posture. Defects in posture can be corrected in preschool children if detected early enough. The teacher should always be alert to poor posture in pupils and take steps to single out cases for special attention. Physical exercise and posture training throughout school and college, and a program of physical exercise in adulthood are important to good health.

Faulty posture may be related to improper clothing and especially to the wrong kind of shoes. A definite relationship between flat feet, twisted spine, and other posture deformities and ill-fitting shoes has been established.

Exercises for Faulty Posture. The following exercises are recommended for correcting ordinary faulty posture.

1. The person with faulty posture should stand in front of a mirror. Another person should place his hand about one inch in front of the flat bone of the chest and push it forward to touch the hand, without swaying the body. He should try not to draw his shoulders back but keep them relaxed. Gradually the distance to which the chest is to be brought forward is increased by holding the hand farther away. Once the person is accustomed to the feeling of this exercise, he can do it without using a mirror. This posture should be repeated until it becomes easy and natural and can be maintained without strain or discomfort. The object is to achieve a proper relation between the thorax and the pelvis.

After this exercise has been repeated twenty times, the following exercises should be performed.

2. Raise arms forward, stretch them upward, rise on tiptoes, and inhale. Lower arms to the sides, slowly press the arms back, and exhale. This exercise, when done correctly, expands the chest, bringing in all the extensor muscles of the back and the levator muscles of the shoulders.

3. Stand with arms down and back, fingers interlocked, and palms out. Extend the neck, roll the shoulders back and turn the forearms so that the palms turn in, then down, and then out. Reverse to starting position and relax. This exercise is valuable for projecting the chest forward, stretching the shortened ligaments, and drawing in the abdomen. Care should be taken to have the chin back when the arms are brought down and turned out. When this exercise cannot be done with the fingers interlocked, a handkerchief tied in a loop may be substituted and held in the fingers.

4. Stand with the arms at the sides. Raise arms, stretch, inhale, bend forward, and rise. Lower arms, exhale. In this exercise the lungs are filled when the chest is in the most favorable position for expansion. The breath is retained when the trunk is flexed, forcing the air into the cells of the lungs, under pressure. The bending and rising employs the extensor muscles of the neck and the retractor muscles of the shoulders.

5. Lie prone on a couch with the feet strapped, or on the floor with the feet caught on the edge of a bureau or other article of furniture. Clasp hands behind the head. Raise

the head and extend the spine, pressing the elbows back. This exercise strengthens the back and shoulders. Follow with a deep breathing exercise.

6. Lie in the same position as in exercise 5, arms at the sides. Raise head, bring arms forward, and imitate the breast stroke.

In this exercise the spine is kept in static contraction, while the retractors of the shoulders are alternately contracted and relaxed.

Additional Exercises. Here are some simple exercises which help to strengthen the muscles of the back and abdomen and thus improve posture.

1. Lie on the back, hands back of the neck. Take a deep breath and raise chest high; keep chest up and exhale by pulling abdomen in.

2. In the same position, bend the knees and pull feet up. Pull abdomen in hard, and then relax.

3. Sit in a chair, trunk bending forward from the hips, keeping spine straight. This exercise may be done standing.

4. Stand with the heels four inches away from the wall but with the hips, shoulders, and head touching the wall; flatten the lower part of the back against the wall by pulling in the abdominal muscles. Holding this position, come away from the wall, with the weight well forward on the balls of the feet.

5. Stand with hands on hips, back flat, and chin in; raise one leg forward without bending the knee; lower it; repeat with other leg.

6. With head forward, clasp hands behind the head. Force the head back against their pressure, keeping chin in. This strengthens the muscles of the back of the neck.

7. Stand tall, holding the back straight. Rise on the toes, with arms extended forward and up, stretching the arms and the body.

PREGNANCY AND PRENATAL CARE. Pregnancy is the state of a woman from conception to childbirth, usually 280 days. During this time, many changes take place in the body of the prospective mother. While the greatest changes take place in the organs immediately concerned with childbirth, every organ is influenced by pregnancy. When pregnancy occurs, the uterus becomes thickened and enlarges with the growth of the prospective child. The breasts begin to develop as early as the second month and in young women who are having their first baby as early as the second or third week. A greater tenderness and fullness of the breasts and a darkening and enlarging of the nipples is apparent. Various glands of the body are affected by pregnancy and produce greater amounts of secretion. The whole rate of chemical changes, measured by basal metabolism, is also likely to be increased.

Certain definite signs indicate to the doctor that a woman is pregnant. In the majority of cases, the regular menstruation disappears after the woman has conceived, and will not recur again during pregnancy. Disappearance of menstruation in a woman whose menstrual periods have always been regular usually indicates that she is pregnant. There are cases, however, in which a woman has had one or even two discharges of blood from the uterus after conception, but the quantity and duration are usually much less than normal. More frequent urination is often a sign of pregnancy. Some women will experience a feeling of sickness, nausea, and vomiting, especially in the morning. These symptoms usually develop during the second month and rarely last past the end of the fourth month, and many variations occur in their appearance, intensity, and duration. Some women are troubled several times a day, and in rare instances the sickness takes place only at night when the woman goes to bed.

Many women become increasingly emotional during pregnancy, with feelings of peevishness, fretfulness, irritability, unreasonableness, and depression. Other women, on the contrary, feel unusually cheerful. The craving for unusual foods is a manifestation of the emotional changes that may occur, as is a change in daily habits. A woman who has been exceedingly clean and meticulous may suddenly become careless and slovenly.

When the expectant mother is twelve to fourteen weeks pregnant, her abdomen will begin to enlarge. At the end of sixteen weeks the enlargement of the abdomen will seem pronounced to her, although other people probably will not notice it for another month. The womb continues to enlarge in order to give room to the growing fetus. Between the sixteenth and eighteenth weeks she is likely to feel a faint fluttering, which is called "quickening." This symptom is not a certain one, because things can occur inside the abdomen that resemble the movement of the fetus but actually stem from other causes. Women who are excessively worried about being pregnant frequently imagine that they feel movements.

Some signs of pregnancy are so positive that they leave no doubt. One is an x-ray picture which shows the presence of the prospective child. Another is its heartbeat, which is audible between the eighteenth and twentieth weeks and occasionally earlier. Laboratory tests are almost infallible. The Aschheim-Zondek tests ("rabbit tests") are highly reliable in diagnosing pregnancy. They are, however, expensive and only required in unusual cases.

Once the condition of pregnancy has been established the expectant mother should talk to the doctor about prenatal care, for her health must be the best possible during pregnancy. Any disease or ailment she has must be known to the doctor to avoid future possible complications for mother and child. Prenatal care is especially significant if she is diabetic or has heart disease.

Fees should be decided in advance in a frank discussion with the doctor or obstetrician. Currently a lump sum for prenatal care, delivery, and postnatal care is common. If the child is to be born in a hospital, arrangements for reserving a bed for confinement should be made well in advance. Some families find that hospitalization and sickness insurance cover most of the expenses. However, financial limitations need not and must not limit or prevent prenatal care. Most hospitals offer classes which instruct expectant mothers, and fathers, in the care of the baby. The prospective mother should also discuss with her doctor whether or not her new baby is to be breast fed or formula fed. If breast feeding is recommended, the doctor will advise her in the care of her breasts.

The expectant mother will see her doctor usually once a month, unless unusual symptoms arise, and more often during the later days of pregnancy. During these visits, he will make a complete physical examination, which includes blood pressure and urine, to determine whether inflammations or diabetes are present. He makes accurate measurements of the organs concerned in childbirth and thus is able to anticipate difficulties which might arise. He examines her blood, one of the blood tests establishing whether or not the blood contains the rhesus factor. Blood containing the rhesus factor is RH positive, blood which does not is RH negative. If the baby's blood is RH positive and the mother's is RH negative, the baby may be born with anemia and require a blood transfusion at birth.

At each visit, the doctor will ask the pregnant woman about symptoms, since certain symptoms may indicate complications. He should always be informed of persistent headaches, bleeding from the vagina, undue swelling of the hands and feet, leakage of water from the vagina, blurred vision, abdominal pains, serious vomiting, fainting spells, scanty urine, and excessive gain in weight. If necessary, he will then determine the cause and significance of these symptoms in order to anticipate and, in most cases, prevent serious complications.

The best way to help prevent complications in labor or delivery is to maintain good health and stamina throughout the period of pregnancy by proper diet and strict attention to the rules and advice of the doctor. The food supply for the baby reaches it through the blood vessels which connect with the mother. If her diet is deficient, food cannot be extracted from her tissues and organs for its growth. Her food intake should be regulated with the needs of the growing child. A good general rule for her is to eat the foods she usually eats, provided she has had a proper diet, but to make certain that she receives sufficient milk, and more fruits and vegetables than she ordinarily would. She should particularly watch her supply of vitamins and such mineral salts as calcium, phosphorus, iron, and iodine. Milk and milk products provide most of the essential calcium, but the doctor may recommend additional calcium in the diet.

Iron is absolutely vital for the building of red blood cells. That many babies are born slightly anemic indicates that the diet of many pregnant women is deficient in iron. They should be sure to eat plenty of iron-containing foods and, if necessary, take extra iron prescribed by the doctor.

Of the mineral salts, iodine is of great significance. A lack of sufficient iodine in the diet may influence not only the mother's thyroid gland but that of the prospective child.

She also requires more protein. Meat is one of the best sources of not only protein but also the B vitamins, such as thiamine, riboflavin, and niacin. Fish, poultry, and eggs also supply protein.

Fats, particularly butter, cream, and cheese, provide vitamin A and should be included in the diet. Sugars and starches, including whole-grain cereals, bread, and potatoes, are needed to provide materials for energy. But since fats, sugars, and starches also supply a substantial amount of calories, they should not be eaten in large quantities. Fried or greasy foods, heavy sauces and dressings, and rich pastries and pies should be avoided.

The pregnant woman should get regular moderate amounts of sunshine, if possible. If not, additional vitamins, A and D, may be prescribed in the form of cod liver oil. Fresh fruits and vegetables, particularly citrus fruits and tomatoes, supply vitamins A, B, and C.

Cigarettes can be smoked in moderation—five or six a day—but alcohol should be eliminated. She can continue to drink coffee and tea during pregnancy unless they cause sleeplessness.

The nausea and vomiting that occur during the early months of pregnancy are sometimes helped by eating small amounts of food every two and a half hours rather than three daily meals. Various new remedies, such as Bonamine, compazine, Dramamine, and Marezine, are available to relieve continuous vomiting.

During the months before the child is born, the pregnant woman should wear comfortable clothing, and be careful not to wear elastic garters that constrict blood vessels and aid development of varicose veins.

Although the pregnant woman's mental condition cannot affect her child's physical condition, she should nonetheless avoid nervous irritation, undue fatigue, and excess emotional reactions, not only for her own benefit but also for the sake of those about her.

Medical care and advice are particularly desirable during the last four or five weeks of pregnancy. Her condition for the confinement will be rechecked. Meanwhile the baby has grown to such a size that it cannot twist and turn in the womb any longer. It has settled into the position of delivery, normally with its head downward. If the doctor finds that these developments are slower than desired, he may attempt to correct the position by manipulation. He will also establish whether or not the space for passage of the baby is satisfactory. He will decide when a Cesarian section is necessary.

A rigid or special program of self-care is seldom necessary for the pregnant woman, but there are some hygiene rules she would do well to follow. She should, of course, keep herself well groomed. Social activites can and should be continued on a moderate scale. Pregnancy is no reason for becoming dull and unattractive. As a rule, shoes with one- or 1½-inch heels are better than higher-heeled shoes which make it more difficult to stand or walk comfortably and thus give an awkward appearance. The doctor may prescribe a maternity corset to relieve stress and strain on the abdominal muscles. It should be well fitted and preferably made of a nonelastic material. Brassieres which lift the breasts upward and inward and do not flatten them are recommended.

The pregnant woman always needs ample sleep and rest, in a well-ventilated room, and especially during the last few weeks. An afternoon nap is desirable. If she cannot sleep, just lying down is beneficial. If she has difficulty resting, the doctor may give her some medication to promote relaxation.

During pregnancy, small amounts of a liquid called colostrum, which later is followed by real milk, may exude and form on the nipples. It must be removed by soap and warm water to avoid irritation.

The pregnant woman should visit her dentist early in pregnancy and follow his instructions for care of her teeth.

She can continue to bathe during pregnancy, although many doctors prefers showers or sponge baths to tub bathing during the last month or two. The best temperature for the water is between 85° and 90° F., even for those who are accustomed to cold or lukewarm baths. Unusual types of baths, like Turkish and Russian sweat baths, ocean baths, or cold showers, should never be taken except on the advice of the doctor.

The amount and kind of exercise that the pregnant woman takes depends primarily on her previous habits, but she should never exercise to the point of fatigue. As soon as she begins to feel tired it is a good time to stop. Walking is the best exercise, except in bad weather. It stimulates deep breathing, brings more oxygen into the lungs and blood, and assists in proper elimination. She should always walk slowly and avoid crowds. Two miles daily is an average amount of walking. Although sun is beneficial, she should avoid too much exposure.

Strenuous activities which require lifting, excessive stretching or reaching are to be eliminated. Particularly undesirable are running, tennis, swimming, skating, skiing, and horseback riding. During the early months of pregnancy, dancing may be enjoyed, but the pregnant woman should avoid crowded dance floors where she can be bumped and pushed.

If she likes to drive, short drives can be continued, avoiding rough roads and bouncing. During the last few months, traveling should not be undertaken if possible.

As the birth of the child approaches, all arrangements for its coming can be checked, such as accommodations, clothing, bassinet or bed, diapers or a diaper service. If there are other children in the family, arrangements for their care should be made.

If this is the woman's first baby, it is essential to be able to recognize the beginning of labor. Slightly painful contractions of the womb will be the first sign. They begin in the lower part of the abdomen and soon spread to the front of both sides. After some time these contractions become more frequent and pronounced. A few drops of blood mixed with mucus may appear or, in some cases, water may flow at the onset of labor.

At the first sign of labor, the woman should notify her doctor, since the time for confinement may have come. A woman bearing her first child, a primipara, usually has a more lengthy labor. When the contractions start to come every few minutes, the birth is approaching delivery. After the first baby, labor, in most cases, will be shorter so that particular care of the time element must be taken. There is no cause for concern if labor does not begin according to expectations. A few days', even ten days', difference in calculation is not unusual since not all pregnancies take the same course.

The expectant mother should prepare to take certain things with her to the hospital, or have them ready for home care. The first few days at the hospital she must wear hospital gowns, but as soon as she can walk she is usually permitted, if she wishes, to wear her own bedclothes, slippers, and gown. Sanitary pads are supplied by the hospital, but sanitary belts are not. She should bring with her toilet articles she will want to use, such as comb and brush, toothpaste and toothbrush, cosmetics, hand mirror, manicure set, tissues or handkerchiefs, watch or little clock, stationery, fountain pen and pencil, and something to read. She should have indicated to her husband which clothes she wants him to bring her for returning home. The baby will need a shirt, a few diapers, cotton pads, a kimono, a sweater, a bonnet, bunting, and a blanket.

If she has the baby at home, she can talk over with her doctor what she will need. Arrangements should be made for the services of a competent person to assist her—if not a private nurse, then a visiting nurse.

Most communities have agencies to help her choose.

At home the mother will need the following articles for the baby:

3 shirts, size 2. Cotton is preferred, since most homes are adequately heated. They should be large enough to slip on easily and not be outgrown quickly. Those open down the front are most convenient, but slipovers provide enough neck space to prevent squeezing the baby's face when put on or removed.

3 dozen or more diapers, size 20 to 40 inches and of good quality (if a diaper service is not used). Paper or cotton-filled diapers are more expensive, but can be used once and destroyed and are convenient for traveling. Knitted soakers are preferable to rubber diapers or pants, but none should be worn constantly because they irritate the skin. The silk-treated soakers are the safest. They should always be washed, dried, and powdered between changes.

3 nightgowns of soft outing flannel, 27 inches long with drawstrings at hem and wrists and open in back.

3 or 4 kimonos of medium weight, knit or flannelette, with little or no trimming. Simple dresses with "gertrudes" are preferred by some mothers, but kimonos are more practical.

1 sleeping bag or baby bunting, which is a sleeveless square slip with hood attached, and zipper or tie front. It is useful

out-of-doors for a baby born in cold weather.

3 pairs of soft, loose-fitting stockings, socks, or booties.

5 blankets, 3 of them cotton receiving blankets and 2 one-yard squares of wool.

2 flannel, wool, or crocheted jackets.

2 quilted pads for lap or bed protectors, or a square of rubber sheeting.

The mattress for the baby bed or basket should be flat and smooth and not too soft. A pillow is not recommended except for use in the carriage with a young baby. Three to six muslin sheets are needed. An upper sheet is advisable to protect the baby against direct contact with the wool blanket, to which he may be sensitive. A rubber or plastic sheet under the regular sheet helps keep the mattress dry and clean. A hamper for soiled clothing and bedding is useful and a covered pan for soiled diapers is essential.

A basket or tray is useful to keep small toilet items together. Toilet articles should include:

soft bath towels and other small soft towels

3 or 4 washcloths

1 cotton bath blanket

sterilized cotton

safety pins (which should, of course, never be left open)

plain unmedicated soap

mineral oil

covered jar containers

ointment and powder in case of diaper rash, as recommended by doctor

Care should always be taken to keep all pins, nipples, soap, and other small items, especially powder, out of the baby's reach. Spilled powder is easily inhaled and can cause difficulty. Feeding utensils should include:

covered kettle for sterilizing bottles

bottle caps and nipples

nursing bottles (the number needed will depend on the number of feedings to be given each day and the frequency of sterilizing. Bottles should be sterilized at least once a day)

4-ounce bottles for water and orange juice

See also Chapter 6, "Prenatal Care and Childbirth."

PRESBYOPIA, a form of farsightedness in which objects close to the eye may be seen only with difficulty. Farsightedness is a change which normally comes with advancing years. First showing itself when the person is, perhaps, in his forties, presbyopia becomes progressively more acute until approximately the age of seventy-seven.

Among younger persons, the lens is elastic so that it can make itself quickly globular in order to see objects close at hand. With age, however, this elasticity lessens, the lens tends to remain increasingly flat, and the nearest point of clear vision becomes farther removed from the eye.

A person whose "point of convergence" is moving gradually farther from his eyes may boast of his ability to read auto licenses a block away but have to hold a book or newspaper at arm's length in order to read it.

In prescribing convex lenses for presbyopia the oculist will take account of the patient's vocation. Thus, a linotypist should be able to see, with ease, at a distance of twelve or thirteen inches, whereas a pianist might require glasses which are not quite so strong.

The lenses, so prescribed, are not permanent and should be changed. The frequency of the changes can, in some instances, be limited, however, by the use of certain exercises suggested by the physician. *See also* EYE.

PRESCRIPTION, a written direction by which a remedy may be prepared and administered. Its four parts include: (1) the superscription, which consists merely of the letter R, with a line drawn across the second leg. This sign is an abbreviation for the Latin word *recipe,* meaning "take." (2) The inscription, which gives the ingredients to be used in preparing the remedy. (3) The subscription, which indicates how the remedy is to be compounded. (4) The signature, often preceded by the letter S, for the Latin *signa.* In this part the druggist is told what instructions to write on the outside of the container for the benefit of the patient.

Prescriptions at one time often contained a large number of ingredients, the doctor having prescribed something to cover all of the patient's symptoms. Today drugs are more powerful and more specific in their action and so the doctor usually limits the number and is likely to include only a few ingredients in a prescription. He is more concerned with controlling the source of the disease than with relieving all of the symptoms.

PRICKLY HEAT, medically called miliaria, an acute inflammatory skin rash, characterized by acute itching, which occurs when the skin fails to adapt itself to an increase in temperature and humidity. Heat rash, as it is also called, affects children more frequently than adults. Newcomers in a tropical locality will often cease to suffer from prickly heat as soon as their bodies have become adjusted to the new environment.

This rash consists of small elevations containing a watery fluid. They are found over pores and occur because the inflamed skin, usually pinkish, prevents the perspiration from emerging in the usual manner. Often these eruptions link with others to form stretches of unbroken rash.

Persons subjected to a hot and humid atmosphere often can avoid prickly heat by observing a few precautions. Heavy clothing should never be worn, especially by children. Frequent baths, followed by the use of a dusting powder, are desirable, and water or other liquids should be consumed in liberal quantities.

If an attack of prickly heat does occur, however, it will ordinarily yield to standard treatments such as the application of cool packs to the area. The skin should then be dusted with an antiseptic and nonirritating powder. Soap should be avoided since it is likely to irritate the rash. For cleansing purposes, a suitable oil is preferable, followed by the application of a soothing lotion.

If the rash persists, the person should consult a physician since the eruptions are a constant invitation to secondary infection.

PROLAPSE, the dropping of an internal body organ from its normal position, or the protrusion of the lining of a body cavity through a natural opening, or of an organ through a wound.

At childbirth, the stretching of the supportive tissues of the uterus may produce prolapse of the uterus, in which the womb falls from the normal position and the cervix is pushed far into the vagina. Severe prolapse can cause the womb to push the cervix through the vagina. This may provoke complications which require surgery. To correct prolapse by other than surgical means, various types of pessaries may be used, depending on the nature of the prolapse.

Prolapse through wounds occurs in the case of the bowels or the lung, when the abdominal or chest wall is penetrated. Another example of prolapse may be associated with a perforated corneal ulcer, where there is danger of prolapse of the iris.

PROSTATE, an organ in the human male located at the neck of the urinary bladder, surrounding the first part of the urethra, the passage through which urine is excreted from the bladder.

The prostate is partly glandular and partly of muscular tissue. It produces a substance called prostatic fluid which is an important part of the semen, the material that transports the male sperm cells into the female during intercourse. Prostatic fluid is produced constantly and es-

capes through the urine. During sexual excitement it increases in volume and is discharged into the urethra and thus into the semen at the time of ejaculation. The exact function of the prostatic fluid is not known, but it is believed to be related to the survival of the sperm in the female vagina.

The prostate is a gland with a minor function in reproduction and does not produce a hormone or other substance required in the body, nor does prostatic fluid enter the blood stream.

Inflammation or infection of the prostate is not uncommon and may be chronic or acute. Prostatic massage affords relief to men with chronic and subacute prostatitis. Acute prostatitis can become extremely troublesome. The desire to urinate increases in frequency and urination is painful. An abscess may form in the gland and not only give great pain at the slightest motion but may break into the urethra or other nearby tissues and have to be treated surgically. Antibiotics and a hot sitz bath each evening are helpful in many cases of the various types of prostatitis.

The most frequent disorder of the prostate is its gradual enlargement in men over fifty. Sometimes this is first noticed in increasing difficulty of urination; in other cases the first sign may be desire, even during sleep, to urinate more often.

As the condition develops, a residue of voided urine tends to remain in the bladder. Eventually this will begin to decompose and irritate the whole bladder, leading to inflammation. One recourse now widely employed is the use of a catheter to assure complete evacuation, another is surgical removal of part or all of the prostate, and a third means is the use of glandular substances which restrain its overgrowth.

One of the most impressive recent advances in medicine has been the improved techniques for treating prostatic conditions. Surgery has advanced from a two-stage operation which had many fatalities to the use of a tube, passed into the prostatic area from outside the body, through which electrical dissection can remove enlarged tissue.

The prostate is especially subject to cancer and some authorities believe it the commonest cancer of men since it accounts for 10 per cent of the deaths from cancer. Cancer arises in the prostate frequently without any symptom or warning, but becomes evident in one of two principal ways. Difficulty in urination, much like that attending simple prostatic enlargement, may occur, and sometimes blood appears in the urine. Neither of these signs is conclusive proof of cancer, but since urinary irregularity may signal a highly dangerous and progressive condition prompt medical attention should always be given.

The other sign of prostatic cancer is pain in the bones of the pelvis and thigh. This is caused by the spread of the original cancer. Medical examination of the prostate gland, a simple procedure, and x-ray pictures of the bones will establish the diagnosis.

Today cancer of the prostate can be treated with great success if it is recognized while still localized—that is, before it has spread. A rather reliable means of insuring that if it does occur it can be recognized in time is regular prostatic examination by a doctor at six-month intervals for every man over fifty. The procedure is simple and quick and is a form of life insurance.

The only real cure of this condition is complete removal of the whole gland before cancer has spread to other areas. However, new methods developed in the past few years make it possible to prolong the lives of those in whom cancer has spread to the bones and to relieve their suffering. Removal of the testicles or administration of female sex hormones or both give many such patients twice the life expectancy they had before, as well as relief from acute suffering.

PROTEIN, one of a group of complex nitrogenous substances of high molecular weight which are found in various forms in animals and plants and are characteristic of living matter. In the chemical makeup of the body, proteins occupy a significant place, being essential in the maintenance of tissue and also a valuable source of energy. In the process of digestion, the complex proteins, which are largely giant molecules, split into simpler forms and finally into amino acids.

Amino acid contains carbon, oxygen, hydrogen, and nitrogen and some contain sulphur. Amino acids replace parts of body protein which are constantly being lost or destroyed through excretion. Some amino acids can be manufactured by the body from other substances but not in sufficient quantity to sustain life, so that the diet must contain essential amino acids if body growth and repair are to continue.

Proteins which furnish essential amino acids in large amounts are called complete proteins. Meat, largely composed of animal protein, contains the most nearly complete edible protein. Plant proteins are generally incomplete, and cannot supply the body with enough of certain essential amino acids. Eggs, fish, and milk are complete proteins.

Proteins have been classified into numerous groups, two of the significant ones being albumins and the globulins. Egg white is largely albumin, but also contains globulin. Blood plasma contains both. The ability of the blood to clot depends on fibrinogen, a globulin. Some of the antibodies which the blood develops to combat disease are also globulins.

Every diet should contain two or more portions of protein foods a day to prevent amino acid deficiency. A diet high in carbohydrates and low in protein fails to supply the body adequately with amino acids and edema can result. *See also* EDEMA; NUTRITION; VITAMINS.

PRURITIS. *See* ITCHING.

PSITTACOSIS, commonly called "parrot fever," a disease not only of parrots, parakeets, lovebirds, canaries, pigeons, ducks, and other birds, but one also readily transmitted to human beings. Occasionally the infection is spread from one infected person to another.

The infection is caused by a virus which can be found in the nasal discharges and droppings of infected birds and which contaminate their feathers and cages. The virus enters the human body by inhalation. Psittacosis usually appears sporadically, but outbreaks have occurred among family groups, employees of pet shops, and laboratory workers.

In birds the liver and spleen are affected, but in men the lungs are usually involved. The disease may be serious, especially in older persons.

Usually the disease begins seven to fifteen days after exposure to the infection with headache, sore throat, chills, fever, and backache followed by a dry cough. In severe cases the temperature may remain high for two or three weeks. The lungs are congested and sometimes a large amount of slightly blood-stained sputum may be expectorated. Convalescence begins with a drop in temperature and is generally lengthy in severe cases.

Psittacosis is one of the few virus diseases which yield to treatment with certain antibiotics. These also can prevent bacterial infections which often follow an attack. Expectorants and inhalants may be prescribed for dry coughs and sputum discharge. A person who has psittacosis is ordinarily isolated and anyone coming in contact with him is protected against discharges from cough or sputum. A wise precaution includes destroying the infected bird, and burning the cage and all materials that have been in contact with the bird.

PSORIASIS, a chronic inflammatory skin disease, and one of the ten most frequent skin ailments. It affects both men and women, and usually appears after the age of fifteen. It is noninfectious, but some families seem to have a tendency to it.

The cause of psoriasis is unknown. Numerous theories have been advanced, but as yet no cause has been definitely established. Some doctors believe it is of nervous origin, others think it may be related to difficulty in digesting fat, or to certain germs and viruses.

The first sign of psoriasis is generally an eruption of pinhead-size, bright red spots which group to form larger ones, finally becoming great patches of reddened skin. The healing begins from the center and leaves a red or reddish brown stain. Also characteristic of psoriasis are thick, silver-white scales. When they are removed, small bleeding spots remain. There is seldom any itching nor is general health affected.

Eruption is usually on the elbows, knees, and backs of the arms and leg; occasionally the chest and abdomen are involved. Sometimes the lesions become infected and form pus. Fingernails and toenails and the palms of the hands and soles of the feet may be affected also.

Treatment requires patient careful management by the doctor and complete cooperation of the patient. Since the cause is unknown, treatment may be varied and tentative until the doctor arrives at the most effective method to treat a particular case.

Psoriasis has been treated by diets, most of which seem to have been ineffective, with the possible exception of low-fat diets. Tar bath treatments have been helpful and many patients have improved with exposure to sunlight or ultraviolet rays following application of special tar ointment.

Fowler's solution of arsenic, formerly used, has largely been replaced. Several special drugs have been developed for treatment of psoriasis. Chrysarobin is often effective when the palms of the hands and soles of the feet are involved.

Hormone injections have been tried; but unless peeling of the horny layer of the skin is excessive and widespread, there is not enough evidence of relation between glands and psoriasis to warrant the use of hormones.

Radiation therapy is often helpful in healing psoriasis, but cannot prevent its recurrence, and this treatment should only be used in special cases and with extreme care, since serious changes in the skin may occur.

Sedatives and tranquilizing drugs have been found effective, especially in those cases which seem connected with emotional stress.

Psoriasis in children must be managed with special care, since there is danger of absorption of the tarry substances or other drugs, such as ammoniated mercury used in treating psoriasis of the scalp. For this type of psoriasis, shampooing with salicylic acid, ammoniated mercury, and other substances is sometimes effective.

PSYCHOANALYSIS, the method developed by Sigmund Freud to determine the patterns and motivations of human personality in order to treat various emotional disorders. Many persons, among them Jung and Adler, have worked in this field, modifying and changing the Freudian psychoanalytic method, so that many types of psychoanalysis are now practiced. The technique is used in the study and treatment of a wide variety of emotional problems, particularly the neuroses.

Typically the patient in psychoanalysis meets with his analyst a minimum of two one-hour periods a week, and talks as freely and fully as possible about anything he chooses. The patient comes to realize more and more what in his past and present life is relevant and significant and to discuss that. Gradually the psychoanalyst and patient come to recognize the roots and patterns of the patient's attitudes and actions. The goal is to create within the patient both an intellectual and emotional awareness of why he thinks and acts as he does. Often an intellectual grasp of the problems precedes an emotional grasp—i.e., he may *know* that he drinks to excess when he is worried, but still not have reached the point where this knowledge will serve to help him. Since neuroses have origins which reach far back into the patient's life, the patient often devotes a large part of his attention to early childhood and adolescence.

Psychoanalysis can take from months to years, the patient deciding when he no longer needs the services of his psychoanalyst.

PSYCHOSIS, a severe mental disorder, which manifests itself in abnormal behavior, reactions, and ideas. The person is no longer able to cope with the demands of his environment. A psychotic person differs from a neurotic person in that the neurotic person has succeeded in making an adjustment to his environment, the nature of the adjustment usually constituting the neurosis. *See also* MANIC-DEPRESSIVE PSYCHOSIS; NEUROSIS; PARANOIA; SCHIZOPHRENIA; and Chapter 22, "Mental Illness."

PSYCHOSOMATIC DISORDERS, illnesses which result from the interaction of mind and body. The emotional factor in sickness has been recognized since ancient times. However, our understanding of the role of emotional factors and their interrelationship with organic diseases has only recently advanced to the point that psychosomatic medicine is now a recognized and widely used term as well as a definite branch of medical science.

Psychosomatic disorders may result from multiple causes where the emotional stimulus is combined with other factors, such as a physical predisposition. In ailments like asthma or colitis, for example, the site of the difficulty may be physically predisposed, while the immediate source is emotional in origin.

Psychosomatic disturbances may take place in any of the involuntary organs of the body, including the digestive tract, the respiratory region, the heart and circulatory systems, the genitourinary system, the endocrine glands, and the skin.

Certain forms of allergy are also greatly influenced by emotional factors. In some instances chronic cases of asthma have been helped by psychotherapy. *See also* NEUROSIS; PEPTIC ULCER.

PTOMAINE POISONING. *See* FOOD POISONING.

PULSE, the intermittent change in the shape of an artery due to an increase in the tension of its walls following the contraction of the heart. The impulses which the beating of the heart sends through the arteries can be felt at various places on the surface of the body. The artery usually selected for examinatioin of the pulse is the radial artery lying over the radius bone at the wrist. A finger is placed on this artery and the number of beats per minute recorded. A machine which measures pulse rate has also been developed.

In adults, the number of pulsations per minute varies from 67 to 72. In infants, the rate is 120 to 140 in the first few weeks of life, slowing gradually to 100 to 120.

Excessive rapidity of pulse rate is called tachycardia, and excessive slowness is called brachycardia. In fever, the pulse rate increases from 8 to 10 beats per minute for each degree of temperature rise above normal. After exertion the rate increases but usually returns to normal within a few minutes. Many long-distance runners have pulse rates as low as 40 to 65.

Normal pulse is regular, the beats occurring in the same intervals. In auricular fibrillation, the pulse is extremely irregular. The force of the pulse may also vary in disorders associated with a depressed physical state and with certain ailments of the blood vessels. *See also* ARTERIO-SCLEROSIS; BLOOD PRESSURE; HEART.

PUNCTURE WOUND. *See* WOUNDS.

PURGATIVE. *See* CATHARTICS.

PURPURA HEMORRHAGICA, a condition caused by a decrease to below normal in the number of blood platelets, which are factors in coagulation. When a shortage of blood platelets occurs, bleeding will begin almost spontaneously, particularly from the mucous membranes in the nose and mouth. Bleeding underneath the skin is frequent, giving the appearance of bruises.

The number of platelets may be lessened as a result of some action on the bone marrow, in which the cells that form the platelets are manufactured. Fewer platelets may result from a decrease of the cells or from a toxic action that destroys these blood cells more rapidly than they are formed. Sometimes it is associated with sensitivity to drugs, such as the sulfonamides, quinine, barbiturates, or with the toxicity that results from the action of certain types of disease, such as measles, tuberculosis, and infectious mononucleosis. In many women, a lessening of the platelets occurs at menstruation.

Purpura hemorrhagica is seen most frequently in persons between the ages of twelve and twenty-five, although it may occur at any age. The condition may develop gradually so that the onset cannot be determined accurately. Some acute cases are so severe that there is danger of bleeding to death within a few days or weeks. In others, the condition may be chronic, varying in severity throughout the person's life.

Many different procedures have been used to treat patients suffering from purpura, often with the hope of at least improving the condition, since a cure is not always possible. One of the simplest and most direct methods is injection of blood into the body, either intravenously, into the muscles, or under the skin. Transfusion of whole blood is one of the most helpful treatments. The use of ACTH, cortisone, or hydrocortisone, in connection with transfusions or alone, has been found to modify rapidly the bleeding tendency in many cases. Sometimes removal of the spleen by surgical operation has been helpful and is now an accepted technique of treatment. Injection of hormones in connection with the operation depends on the individual case. In many instances, a new chemical, vitamin K_1, supplements other supportive measures, such as replenishment of iron.

Most of the management of treatment of purpura hemorrhagica is considered experimental for the individual case, and for each patient a study should be made to determine the presence of an allergy to a protein, and whether or not the disturbance in platelet production is related to such sensitivity. The removal of allergens and use of antihistamines and other supportive measures has generally been helpful in the treatment of disorders caused by allergies.

PUS, the thick, creamy, yellowish product of inflammation, found in abscesses. It consists chiefly of serum and white blood cells. The color varies with the causative microorganism. A discharge containing or forming pus is called purulent.

PYELITIS, an inflammation of the pelvis or lower part of the kidney. In pregnancy, chills, fever, and pain between the hips and ribs may be indicative of pyelitis. *See also* KIDNEYS; NEPHRITIS.

PYELONEPHRITIS, the most common type of kidney infection, involving both the pelvis of the kidney and the kidney itself. *See also* KIDNEYS; NEPHRITIS.

PYEMIA, an infection due to the presence of pus-producing germs in the blood stream and the formation of abscesses where these organisms lodge. *See also* BACTEREMIA.

PYLORUS, the valve which releases food from the stomach into the duodenum and into the small intestines. Ulcers may form in the pylorus with subsequent scarring and constriction. Babies are sometimes born with an enlargement of the muscles which forms the pyloric valve. This causes obstruction of the passage of food and spasms which result in vomiting. The child will lose weight rapidly since he cannot retain food. The usual treatment for a congenital malformed pyloric valve is a surgical division of the muscle.

PYORRHEA, usually refers to an inflammation of the gums and outer covering of the roots of the teeth when it reaches the purulent stage. It is easier to prevent than cure and rarely occurs when good general care is taken of the teeth and gums. Beginning with tender bleeding gums the inflammation advances until the teeth become loosened from the supporting gum. The dentist follows a regular course of treatment. If started early enough, treatment is effective, but when there is extensive bone loss and shifting of teeth in their sockets little can be done, and removal of the teeth affected is advised in order to save the rest. *See also* GINGIVITIS; TEETH.

Q FEVER, often called nine-mile fever, an infection which resembles influenza or virus pneumonia. It is caused by a rickettsial organism, a microorganism smaller than bacteria but larger than a filterable virus, and is transmitted to man by ticks that live on infected animals. Q fever was first recognized in Australia, where it occurred among workers in packing houses and dairies and among foresters. Almost at the same time, a group of laboratory workers in Montana contracted it. The outbreaks were apparently due to inhalation of dust contaminated with rickettsiae or by dried feces of infected ticks.

Q fever begins with fever, headache, chills, malaise, and weakness. Mild cases last a few days, but more severe attacks may persist for two to three weeks; the condition usually ends in complete recovery. Treatment ordinarily consists of good nursing care and use of appropriate drugs early in the course of the illness.

Q fever can also be acquired by contact with infected milk or dairy products, and proper pasteurization of milk is a significant factor in preventing the spread of Q fever.

QUACKS, persons who falsely claim to possess medical knowledge which enables them to cure or treat disease. Fortunately today legislation has been passed which limits their activity, whereas formerly they had complete freedom to advertise through newspapers and radio, and to prepare and sell medicines.

Persons suffering from illnesses for which medical science does not guarantee a cure seem especially susceptible to the claims of medical quacks, who will promise to cure arthritic conditions or cancer—in fact, anything. Modesty is never one of their strong points, and usually there is nothing they will not claim to accomplish. Their fees are often exorbitant, but thousands of persons, out of fear and gullibility, succumb to their wiles. Quacks can truly be said to exploit and live off the suffering and fear of others.

QUARANTINE, the limitation of freedom of movement of persons or animals who have been exposed to a communicable disease, for a period of time usually equal to the longest incubation period of the disease to which they have been exposed. The word quarantine comes from the Italian word for forty. During the Middle Ages, ships were detained for forty days before entering port in an attempt to avoid spread of the plague.

Today most countries are constantly on the alert to guard against disease-bearing persons or animals entering the country. For example, in England and Hawaii a dog cannot be brought into the country until after a quarantine period to assure that the dog does not have rabies.

Persons actually sick are isolated, not quarantined. Every infectious disease has a particular period of quarantine and of isolation. For example, a child with scarlet fever is isolated, and members of the family are quarantined.

QUICKENING, the first feeling of fetal movements by a pregnant woman. These first noticeable movements of the unborn child usually appear during the sixteenth to eighteenth week of pregnancy.

QUININE, an alkaloid obtained from the bark of the cinchona plant, is a drug used specifically in the treatment of malaria. In solution quinine may be taken orally, in another form it may be injected but usually it is taken as a salt, quinine sulphate, in the form of capsules, pills, or tablets. It is also used as a tonic and as bitters, and has been helpful in cases of neuralgia and certain forms of muscle weakness.

Quinine should be taken only under a doctor's supervision, as overuse may have a toxic effect. Atabrine, a substitute, is also prescribed as a specific against malaria.

Another derivative of the bark of cinchona is quinidine, a drug that is valuable in treating heart ailments in which rapid or irregular beating of the heart is a symptom. It slows down heart action and lengthens the time of conduction of the heartbeat. It has been found particularly beneficial in treating fibrillation of the heart muscle.

QUINSY, a sore throat caused by an abscess in the tissues around the tonsils. Pain is generally localized on one side. The person has great difficulty in swallowing and talking, the breath becomes unpleasant, the tongue thickly coated, and the sense of taste and smell may be affected and almost lost.

Rest in bed is imperative and the physician will prescribe antibiotic drugs at once to relieve pain and control infection. Sometimes he will incise the abscess to release the accumulation of pus. *See also* TONSILLITIS.

RABBIT FEVER. *See* TULAREMIA.

RABIES, or hydrophobia, an acute infectious disease of animals, caused by a filterable virus, and transmitted to other animals and human beings by the bite of an infected animal. It occurs in dogs, cattle, horses, wolves, cats, bats, and other animals. The dog is most often attacked by rabies, as well as being the most frequent transmitter of the disease to human beings.

The first signs of rabies in a dog are irritability and restlessness, followed by difficulty in swallowing and paralysis, which makes the mouth hang open and causes drooling of saliva. In the final stages of rabies, an infected dog will howl, snap, run about, and bite. Eventually it becomes paralyzed, has convulsions, and dies. The disease rarely reaches the last stages, since the animal is usually spotted before and disposed of.

Rabies is caused by a virus which appears in the saliva of an animal several days before it has serious symptoms. When this virus enters the body of a human being, either from the bite of an animal or in another way, the virus affects the nervous system and eventually reaches the central nervous system, including the spinal cord and brain. Bites on the face, lips, and hands are more serious because the point of inoculation of the virus is nearer the brain.

Epidemics of rabies have appeared in the United States from time to time. Reports of cases of rabies resulting from the bite of bats led recently to the discovery that many of the millions of bats inhabiting the Carlsbad Caverns of New Mexico either are or have been infected with rabies.

Because of the terrible possibility of rabies, a definite course should, if possible, be followed after any dog bite. The animal should be kept confined for at least ten days and watched for signs of rabies.

As a first-aid measure, a wound incurred from a dog bite should be washed immediately with a strong warm soap solution. Punctures and lacerations should be washed to the depth of the wound, using a blunt-tipped syringe. If a person is bitten on the face or hands, the doctor will begin to give antirabies vaccine at once, since the rabies virus reaches the brain and nervous system so rapidly. The vaccine most commonly available is the Semple vaccine. Sensitivity reactions to serum must be guarded against, however, and a valuable adjunct to vaccine treatment is antirabies serum, especially for bites about the head, or severe wounds of the hand. Vaccine is also given when visible wounds are known or suspected of having been made by the teeth of the animal, when pre-existent cuts and sores may have been contaminated by fresh saliva, and when small children who have had contact with the animal are too young to give reliable testimony.

The doctor will usually discontinue treatment if the biting animal is alive and well after seven days of observation. The onset of rabies usually follows the bite of the infected animal in from twenty to ninety days, and during this period the symptoms may include restlessness, apprehension, and irritation and tingling at the site of the bite. When the disease begins, a slight huskiness of the voice is followed by a sense of choking, since the muscles of swallowing and breathing go into spasms. The infected person may refuse to drink water, because of the pain that accompanies swallowing. Once the disease has developed, it is almost certainly fatal in from two to ten days, the average being three days.

The best general measure to prevent rabies is to have all puppies receive rabies inoculation as soon as possible. Most cities and communities have strict regulations regarding this, as well as a rule requiring that all dogs outside their home be on a leash.

RADIATION, the therapeutic use of roentgen rays or radium. The term is also used to denote divergence from a common center of sensations and stimuli.

Radiography describes the use of x-ray as well as roentgenography, which derives its name from Wilhelm Roentgen, the inventor of the x-ray.

Radiation treatment is widely used in medicine and includes the exposure of part or all of the body to x-rays, or specific spots to radium and newer radioactive isotopes.

The advent of atomic energy and use of radioactive materials in industry and medicine has posed many new problems because of the possible disastrous effect of radiation on living tissue. The United Nations Scientific Committee on the Effects of Atomic Radiation has been established to study this problem. *See also* x-rays.

RADIUM, a highly radioactive element found in pitchblende and other mineral deposits; it was discovered in 1898 by Pierre and Marie Curie. The rays which radium gives off have an effect on the growth of human tissue, and radium has been effectively used in treatment of skin diseases of various types, including cancer, tumors, growths on the skin, and in hemorrhage and infections.

Radium is generally employed in the form of one of its salts, since they are more stable than the element itself. Various types of tubes are required for the insertion of radium into body cavities and tumorous tissue. Platinum or gold needles may be used, or tiny glass tubes, called "seeds," which are filled with radon, a gaseous emanation of radium, and inserted into tumors, in some cases permanently.

RALE, a French word meaning rattle and referring to the various sounds that are heard in the lungs when the doctor examines them with a stethoscope. Many adjectives have been employed by doctors to describe these sounds, such as coarse, medium, fine, moist, and dry.

RAT-BITE FEVER, an infection, characterized by fever, nervous symptoms, malaise, and serious disability, which is contracted from the bite of a diseased rat, or, less commonly, a cat, dog, weasel, squirrel, or pig, which injects a spiral bacillus into the body of the person bitten. The bacteria live in the noses and throats of rats without disturbing them, but cause a variety of febrile diseases when injected into human beings.

Another condition like rat-bite fever is Haverhill fever, so named because the first epidemic which was studied occurred in Haverhill, Massachusetts. Since that time, other cases have been reported in different parts of the United States. It is also caused by the bite of a rat or sometimes, by food contaminated with an organism similar to that transmitted through the bite.

Rat-bite fever has been found in practically every part of the world, and occurs most often in infants and children. Not every rat carries the infection. In the United States the large and vicious Norway or sewer rats are the most frequent carriers.

The incubation period of rat-bite fever ranges from one to four weeks. When the disease begins, fever comes and goes, fluctuating from time to time, and occasionally a skin rash appears. Haverhill fever has a much shorter incubation period and the fever does not increase and recede. The joints are involved, but if any skin rash is present, it is minor.

Rat-bite fever is treated with penicillin, streptomycin, or the tetracyclines. Other drugs are given to relieve headache and malaise. Most patients recover, particularly if the condition is diagnosed early and the treatment is prompt. Anyone bitten by a rat should immediately have the wound treated by a physician, who will cauterize the wound and treat it with a strong antiseptic. In case of abscess, he will incise and drain the wound; and if the puncture is deep, he may take prophylactic measures against tetanus.

RAT CONTROL. Rats cause tremendous property loss each year, as well as being carriers of diseases, such as rat-bite fever, bubonic plague through the rat flea, Weil's disease or hemorrhagic jaundice, tapeworm, ringworm, food-poisoning through bacteria, and a form of typhus. The elimination of rats is therefore an essential part of any public health program and of concern to the private home owner or building proprietor. The best means of preventing rats is to make a building rat-proof by plugging openings, clearing away debris, and other measures. Once rats are established, they may be hunted or trapped, but use of poison is usually the most practical means of getting rid of them.

The ideal poison is one that will kill rats but which is harmless to animals and man. Many poisons have been tried, with varying degrees of success. A compound known as ANTU is effective. It affects dogs, cats, and other pets only mildly; a single dose will kill a half-pound rat quickly, but have little effect on a dog weighing ten pounds. One pound of ANTU is sufficient to kill 200,000 rats. Finely ground corn or wheat is mixed with ANTU and sprayed or dusted on cut-up vegetables, tomatoes or potatoes, as bait. After the rat has taken a small quantity of the poison, its lungs fill up with body fluid and it dies by suffocation.

Other poisons, more or less toxic, are also employed, such as zinc phosphate and thallium sulphate. However, rats quickly learn to be wary of food containing these poisons and will eventually avoid it.

Two newer poisons have been developed, warfarin and a related compound, toumarin. They are also mixed with edible bait and when ingested by rats the poisons attack the blood and act as anticoagulants. The rats bleed to death internally in from five to six days. *See also* RAT-BITE FEVER.

RECTUM, the lowest segment of the digestive tract, about six to eight inches long, terminating in the anus or lower opening through which solid waste matter is evacuated from the body. The large intestine, immediately above the rectum, first acts on the indigestible residue which remains when food has been digested and passes it on into the rectum. When this occurs, the body, by a specific mechanism, indicates to the brain that expulsion of the waste through the anus is ready. This is the urge for movement of the bowels. *See also* DIGESTIVE SYSTEM; INTESTINES.

RED BLOOD CELLS. *See* BLOOD.

REDUCING DIET. *See* DIET, REDUCING; OBESITY; and Chapter 4, "Diet and Health."

REFLEX, an involuntary movement or reaction to a stimulus, removed from the point of action. Many reflex actions take place in the body as part of its ordinary functioning or in connection with disease. The knee jerk, an example of a reflex action, is absent in many diseases of the brain and spinal cord. The oculo-cardiac reflex is a slowing of the heartbeat that follows compression of the eyeball. A slowing of five to thirteen beats per minute is the normal decrease. When a substance is put on the back of the tongue, the swallowing reflex takes place. Laughter is a reflex to tickling, and when an infant starts on hearing a loud noise, a startle reflex is provoked.

RELAPSING FEVER, one of a group of specific infectious diseases caused by spirochetes; it is characterized by recurring attacks of high fever. The disease is transmitted by the bite of ticks, lice, and sometimes bedbugs.

Usually relapsing fever begins with sudden chills followed by a fever which may go as high as 105° and remain at a high level for several days, and headache and weakness may occur. At the crisis there is often danger of collapse. After a few days the patient suddenly recovers, but in a week or so will again be ill.

To treat relapsing fever, bed rest is essential, particularly during the period of high fever. Sponge baths and the use of salicylic acid and sedatives help make the patient more comfortable. Antibiotics, such as Aureomycin, Terramycin, and Chloromycetin, have been found the most effective drugs in controlling this disease.

REPRODUCTION SYSTEM. The human reproduction system, which consists of the generative apparatus, is discussed here with reference to its anatomy and to conception.

Anatomy. One of the basic sex organs in the male is the scrotum, or bag, which contains the two testicles. These produce not only the sperm cells, which fertilize the female egg, but the cells which give a man his secondary sex characteristics, the deep voice, beard, heavier bones, narrow pelvis, rough skin, and flat breasts.

Each testicle has a long tube which leads to a separate semen reservoir. The sperm cells pass through these tubes to the semen reservoirs, in which there is a sticky white fluid provided by the neighboring prostate gland. This combination is known as semen.

In sexual intercourse, the external organ, the penis, becomes rigid and is inserted by the male into the female's vagina. At the climax of this relationship, the semen is shot through the penis into the vagina, close to the opening into the womb.

The male and female sex organs are curiously similar. For example, the ovaries of the female resemble the testicles of the male. The female egg cells originate in the ovaries and pass into the Fallopian tubes, which resemble the semen reservoirs in the male. The eggs remain in these tubes a few days and then, unless fertilized, go down into the womb, or uterus. The uterus is a small empty organ which can be greatly expanded. From there the cells leave the body by way of the vagina during the female menstrual period.

The entrance to the vagina resembles a small pair of vertical lips. Outside these is a larger pair of lips which encloses not only the entrance to the vagina but also the mouth of the urethra, through which urine is expelled, and, in front of that, the clitoris. The clitoris is a small fleshy projection which, in sexual excitement, may become erect, like a tiny penis. The external female sex organs are known as the vulva.

Conception. Conception of a human being is an intricate event. In intercourse, the sperm cells are deposited near the mouth of the womb. These sperm cells may travel further, enter a Fallopian tube, where one of them may meet with and fertilize one of the female egg cells. At once, by process of self-division, the egg cell will begin to grow, feeding mainly on the food which it finds within itself.

Leaving the Fallopian tube, this fertilized egg cell fastens itself to the inner wall of the womb. Soon, between the wall and the cell, the placenta develops. This is the channel of communication between mother and child, but the blood of the two never intermingles. Each, in the placenta, will have its own separate blood vessels. Other materials, however, such as fluids and gases, are passed from mother to child through the walls of these blood vessels, a process known as osmosis, which permits the mother to supply the child with such essentials as food, water, and oxygen. The child may also use this channel to rid itself of waste.

The placenta, together with membranes developed during pregnancy, is eliminated after the birth of the child, in the "afterbirth."

The new human being may be said to exist as soon as the sperm cell has fertilized the egg cell, at which time the sex is determined. The best established theory maintains that every cell in the body of a female contains two chromosomes, or sex determiners, whereas each cell in the body of the male has only one. However, when the female produces egg cells, only one determiner will be found in each. When the male develops sperm cells, half of them contain one determiner each, while the rest do not contain any. If the sperm cell which fertilizes the egg cell happens to contain a determiner, the result will be a fertilized egg cell with two determiners and the child will be female. However, if the fertilizing sperm cell does not contain any determiner, the child, possessing only the one determiner, will be male.

This theory is generally accepted. Therefore, neither parents nor doctors could ever conceivably control the sex of the child. Moreover, as yet, there is not a scientific means of determining, before birth, whether or not the child is male or female. *See also* CERVIX; CONTRACEPTION; OVARIES; PREGNANCY AND PRENATAL CARE; TESTICLES; UTERUS; and Chapter 6, "Prenatal Care and Childbirth."

RESERPINE, a new alkaloid drug which has proved useful against high blood pressure and in relieving the symptoms of acute mental disorders. The substance is derived from rauwolfia serpentina, a root from which extracts have been used in India for many centuries for a variety of medical purposes. Reserpine is a specific substance isolated from the root and believed to be the active principle to which the therapeutic effects are due. In India rauwolfia is a widely used sedative and was employed against snakebite and other conditions many centuries ago. *See also* BARBITURATES.

RESPIRATORY DISEASES, those disorders which affect the act of breathing with the lungs or the apparatus, the organs, tissues, and membranes, involved. The respiratory system in the human being is chiefly composed of two lungs and the air passages which lead to them. *See also* COMMON COLD; LUNGS; PNEUMONIA; TUBERCULOSIS; and Chapter 15, "Respiratory Diseases."

RESUSCITATION, the prevention of asphyxial death by artificial respiration. Unconsciousness is always an emergency situation. It can occur from inhalation of carbon monoxide, drowning, poisoning, electric shock, and other causes. Although various devices for artificial respiration are effective, manual artificial respiration is usually the most readily available, and unconsciousness requires immediate first-aid treatment.

The average person breathes from sixteen to twenty times a minute. However, most authorities believe that in artificial respiration a greater number of movements are necessary, since the patient will take in less than the normal amount of air in each breath. Some recommend that the rate be between twenty-four and forty movements per minute.

Until recently the most commonly practiced method of resuscitation was the Schaefer technique, named for the British physiologist who devised it. Another method, the Holger method, was then adopted by the American Red Cross, the American Medical Association, and other agencies. This procedure has now been replaced by mouth to mouth resuscitation.

The Holger method. The unconscious person is placed face down, with the hands on top of each other, the forehead resting on the hands with the face turned slightly to one side, and the elbows extended outward. The operator kneels on one or both knees in front of the head of the victim. He places his hands under the victim's arms, above the elbow, and rocks backward, drawing the arms upward and toward himself. The arms are elevated until firm resistance is met, then replaced on the floor. The operator then moves his hands to the back, just below the shoulder blades, and rocks forward, exerting pressure on the back. The operator's arms are kept straight during both the lift and the pressure phases, and the complete cycle is repeated about ten to twelve times a minute.

Hip lift. The unconscious person is placed in a prone position face down. The operator kneels on one knee near the victim's hip, straddles the victim, and places the other foot near the opposite hip. He places his hands under the hips, and raises the pelvis vertically upward four to six inches. The hips are then replaced on the ground and the cycle is repeated. The hip lift is performed twelve times per minute. Lifting the hips produces active inspiration, as a result of several mechanisms: (1) When the hips are elevated, the abdominal contents sag downward toward the floor and result in an intra-

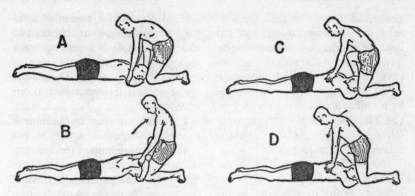

Arm lift-back pressure method of manual artificial respiration (after Holger Nielsen). A, placing hands for arm lift. B, arm lift. C, placing hands for back pressure. D, back pressure.

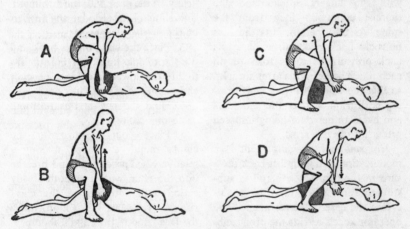

Hip lift-back pressure method of manual artificial respiration. A, placing hands for hip lift. B, hip lift. C, placing hands for back pressure. D, back pressure.

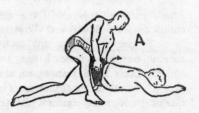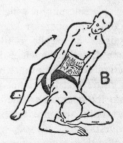

Hip roll-back pressure method of manual artificial respiration. A, side view of hip roll. B, front view of hip roll.

abdominal negativity that tends to draw the diaphragm downward. (2) Because of the ligamentous attachments between the viscera and diaphragm, the downward movement of the abdominal organs is followed by a similar action of the diaphragm. (3) Elevating the hips hyperextends the spine and increases the intercostal spaces of the lower ribs.

Hip lift-back pressure. The hip lift-back pressure method combines alternate lifting of the hips, as described, with pressure on the midback just below the shoulder blades, with the fingers spread and the thumbs about an inch from the spine. As the operator lifts the hips he rocks backward, and as he exerts back pressure he rocks forward. In each phase he keeps his arms straight, so that the work of lifting and pressing is distributed over the shoulders and back, rather than being imposed primarily on the arms.

Hip roll-back pressure. This is a modification of the hip lift-back pressure method in which a roll is substituted for the lift in order to increase the ease of performance. The operator kneels astride the prone subject as described for the hip lift method. Instead of lifting both hips, he uses the knee on which he is kneeling as a fulcrum on which to roll the victim. The operator keeps his arms straight, and rolls himself in the same direction in which he rolls the victim. Great care must be exercised to insure that the victim is rolled up onto the operator's knee or thigh, so that both hips are raised from the ground.

Mouth-to-mouth method. The Red Cross has recently revived an ancient method of artificial resuscitation as the best way of reviving infants and children whose breathing has stopped. This method is known as mouth-to-mouth resuscitation, and replaces the back pressure-arm lift method.

Following are steps in the mouth-to-mouth technique.

1. Clear the mouth of foreign matter with the middle finger of one hand, and with the same finger hold the tongue forward.

2. Place the child in a face-down, head-down position, and pat him firmly on the back with the free hand. This should help dislodge any foreign object in the air passages.

3. Place the child on his back and use the middle fingers of both hands to lift the lower jaw from beneath and behind so that it "juts out."

4. Hold the jaw in this position, using one hand only.

5. Place your mouth over the child's mouth and nose, making a relatively leakproof seal, and breathe into the child with a smooth steady action until you observe the chest rise. As you start this action, move the free hand to the child's abdomen, between the navel and the ribs, and apply continuous moderate pressure to prevent the stomach from becoming filled with air.

6. When the lungs have been inflated, remove your lips from the child's mouth and nose and allow the lungs to empty. Repeat this cycle, keeping one hand beneath the jaw and the other hand pressing on the stomach at all times. Continue at a rate of about twenty cycles a minute. If at any time resistance to breathing into the child is felt and the chest

does not rise, repeat second step, then quickly resume mouth-to-mouth breathing. *See also* Chapter 28, "First Aid."

RETINA, the light-receptive layer and terminal expansion of the optic nerve, the eye. Vision is accomplished through the passing of light rays through the human eye to the nervous tissue at the back of the eye, called the retina. A serious disorder of the retina is detachment of the retina, a condition in which small areas of the retina separate from the underlying coats, usually as the result of injury, infection, or tumor and, sometimes, as a result of a disease, such as tuberculosis. An operative procedure has been developed in retinal detachment.

Inflammation of the retina is called retinitis, which may be due to infection, hemorrhage, or other types of injury. Sometimes it is associated with inflammation of the kidneys or hardening of the blood vessels.

Retinoblastoma is a malignant tumor of the retina, occurring in infancy or early childhood. In some instances tumor of the retina is present at birth. This disorder rarely occurs in persons more than ten years old. *See also* EYE.

RHEUMATIC FEVER, a febrile disease characterized by painful migratory arthritis and a predilection to heart damage leading to chronic valvular disease. It most frequently attacks young people between the ages of six and nineteen and, although no longer the leading cause of death in this age group, is among the foremost health problems. In at least one-fifth of all cases of rheumatic

fever the most serious associated condition is the attack on the heart. Rheumatic fever usually appears following infections of the nose and throat, but it may also be associated with ear infection, scarlet fever, St. Vitus' dance and other similar ailments related to streptococcal infection.

Great progress has been made in understanding and controlling rheumatic fever with the advance in control of infection and the near-conquest of streptococcal disease. However, the exact cause has not yet been determined nor the primary problem of prevention solved.

When rheumatic fever involves the heart, inflammatory changes occur in the muscles which affect the strength of the heart and cause it to dilate, and thus the heart does not function properly. Often rheumatic fever develops insidiously. The so-called rheumatic lesions may affect the joints, producing symptoms similar to "growing pains," and sometimes severe pain related to infection of the lymph glands is present. Mild fleeting pain may be felt in the tendons or muscles and pain in the heels is not infrequent. Twitching and mental hallucinations such as accompany St. Vitus' dance are sometimes symptoms.

More than half of the patients with rheumatic fever have had tonsillitis or sore throat from one to four weeks before the rheumatic symptoms appear. These symptoms may appear gradually or suddenly, and are usually associated with overexertion or chilling. The temperature rises to 102° to 104°, the pulse becomes rapid, there is profuse sweating, pain in the joints, and prostration. Joints most subject to stress and strain are affected first and pain seldom begins in all the joints at once. Sometimes the joints swell because of the accumulation of fluid.

Pain and the other symptoms can usually be controlled by a doctor. The detection of the first signs of the heart disease associated with rheumatic fever is somewhat more difficult. When patients come under hospital care early, electrocardiograph tests will show at once transient abnormalities in the heart. The obvious signs of heart damage, such as irregularity, rapidity, pain, changes in size, and accumulations of fluid in the heart sac, appear later and are easily detected by the doctor. When the heart enlarges and its action is impaired, the sounds of the heart change and the pulse generally reflects the condition of the heart. Also typical of rheumatic condition are nodes which appear under the skin and an outbreak of rash.

The valves of the heart may be affected. Small nodules form on the valves and interfere with normal function. The nodules eventually disappear, leaving scars and causing the valve to develop unusually large numbers of blood vessels. If attacks of rheumatic fever recur, the patient may develop hardening of one of the valves. The blood is also affected. The white cells increase with the infection and the sedimentation rate of the red blood cells mounts, receding as the patient improves. Sometimes infection of the kidneys and the intestinal tract or severe pain similar to that of an attack of appendicitis accompany rheumatic fever.

At a point in an attack of rheumatic fever, the activity lessens and the infection becomes relatively inactive. When the condition becomes stabilized, the doctor usually re-examines the blood and heart and retests the white blood cell count and the rate of sedimentation of the red blood cells. Electrocardiograph tests are given and the vital capacity of the patient checked to determine the condition of his lungs. The doctor decides whether or not the patient can undertake mild activity. If the pulse rate continues high, even when the patient is asleep, or if the pulse does not return to its normal rate promptly following slight activity, it is too soon for the patient to resume activity. These tests also indicate the likelihood of partial or complete recovery.

The child with rheumatic heart disease or with any congenital ailment is especially susceptible to secondary infection, and continued treatment with antibiotics is essential. At present, persons with rheumatic fever are treated during the active stage of the disease by a variety of procedures. While these procedures are palliative, few are absolutely specific against rheumatic fever. Sulfa drugs, penicillin, ACTH, and hydrocortisone have all been used, but it has not been proved that any of these alone or in combination have conquered rheumatic fever.

Drugs of the salicylate group are especially useful in controlling such symptoms as fever, pain, and swelling in the joints. However, although these drugs do relieve the painful symptoms, they do not cure the disease itself. ACTH and cortisone have been lifesaving in controlling inflammation.

When the heart is especially involved, extra care must be taken to avoid every possible strain. Continuous bed rest, for weeks or even months, for the duration of the active stage is absolutely imperative. It is the one treatment of which doctors are certain.

Gradual resumption of physical activity must be carefully controlled. For example, the person is allowed to sit in a chair half an hour twice a day for one week; the next week, fifteen minutes more a day, if there have been no untoward symptoms; and, at the end of two weeks, perhaps he may be permitted to go to the bathroom by himself. Then moderate exercise may be allowed for fifteen minutes a day for two or three weeks; and perhaps, after five or six months, normal activity can be resumed, if the person's condition permits.

Unfortunately rheumatic fever has a tendency to recur after it has apparently gone. The doctor must determine, after the active stage has passed, whether or not the heart has been permanently damaged, and the person must continue to be reexamined at regular intervals to make certain that new activity has not begun and that he is in good health. For example, every sore throat should be treated immediately with antibiotics and sulfonamides.

Since complete bed rest, preferably outdoors in an open pavilion or on a protected porch, is so vital, children with rheumatic fever are best cared for in special sanatoriums where they may remain as long as necessary under the best possible conditions of ventilation, rest, sunshine, and nutrition.

If the person with rheumatic fever is anemic, special diets may be given which are high in protein, minerals, and vitamins. Infected tonsils and adenoids should be removed during the quiet periods of the rheumatic fever. All such operations are implemented with sulfa drugs or penicillin or other drugs to prevent secondary streptococcus infection.

The vast majority of children with rheumatic heart disease can and should attend regular schools and engage in a normally active life. In many large cities special schools are maintained for children with handicaps of the heart. In a recent report on the care of rheumatic fever, the following recommendations for treatment of children with inactive cases of rheumatic fever were made.

1. Take measures to improve the general health and resistance of the child.

2. Observe the patient regularly for signs of recurrence and for alterations in cardiac status.

3. Encourage physical activity to the limit of the child's capacity. Only a small percentage of children at adolescence are found to have sufficient permanent heart disease to preclude normal activity.

4. Provide vocational guidance and occupational training for the relatively small group who cannot engage in normal physical activity.

5. Discourage parents and teachers from making a chronic invalid of the child. Educational authorities should

learn that the vast majority who attend regular school when the disease is inactive can and should engage in normal school life.

6. Minimize exposure to upper respiratory infections, if possible, by improving living conditions—for example, by avoiding overcrowding in the home, particularly in bedrooms —and by controlling the spread of infection through school and family contacts. *See also* Chapter 8, "Congenital Heart Disease in Children."

RHEUMATISM, an overall term used to indicate diseases of muscle, tendon, joint, bone, or nerve resulting in discomfort and disability. About 7,500,000 people in the United States are affected by it, which makes it the most widespread chronic disease and 10 times more frequent than tuberculosis, diabetes, or cancer. Of those affected, 400,000 are completely helpless; 800,000, despite treatment, are partly crippled; and the rest have chronic pain and discomfort. Rheumatism has been called one of the principal health problems in the United States.

The most common form of rheumatism is rheumatoid arthritis. Other forms are degenerative joint disease, spondylitis, bursitis, fibrositis, myositis, neuritis, lumbago, sciatica, and gout. These are all primarily afflictions that affect persons after the age of forty; Rheumatic fever, which often involves the heart, is essentially a disease of childhood, attacking children between the ages of five and fifteen. *See also* names of specific diseases mentioned above; and Chapter 8, "Congenital Heart Disease in Children"; Chapter 24, "Arthritis and Rheumatism."

RH FACTOR. *See* BLOOD TYPES.

RHINITIS, any inflammation of the nasal mucous membrane. One of the chief forms is the common cold. Rhinitis is largely the result of infection, but may be due to sensitivity to various substances. *See also* COMMON COLD; HAY FEVER; OZENA.

RHINOPHYMA, a form of acne, involving the blood vessels and sebaceous glands in the nose, which results in swelling and formation of great nodules. Rhinophyma is a disfiguring condition, sometimes called "toper's nose" or "whiskey nose." Little can be done to alleviate it, except by plastic surgery.

RHINOPLASTY, a plastic operation on the nose.

RHUBARB, an herb which contains certain substances which act as a purgative. It was once widely used medically as a laxative in certain forms of constipation involving the intestines. As a purgative it is still popular because of its action of first cleansing the bowels and then checking any tendency to diarrhea. The mixture of rhubarb and soda is a rather widely known home remedy.

RIBOFLAVIN, the scientific term for the vitamin commonly called vitamin B_2. A deficiency of riboflavin may produce general body weakness and various skin disorders. The tip and margin of the tongue become sore and inflamed, painful cracks and fissures occur at the corners of the lips, and the face becomes greasy and scaly. The eyes are particularly sensitive to riboflavin deficiency and the cornea becomes cloudy and ulcerated, the mucous membranes inflamed, and the vision may be permanently impaired.

Management of riboflavin deficiency demands that the patient be given preparations containing large amounts of all major vitamins since a diet deficient in riboflavin is almost always deficient in all vitamins. The diet should then be permanently modified to contain adequate amounts of high riboflavin foods, such as liver, yeast, milk, eggs, whole-grain cereals, and greens. *See also* NUTRITION; VITAMINS.

RIBS, the curved, elongated bones which extend from the backbone around to the front of the chest. There are twenty-four ribs, twelve on each side of the rib case. The upper seven are directly attached to the breastbone and are known as the true ribs. Of the remaining five, or false ribs, each of the upper three is attached to the rib above. The last two, called floating ribs, are not attached to other ribs.

The ribs act as a protective case for the organs in the chest. They may be injured by direct violence, such as blows, but are often fractured by the chest, under compression, as when a vehicle runs over the body. Frequently a fractured rib heals, simply by being properly strapped in place. An x-ray should be taken in every case where there is even a suspicion of a broken rib. Acute pain, increased by breathing, is usually a sign of a broken rib.

In some cases an extra rib, found high up on the chest, may cause pain because of pressure on the tissues. This is known as a cervical rib.

RICKETS, a deficiency disease that affects infants and children and is characterized by a failure of calcium salts to be deposited in sufficient quantity in growing cartilage and newly formed bone in the body. Deformities and other symptoms result from the failure of the bones to develop properly; they include growth of nodules on the ribs, development of potbelly, and bending bones. The child with rickets often sits with his thighs slightly spread apart, with one leg crossed over the other. The hands are placed on the floor or on the thighs, to assist the backbone in holding the body erect. The pull on the tissues by the muscles and the ligaments plus the softness of the bones cause bending, so that bowlegs and knock-knees are characteristic. Rickets also leads to delayed eruption of temporary teeth, and to deformities of the unerupted permanent teeth.

Since rickets is caused by insufficient amounts of vitamin D, calcium, and phosphorus during the age when growth is rapid, and since the failure to receive sufficient amounts of one vitamin is likely to be associated with the failure to receive sufficient amounts of other vitamins and minerals, treatment involves a proper diet which includes them.

Parents should make certain that children, even in the nursing period, receive sufficient amounts of vitamins A, C, and D. They should also receive adequate amounts of calcium in the diet, best taken as milk, to insure proper and healthy growth. Cod liver oil, cod liver oil substitutes, vitamin D milk, and other dietary supplements are successful methods of preventing development of rickets in children and infants.

In severe cases of active rickets, large doses of vitamin D are administered, and in cases that do not yield rapidly massive doses are given. The extent of rickets can be diagnosed, and the progress of treatment checked by x-ray. The diet must also contain sufficient amounts of calcium and phosphorus, which are necessary for the body to properly use vitamin D. *See also* NUTRITION; VITAMINS.

RICKETTSIAL DISEASES, illnesses caused by one of the Rickettsial organisms. Rickettsiae are a family of microorganisms which have characteristics in common with both the filterable viruses and true bacteria. Under the microscope they have many shapes, but most of them resemble tiny rods. They were named after Dr. H. T. Ricketts of Chicago, who first isolated such an organism while he was studying Rocky Mountain spotted fever and epidemic typhus fever. In the course of these experiments Dr. Ricketts contracted typhus and died.

The rickettsiae are transmitted from man to man by an intermediate host, usually blood-sucking ticks, lice, or fleas. They generally pass into the blood stream of man through the bite of the insect, but infection may also be caused by excrement of the insect deposited on the skin.

The organism is responsible for at least four groups of diseases in human beings: typhus fever, the Rocky Mountain spotted fever group, scrub typhus, and Q fever. A person who has had a disease in a particular rickettsial disease group will have complete immunity to other diseases of the same group but will not be immune to those of the other groups.

Treatment, prevention, and control of the rickettsial diseases have made great strides with the recent development of large-scale antirickettsial vaccines, improved methods for mass delousing with DDT and other new insecticides, and with some of the newer antibiotics. *See also* names of specific diseases.

RICKETTSIALPOX, a disease caused by Rickettsia acari, a mild infection first identified in New York City in 1946. Since that time, 140 to 180 cases have been reported there each year. No cases have been reported anywhere else.

The infection is transmitted by a small colorless mite which infests house mice and small rodents. About a week or two after the bite of an infected mite, a firm reddish blister appears at the site of the bite. It dries, forms a small black ulcer, and in two or three weeks the scab drops off, leaving a small scar. It is not painful. Rickettsialpox is characterized by fever, chills, sweats, headache, muscle pains, and loss of appetite, which last about a week. The eyes are sensitive and light hurts them. A rash appears on the body, sometimes involving the mucosa of the mouth, which also disappears in about a week.

Rickettsialpox is sometimes confused with chickenpox. However, it is not a childhood disease, and may occur in all age groups. Eradication of house mice and consequently the carrier mites helps to control the disease. *See also* RICKETTSIAL DISEASES.

RINGWORM, a ring-shaped infection, the most common of the superficial fungus diseases, once believed to have been caused by a worm, and hence formerly called tinea, the Latin word for worm. The infection is also found in dogs, cats, and other domestic animals, and is spread by contact with infected sources.

Normally the skin carries several species of fungi which remain inactive until they are aroused by conditions favorable for their growth, such as lowered resistance, excessive perspiration, heat, moisture, or friction. The fungi then attack the hair follicles of the scalp or beard, the nails, and certain nonhairy skin surfaces. The infection results in unsightly troublesome sores which stubbornly resist treatment.

Ringworm usually starts with small, red, slightly raised, round or oval sores which gradually enlarge and become redder. Blisters often follow, with some itching and burning. They generally start healing in the center, while the infection spreads outward in circular fashion.

Many ringworm infections, especially those found in children, are highly contagious. Public schools and children's hospitals take the utmost precautions to prevent the spread of the infection when a case is reported.

Ringworm of the scalp, or tinea capitis, is a common highly contagious infection, found most frequently in children. The hair loses its luster, becomes brittle and breaks off easily. The scalp becomes covered with grayish scaly patches and short stumps of diseased hair. The more severe forms consist of boggy inflamed sores which contain pus. Temporary baldness in stubborn cases may become permanent.

Treatment is directed primarily toward preventing the spread of the infection. The involved areas must be kept clean and dry and protected from any friction. The scalp should be shampooed daily with tincture of green soap and a good fungicide. The hair should be clipped short and the cuttings burned. In resistant cases the hair and its roots are removed by a physician. Combs, brushes and caps used during this period should be sterilized or destroyed and the fingers and nails of infected persons kept clean to avoid a secondary infection and to prevent spreading the ringworm by scratching.

The sooner a ringworm infection is recognized and proper treatment begun, the more rapidly will the spread of the infection be halted and the disease eradicated.

Ringworm of the groin, or tinea cruris, an eruption which generally affects the skin of the inner thighs or under the arms, may be found in both sexes, though more commonly in males. The eruption varies from light brown scales in mild cases to bright red patches in the active stages, with well-defined raised borders. There is intense itching, which is worse at night, and the condition is aggravated by obesity, excessive sweating, and lack of cleanliness.

Ringworm of the groin is one of the most common fungus diseases in the tropics where it is known as dhobie itch. During World War II it was prevalent, particularly in Egypt and East Africa. The disease is sometimes contracted around swimming pools and bath houses from infected clothing and towels. The eruption often subsides during cold weather, the infected skin becoming dry, flaky, and stained. Usually, however, it recurs with warm weather.

As in all cases of ringworm, the utmost precaution should be taken to prevent the spread of the infection. Frequent bathing, following by liberal use of dusting powder, and daily change of underclothing are essential. The infected person should sleep alone, and bed linens and personal laundry should be sterilized.

Treatment depends on the acuteness of the condition. For chronic cases the specialist often prescribes ointments containing bismuth or salicylic acid. The infected area must be kept clean and dry at all times, and reinfection by scratching or wearing contaminated clothing must be avoided.

Ringworm of the body, or tinea circinata, is another form of the infection, found in the nonhairy skin. This eruption begins as a small red sore and enlarges outward. The dry type tends to become scaly and the moist type forms little blisters or pus sacs. It usually begins on the exposed parts of the face and neck and later spreads to the trunk, forearms and legs. It is generally acquired from household pets.

This type of ringworm yields readily to treatment. The infected area is scrubbed with tincture of green soap to remove the crusted debris, and mild ointments of sali-

cylic acid and sulphur are sufficient to control the condition.

Favus (tinea favosa). Although favus, another type of ringworm generally attacks the scalp, and is often limited to that region, it is caused by a different fungus than the one responsible for tinea capitis. Favus is caused by a vegetable parasite known as Trichophyton schoenleini, named for the German physician who first discovered it, Johann Lukas Schönlein. Climatic and social conditions may be factors in the transmission of this disease. It is relatively rare in the United States, but occurs commonly in China, Central Asia, the Balkans, and Germany. Children are much more susceptible to the infection than adults.

Favus begins as a small, scaly, inflamed sore which is soon covered with a sulphur-yellow, cup-shaped adherent crust, or scutulum, through which sparse short hairs project. The hairs are brittle, dull, and lusterless, and break off easily. A "mousy" odor is usually present.

If the condition is treated early, little permanent baldness or scarring results. Cases of long duration may occasionally show large patches of slightly reddened and scaly areas of baldness.

Treatment is similar to that for tinea captis. The hair is closely clipped, the crusts removed, and the scalp thoroughly shampooed. Antiparasitic ointments and lotions are applied, and the infected hairs are pulled out. The hair should be kept short and local treatments continued for at least a month after the scalp seems to be cured.

Ringworm of the nails, tinea

unguim, or onychomycosis, may be associated with infection of the hair, as in favus, or it may appear independently. It is not uncommon among nurses, who acquire the infection by contact. The condition begins on the undersurface of the nail, which becomes dull and ridged, and is raised off its bed by a cloudy grayish patch extending toward the nail root.

Treatment consists of removing the infected nail and applying antiparasitic medication during the entire period of growth of the new nail. Recurrences are common, especially among those whose work necessitates wetting the hands often, for example, washers, soda dispensers, fur skinners, canners, and housewives.

For ringworm of the beard *see* BARBER'S ITCH.

See also ATHLETE'S FOOT.

ROCKY MOUNTAIN SPOTTED FEVER,

an infectious condition caused by a rickettsial organism similar to the one that causes typhus, and transmitted to man by the bite of the wood tick or the dog tick. Spotted fever was known to the Indians of Montana and Idaho long before white settlers came. It has appeared, in recent years in most parts of the country. Similar tick-borne diseases are the boutonneuse fever of the Mediterranean, South African tick-bite fever, and other varieties found in Brazil, Colombia, Mexico, and Canada.

Three species of man-biting tick carry spotted fever in this country: the common wood tick of the northwestern states, the dog tick in the East, and the Lone Star tick of Texas. The ticks, which attach themselves to

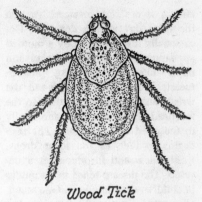

Wood Tick

The wood tick is a virus carrier. Certain kinds of wood ticks can infect humans with Rocky Mountain spotted fever.

animals in wooded areas, pick up the rickettsiae and remain infected for life. The eggs and newly hatched ticks also carry the parasite and pass it on from generation to generation. Human beings are infected by the tick bite or from a skin wound contaminated by crushed ticks or tick feces. People have been known to be infected by crushing ticks with their fingers while removing them from dogs. In the West, where the wood tick is the carrier, more men have contracted the fever than women. In the East, where the infection is transmitted by the dog tick, women and children are more often affected.

About two days to two weeks after a person has been infected, the symptoms appear. A few days of malaise, chilly sensations, and loss of appetite are followed by headache, chills, severe pains in the back and muscles and the large joints. The face is flushed, the eyes are sensitive to light, a dry cough often develops, and the temperature may rise to 105°

and in severe cases even higher. On the third day a rash develops. Occasionally it is preceded by a mottled appearance of the face, neck, and upper chest, almost like that in measles. The rash spreads to the wrists, ankles, and back; then to the forehead, arms, and legs; and finally to the chest and abdomen. The rash begins to fade as the fever drops. Restlessness and insomnia often develop. The disease tends to be milder in children than in adults. One attack of spotted fever generally gives immunity for a long period. Second attacks may occasionally occur after a lapse of eight years or longer.

Early diagnosis and treatment with antibiotics can reduce the fever in a few days and prevent or minimize the more severe disturbances which follow the fever.

The most effective protection for persons exposed to spotted fever is vaccination, preferably in the spring, before the ticks become numerous. A series of three injections establishes immunity for about a year, but must be repeated annually. People in tick-infested areas should wear one-piece outer clothing and high boots. The entire body should be inspected daily for ticks, especially about the hair-line of the neck and the pubic hairs. The tick is slow to attach itself, and starts feeding only some time after it has become attached. Children should be examined twice daily, since in their play they may become especially exposed. Ticks should be removed with great care, to avoid crushing them and thus contaminating the spot to which they have become attached. The site of attachment should be disinfected with soap and water, and the wound swabbed with a toothpick dipped in crude phenol or the most potent household antiseptic available. A dab of ether, chloroform, or acetone will usually cause the tick to drop off. If not, forceps or tweezers should be used gently, with care taken not to leave the mouth of the tick embedded in the skin. Ticks should never be removed with the bare fingers. Dust sprays containing an insecticide may be used to remove ticks from livestock and dogs, but should not be applied to cats, which lick their fur and may be poisoned. DDT and chlordane, applied directly to the ground and to low vegetation, are both effective in controlling wooded areas infested by ticks.

ROUNDWORM. *See* WORMS.

RUBELLA, another name for German measles. *See* GERMAN MEASLES.

RUPTURE. *See* HERNIA.

SACROILIAC, the joint at the base of the spine, between the sacrum and the ilium.

SACRUM, a triangular-shaped bone formed by the five sacral vertebrae fused together at the lower end of the spine. Inflammation of the joint between the sacrum at the back and the pelvis at the front produces pain which is sometimes mistaken for sciatica.

SADISM, a sexual perversion in which a person derives pleasure from inflicting cruelty or pain on others. The word sadism is derived from the Marquis de Sade, a Frenchman who lived about 1800 and wrote several books about sexual cruelty.

ST. VITUS' DANCE. *See* CHOREA.

SALIVA, the opalescent, tasteless, weak alkaline fluid secreted chiefly by the salivary glands which open in the mouth under the jaw in front of the ear and under the tongue. The lining of the mouth also secretes saliva.

Saliva contains an enzyme which acts in the digestion of starch to change it into sugar. It serves also to moisten and soften food in the chewing process, and to keep the lining of the mouth moist.

SALK VACCINE. *See* POLIOMYELITIS; and Chapter 23, "The Neuromuscular and Neurological Disabilities."

SALPINGITIS, inflammation of the uterine or Fallopian tubes, due to infection. *See also* FALLOPIAN TUBES.

SALT, chemically a substance resulting from the combination of an acid and a base. In nontechnical usage, however, it usually refers to the white powdery condiment, sodium chloride, commonly used to season foods.

The average person consumes about half an ounce of salt daily. This is usually adequate; but in extreme heat, when perspiration is heavy, more than the usual amount of salt is lost by the body and a deficiency can result, characterized by weakness, cramplike pains, and nausea. The increase in salt consumption necessary to relieve the deficiency is small— one extra pinch of salt is usually enough.

About three ounces of salt are present in the body of an adult person at any one time. The body's use of salt and its elimination are believed to be regulated by the cortex, or outer layer of adrenal glands, the small bodies which secrete cortisone.

The human body uses salt to supply the chlorine required to synthesize hydrochloric acid, a significant digestive substance secreted by the stomach. Pepsin performs its digestive function only in the presence of hydrochloric acid.

The amount of salt in the diet may be related to various conditions which affect the kidneys and blood pressure, and low-salt and salt-free diets are prescribed in such cases. A reduction in salt, perhaps the usual half ounce decreased to a tenth of an ounce, may be desirable in dropsy or edema, in which fluid accumulates in the tissue.

Sodium chloride has various medical functions. Salt is injected when fluid which has been lost from the body by bleeding must be replaced. A strong salt solution is a good emetic and a weak solution is a mild gargle.

SANDFLY FEVER, an infectious viral disease, resembling dengue fever in many of its symptoms. It is of short duration and occurs most frequently in the Mediterranean area. It is caused by the bite of the sandfly, Phlebotomus paptasii. The condition is also known as pappataci fever, three-day fever, and phlebotomus fever. *See also* DENGUE.

SARCOMA, malignant tumor, most frequently involving nonepithelial tissue, which includes fibrous and connective tissue, cartilage and bone.

Cancer in the skin, arising from the layers below the epidermis, occurs only in children. Sarcoma of the nerve cells is known as fibroneurosarcoma. It is also found in lymphoid and fatty tissue. Sarcoma may be detected and diagnosed by microscopic examination of a piece of the tumor, a procedure called a biopsy. *See also* CANCER.

SCABIES, popularly known as "the itch," or "seven-year itch," follows invasion of the skin by the microscopic itch mite, which is no more than a fiftieth of an inch long, and whose scientific name is Acarus scabiei.

The mites live on the surface, but the eggs of the female are laid under the skin. The female mites burrow under the skin and may remain for a long time, traveling along a tunnel of some length and laying eggs in the burrow. The young develop within a few days, then come to the surface where they repeat the cycle.

Several areas of the body seem to be favored by the mites. Most often they burrow on the inside of the fingers, near the webs. Other locations are the insides of the toes, the ankles and knee joints, the front of the armpit, the breasts of girls and women, and the outer sex organs of boys and men. The face never seems to be attacked.

The body becomes sensitized to the insects and intense itching results. Numerous blisters may form, and scratching may result in infection.

To rid the body of the itch mites, the most effective treatment includes bathing in hot water every day, followed by the use of sulphur oint-ment. For patients sensitive to sulphur, ointments containing other drugs, including benzene hexachloride which is less irritating than sulphur, may be prescribed.

Underclothing and bedding must be changed daily until all danger of further hatching of the eggs is removed. Extreme care must be taken that the infested person not infect other persons with whom he comes in contact.

SCARLET FEVER, an acute infectious disease characterized by a scarlet skin eruption. It occurs most frequently in fall or winter, and in children between the ages of five and twelve. Children less than one year old seldom contract it, probably because they have received antisubstances in their blood from the mother which afford protection.

The period of incubation is approximately three days following contact with an infected person. The symptoms are a painful sore throat, chill, nausea, and vomiting. The pulse rate increases, the temperature may rise as high as 104°, and the child may suffer a severe headache.

The rash first appears in pinpoint spots of bright red, usually on the chest and neck, and then gradually over the rest of the body. Although this rash attacks the body more often than the face, the face often shows red spots, if only because of the high fever. Although the rash may continue only two or three days, it will take a week or more before the skin regains its normal color. Ten days to two weeks after the onset of scarlet fever, peeling of the skin begins. Large pieces of skin may come away from the feet and hands or drop off in scales, and other parts of the body can be affected, such as the teeth, fingernails, and sometimes the hair. The tongue develops a pitted scarlet appearance which gives it the name strawberry tongue.

Although scarlet fever often proves to be a relatively mild infection, it may have serious complications. The kidneys are frequently involved, or the ears, glands, and joints, so that this disease can do serious damage.

Scarlet fever is occasionally contracted by drinking milk or by contact with wastage thrown off from an infected person. The peeled skin is harmless, unless it happens to carry secretions from the nose or throat of the patient.

Many persons may have had the disease in a mild form at an earlier time, when it was erroneously diagnosed or ignored, and thereby gained immunity. This may help to explain why scarlet fever appears to be only mildly contagious. One attack of the illness seems to assure almost certain immunity.

Scientific understanding of scarlet fever has advanced greatly in recent years, and both diagnosis and treatment have improved. The streptococcus is the cause of the disease, and wherever the germ grows, poison or toxin is produced. If this poison is injected into the skin of someone who has never had scarlet fever, a severe reaction will be noted. In those persons who have had the disease and are immune, there will be no reaction.

When a small amount of this poison is rendered harmless and is injected into a person who has never been infected, he will then be able to resist the disease. However, this preventive toxoid is administered only to a person who has been exposed, or who works in the vicinity of people with scarlet fever, or during epidemics. The most effective technique to prevent spread of scarlet fever is to avoid contact with infected persons, particularly when discharge from the nose, throat, or ears is active.

As long as the fever persists, a mild diet is recommended. Once the fever has subsided, however, soft foods are usually given until the peeling period begins, when milk and fresh vegetables are added as well as food rich in vitamins, minerals, and protein.

Treatment demands that particular attention be given that as little effort as possible be placed on the kidneys and heart, since they are already receiving from the toxin itself an attack almost greater than they can endure. Ordinarily the patient is required to remain in bed at least three weeks and must be protected from chill and cold. Sponge baths of tepid water may be given. A mild gargle may relieve sore throat, and one of the newer antibiotics will be even more effective. The person who cares for the patient should preferably be someone who has already had the disease, since he is directly exposed to germs. Reactions of the heart and kidneys and ears must be carefully watched. Occasionally when the ear is infected the ear drum is punctured so that the pus can be drained before the internal ear is involved.

Since the advent of sulfa drugs and penicillin, serious complications from scarlet fever have become rare.

The drugs are also highly effective against the germ itself so that scarlet fever is no longer a serious threat. *See also* Chapter 7, "The Process of Infectious Diseases and Immunization of Children."

SCHIZOPHRENIA, a severe mental disorder, a major psychosis, which involves a loss of contact with reality and a temporary or permanent disorganization or disintegration of personality. "Schizo" means splitting, "phrenia" means mind, and the term refers to a splitting away of the mind from reality. Schizophrenia is the most common form of mental illness and one-fourth of all hospitalized mental patients fall into this category.

The schizophrenic person rejects the outside world and turns to his own self-created world. His actions are made in accordance with this imagined world and so are difficult to interpret. His speech may be garbled and unintelligible and his actions completely inappropriate to his external situation, since they are motivated by his fantasy world and his inability to perceive reality in the normal way.

Schizophrenia is not one disease but rather a set of complex symptoms which encompass many forms of mental disorder. The causes are extremely difficult to treat. Factors which would appear pertinent in some cases do not apply to others. The schizophrenic is a person who has apparently been unable to find a way of adjusting to some painful situation and so has rejected the outside world in favor of his own inner version. Organic factors are also believed to be related to schizophrenia.

In the past few decades, understanding and treatment of schizophrenia has greatly improved and the rate of partial or complete recovery is higher. Expert psychiatric care is essential, preferably as soon as possible. *See also* Chapter 22, "Mental Illness."

SCIATICA. *See* SCIATIC NERVE; SCIATIC NEURITIS.

SCIATIC NERVE, the large long nerve which supplies the muscles of the thigh, leg, and foot and the skin of the leg. It runs the entire length of the leg with many branches and subdivisions. The nerve can be irritated or compressed at any point. *See also* SCIATIC NEURITIS.

SCIATIC NEURITIS, also frequently called sciatica, inflammation of the sciatic nerve, the longest nerve in the body, which passes from the lower part of the spinal column downward to the leg along the rear of the thigh. The word sciatica is often applied to cover a variety of ailments having no involvement with the sciatic nerve. True sciatica is sciatic neuritis, and pain is felt in the thigh and other areas associated with the sciatic nerve. Sciatic pain accompanies numerous conditions, and may be due to a number of factors which adversely affect the sciatic nerve.

The part of the spinal cord where the nerve originates may be disturbed, for example, by a slipped or ruptured disc, or by an inflammation in the vertebral bones. An abnormal condition in a nearby blood vessel may cause it to press on the nerve. Acute and prolonged constipation is some-

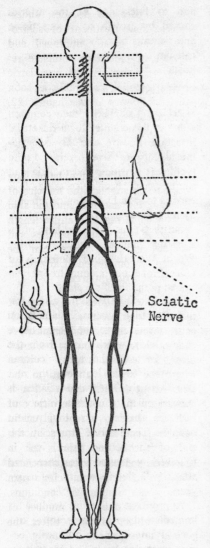

Sciatic
Nerve ←

The site of the sciatic nerve.

may precipitate a sciatic disturbance, such as a bad fall or severe contortion of the body, or prolonged exposure to cold and dampness.

Because of the number of possible causes and the numerous possible ramifications which sciatic neuritis may have, it is, like headache and backache, an apparently simple discomfort which masks a potentially complicated situation. Diagnosis of the specific cause of a particular case of sciatic neuritis demands the attention of a skilled physician. The pain is only a symptom and the source of it must be determined before proper treatment can begin. The physician will first ascertain whether the pain involved is due to a sciatic condition or some other cause. He will check the sacroiliac joint, the spine for curvature, the back for bones out of position, the legs for muscle spasms or disordered muscles and tissue.

Treatment may begin with simple measures to relieve the immediate discomfort: bed rest, placing the body in the position with the least possible strain on affected parts, or use of heat to reduce pain. The doctor will examine the patient's diet and his daily activities, making sure that the diet is nutritionally adequate and that the patient's job, exercise, and general environment do not aggravate his condition. He may, for example, recommend that a patient who works in a cold damp place change his job. Injection of one of a variety of medicinal substances into the sciatic nerve or the surrounding areas is sometimes advisable and may bring good but not permanent results. Other measures are available for specialized treatment. *See also* SLIPPED DISC.

times responsible because the accumulation in the bowel exerts pressure on the nerve or because the body absorbs unexcreted toxic substances to which the nerve reacts. External conditions or occurrences

SCLERODERMA, a disease in which all the layers of the skin become hard and rigid. A serious affliction, scleroderma attacks women more often than men, usually between the ages of twenty and forty. Localized scleroderma often appears and disappears spontaneously in children.

Before the disease becomes apparent, the victim may for some time have complained about alterations in the circulation of his blood. Soon the hands and feet take on a bluish tinge, which changes later to white or yellow. At the same time the tissue itself becomes increasingly hard and rigid. Eventually both arms and legs—and even the entire body —may become hard as stone.

Almost nothing is known about the cause of scleroderma. Obviously serious damage is done to the tissues, as well as to the superficial blood vessels, but the nature of the toxin is unknown. Some authorities have suggested that the cause may be traced to glandular changes and others believe that the nervous system causes the condition.

Treatment has included use of the electric needle, use of ointments and massage, and a change of climate. Modern drugs have been tried, such as sodium paba, cortisone, and ACTH. Little success has been recorded, however, either in the control or the cure of this serious and strange disease.

SCLEROSIS, a hardening of part of the body due to overgrowth of fibrous tissue. The term is applied particularly to hardening of the nervous tissue from atrophy or degeneration of the nerve elements, and to thickening of the arteries caused by growth of fibrous tissue and deposits of fatty substances and calcium salts. *See also* ARTERIOSCLEROSIS.

SCOLIOSIS. *See* SPINAL CURVATURE.

SCRUB TYPHUS, the common name in this country for a rickettsial infection known also as tsutsugamushi, Japanese river fever, and mite typhus. It is widespread in Asia and southwestern Pacific areas, and is carried to man by field mice infected by mites or chiggers.

Scrub typhus was a serious problem for military medicine during World War II, when thousands of cases broke out among troops stationed in the Pacific region.

The illness follows the course of the rickettsial infections, with headache, fever, chill, and insomnia. A characteristic symptom is the small ulcer, or eschar, which develops where the mite is attached to the skin. About the fifth day a red rash appears on the trunk. The ulcer and rash are generally absent in Asiatic peoples. Temperature drops by the end of the second week, and is followed by slow convalescence. One attack will give immunity for many years.

Appropriate antibiotics produce an immediate drop in temperature, and general improvement ordinarily occurs in twelve hours. Vaccines have not yet been developed to prevent the disease. Mite repellents such as phthalates, or benzyl benzoate, smeared by hand on clothes and exposed skin surfaces, are effective. These drugs should not be used on or around sensitive skin areas such as the eyes or the crotch. *See also* RICKETTSIAL DISEASES.

SCURVY, a nutritional disorder caused by a lack of vitamin C. It is characterized by extreme weakness, spongy gums, and a tendency to develop bleeding under the skin and from the mucous membranes and bone coverings. *See also* NUTRITION; VITAMINS.

SEASICKNESS. *See* MOTION SICKNESS.

SEBACEOUS CYST. *See* WEN.

SEBORRHEA, a functional disease caused by excessive secretion of the sebaceous or oil-producing glands in the skin. The condition may vary widely, from nothing more than dandruff, the commonest form, to seborrheic dermatitis, in which the whole scalp and sometimes the face and other parts of the body develop a greasy kind of crusting and scaling, accompanied by red irritated areas.

In some cases, dandruff begins in childhood as a simple scaling of small white bits of skin from the scalp and then continues as a mild annoyance for many years. Often, however, the process gradually becomes more and more involved with greasy discharges from the scalp and skin of the face, and "oily" seborrhea may develop, sometimes with so much discharge that drops of oil actually collect on the skin.

Physicians attribute these symptoms to a variety of causes. Some feel that these phenomena are the result of a constitutional predisposition to a kind of skin which is subject to excessive growth of oil-producing glands and enlargement of pores.

Others believe that actual infection by some microorganism is involved. Changes in behavior of various internal glands of the body and such factors as faulty diet and chronic intestinal disorder are also blamed. Many feel that in all likelihood more than one of these factors, and possibly all of them, may be involved.

Treatment of troublesome dandruff should be under a doctor's direction, but the person who has seborrhea will find that more than the usual participation by the patient is required. Success depends largely on his willingness to take frequent shampoos, massage the scalp with prescribed lotions and ointments, and brush the hair daily.

The doctor has other measures which he uses to shorten the treatment time. A new preparation, derived from selenium, has proved effective against many of the annoying symptoms but should not be used without a doctor's advice.

The patient's general health is significant, and rest, exercise, and proper hygiene are essential. Excessive fatigue, lack of sleep, anxiety and emotional strain may be involved in inducing the state which is conducive to the development of seborrhea. If necessary, the blood should be brought to normal by dietary supplements such as vitamins and iron.

In cases in which nothing more serious than some scaling of the scalp is involved, a direct attack on the dandruff alone may be all that is required. The dandruff-prone person should shampoo his hair and scalp thoroughly at least once a week, bathe daily, and avoid wearing clothing that overheats and softens the skin.

If the oily condition becomes severe, the doctor may require special shampoos of olive or similar oils and glycerin to remove the fatty covering of the scalp and make it accessible to treatment. Following this, alkaline rinses of diluted borax and ammonia may be applied to reduce the oiliness, although these rinses must be followed by an oily application to prevent irritation of the scalp.

Seborrheic dermatitis, the most severe form of seborrhea, is ordinarily a sequel to oily dandruff and skin. Treatment is difficult and must be varied to meet the particular condition encountered. A good daily hygienic routine is essential, with ample sleep, bathing, and a diet rich in protein. Vitamin B complex or vitamin B_{12} may also prove beneficial. The doctor may use various special ointments, and antibiotics will help control infection if it occurs.

SENESCENCE, the process of aging. As people grow older, their bodies undergo changes. The cells of the body begin to lose their power of repair, and the glands tend to function less efficiently. Digestion becomes disturbed, and the senses of taste, smell, sight, and hearing often weaken or begin to fail. In the aging process of the human body, the condition of the blood vessels is the most significant single factor. Hardening of the arteries, the wearing out of the muscular tissues of the blood vessels, and heart failure are the result of degenerative changes in the tissues. As the consequence of these changes,

the body may either lose bulk or become corpulent. The bones are harder and more brittle, the hair grays and often falls out, the capacity for muscular and mental effort decreases, and diseases affecting the circulatory system, heart, kidneys, lungs, and other organs begin to manifest themselves.

Within the limits imposed by aging, medical science can do much for these disorders, and older persons should be examined by a doctor at frequent intervals.

Many of the changes in the vision of older persons are due to changes in circulation, including hardening of the arteries. The pupil of the eye becomes smaller and less movable, and the color of the eyes becomes lighter. The lens of the eye grows and increases in weight throughout life, and a reduction in elasticity promotes the condition known as presbyopia, which is due to a loss of accommodation in the lens. Sometimes a cataract, typical of old age, forms. The exact cause is not known, and the decision whether or not to remove a cataract depends on many factors related to the person's mental and physical condition, as well as the actual condition of the eye.

The eyelids of an older person develop wrinkles, and he seems to cry more easily, sometimes suffering from an excess of tears. This is often due to relaxation of the tissues of the eye, which do not hold the material as well as do the tissues of younger persons. With surgical advances, techniques have been developed for maintaining the normal relationship between the tissues and overcoming the excess of tears.

Like the rest of the body, the teeth and jaws are subject to change in old age. The jaws change shape and the teeth tend either to fall out or require extraction. Artificial dentures often replace the loss of teeth.

The functioning of the digestive system becomes less efficient as a person grows older, and frequently a simpler, more easily digested diet is preferred. Three meals a day should still be eaten, but they can be smaller. The diet, of course, should continue to be balanced, and vitamin or mineral supplements taken if necessary. Less protein is required for tissue repair, although foods which supply energy are still essential in sizable amounts.

During late maturity, a thorough physical checkup is a wise precaution against disease in old age. Although aches and pains may multiply as one grows older, there are no diseases specifically caused by old age, and many maladies to which older persons are subject result from chronic diseases which occurred years before. The diseases that take the greatest toll of life among the aged are heart diseases, cancer, and cerebral hemorrhage. Other afflictions are arthritis, rheumatism, diabetes, prostatic enlargement, kidney diseases, hardening of the arteries, high blood pressure, and nervous and mental conditions.

With the general advance in medical science, more people are living longer. Thus older persons are coming to constitute an increasingly larger percentage of the population, and their particular problems are becoming of concern to more and more people. See also GERIATRICS; SE-NILITY; and Part VIII, "The Later Years"; Chapter 27, "Medical Statistics."

SENILITY, the extreme stage of cerebral arteriosclerosis, which produces in the aged symptoms approaching dementia. The mind of the senile person becomes feeble and he may be so confused that he requires constant care and attention, and cannot be left alone. This condition is also marked by extreme forgetfulness. In such moments, he may begin to do something in one part of the house and then suddenly go off to another room, forgetting what he had started out to do. In other instances, the senile person may wander away from his home and walk confusedly about, not even having presence of mind to ask directions.

Often the rest cycle is reversed, and the senile person sleeps during the day instead of at night. He will be active all night, moving about from room to room while the rest of the household sleeps. At daybreak, drowsiness sets in and he may sleep and doze the rest of the day.

In the most advanced stages of senility, all touch with reality may be lost and symptoms of dementia manifested. Coherent communication with others becomes impossible and helplessness, incontinence, and loss of brain function are noted. At this stage, hospitalization is often the best solution, and a large percentage of beds in mental institutions are devoted to senile persons.

In treating senility, the doctor will check and prescribe accordingly for high blood pressure, overweight, and diabetes. Any correctable illness or condition will also be treated, including diet deficiencies and anemia, both fairly common among senile persons. In most cases, the teeth and digestion of the aged will be in such poor condition that a bland diet of chopped meats and strained and puréed vegetables will be advised. An effort should be made to cater to the special tastes and preferences of the individual, who may be "cranky" about his food. In treating the reversed sleep cycle, a combination of a mild stimulant in the morning and a moderate sedative at night is effected in most cases, although the situation may be fairly difficult to control. Tranquilizing drugs, among other measures, have been found effective in treatment of the extremely confused. Much remains to be learned and done in the care and treatment of senility. *See also* GERIATRICS; SENESCENCE; and Chapter 26, "Geriatrics."

SEPTICEMIA, another word for bacteremia or blood poisoning. *See* BACTEREMIA.

SEPTIC SORE THROAT, an acute infection of the throat caused by an organism, streptococcus hemolyticus. It is the most severe of all sore throats, and serious complications may ensue if treatment is not prompt.

Ordinarily the condition develops rapidly, starting with chill and fever that may go as high as 105° F. Swelling and soreness in and around the throat make it painful to swallow or even to move the head. As the infection spreads downward, the voice becomes hoarse, the breath short, and coughing begins.

The most immediate danger is ulceration within the throat at the point of infection, or the formation of abscesses in the neck glands where the disease causes inflammation and swelling. Not infrequently the infection may go considerably further, invading the heart or abdomen and causing acute specific illness in those areas, or in other parts of the body.

The disease is sometimes called epidemic septic sore throat, because it may be spread by sources of infection, such as contaminated milk, which affect numbers of people in a community. Adequate pasteurization will prevent this, but any defect in the pasteurization process may let through a batch of milk infected with the microorganisms which cause septic sore throat, as well as other diseases. This particular streptococcus infects cows and when it does is found on their udders. An infected milker may spread the disease, and milkers should always wash their hands before going to work and preferably also during the process. Infected ice cream has been found to be the source of at least one epidemic. When a number of cases of septic sore throat are reported in a community, health authorities suspect a common source of infection and often are able to trace it to one milk route and even to a particular herd of cattle.

Antibiotics, such as penicillin or aureomycin, are effective against the infection. Immediate bed rest for the duration of the illness is advised. Hot wet packs on the neck may help to combat the infection. Sprays, gargles, and other preparations applied directly to the throat are of little help.

If swelling of the throat begins to interfere to any considerable extent with breathing, oxygen may be given. Despite its severity, fatalities from septic sore throat are infrequent because of the accessibility of the infection to medical care.

SHINGLES. *See* HERPES ZOSTER.

SHOCK, the condition caused by acute failure of the peripheral circulation, the circulation of the blood in the veins and in the capillaries farthest from the heart. The essential functions of the body are diminished. Shock may occur during times of great emotional stress, injury, pain, sudden illness and accident, such as burns, and has been one of the most difficult emergencies to confront physicians.

It is believed by most doctors that loss of blood is the cause of shock in most cases, and therefore treatment of shock emphasizes maintaining the blood supply through use of blood plasma by transfusion.

The first change that occurs in shock is dilation of the blood vessels on the surface. When this happens, the person begins to sweat, while his skin is relatively warm. His blood pressure falls and his pulse becomes slow and feeble.

The victim of shock should first of all be placed with his head low, since a loss of blood from the brain may result in failure of the brain to function. If the state of shock continues over a period of even a few hours, it may be fatal or cause permanent impairment of the brain. He must be kept comfortably warm. Pain, which may be a contributing

factor to the intensity of shock, is relieved by sedative drugs.

A secondary shock due to damage of the tissues follows the initial shock from a wound or injury, and may be apparent an hour or more after an injury. A person in secondary shock is pale, weak, exhausted, and, if conscious, may complain of thirst. His perspiration is cold and clammy, pulse rapid and thready and breathing rapid and shallow, blood pressure low and the superficial blood vessels collapsed. Secondary shock is seen mainly after severe burns or as a late manifestation of a surgical operation.

In shock following burns, the patient, if conscious, should be given salt and soda in water (1 quart of cold water, 1 teaspoon of salt, and ½ teaspoon of baking soda) to replace the salty fluids lost from the tissues. This is only a first-aid measure to be taken until the doctor arrives.

Patients suffering from diabetic or insulin shock require special treatment which only a doctor can administer.

In surgery, continuous transfusion of blood or plasma is sometimes a part of the operative procedure. It greatly lessens the incidence of shock. *See also* INSULIN SHOCK THERAPY.

SHOCK TREATMENT. *See* ELECTRIC SHOCK TREATMENT; INSULIN SHOCK TREATMENT; and Chapter 22, "Mental Illness."

SHOULDER, a joint of the ball-and-socket type, constructed of bones held in position by powerful muscles, tendons, and ligaments. Because of its unique structure, it has a greater range of movement than any other joint in the body. However, the shoulder is unsupported from beneath and is therefore subject to dislocation in this direction.

The shoulder joint is easily injured and may become stiff and painful from a number of causes. When this occurs, the person usually must cease all activity for a time, as further movement will intensify the injury. Frequently a torn tendon may cause pain and stiffness. The tendon may be torn as a result of dislocation, fall, or strain. Infection of the bursa, or sacs, in the shoulder region may produce inflammation which inhibits movement of the shoulder.

Fractures of any of the bones in the shoulder require surgical treatment. Dislocation demands setting of the bones and immobilization by means of bandaging or placing the shoulder in a cast. Immobilization is also essential in case of intense pain due to sprain, severe infection, or torn ligament, and usually it is expedient to place the arm in a sling which will enable it to be supported close to the side. In most cases, this is all the treatment required. A splint and plaster cast to hold the arm raised and away from the body, the abductor position, may be desirable in other cases. After removal of splints and casts, heat, massage, and exercise will help prevent loss of function and restore mobility. Recurrent dislocation of the shoulder is fairly common, especially among athletes, and surgery is practically the only conclusive treatment for this condition. Subsequently the shoulder must be placed in a cast and after its removal appropriate exercise is required to restore normal function.

"Frozen shoulder" is a disorder involving the bursas and tendonous tissue, and it produces extreme pain and stiffness. Rest is of utmost significance and application of heat is often helpful. When calcium is deposited in the area, hydrocortisone or similar drugs may be injected. Gentle exercise and heat help to restore normal function, and in some cases such treatment is required for a long time. *See also* ARTHRITIS; BURSITIS; DISLOCATION; JOINTS AND JOINT DISEASES.

SINUSES, cavities or channels within bones. Those in the head which connect with the inside of the nose by narrow passageways sometimes cause trouble. The sinus in the cheekbone is called the antrum, the one above the eyes is the frontal sinus, and deeper behind the nose is the ethmoid sinus, which is actually a series of small sinuses, varying from three to more than fifteen in some cases.

The membranes of the sinuses are susceptible to infection. If the opening of the sinus into the nose becomes blocked, the infectious matter will cause symptoms of sinusitis, which include headache, pain, and, when the infection is absorbed into the body, high fever. An ordinary cold may end in a few days, but if the sinuses become infected the symptoms may last for many weeks. Eventually the sinus disorder may become chronic, with an increase in the intensity of the original infection.

The doctor usually treats an infection of the sinuses by cleansing the nose and shrinking the membranes by applying vasoconstrictors such as epinephrine. He then determines whether or not the infectious material is draining from the sinuses into the nose. X-rays will indicate whether there is any blocking or polyps or tumorous growth. Infection may be controlled with drops, sprays, or application of medicinal packs. Drugs may be given orally, or applied directly to the nose by washing out the sinuses. Sometimes surgical procedures are advisable. Current treatment with drugs, such as the sulfonamides, penicillin, and other antibiotics, has practially eliminated surgery. Occasionally, however, certain complications may necessitate operation to improve drainage or destroy an abscess. When polyps are growing in the sinuses, ACTH, cortisone, and similar hormone products have been successfully used.

Allergenic substances are sometimes responsible for sinus disorders, and the doctor may prescribe antihistaminic drugs. In chronic sinus infections, vaccines have been helpful once the particular type of germ responsible has been determined. In time, resistance to the infection will develop.

Persons with acute or chronic infections of the sinuses should avoid swimming, diving, and strenuous outdoor exercise. Particularly obstinate cases of sinus infection may improve in a hot dry climate.

SKELETON, in the human body, is the bones or the body framework which support the soft tissue and protect the internal organs. The body's bony framework may be described as consisting of axial and appendicular sets of bones. The head, the ribs and breastbone, and the spinal column form the axial part, and the arms and legs are the appendages. Two bony girdles, the shoulder and the pelvic girdle, connect the axis and the appendages.

The two innominate bones form the pelvic girdle, which is actually made into a rigid girdle by the sacrum. The shoulder girdle, which is formed by the scapula and the clavicle, is incomplete in front and behind, but supported in front by the uppermost part of the sternum, the breastbone.

The upper limb is attached to the axial skeleton by the clavicle and scapula. The lower limb is attached by the innominate bones, which are jointed in front to one another and at the back to the sacrum, the lower end of the spine.

These elements, with their component bones, comprise the skeleton. Altogether 206 bones form the adult human skeleton, including the tiny bones of the middle ear. The skeleton is a complex structure of bones and joints, and its movements are made possible by the skeletal muscles which are attached to their respective bones by tendons. Tendons anchor muscles to bone by means of connective tissue fibers which enter the bone structure. Together the skeleton and muscles have a great part in body function, since every body movement, voluntary and involuntary, depends on the skeletal and muscular systems.

Disorders of the skeleton embrace the various infections, inflammations, and diseases, including cancer, that may attack the bones. Sprains of the ligaments binding bones together may occur, debility as in foot strain or flat feet, or dislocations and fractures of bones or joints. Arthritis and rheumatism may attack the bones and joints. Various mechanical defects, such as curvature of the spine, can develop, or congenital deficiencies may present difficulty later in life. *See also* ARTHRITIS; BONES; DISLOCATION; FRACTURES; JOINTS AND JOINT DISORDERS; SPINE; VERTEBRA; and Chapter 3, "The Body and its Functions."

SKIN, the largest single organ in the body, forming a protective covering over it. The skin of an adult person weighs about six pounds and if spread flat would cover an area of about 16 to 20 square feet.

Externally the skin is furrowed. The furrows are formed by the attachment of the skin to the structures beneath and by the movement of the skin, and remain constant for each person. Between the furrows are ridges which are dotted with the openings of the pores which release perspiration through the skin.

The skin of the palms of the hands and the soles of the feet is thicker than the skin on other parts of the body. The lines on the fingers which form an impression called a fingerprint consist of rows of papillae in the true skin projecting into the epidermis. If part of the epidermis is lost, the new epidermis that forms will show exactly the same arrangement of lines as before.

The structure of the skin is composed of three layers: an outer layer called the cuticle; the next layer which is the true skin; and the lowest layer where the blood and lymph vessels and similar structures vital to the health and life of the skin are located. Here, also, are some of the glands and roots of hair follicles. The skin receives one-third of all of the blood that circulates.

The skin is constantly renewing itself from birth to death. The outermost layers are detached as the lower layers produce new cells. Billions of new cells are produced every day while billions of horny dead cells are shed by the body. There are thirty layers of cells which are constantly being added to from below and shed from above.

One of the chief functions of the skin is to maintain a constant temperature through evaporation of heat from the body. The amount of heat radiated depends on the external temperature. Other glands in the skin secrete an oil which maintains the skin in a flexible condition. Each square inch of surface on the palms of the hands has more than 5,000 sweat glands. The skin also excretes waste material, helps prevent loss of body fluids, and is the fundamental sensory organ. Hair on the body originates from hair follicles embedded in the skin.

The skin is an organ of the body as much as the liver, heart, or lungs. When the flow of blood to the skin is hindered for any reason, the skin becomes harder, thicker, and loses its normal appearance. In old age, when blood circulation to the skin decreases, the skin loses its youthful appearance, wrinkles form, and the color changes.

The color of the skin is determined largely by melanin, a dark pigment. The amount of melanin varies with each person, but depends largely on heredity. The action of sunlight also is significant because exposure to the sun stimulates a greater production of melanin in the skin which causes tanning, or freckles if unevenly distributed. The circulation of blood through the skin gives it a pink or "flesh" color. A person may appear pale when anemic or ruddy when the amount of blood in the capillaries is increased.

Fingernails and toenails are actually modifications of the skin, and the mucous membranes found in body cavities such as the mouth, nose, digestive tract, and eyes are also modified skin. Mucous membrane differs from outer skin in many ways, principally in the secretion of mucus.

Any inflammation of the skin is called dermatitis. Although some forms of dermatitis are due to serious internal causes, 95 per cent of the cases of disturbed skin are simple irritations due to infection or some external cause.

A change in the skin is a characteristic of many deficiency diseases. Vitamins have a definite relationship to the skin and at least six skin conditions are connected to vitamin deficiencies. For example, a vitamin B_2 (riboflavin) deficiency will cause blisters and cracking at the corners of the mouth. A deficiency of vitamin C leads to scurvy with hemorrhages in the gums and skin. A vitamin A deficiency results in dryness of the skin and hair, although most people who have dry skin and hair do not have this deficiency. Practically every skin disease has at one time or another been treated by some kind of diet. Psoriasis, for example, has been treated with doses of vitamin D, but it is a stubborn ailment and its cause is not yet known. Urticaria and various forms of eczema which are allergies to certain proteins are definitely related to diet.

Many different diets have been tried in treatment of blackheads, pimples, and acne—for instance, diets without meat, without sugar, or without fats. At present most skin specialists agree that a low-fat diet is beneficial, since in many cases of acne an overactivity of the oil glands of the skin is present. Many cases of acne, however, are unaffected by foods. Particular foods seem to aggravate some acne, most frequently chocolate, nuts, shellfish, peanuts, pork and pork products, milk and milk products and sharp cheese. The only conclusion that may be drawn is that acne cannot be controlled by diet alone, but that a well-balanced diet is certainly an important part of maintaining healthy attractive skin.

Certain illnesses induce various abnormalities of skin structure known as primary or secondary lesions. The primary lesions include papules, vesicles, pustules, bullae, and scales. The secondary lesions, which result from a primary condition, include atrophy, pigmentation, sclerosis or hardening, ulceration, crusts, and lichens.

Normal skin will thrive well with nothing more than a reasonable amount of cleanliness. The skin of a baby requires more care than that of an adult, since it is more easily irritated. Women, especially, are concerned with the appearance of their skin and are often susceptible to the advertising claims of various products for the skin. However, no substance applied to the skin can "feed it," and any benefit derived is only superficial and temporary. A substance powerful enough to actually alter the skin would be completely unsafe to use. *See also* ACNE; ACNE ROSACEA; COSMETICS; DERMATITIS; ECZEMA; NAILS; PIGMENTATION; PSORIASIS; RINGWORM; TATTOOING; and Chapter 20, "Diseases of the Skin."

SKULL, the entire bony framework of the head, consisting of the cranium and the face. The cranium is made up of the frontal bone, the front part of the cranium, the occipital which lies behind, and the sphenoid, temporal, and parietal bones at the side. The roof or vault is formed by the frontal and parietal bones, and the base of the skull by the occipital, temporal, sphenoid, and ethmoid bones.

The occipital bone has a large opening through which the brain is connected with the spinal cord; in addition, other openings provide for the passage of numerous nerves and blood vessels.

The bones of the face fit closely beneath the orbits of the eyes, around the nasal cavities and mouth, and in the cheek.

The skull of a baby is thin and soft. The bones that form the vault of the newborn baby's skull are separated and the membranous space between is called fontanelle. The movement of these bones affects the shape of the head, which may be temporarily altered by molding during birth.

Various diseases may provoke changes in the shape of the head, such as rickets, hydrocephalus, acromegaly, and osteitis deformans, and some birth injuries and congenital deformities also affect the shape.

The skull is subject to fractures of two types: the closed or simple fracture, and the open or compound fracture. Simple fractures vary from a small fracture line to extensive cracking of the bones throughout the skull. Simple fractures may be complicated if one of the pieces of bone presses on the brain. Other complications occur when the fracture crosses a major artery or vein or involves a cranial nerve. In most simple fractures, healing progresses without much treatment, but special surgery is usually imperative in cases of fracture across a major artery. Compound fractures of the skull are more serious and care must be taken to guard against meningitis. Sulfa drugs and antibiotics have been helpful in reducing the incidence of this infection in skull fractures. *See also* BRAIN; CONCUSSION; HEAD INJURIES.

SLEEP, the periodic state of rest during which there is a noticeable decrease of consciousness and activity. The average person requires sleep just as he does food, and the demand for sleep is as regular as that for food. During sleep, the body has an opportunity to repair itself, to get rid of wastes that have accumulated in the tissues during the day. The rate of metabolism during sleep is at its lowest point, being sufficient only to keep the vital parts of the body in operation. Blood pressure drops, the pulse rate slows down, breathing is irregular and slackened. The body is less sensitive to pain, light, and sound. Even the temperature is somewhat lower than during waking hours.

An infant sleeps almost all of the time, awakening usually only for feeding. A child of two or three years of age should sleep twelve or thirteen hours a day. Seven or eight hours of sleep is usually adequate for an adult. More hours of sleep are required in the early years of life, since the body tissues build reserves of energy during sleep necessary to meet the greater demands of the growing body. The aged person usually sleeps only about six hours at night; occasionally four hours' sleep seems to be adequate. The amount of sleep needed varies among people, but everyone should have enough to awaken rested and refreshed. *See also* NARCOLEPSY; SENILITY; SOMNAMBULISM.

SLEEPING SICKNESS. *See* ENCEPHALITIS.

SLEEPLESSNESS. *See* INSOMNIA.

SLIPPED DISC. The backbone as an integrated system is so designed and put together that it breaks only under the most extraordinary and violent shocks. It can support a weight far larger than that of the body of which it is a part, and can move this body in practically any direction. In addition, the backbone is capable of a range of movements extending from a stevedore's lift to an acrobat's contortions and a ballet dancer's delicacy and discipline.

The intervertebral disc, a little cushion of cartilage that lies between every second vertebra of the spinal column, makes all this possible. The center of each disc is composed of a special material called nucleus pulposus, which tends to move about slightly in correspondence to movements of the body. These discs cushion the body and especially the head against direct impact of the shock of walking which a solid bone would transmit. They also permit an ease and degree of rotation of the vertebrae which would otherwise be impossible.

The functions and changes in these discs have only recently been comprehended. The "jeep disease" of World War II, a severe and persistent back pain associated with constant riding in a jeep over rough roads, led to medical investigation which proved that the pain was caused by dislocation of one of the intervertebral discs which had been squeezed or bumped out of position by violent movement. Sometimes the nucleus pulposus ruptures, loses liquid, and contributes to the squeezing that displaces the disc.

Occasionally a disc is displaced during common experiences of everyday life. An automobile accident may throw a sudden and excessive shock on the spine and cause an injury at first not apparent. A bumpy airplane landing may have the same effect. Many forms of athletic exercise involve some risk of injuring a disc. Activities, such as football, baseball, and gymnastic work which subject the spine to frequent sharp heavy shocks while the back is in an unusual position tend to do this most frequently.

The detection of a dislocated disc is not a simple matter and may require prolonged study. The injury is not apparent through simple exploration with the fingers. X-ray and careful review of the symptoms will help the doctor make a diagnosis.

Rest, wearing braces, and surgery are all alternative remedies for the condition. The doctor's judgment alone can determine the best treatment.

SMALLPOX, or variola, a contagious infectious disease, often fatal, with fever followed by a papular eruption which produces pitted scars. The introduction of vaccination, developed by the English physician Edward Jenner in 1796, and the more recently improved techniques for quarantine and isolation have brought smallpox almost completely under control and it is now comparatively rare. It still occurs in the Far East and in some tropical countries. In 1947 an imported case in New York City spread to eleven people before it was controlled.

The virus of smallpox is present in the discharge from the nose and throat, in blisters on the skin, in the scabs that eventually fall off, and in the excretions from the body. The disease may spread from any of these sources, which accounts for the ease and rapidity with which the disease infects anyone who is not immune.

The incubation period is generally eight to twelve days. Smallpox begins with violent headache, chill, pain in the back and limbs and a high fever, and, in children, convulsions and vomiting. Within three or four days small reddened pimples appear over the face and wrists and spread rapidly to the arms and chest. These form blisters in a day or two and in about eight or nine days begin to dry, leaving a blackish crust.

The face swells and feels irritated and the rash, particularly on the face, can be agonizing. The eyelids may be swollen shut. After three or four weeks the crusts fall off and the characteristic pitting scars or pockmarks of smallpox remain.

Complications caused by bacterial infection result in bronchopneumonia, conjunctivitis, or more serious damage to the eyes or middle ear.

Since smallpox is one of the most contagious diseases known, isolation and strict quarantine are essential. It can spread not only during the course of the illness but also during the long convalescent period which follows. Clothing, bed linens, and any object which the patient has handled carry the infection. Any person who has been in contact with a smallpox patient should be vaccinated, unless he has had a vaccination during the previous five years. Vaccination may even protect the patient if it is done during the early incubation period, and may, if effective, result in milder symptoms. One attack of smallpox gives lifelong immunity.

The immunity gained by vaccination is temporary and vaccinations must therefore be repeated at five- to seven-year intervals. The first vaccination is generally given between the ages of three months and one year and is repeated between the ages of seven and eleven years, especially if an epidemic is present or if travel is planned to areas where the disease is more common than in the United States. *See also* IMMUNITY; IMMUNIZATION; INFECTION; INFECTIOUS DISEASES; VACCINATION; and Chapter 7, "The Process of Infectious

Diseases and Immunization of Children."

SMELL, the perception of odor. The degree of perceptiveness varies among persons, some having a highly developed sense of smell and others having very little. Sense of smell appears to be less significant to persons than, for example, sense of sight or hearing, and a total loss of the olfactory sense usually requires little adjustment.

To test olfactory sensitivity, well-defined odors are used. A person with a high sensitivity can detect camphor in a solution of 1:30,000,000 and vanilla in a solution of 1:10,000,000. Apparently the strongest odor is that of mercaptan, a derivative of alcohol in which oxygen is replaced by sulphur. It can be detected when 1/23,000,000th of a milligram is present in a quart of water.

Loss of the sense of smell is called anosmia. *See also* ANOSMIA; NOSE, DISEASES OF; OZENA.

SNEEZING, a natural reflex action involving a deep intake of breath followed by closure of the glottis; the mechanism is similar to that of a cough. A violent expiration effort ensues, the glottis opens, a blast of air is sent out through the nose, taking with it mucus and other material. Frequently the eyes water immediately following a sneeze.

Paroxysms of sneezing and watering eyes are characteristic of hay fever and other allergic conditions. A sneeze may occur without an irritant, such as when a person stares at a bright sky or stands barefoot on a cold floor. Sneezes can often be suppressed by placing a steady pressure between the nose and lip with one or two fingers.

Sneezing can be a symptom of a common cold or of some respiratory disease such as influenza. Since a sneeze disseminates virus or bacteria, it should always be covered with a handkerchief or tissue.

In cases of persistent sneezing the nose should be examined by a doctor, since a disordered septum or other source of irritation may exist which requires special attention. Treatment of sneezing always involves treating the underlying condition.

SNORING, the rough audible sound made by breathing through the nose in such a way as to cause a vibration of the soft palate. The noise made by snoring is due to the intermittent passage of air at places in the mouth where there may be partial obstruction. Adenoids sometimes cause snoring, especially in children.

Snoring can occur in several ways. During sleep a partial relaxation of the muscles holding the vocal cords may occur so that they fall closely together and interfere with the passage of air. Or, when a person is sleeping deeply or is unconscious, and lying on his back, the tongue may fall back and partially close the opening through which air passes. This is what causes the noisy breathing called stertor which occurs in concussions and apoplexy.

Sometimes, because of irritation or inflammation, mucus may collect in the nose or in the passages behind the nose, or the muscles associated with the nose and throat may be abnormally tense and interfere with passage of air. If the nose is blocked and the lips are held tightly together, a whistling sound occurs as the air passes out.

Snoring sounds seldom disturb the person snoring. Often he will stop snoring if, when he is lying on his back, he is turned to the side. Closing his mouth, or pushing the lower jaw forward and with it the base of the tongue, is sometimes effective.

SODIUM BICARBONATE, also known as baking soda, a white crystalline powder. Given as an antacid, it overcomes excess acidity of the juices of the stomach and excess acidity of the body generally. In cases of acidosis, which may be due to diabetes or another condition, large doses of baking soda may be taken orally. Because it can liquefy mucus, a sodium bicarbonate-water solution is sometimes used to cleanse the nose and other mucous surfaces. A lotion made of a teaspoon of baking powder to a pint of water helps to relieve itching, and a baking soda bath may be beneficial in helping similar conditions.

SOMNAMBULISM refers to a sleep or sleeplike state during which walking or other activities are performed. It is fairly common in children. In adults it is rarer and of more serious significance. Usually sleepwalking stems from some conflict in the mind which is unresolved and continues to stimulate the person even during the period of sleep. Usually when the person's doubt or fear is removed—which, in serious cases, may require psychiatric help—the sleepwalking ceases. A person awakened during sleepwalking is usually perplexed and distressed. He should not be criticized or scolded, but consoled and returned to bed.

SORE THROAT refers to inflammation of the pharynx, called pharyngitis, or of the tonsils, called tonsillitis. In a common cold, the soreness is usually in the back wall of the upper throat and affects the nasopharynx and the palate. *See also* COMMON COLD; HOARSENESS; LARYNGITIS; PHARYNX; QUINSY; SEPTIC SORE THROAT.

SPANISH FLY. *See* CANTHARIDES.

SPASM, an involuntary sudden contraction of a muscle. The usual cause is irritation of the nerve cells or nerves which supply the muscle. A sustained contraction is called tonic. If contraction and relaxation rapidly alternate, it is a clonic spasm. A general spasm over the body is a convulsion or fit. Massive spasms are characterized by sudden movements which involve most of the body musculature and last from a fraction of a second to several seconds. They may affect infants and young children. The commonest form of spasm is one in which the limbs and trunk are suddenly flexed, followed by relaxation. Similar attacks may occur in series.

Almost anyone can at some time have a muscle spasm. Sudden chilling of the body during swimming may cause a muscle spasm, or whenever the circulation of the blood in any part of the body is greatly diminished sudden involuntary contractions may occur. Disorders in the nervous system—for example, the death of a nerve cell in the interior portion of the spinal cord—may result in paralysis of the muscles with spasm of the opposing muscles.

Sometimes children develop habit spasms—not to be confused with chorea or St. Vitus' dance. The movements of habit spasm are quicker and always repeated in the same way, whereas the movements of chorea are irregular and variable. Spasms in children may sometimes occur as a result of distress, such as fear of punishment.

Whenever a spasm of the muscle occurs, examination by a doctor is necessary to determine the source. If it is a condition affecting the nerves, medical or surgical management may be required. In some instances, injection of one of various substances around the nerves of the area involved is the only treatment to stop a spasm. *See also* CHOREA; CONVULSION; HABIT SPASM; TIC DOULOUREUX.

SPEECH, the faculty of uttering articulate sounds to express thought. The centers of the brain involving the capacity for speech are in the cortex. An injury or disease that interferes with cells of the cortex or with fibers that link them, as in aphasia, hinders the thought processes of speech.

Sound is produced by vibrations of the vocal cords as air rushes through the larynx. In laryngitis, the vocal cords are affected and the voice becomes a whisper. Paralysis of the cords causes complete loss of voice, or aphonia. The voice may be suddenly lost in hysteria. Here the cords remain normal and the cause is emotional.

Sound produced by the larynx is modified by articulation, which involves alterations in the shape of the mouth and pharynx and movements of the teeth, tongue, and palate. The nerve centers which control articulation are in the medulla and are connected with the speech centers in the cortex. Articulation may be affected wholly or partially by damage in these areas.

Lisping, stammering, and stuttering are speech defects which can be corrected by training and various exercises. Speech defects caused by harelip or cleft palate may be corrected by surgical treatment, or prosthesis. Surgeons, psychologists, otolaryngologists, speech therapists—all can help in the correction of faulty speech.

Learning to talk is a sign of a child's mental development, but delayed speech should be no cause for alarm unless it is due to mental defect or deafness. If a child still does not speak by the age of one year, he should be taken to a doctor so that his hearing and general intelligence may be tested. Children learn to speak by imitation and will adopt the accents, inflections, and mannerisms of those around them. The best way to encourage correct speech in a child is to listen with interest to what he has to say, making as few corrections in his speech as possible, and speak to him in a modulated, articulate, and correct way.

Here are seven rules which parents should follow in developing habits of good speech in their children:

1. Do not correct the child's pronunciation or enunciation. Praise

that which is correct, but do not stress that which is wrong.

2. Do not imitate the child's baby talk. By doing this, you simply confirm him in his error. If you speak good English, he will imitate it as soon as he can.

3. Never "talk down" to babies and little children.

4. Do not nag, coax, or raise your voice in an effort to get the baby to talk. Speech will come naturally.

5. If any of the baby's relatives or playmates or you stammer, give the baby an opportunity to learn to talk from someone else. Children imitate what they hear.

6. Give the child a chance to learn to talk and listen to him when he talks. This will encourage him.

7. Tell the child to listen. However, do not ignore him but include him whenever possible in the conversation.

See also APHASIA; STUTTERING AND STAMMERING.

SPINA BIFIDA. An essential step in the development of the human embryo before birth is the growing together of two sides of the original channel in the back, thus forming the space where the spinal cord will lie. Failure of these to grow together results in a structural condition known as spina bifida, meaning literally a split spine.

This condition occurs in approximately one in every 1,000 births, but the specific form of the defect always varies. Ordinarily spina bifida will be only a gap in the coverings which should enclose the spinal cord. In other instances, however, one or more vertebrae may be absent. This deformity may be accompanied by a bulge in the sheathing of the spinal cord projecting to the exterior, as in a hernia. This creates in the back a bulbous body filled with liquid.

Some cases of spina bifida are accompanied by what is called hydrocephaly, derived from words meaning water and head. In this condition the fluid which is normally required within the membrane containing the brain increases inordinately in quantity and the skull bones expand to compensate. The size of the head becomes grossly disproportionate to that of the body.

Immediate medical attention should be given to every such case. Exposure of any part of the nervous system, as occurs in spina bifida, is extremely serious. Surgical repair will benefit at least half the children affected by the condition but must be undertaken as early as possible to obtain the greatest benefit. The elimination of the bulge in the back often will accomplish much for the patient.

If the condition is left unattended, the distortion of the spinal nerves and the strain to which they are subjected will disturb their function. When the abnormality occurs in the lower spine, the defect may cause paralysis of the legs and loss of normal control over bladder and bowel action. If the nerve supply of the skin is inadequate, ulcers may develop.

SPINAL CORD, the relatively large branch of nervous tissue that extends from the brain down through the vertebrae. The brain and the spinal cord together constitute the central nervous system.

The spinal cord is the medium for communication between the brain and many other parts of the body, and also effects numerous reflex actions. Some of these are: reflexes controlling many essential muscular movements, such as those jerking the body away from sources of pain; reflexes partly controlling the bowel and urinary bladder, and movements in the digestive and circulatory systems and other organs. The spinal cord transmits sensations of touch to the brain.

The cord is about eighteen inches long and approximately the thickness of the little finger. Branching from it to the left and right, into the body itself, are thirty-one pairs of nerves. The vertebral column, or backbone, is much longer than the eighteen inches of the spinal cord. Consequently many of the projecting branches which serve lower parts of the body, and so leave the vertebral column lower, must extend through the rest of the column down to the point where they branch out of it.

The spinal cord may be disordered in a number of ways. In myelitis, such as poliomyelitis, it is inflamed. Sclerosis, in which tissue associated with nerves hardens and damages them, may affect the spinal cord. Meningitis is inflammation of the membranes which encase both the brain and the spinal cord. The cord may be affected by concussion, inducing temporary paralysis, or it may be directly injured, as when the vertebral column itself breaks.

SPINAL CURVATURE. The spine is one of the most fundamental structural elements of the body and forms a basis around which other essential parts are arranged. Seen from the side, the spine has a modified S shape, giving it a springiness and elasticity that protect the delicate organs in the head and elsewhere from constant bumps and shocks. Seen from the front, it is a straight line. When this line loses its straightness and becomes a looplike curve, either to the right or to the left, the resulting condition is scoliosis, or curvature of the spine.

This curvature frequently is a symptom or a sequel of another disorder rather than a disorder itself. Usually the backbone is extraordinarily protected by the system of muscles and ligaments that combine with the spine to give the body its normal erectness. However, an inadequacy may occur in these muscles which permits the spine to curve toward either side. One or more bones, rather than the muscles, may suffer breakdown, and thus throw other bones and tissues out of place.

Scoliosis may occur from habitual bad posture. At first, only the positions of the parts are abnormal and the tissues remain unaffected. Later, however, if the fault is not corrected, tissue changes do occur and the curvature will become more or less permanent.

Correct posture is especially essential for children, and parents should keep careful watch to insure the child's correct posture and eliminate any postural defects promptly to avoid any permanent deformity. Often special exercises aid in developing muscular strength, which may be lacking, to hold the spine in its natural erect position.

The structural significance of the spine makes almost inevitable the displacement of other parts of the body when spinal deformity occurs. The lung of the side opposite the curvature may become overcompressed; one or more nerves may suffer undue pressure. Frequently the lower rib or ribs will be thrown down against the thigh with no apparent spinal displacement.

Such disorders should be examined by the doctor to determine whether or not the displacement observed is originating with a curvature in the spine which has hitherto escaped notice and diagnosis. The patient is observed standing in his habitual relaxed position and then attempting to straighten his back as fully as possible. The doctor may check the form of the spine against a straight vertical standard such as a plumb line.

Orthopedists, who specialize in correcting deformities, can correct bad posture and support weak bodily structures with external mechanical means such as braces and casts. Ordinarily, however, this is a last resort and emphasis is first placed on training by exercises.

SPINAL FRACTURE, any break of the bones of the spine. It is a serious injury since the spine is the structural foundation for most of the body and is the intermediary for communication between the brain and the body. Before the advent of x-ray, the only positive sign that a back was broken was usually paralysis in one or more parts of the body. X-ray enables a much more thorough and certain diagnosis. Treatment of such fractures has also improved.

Serious injury to the spine results from a violent shock or blow. Since the spine is well protected by its structure and surrounding tissues, it must be struck or strained with unusual force to break. Spinal injury can occur in automobile accidents, falls, in excessive efforts to move or lift a heavy load, or from a sudden violent jerk. The most severe breaks in the back occur in the region of the neck, where there are a greater number of nerves affecting other parts of the body than at a lower point of the back. The most serious consequences come from a fracture which invades or tears the spinal cord or causes a hemorrhage into it. Occasionally the cord may be injured as seriously as from a break when two or more vertebrae, the bones which make up the spine, are forced apart without actual fracture to the bones themselves.

Spinal fracture, or any injury to the spinal cord or back or spine that seems to involve the nervous system, requires the immediate attention of a neurologist. X-ray study of all bones involved is essential.

Restoring the bones affected to their normal position is a primary expedient, usually done by a surgeon or orthopedist, a specialist in correction of deformities of the back and limbs. Supports to hold the bones in place while they are healing will then be applied. In some instances when nerves associated with the excretory functions have been damaged, the patient will need assistance with bladder and bowel action.

When there is any possibility that a person has a broken back, the person should be moved as little as possible and a doctor called immediately. Under the supervision of the doctor, the injured person will be placed, with a minimum of movement, onto a board for transport to the hospital. If the neck is broken, it is essential that the head be kept motionless. Deadening of sensation in parts of the body below the point of injury and loss of bowel and bladder control are signs of serious damage. Serious spinal injury will probably produce shock and the victim must be kept warm and, if it can be done without moving him, the head placed lower than the rest of the body.

SPINE, the column of small bones, called vertebrae, and associated tissues which maintains the body in its erect posture. The spine or backbone is a kind of natural spring, elastic in character and shaped like an S, which prevents the body from suffering the incessant shocks it would get if the spine were a single solid bone. Between the vertebrae are cartilaginous discs, which have further shock-absorbing action and which permit turning and twisting motion without friction among the vertebrae.

The spine also carries the spinal cord and its extensions, which provide not only intercommunication between the brain and much of the body but regulate many reflex functions.

The spine, made up of such heavy bones and so well protected by associated muscles, is one of the most secure parts of the body. *See also* BACKACHE; CHIROPRACTIC; SLIPPED DISC; SPINAL CORD.

SPLEEN, a large, ductless, gland-like organ which lies in the upper left part of the abdomen, just below the diaphragm and toward the rear of the body.

Although the functions of the spleen are known to have significant relationships to the character and circulation of the blood, they are not fully understood. One unanswered problem concerns the dissolution and disposal of red cells of the blood which have exhausted their usefulness, and another surrounds the production of new blood cells. Since such cells are intimately concerned in combatting infection, the spleen is further implicated in the control of disease.

At times the spleen contracts, discharging a quantity of blood into the general circulation. Therefore, when an animal or human being exercises intensively, the spleen is believed to maintain the proper volume of blood circulating in the blood vessels.

Animal experiments have provided some interesting information regarding the spleen. The organ itself evidently does not experience pain. Thus, by operation, a celluloid window can be inserted in an animal's abdominal wall and the behavior of the spleen can be watched directly. The spleen can also be transplanted to a location outside the abdomen. When this is done, skin rapidly grows over the spleen, and its expansion and contraction can be observed directly. Dr. Joseph Barcroft, well-known physiologist and investigator, has done valuable work in this field.

An ancient idea, that the spleen

is related to emotions, is expressed in the phrase, "venting your spleen." Barcroft's experiments on a dog tend to justify this. A dog which was a confirmed cat chaser was trained to lie motionless on a table. Then the doctor would put before the dog's nose, alternately, first a duster which had not touched a cat, then a duster which had been in a basket with a cat. Although the dog continued to lie motionless when it smelled the second duster, its spleen could be observed to contract. Smelling the other duster left the dog's spleen unaffected.

Other animal experiments have revealed the contraction and discharge of blood under the influence of exercise. When the exertion is intensive enough, the kidney may become so depleted of blood that it suffers actual damage. Evidently, then, the activity of the spleen in maintaining evenness of blood circulation helps to protect other organs which might be adversely affected without this supplement.

Enlargement of the spleen is a disorder of variable sources. Sometimes enlargement is due to splenic destructive activity against worn-out blood cells and disease-creating organisms which are retained within the spleen. Sometimes a fatty material enlarges the spleen. Enlargement of the spleen appears in several major infectious diseases, among them malaria. Among primitive people of tropical areas, where malaria and consequently enlarged spleen are practically universal, a favorite stratagem of hand-to-hand combat is to club the opponent about the spleen in an effort to rupture it, which can be fatal.

Other conditions which tend to chronic splenic enlargement are Hodgkin's disease, splenic anemia, pernicious anemia, leukemia, and hydatid and amyloid diseases. Furthermore, acute enlargement may accompany enteric fever, anthrax, pyemia, septicemia, and other infections.

Rupture may occur either because of external injury, as in an automobile accident, or spontaneously in connection with a massive enlargement. Hemorrhage is then intense, because the extensive blood supply which normally passes through or is bound in the spleen pours into the abdomen. If delay is not protracted, the condition can be treated surgically.

Splenic enlargement may accompany leukemia or a condition known as Banti's disease, in which severe anemia occurs.

An enlarged spleen is not always explicable, and if an adequate cause is not ascertained the organ must be removed. In such cases a lymphoma or tumor of lymphoid tissue may be responsible. In certain specific diseases, such as purpura hemorrhagica or thrombocytopenia, a clotting disorder of the blood, removal of the spleen is considered beneficial. In the case of Banti's disease, splenectomy is not generally recommended. The spleen is not essential to life—as is, for example, the liver —and its removal rarely produces adverse effects.

SPLENIC DISEASE. Primary disorders of the spleen are so rare that the spleen has been considered an anticancerous organ, although secondary cancer of the spleen does occur. However, like other tissues of the body the spleen is liable to injuries from falls, wounds, and accidents. In some disorders the spleen fills the entire left side of the abdomen and weighs many pounds. Disturbance of circulation of the blood in the spleen is characterized by acute abdominal pain and a sudden increase in the size of the organ.

Among unusual conditions affecting the spleen are the appearance of accessory spleens scattered through the abdomen; and floating or wandering spleen, in which the tissues which hold it in place become relaxed and the organ moves from position, a condition far more frequent in women than men.

Often the spleen is enlarged in malaria, leukemia and other blood disease, and can be a symptom of many generalized diseases. In Banti's syndrome, extreme enlargement of the spleen is associated with severe anemia.

Sometimes surgical removal of the spleen is considered helpful—for instance, in severe cases of purpura hemorrhagica or thrombocytopenia, a condition in which the blood does not clot easily. The spleen may also be removed when tumors are present.

Steroid hormones, ACTH, and cortisone are valuable in splenic disease to lessen the destruction of red blood cells. ACTH and cortisone may be employed before an operation for removal of the spleen, often in connection with transfusions of whole fresh blood. *See also* SPLEEN.

SPONDYLOLISTHESIS, or slipped vertebra, a condition in which an exaggerated lumbar curve is formed when the fifth vertebra is so affected as to slip forward toward the front of the body. This abnormality is caused by defective growth of bone in the neural arch. Because support is lacking, the condition causes backache, which disappears when the person rests. The pain reappears on exertion and is felt down the thigh and leg.

SPOROTRICHOSIS, an infection of the skin and mucous membranes, caused by a fungus, the Sporotrichum schenckii, which grows on plants and brush. Persons exposed to vegetation, such as gardeners or farmers, are most apt to become infected, usually by acquiring the fungus on the skin or a break in the skin. Sporotrichosis has also been found in horses, dogs, and cats.

About twenty days to three months after contact with the fungus, a hard rubbery growth appears at the site of injury. The growth hardens, becomes inflamed, and gradually breaks through the skin, discharging a small amount of thin pus. The surrounding skin becomes discolored and finally turns black. The infection may spread to other skin areas, but rarely affects any internal organs.

Potassium iodide has been used successfully to treat sporotrichosis and is often continued for at least a month after apparent recovery as a safety measure. Abscesses which are slow in healing may be drained to hasten recovery and then treated with the iodide.

SPRAINS, injuries in the area of a joint, in which a sudden movement or a fall will stretch or overstrain connective tissue fibers belonging to the ligaments, muscles, or tendons so that they are torn or ruptured. Fluid or blood then gets into the joint. Sometimes a sprain is so severe that a bone is broken. For this reason every severe sprain should be x-rayed. The opening of the football season and the onset of winter produce a sudden increase in the number of sprains, particularly of the ankle.

It is advisable to treat the injury as soon as possible. A firm bandage should be applied evenly and smoothly over the joint in order to limit internal bleeding. If materials are available, the sprain may be treated by putting a layer of cotton wool about an inch thick over the joint, and for an inch or two beyond it on either side, and bandaging as firmly as possible without causing discomfort.

First-aid measures are helpful, but most sprains require medical attention. Ordinarily a simple sprain is treated by rest, elevation of the leg and ankle, and the application of an ice bag. The doctor will immobilize the joint by strapping or he may use adhesive materials or even apply a plaster cast. Current treatment, however, recommends movement of the joint as soon as possible. In order to control accompanying pain, the physician may inject an anesthetic substance into the injured area, thus permitting the patient to use the foot or hand.

Movement is difficult in a joint which has been fixed in one position for a long time, particularly if inflammation and swelling are pronounced. In such cases movement is not attempted immediately, but gradually. The bandage may be removed for a short time, and the joint gently massaged to aid softening of the tissues and relaxation of the stiffness. Heat should not be applied to a sprained ankle until the danger of congestion and hemorrhage has been controlled. The value of heat is greatest in the final stages, when repair has begun, in order to encourage circulation and absorption of excess fluid. *See also* JOINTS AND JOINT DISORDERS.

SPRUE, a feverless chronic disease. Sprue comes from the Dutch word that describes an inflammation of the mouth. The disease, known for more than two thousand years, is generally considered to be a tropical ailment, although it will occur in persons who do not live in the tropics. Both tropical and nontropical sprue are probably nutritional deficiency disorders of the small intestine, marked by impaired absorption of food elements, particularly fats. However, the exact cause is unknown.

Symptoms of sprue are diarrhea, cramps, and distended stomach due to gas. The material from the bowels is pale, greasy, unformed and foul, and occasionally watery. The person with sprue becomes emaciated, muscles and fat waste away, and, in advanced cases, recovery is difficult. Clubbed fingers and spotted skin may develop. When the person also suffers from a vitamin B complex deficiency, fissures develop at the corners of the mouth and the tongue is smooth and fiery red.

In the past, many different kinds of diets were tried in treating sprue. Currently liver preparations and folic acid have produced favorable results. In sprue, treatment also involves a careful control of the diet, which should be moderately bland, low in fat, and high in proteins. Calcium intake can be increased with skim milk and calcium lactate tablets, and ripe bananas, vitamin B_{12}, and iron supplements have been found beneficial. Occasionally antibiotics and cortisone have been temporarily successful, but their prolonged use presents certain problems. Sometimes small and repeated blood transfusions have been helpful, even life-saving, in critical cases of sprue.

SQUINT, or strabismus, failure to focus both eyes on the same point. In the most common form, one eye looks toward the object while the other is turned from it.

There are many kinds of squints, caused by a large number of disorders and diseases in the eye, the muscles that move it, the nerves supplying them, and the brain which controls and coordinates the nerve impulses.

An eye specialist or ophthalmologist can determine the exact type of squint a person has and then prescribe treatment. Frequently a squint may be cured by wearing special glasses. Sometimes the squinting eye must be trained and special exercises with certain instruments are prescribed. In some cases surgery on the muscles of the eyeball may be advisable.

Treatment is generally effective, but requires the cooperation of the patient. When a child has a squint, sympathetic attitudes on the part of his family and persons around him can be of great help.

STAMMERING. *See* STUTTERING AND STAMMERING.

STANFORD-BINET TEST. The Stanford-Binet "I.Q." or Intelligence Quotient test is a revision of the Binet-Simon tests which were originally conducted in France by two French psychologists, Binet and Simon, who had been commissioned by the French government to study the conditions of mentally defective persons. They did extensive research to determine what the normal child should be expected to do at any particular age.

No test has yet been developed which can conclusively measure someone's intelligence, but many different methods have been tried, with varying degrees of success. The Stanford revision of the Binet-Simon test is one of the most widely used at present. The "I.Q.", a numerical rating, is determined by dividing the chronological age of the child tested into the age level the child achieves on the test and multiplying the result by 100. For example, a ten-year-old child who has the capacity of a twelve-year-old child, according to the standard of achievement for each age group, has an I.Q. rating of 120. The average child is therefore rated at 100. Only one quality is tested, the reasoning intelligence. According to this scale, a person scoring below 70 is a moron; below 50, an imbecile; and below 20, an idiot. Out of a total of 500,000 mentally deficient persons in the United States, 30,000 are classified as idiots, 100,000 as imbeciles, and the rest as morons.

STERILITY, the incapacity to produce children, is a complex phenomenon involving a variety of factors. Chief responsibility may be borne by the woman, the man, or both. Even when one or the other is specifically accountable, sterility may apply only to a given set of circumstances; in another situation the same person might not be sterile. Because of its variability, sterility may properly be regarded as characteristic of a particular union of two persons, rather than of either the man or the woman separately. Scientists have determined that circumstances pertaining to the marriage relationship may cause sterility.

Some marriages are deliberately childless, the husband and wife having decided to take measures to assure this. Other marriages, childless for other reasons, constitute 10 per cent of all marriages in the United States and Great Britain, according to investigators.

In the past, a childless marriage was often assumed to be solely the responsibility of the wife. However, medical statistics indicate that men are responsible for 30 to 40 per cent of all instances of childlessness. Diagnosis of the condition and endeavors to correct it demand first an examination of the husband. If the results indicate that he is responsible, the general physical condition of the wife is determined. A frequent cause of sterility in men is some disorder associated with the male germ cell,

the sperm, one of which must fertilize an ovum, or female egg cell, before conception occurs. These male cells are produced in the testes, the two male sex glands, and stored in the seminal vesicles, higher in the body.

Such disorders may involve various organs or tissues. The glands may not produce sperm cells even though otherwise the man appears to be sexually normal. The sperm cells produced may be weak or malformed, so that they cannot function properly and carry the fertilization process to the final stage. Furthermore, there may be insufficient numbers of them; although only one sperm can fertilize a given egg cell, a normal male provides three to four million of them on each ejaculation. Any of these conditions may be responsible for the woman's failure to conceive, and the doctor has means for testing to find out whether or not such a condition is present.

Conditions in the woman which prevent conception are even more varied than in the man. Among the simplest are infection, inflammation, or injury of the parts of the body involved. Sometimes the cause is blockage of a passage through which the sperm cells should travel. Occasionally congenital deformities of the sexual organs may cause such occlusion or otherwise render conception impossible. In a few instances the uterus may be undeveloped or missing entirely.

A frequent cause of sterility in women is some irregularity in the system of glands of internal secretion, the endocrine glands, or of their products, the hormones. The sex glands are a significant part of the whole glandular network, and a mishap in the latter can affect the female sexual cycle at one of several points, making conception difficult or impossible.

Other conditions which can induce sterility include faulty diet, a subject not yet thoroughly understood, and emotional or mental disturbances which can react upon physical factors.

That a woman has not attempted to prevent conception and still has not conceived does not necessarily mean that pregnancy is impossible for her. The condition may continue for years and then terminate in a normal pregnancy and delivery.

Complete physical examination of both husband and wife by a doctor is essential for the couple who seem sterile and wish to correct it. Such an examination will include studies of sperm cells of the husband and examination of the wife's sexual organs to determine their condition and whether or not the necessary tubes are open and functioning properly. A complete record of the sex experiences of both husband and wife is also imperative. The cause or causes that the physician finds operative will determine the recommendations. Often a previously sterile couple can achieve conception by careful use of knowledge of the alternating periods of fertility and infertility in the female, regulated by the menstrual cycle. When a disease has closed one or both of the Fallopian tubes within the woman, attempts to free them by surgery or forcing a passage of air through them are only rarely successful.

STOMACH, the portion of the alimentary tract, the digestive tube, which extends from the lower end of the esophagus or gullet, the canal extending from the pharynx to the stomach, to the beginning of the duodenum or first part of the small intestine. The normal stomach is J-shaped with a bulge above and to the left of the junction with the esophagus. The shape varies according to its fullness or emptiness and the position of the person.

The stomach narrows to join the small intestine, forming the pyloric canal which has a thick muscular valve called the pyloric sphincter. Three muscular coats in the wall of the stomach are covered inside by a layer of mucus and a submucous lining containing blood vessels, lymphatics, and nerves. The internal surface of the stomach contains the minute gastric glands which manufacture hydrochloric acid and certain ferments which digest food into simpler substances. The muscular walls grind and mix the food with the gastric juices. About every twenty seconds, a wave of contraction passes along the stomach from the upper part to the pylorus. During digestion, the contractions also cause partially digested food to pass into the duodenum in the form of chyme, a thick fluid.

Various congenital deformities may affect the stomach, such as enlargement of the muscle of the pyloric valve. Gastroptosis or dropped stomach may occur later in life. Surgery is generally successful in correcting congenital abnormalities when they are known.

Inflammation of the lining of the

stomach is a common disorder, occurring in various forms and at any time throughout life. Peptic ulcers are another common stomach disorder, resulting from action of the gastric juices on the stomach wall. An increase in the amount or concentration of gastric juice causes acidity.

Cancer of the stomach is responsible for a great number of deaths each year in the United States. It usually occurs in late middle age and more often in men than women, men past forty-five being the most frequent victims. Cancer of the stomach is of several types, including ulcerating cancer, tumor growing in the stomach cavity, and a diffuse thickening of the stomach wall. Loss of weight, appetite, and general normal health are symptoms of stomach cancer, but unfortunately the cancer is often too far advanced before it is detected to be effectively treated and may have spread to regional lymph nodes and other organs. Because of the danger of stomach cancer, any form of stomach "upset" after middle age should receive immediate medical attention. If the cancer is discovered soon enough, an operation to remove the cancer with a portion or even all of the stomach can be successful in curing the condition, and so it is imperative that it be diagnosed at the earliest possible time. Cancer of the stomach is too often a hopelessly fatal disease because of a late diagnosis. *See also* DIGESTION; FISTULA; FOOD POISONING; GASTRITIS; INDIGESTION; PEPTIC ULCER; and Chapter 18, "Disorders of the Digestive System and Diet in Digestive Disorders."

STOMACH ACHE. *See* ABDOMINAL PAIN.

STOMACH ULCER. *See* PEPTIC ULCER.

STREPTOCOCCUS, a genus of bacteria which grows in chains, resembling tiny strings of beads when viewed under the microscope. Streptococcus germs are present in infections such as erysipelas, scarlet fever, subacute bacterial endocarditis, puerperal fever, subacute sore throat, streptococcus throat, and certain forms of enteritis and rheumatic fever.

STREPTOMYCIN, an antibiotic drug obtained from the moldlike microscopic plant, Streptomyces griseus. It is similar to penicillin in its antibacterial action and method of manufacture, and has been found particularly effective against many disease-producing germs that penicillin also attacks. In addition it is a powerful agent against some diseases that are not affected by penicillin, such as tularemia, a severe infectious disease acquired in handling infected rabbits.

Streptomycin is also effective in treating certain types of blood and urinary infections which are not helped by other drugs. Reports indicate that it may cure tuberculous meningitis, and it has been successfully used in diseases produced by the common colon bacillus. Pneumonia, streptococcus infections, staphylococcal pneumonia, and staphylococcal meningitis are among the many diseases in which streptomycin has been effectively used.

Streptomycin is taken orally or injected directly into the blood stream, as the condition dictates. In cases of meningitis, it is injected into the spinal fluid. *See also* ANTIBIOTICS.

STROKE, a sudden and severe seizure or fit of disease. The term is generally used for apoplexy, and in connection with sunstroke and heatstroke. *See also* APOPLEXY; HEAT SICKNESS; and Chapter 12, "Diseases of the Heart."

STUTTERING AND STAMMERING, may be described as spasmodic speech defects, resulting in a sudden check in the flow of words, or a rapid repetition of a consonant or consonants with which the person has difficulty. Usually the difficulty is with the sounds *p, b, m,* and *w,* which are sounds made by the lips. The stutterer or stammerer does not, however, always have difficulty with the same sounds. His emotional state at the time of speaking may be a factor in how he speaks.

Stuttering or stammering are almost never due to any organic weakness, either in the organs used in speaking or in the nerves and nerve centers which control them. Physical factors may, however, sometimes aggravate it. The doctor will first make sure that inflammation of adenoids, abnormal length of uvula, abnormal size of the tongue, and improper development of the mouth are not involved.

Often children who stutter develop behavior changes; a fear of appearing ridiculous produces a subsequent lack of confidence. Persons naturally left-handed but trained to use their right hand stammer more frequently than others, and males more often than females. Anyone acutely embarrassed or terrified is likely to stammer, until his emotion is under control. Stammering is usually an expression of self-consciousness, shyness, or fear. In an eager youngster, however, it may be nothing more than failure to keep up with his rapid flow of thought; words and thoughts are conceived faster than they can be expressed. Stammerers almost always can sing and talk to themselves quite fluently.

Because stuttering and stammering are primarily conditions which have emotional causes, treatment is directed toward the person's mental conflicts. When the conflict is resolved, the person will probably regain self-confidence and the speech defect disappears. The person with a speech defect may benefit from special speech correction classes. A class is often preferable to personal instruction since the person will be encouraged by the progress of others and the realization that he is not alone in his problem. His family and friends must be patient, tolerant, and confident; anger and impatience will only aggravate the situation.

STY. *See* EYE.

SUFFOCATION. *See* ASPHYXIA.

SULFONAMIDE DRUGS, or "sulfa" drugs, are derived from or are compounds of sulfonamide, and their introduction into medicine marked a turning point in the treatment of disease. Among the sulfonamide drugs are sulfadiazine, sulfapyridine, Gantrisin, Kynex, and others. These drugs act effectively on diseases caused by staphylococcus, meningococcus, streptococcus, and organisms of the dysentery group.

Before sulfa drugs, treatment of such diseases as lobar pneumonia and spinal meningitis depended on serums, which were only moderately successful. Management of infections of the middle ear was so ineffective that loss of hearing and mastoiditis often followed. Treatment of gonorrhea depended on repeated and frequently unsuccessful urethral injections. The use of sulfa drugs virtually revolutionized treatment of these and other conditions.

The sulfonamides differ in degree of activity, rate of absorption or metabolic and toxic effects, and should only be taken under the supervision and recommendation of a doctor. In some persons they cause undesirable side effects, such as rash, fever, and a lowering of the number of white cells in the blood. While these complications are infrequent, care must still be exercised in use of the drugs.

Penicillin and other antibiotics have superseded sulfa drugs in many cases, or the sulfa drugs are used in combination with antibiotics as antiinfective systemic drugs to combat bacterial infection.

SUNBURN, known medically as erythema solare, discoloration or inflammation of the skin, developing from overexposure to the sun. It may be as simple as a slight reddening of the skin or severe enough to cause blistering, fever, and nausea. Practically everyone has suffered at least a slight sunburn with red, dry, hot skin. Ointments, lotions, or creams help to relieve the discomfort, which results from exposure of the nerve endings.

More severe sunburns, involving blisters, dizziness, headache, fever, vomiting, and other symptoms of constitutional disturbance due to the secondary toxic effects of the burn, should be treated as if the burn had resulted from other causes, such as fire or hot water. A burn from the sun is a burn fully as much as any other, and the victim should consult a physician.

Danger from sunlight is chiefly due to the effects of ultraviolet rays, the short heat rays. More ultraviolet light penetrates near the water than inland, and a cool day with brilliant sunshine is more scorching than a hot but hazy day. The burning effect of bright sunlight reflected from snow is well known.

The skin of an infant is much more delicate than that of adults and will burn and become inflamed more promptly. Special care should therefore be taken to avoid overexposure of an infant to the sun. Blonde or red-haired persons with fair skin are particularly susceptible to burning, but everyone should acquire resistance to sunburn by gradual exposure, beginning with perhaps only five or ten minutes in the direct sun.

SUNSTROKE. *See* HEAT SICKNESS.

SUPPURATION refers to the formation of pus.

SWEAT. SEE PERSPIRATION.

SWIMMING POOLS. The chief disorders transmitted through swimming pools are inflammation of the eye, boils, ear infections, chronic inflammation of the nose and sinuses, sore throat, various skin infections, particularly ringworm and athlete's foot, and infections of the bowels, and dysentery. As a precaution, most public swimming pools require that all persons take a shower and walk through a footbath before entering the pool. No one with any ailment or infection should ever swim in a pool with other persons.

To keep the water in the pool clean and safe, chemicals are usually added. Ultraviolet rays are sometimes used for this purpose. Filter systems help remove sediment and infectious materials and pools are usually drained regularly.

Private pools should maintain the same strict sanitary conditions that most public pools do. Usually filters, chemicals, and purifiers are sold along with the pool, and in some places a special service will regularly clean and purify the pool.

SYMPATHETIC NERVOUS SYSTEM, or autonomic nervous system, supplies and exerts a regulatory activity to most of the involuntary organs of the body—glands, heart, blood vessels, for example—and involuntary muscles in the internal organs.

The system consists of a network of nerves and a series of nerve cell collections called ganglia. Some ganglia are connected to the spinal cord by fibers. Meshworks of fibers are sent out by the vertebral ganglia to the organs located in the abdomen and pelvis. Ganglia also arise within the brain and supply the tear and salivary glands and the pupils of the eye, and are connected with nerves that affect the ears.

Impulses through sympathetic nerve fibers cause dilation of the pupil, sweating, quickening and augmentation of the heartbeat, stoppage of the flow of gastric juice, contraction of arteries, and many other body actions. All these functions are automatic or involuntary.

In contrast, the action of the parasympathetic nervous system, that division between the cranium and the sacrum, is somewhat antagonistic to the sympathetic action. Thus, it slows the heart and stimulates the flow of gastric juices.

The blood supply to any part of the body can be increased by interruption of the sympathetic nerves that pass to that part. In hypertension, sympathectomy—cutting off the sympathetic nerves by surgery—is sometimes employed to increase the flow of blood into the abdominal area and lower limbs and thus decrease the blood pressure. Currently drugs are preferred to surgery to block the sympathetic nerves. Interruption or treatment of the sympathetic nervous system has occasionally been used in heart conditions such as angina pectoris, in cases of severe pain involving the urinary tract, to control serious disorders of the sweat glands, and to aid movement of the bowels.

The sympathetic nervous system is responsible for the physical sensations that accompany emotion. For example, suppressed resentment may cause overactivity of the muscles and glands of the stomach, and actual pain can result. In some psychotic or neurotic conditions, the system is involved and changes can occur in affected organs.

SYNDROME, a set of specific symptoms which occur regularly in the same combination and constitute a specific disease. Dozens of disorders are known as syndromes, a large number of them bearing the name of the first doctor to note the syndrome, connect it with the underlying disease condition, and call attention to it. Well-known syndromes are Cushing's syndrome, indicating tumor in certain parts of the brain; Korsakoff's syndrome or psychosis, associated with chronic alcoholism; and Addisonian syndrome, a condition caused by insufficiency of the adrenal glands.

SYNOVITIS, inflammation of the synovial membranes, those membranes which line the joints. The chief manifestation is an outpouring of fluid into the joint cavity. It may occur as a reaction to injury or as a result of infection somewhere else in the body.

"Water on the knee" is a typical instance of synovitis. A combination of rest and gentle pressure from bandaging will help to induce absorption of the fluid. *See also* JOINTS AND JOINT DISORDERS.

SYPHILIS, a contagious venereal disease which can infect any of the body tissues. It is characterized by a variety of lesions, of which the chancre (primary lesion), the mucous patch, and the gumma are the most distinctive. It is caused by a spirochete, Treponema pallidum.

The origin of syphilis is not known, but it has been claimed that Columbus's crew first introduced it into Europe after their return from the New World. A few of the crew members were with Charles VIII of France when he invaded Italy in 1495, and a terrible epidemic of syphilis broke out there, rapidly spreading over all of Europe. Today syphilis is world-wide and still one of the major scourges of mankind. Figures released by the Venereal Disease Program of the U. S. Public Health Service in 1957 reveal that of 266,000 persons examined and found to have syphilis, 55 per cent were teen-aged and young adults.

The vast majority of adult cases of syphilis are acquired through sexual contact. Treatment usually seems to render the infected person incapable of transmitting the disease, but there is some evidence that persons presumably cured can still infect others.

A few hours after exposure, the syphilis spirochete penetrates the skin or mucous membrane and enters the blood stream and tissues. The "hard chancre," the primary stage of the disease, does not appear until ten to ninety days later, three weeks being the average time. Usually the chancre is found on the genitals or in the mouth, but it may appear elsewhere and occasionally not at all. The fluid from the chancre is highly infectious.

Even without treatment, chancres generally disappear in ten to forty days, and the secondary stage, small raised red areas on the skin or small mucous patches in the mouth or on the reproductive organs, begins two to six months later. Generally lymph nodes throughout the body become enlarged. These lesions of secondary syphilis heal by themselves in three to twelve weeks, but may recur later.

The third stage of syphilis develops almost immediately after the secondary symptoms have disappeared, or, in some cases, may be delayed for years. Ulcer-like draining lesions appear on the skin; hard nodules or gumma occur in the internal organs or tissue under the skin. The blood vessels and heart are often damaged and the lungs may be affected during this stage.

Neurosyphilis or syphilis of the central nervous system can accompany either the second or third stage of syphilis, although more commonly the third. When the spinal cord is involved, loss of coordination of limbs may ensue. In general paresis, the brain is infected and mental faculties deteriorate and the limbs become paralyzed.

Syphilis is the only venereal disease that may be acquired congenitally by the passing of the spirochete from the mother to the unborn child. Syphilitic infection may cause abortion or stillbirth. Infants who are born with syphilis may soon die; or, if they survive, may later develop blindness, deafness, paralysis, deformities, or even mental disturbances. Because of these terrible consequences, every prospective mother should be examined for syphilis so that, if she does have it, treatment can begin immediately. Even if treatment is delayed until the fourth or fifth month of pregnancy, the child may still be born healthy. If, however, treatment has been inadequate or absent, the newborn child should immediately be given penicillin. The amount given to children depends on the age the treatment begins; children over two years receive the same dose as adults.

Usually the first symptom of syphilis is a sore at the point where the germ has entered the body. The doctor makes his diagnosis by studying the material from the sore under a microscope. In the Darkfield method, the germs appear light and the rest of the slide dark. He will also give the patient a Wassermann, Kahn, or one of the standard serological tests for syphilis.

When the syphilis germ enters the body, it multiplies quickly and gradually invades every organ and tissue, certain germs being limited to certain parts of the body, and syphilis can therefore imitate a wide variety of diseases.

Current treatment of syphilis with penicillin and other antibiotics has largely replaced former methods of treatment. These drugs can halt the spread of the disease within a few days. Penicillin is used not only for early syphilis but to alleviate the symptoms of neurosyphilis and in congenital syphilis. Because of the notable success, it was at first thought that penicillin and the antibiotics might completely wipe out syphilis, but recent figures compiled by the Venereal Disease Program showed an increase in primary and secondary syphilis in eighteen states. This increase occurred among both sexes.

A person who has syphilis should lead a healthy life, with proper diet and adequate sleep. He should sleep alone and not have sexual intercourse until his physician is sure he is free of contagion. Intercourse will not only interfere with the cure of the disease, but is likely to transmit the disease to the other person. In many states syphilis is a bar to marriage and a physician's certificate or affidavit is required from applicants stating that they are free from venereal disease. Other states require only that the applicants be tested for syphilis, as a mutual warning. Needless to say, anyone with syphilis should postpone marriage until free of contagion. The syphilitic person should be especially careful that others are not exposed to the disease from contact with his personal articles, such as towels, drinking glass, toothbrush, etc. Anything that touches the open sores should be disinfected or destroyed.

It cannot be too strongly urged that anyone who suspects that he has syphilis see a doctor immediately. Some people through false shame or modesty permit the disease to spread to a critical point before seeking medical aid. The fact that a person has once had syphilis should always be mentioned when he later sees a doctor or dentist for other reasons, since it may furnish a clue to treatment. *See also* CHANCRE; PARESIS.

SYRINGE, an instrument used to inject fluid beneath the skin or into a cavity. It consists of a nozzle, barrel, and plunger or rubber bulb. There are various special types of syringe, the rectal syringe, and the urethral syringe.

TABES, a wasting or degeneration. Although there are many types of tabes, the word usually designates tabes dorsalis, also known as locomotor ataxia. *See also* LOCOMOTOR ATAXIA.

TACHYPHAGIA, the habit of rapid eating. The tachyphage is one who gulps his meals without stopping to sit down, or eats so fast he does not relax or enjoy his food.

The tachyphage does not improve his digestive apparatus by this mode of life. The state of his stomach is usually so troublesome that none of the normal pleasures of life, eating, drinking, or even the esthetic and intellectual joys, are ever his.

Fortunate is the tachyphage who, discovering his folly early, can take the necessary corrective measures while he is still in relatively good health. These include regular hours for meals, the use of a proper menu, the exclusion of shop talk from the table and, above all, slow eating.

TALIPES, any one of a variety of deformities of the human foot, especially those of congenital origin, such as clubfoot. *See also* CLUBFOOT.

TAPEWORM. *See* WORMS.

TATTOOING, the production of permanent color in the skin by introducing foreign substances, by pricking in coloring matter, or by making scars. Tattooing, Polynesian in origin, dates from primitive times when savages pigmented their skin and tattooed the body, usually in connection with religious worship. Ritual tattooing is still practiced by native tribes in Africa and in other parts of the world.

In tattooing, mineral and vegetable pigments are carried by needles directly into the true skin. Tattooing of the skin may sometimes occur accidentally, as when particles of powder are deposited in the skin and leave permanent stains. Miners occasionally have permanent discoloration due to the imbedding of coal dust in scratches. Silver and iron have an effect of tattooing when deposited in the skin.

The tattooer will sometimes use his own saliva as the moistening agent in tattooing, and various diseases, including tuberculosis, erysipelas, bacterial infection, viral hepatitis, and even venereal diseases have been transmitted in this manner. Occasionally tattooing produces reactions in the skin which result in the development of tumors.

One of the methods to remove a tattoo is peeling the skin with a caustic substance. This is quite dangerous and even specialists in diseases of the skin hesitate to attempt it. It is also possible to cut away the entire tattooed area, if it is not too large, and graft new skin from another portion of the body over the area. A new and successful method involves sterilizing the area with antiseptics and then sandpapering the tattooed skin off its base. Bleeding is controlled and prompt healing encouraged. Recently special burrs and emery wheels powered by motors have been used for planing. The skin is first made insensitive to pain by freezing it with "Freon."

TEAR GLANDS. The little indentation at the inner end of the eye is known as the tear gland and serves as a kind of reservoir for tears. From this reservoir several small tubes, called tear ducts, carry the tears to the eyes.

Another tube, the nasal duct, carries a similar fluid to the nose. For this reason, whenever a person sheds tears, he will also find it necessary to blow his nose.

The tear glands, as well as the ducts, may occasionally become infected. When this occurs, a swelling is seen at the corner of the eye and a small amount of pus will form. Often a person with this condition will press out the pus and apply a commercial medication without consulting a doctor, but professional assistance is always recommended since the infection may in some cases be serious enough to require the cutting or even the removal of the gland. *See also* EYE.

TEETH, the calcified organs supported by sockets and gums of both jaws. Their chief function is to grind food into small enough pieces to be easily swallowed and digested. The teeth help to form words and also give expression. Their loss is usually associated with old age, and loss of teeth in a young person may require a major emotional adjustment. Sound teeth contribute to health, while decayed teeth and diseased gums permit germs to enter the body. Thus the teeth may become focal points of infection and lead to other disorders.

Anatomy of teeth. Teeth are composed largely of mineral salts, chiefly calcium and phosphorus, and also magnesium, fluorine, and other minerals. A tooth consists of a crown, a neck, and one or more roots. The roots contain dentin, an ivory-like substance which is also found beneath the crown, surrounding a hollow, known as the pulp cavity, which is in the center. The pulp contains blood vessels, nerves, and loose connective tissue, including specialized nerve cells.

The crown, composed of the intensely hard enamel which caps the tooth, may have two or more cusps, or points, on its biting surface. Enamel is derived from the same substance as hair and nails. If the enamel is damaged by accident or disease once the tooth has erupted, natural repair is not possible, nor can decay on the surface or in fissures in the enamel be helped by drugs, vitamins, or nourishment from the blood stream. However, this is not true for the rest of the tooth.

The root of the tooth is covered by cement which in its structure resembles bone. The periodontal membrane is the membrane that holds the tooth within the jawbone, and the alveolar bone supports the tooth and anchors it to the jaw. The alveolus also supplies calcium salts to other parts of the body and acts as a kind of reservoir. Alveolar bone is therefore easily affected by any disease that interferes with the calcium metabolism of the body.

The gums are the soft tissues that cover the alveolar bone, and are continuous with the mucous membranes of the mouth, lips, and cheeks.

Dentition. The process of cutting teeth is ordinarily called teething or dentition. There are two dentitions; the first produces the primary teeth, also known as the deciduous, temporary, or milk teeth, and the second produces the permanent teeth. There are twenty primary teeth: four incisors, two canines, and four molars in each jaw. The incisors are the front cutting teeth; the two in the middle are called central incisors,

and those on either side are called lateral incisors. Outside these are the canine teeth which are sharp, pointed, and able to tear food. Beyond the canines are the molars or grinding teeth. The arrangement of teeth is the same in the upper and lower jaws and on the right and left sides.

The second permanent set of teeth contains thirty-two teeth. Twenty of these gradually replace the primary dentition, which starts at about six or seven years of age and finishes at about twelve years or older. This dentition begins with the appearance of the first permanent molars, and afterward other permanent teeth are cut, including the central and lateral incisors, the first and second premolar, the canines, and the second molar. The premolars which replace milk molars have two cusps on the crown and are also known as the bicuspids. The third molar teeth, the wisdom teeth, may appear between the ages of seventeen and twenty-five or later, or not at all.

Disorders and diseases of teeth. The first teething is sometimes painful and the gums swollen, hot, and tender. The child may be generally upset, and colds, earache, and fever are not uncommon during this period. The second dentition rarely causes any trouble, with the exception of aching which may accompany eruption of the wisdom teeth.

Sometimes malocclusion, or irregularity in placement of teeth, may be found in the deciduous and the permanent dentitions. A special branch of dentistry, orthodontia, has been developed to correct malocclusion, and the earlier the condition

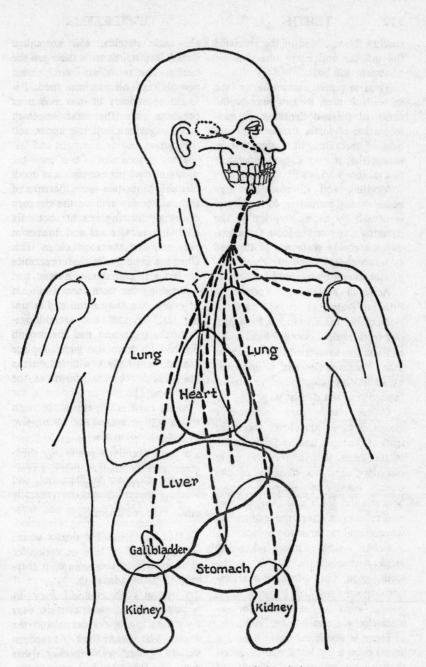

Abscessed teeth can affect many of the vital organs.

reaches the attention of the specialist the quicker and more effective the treatment will be.

Total or partial anodontia, or lack of teeth, is rare. Rickets may be the cause of delayed dentition or malformation of teeth. Premature eruption of teeth has little significance, except that it may cause discomfort to a mother who is still nursing.

Mottling and discoloration may occur during formation of teeth, and is caused by excess fluorine in the drinking water or the food. Occasionally the child's teeth are malformed or incompletely calcified. These conditions should be treated by a dentist.

A small amount of fluorine in drinking water, about one part per million, has been found to help protect teeth against decay. Fluoridation of water has been tried successfully in many communities and is approved by all leading scientific organizations in medicine and dentistry.

Unless teeth are adequately cleansed, tartar may form about the neck of the tooth and lead to infection of the gums, to pyorrhea and other disorders, and to diseases of the mouth. Food may adhere in spaces between the teeth and ferment, and acid substances attack the enamel and cause dental caries or tooth decay.

Dental health. Although heredity helps determine the health of the teeth, good diet, adequate mastication, good mouth hygiene, and regular visits to the dentist for examination and cleaning are important.

There is no single diet which can insure good teeth, but a well-balanced diet, containing proper amounts of proteins, carbohydrates, fats, minerals, and vitamins, will encourage dental health just as it will general health. The teeth particularly need phosphorus and calcium, which is found abundantly in milk and milk products especially, and in leafy green vegetables, whole-grain cereal, and fish.

Dentists recommend that teeth get plenty of chewing exercise, and every diet should include enough crisp and textured foods which require vigorous chewing. Chewing benefits not only teeth but jaws, nasal and breathing passages, and the stomach as well. Chewing crisp fruits and vegetables also helps to keep the teeth clean.

Brushing the teeth should be part of everyone's daily routine. The upper teeth should be brushed down from the gum, and the lower teeth brushed up from the gum. Regular use of dental floss will help keep the areas between the teeth free of food deposits.

Small cavities appear in the teeth which will grow larger if not treated. The dentist should be consulted and the teeth examined preferably three times, and no less than twice, a year. *See also* DENTAL CARIES; DENTIFRICE; FLUORIDATION; ORTHODONTIA; PYORRHEA; VINCENT'S ANGINA.

TEMPERATURE, the degree of intensity of heat of a body, especially as measured by the scale of a thermometer. The normal temperature of the human body is 98.6° F., with occasional variations during the day, amounting to no more than one degree. The temperature is generally slightly higher toward evening, when it may be 99.1°, and in early morning it may fall to about 97.3°.

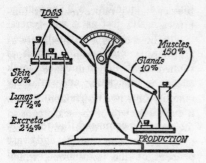

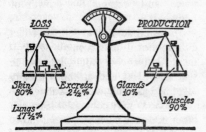

The heat produced by muscles and glands is normally lost through the skin, lungs and excreta. In fever the loss is unable to keep up with production.

A strict balance must be kept in the body between heat production and heat loss. To maintain a normal temperature, excess heat is expelled from the body or extra heat produced.

Heat is lost chiefly through perspiration and through the air and vapor expelled from the lungs. Heat is produced by chemical action in the muscles and in the glands, especially in the liver. Shivering, an involuntary muscular action, produces heat.

The sensation of heat or cold is not due to a change in body temperature but to a change in the temperature of the skin. When the skin feels cold or hot, a message is sent to the brain, the site of a mechanism which controls temperature. This mechanism is set into action with a corresponding drop or rise in temperature.

Disease may disturb the heat-regulating mechanism and cause the temperature to increase or decrease. The temperature of a person sick with a fever may rise to 104° or even higher. In severe cases, such as at the time of death, the fever may reach as high as 107° to 109°. The average fever thermometer has a maximum of about 110°, above which death usually occurs. Cases have been recorded of death from heatstroke in which the persons had temperatures of over 110°.

A temperature below 96° may represent collapse. In certain diseases and operative procedures, body tem-

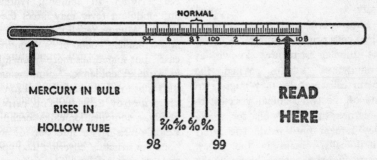

"Normal" body temperature is between 98 and 99 degrees Fahrenheit.

perature may be considerably below this figure for a period of time.

Chilling of the body ordinarily is considered harmful to health. Chilling is more serious for a person with a chronic infection of the nose and throat than for one in good health, and the response to chilling may be congestion in the nose and sinuses and the appearance of a condition like a cold. Some people are more susceptible to chilling than others, or are so sensitive to either heat or cold that symptoms of allergy are manifested. *See also* CHILBLAINS; FEVER; FROSTBITE; HAZARDS OF COLD; THERMOMETER.

TENDON, or sinew, a fibrous band of connective tissue which unites a muscle with another part of the body, and transmits the force exerted by the muscle. *See also* ACHILLES' TENDON; BURSITIS; MUSCLE.

TESTICLES, or testes, the two male sex glands which hang outside the body in a small sac of skin called the scrotum. They perform two significant functions: they produce both the male reproductive cells, the sperm, and the male sex hormone, the internal secretion which causes the body to assume the attributes of masculinity.

Both sperm and so-called interstitial cells originate within the testes, the tubular structures known as seminiferous tubules. When the sperm cells mature, they migrate to one of the two seminal vesicles located near the urinary bladder, where they remain until used. The interstitial cells remain in the testes, occupying the spaces between the tubules, and produce male sex hormones.

The hormone known medically as testosterone has been extensively studied and found to have many effects in the body. Appearing in quantity only as puberty approaches, it evokes growth of the sex organs to their adult size. Stronger and heavier male bones and muscles are dependent on the testosterone, which also causes the vocal cords in the larynx to enlarge, resulting in the characteristic low pitch of the male voice, and prompts the growth of body hair.

Testosterone has a definite effect on emotional and mental development, influencing adult interest in sex, and ideas and attitudes usually identified as adult and masculine.

The body may contain at least one other male sex hormone, if not more, but this has not as yet been scientifically established.

The term eunuch signifies a male deprived of the testicles or of the external male genitals. Such men tend to lose many or most typically male characteristics.

Disorders of the testes include infection, damage from mumps, cancer, or failure to descend normally into the scrotum. In addition, typhoid and undulant fever may affect these organs. Mumps reach the testicles in approximately one in a hundred cases, but sometimes more frequently in a major epidemic. Mumps cause the testes to swell painfully and sometimes destroy their function permanently, a complication called orchitis. Epididymitis is an infection of the hoodlike structure covering the upper end of each testicle. The sulfa and antibiotic drugs are used advantageously in testicular infections.

The testicles normally descend from within the body to the scrotum by the time of birth. However, this does not always occur. Since the internal temperature of the body is too high to permit the organs to produce sperm cells, the glands cannot develop and function properly. Therefore, when the testes do not descend, some of the male characteristics may be latent. Treatment by hormones alone may be sufficient, but often surgery is indicated to correct this condition, called cryptorchism.

Cancer of the testes is rare. The first sign of it is usually in the lymph nodes about the neck. Pain or other symptoms in the testicle itself occur later. *See also* ORCHITIS; REPRODUCTION SYSTEM; UNDESCENDED TESTES.

TETANUS, or lockjaw, an infectious disease, often fatal, which especially attacks the muscles of the neck and lower jaw. This disease is caused by the tetanus bacillus, a germ which ordinarily infests the intestines of cattle, horses, or men, and which is also found in the earth. The germ invades human beings primarily through wounds. Since it thrives best without oxygen, it is found most abundantly in deeper wounds, especially those which contain soil or foreign refuse.

About seven days after the invasion of the germ, the person infected is likely to feel a kind of pulling pain in the wound. This is accompanied by a spasm of the muscles. He may develop chills and

fever, a painful headache, and probably a general feeling of irritability. Stiffness is first evident in the muscles of the jaw and neck, and a series of violent convulsions and spasm may soon follow. Sometimes occurring as frequently as every minute, these spasms may be so extensive that every muscle in the body is involved.

The tetanus bacillus engenders an exceedingly strong poison which may be fatal. Prevention of the disease consists of injecting an antitoxin under the skin as soon as a wound has been inflicted. The wound is then opened wide, thoroughly cleaned of foreign matter, and cleansed with antiseptic. This preventive technique is so efficient that not one death from tetanus was recorded among the U.S. forces during World War II. *See also* IMMUNIZATION.

TETANY. *See* PARATHYROID GLANDS.

THERMOMETER, in medicine, the instrument used to take the temperature of the body. In the United States, the Fahrenheit scale is most frequently used, usually graduated between 94° and 110°. The normal body temperature, 98.6°, is generally indicated by an arrow. The centigrade thermometer is used in Europe.

Before taking a temperature, the mercury must be shaken down below the normal mark. This is done either by firmly grasping the stem between the thumb and forefinger and shaking the thermometer forcibly in the air, or by holding the stem in the same way and striking the inner side of the wrist on the knee.

The temperature can be taken in the mouth, armpit, groin, or rectum. Before placing a thermometer in the armpit or groin, the part should be thoroughly dried and the thermometer placed between two skin surfaces, care being taken that clothing does not come between the bulb and the skin. For rectal temperatures, the bulb of the thermometer is smeared with a little petroleum jelly and then gently manipulated into place. The thermometer should remain in the mouth or rectum for three to five minutes, and in the armpit or groin for seven to ten minutes. After use, the thermometer should be thoroughly cleansed, sterilized, and stored in a safe place.

THROAT. The inside of the throat includes the larynx, the pharynx or voice box, the upper part or fauces, which is the space surrounded by the soft palate, a group of muscles used in swallowing, the palatine arches and the base of the tongue. On the outside, the front part of the neck is also described as the throat.

A sore throat is an inflammation of part of the throat. Inflammations are manifested by redness, swelling, and excessive discharges of mucus due to many different sources. Most common is exposure to cold, an extension of inflammation from the tonsils, adenoids, or the nose.

One form of sore throat, pharyngitis, may be an entirely separate disease or the symptom of another ailment, such as scarlet fever, influenza, measles, or smallpox.

Excessive use of tobacco, exposure to large amounts of dust, smoke, irritating fumes, and sudden changes in temperature or excessive dryness and similar atmospheric conditions may cause irritation of the throat.

Persons who are sensitive to certain food substances frequently react with blisters on the tissues of the throat, which become infected and produce irritations and inflammation. Swelling and inflammation of the throat may produce pain in the ears, because of blocking of the tubes which pass from the nose to the ear. A sense of fullness or obstruction, with much spitting and hawking, can also develop.

In "strep" throat, which is septic sore throat caused by the streptococcus germ, a membrane, a thin layer of tissue, sometimes appears in the throat, the glands may swell, and the temperature may rise as high as 105° F. Penicillin generally cures this condition.

Application of an ice pack may relieve the pain of an inflamed throat. Most doctors feel that gargles are ineffective since they seldom reach into the throat, although they may help to remove mucus and to wash out infected material. Direct application of an antiseptic to the throat gives a specific effect. Either an atomizer or a cotton swab may be used. To be sure that the antiseptic reaches the back of the throat, it may be necessary to hold the tongue or use a tongue depressor or atomizer.

The primary purpose of a mouthwash or throat wash is to clean and soothe. A good cleansing mouthwash is salt solution, made by adding a fourth of a teaspoon of salt to half a glass of warm water. If mucus is profuse, the addition of a quarter of a teaspoon of bicarbonate of soda, ordinary baking soda, may be beneficial. *See also* LARYNGITIS; QUINSY; SEPTIC SORE THROAT; SORE THROAT.

THROMBOSIS, a clot formation inside a blood vessel; the clot is called a thrombus. Thrombosis is caused by failure of the mechanism in the blood which keeps it fluid. Such a disorder usually occurs in veins in which the flow of blood is slowed, as in a varicose vein of the leg, or in a leg vein of a person who must lie in bed for a long time. In some cases, thrombosis is associated with bacterial infection in the area affected, or in an actual inflammation of the vein, as in thrombophlebitis. Thrombosis may also occur in narrow arteries through which the blood passes with difficulty, but arterial thrombosis is much rarer than venous thrombosis.

Thrombosis does harm by obstructing the flow of blood to and from the part supplied by the vessel and as a source of traveling fragments of clots, or emboli. An embolus is especially dangerous when it affects the lung, and there is always danger of sudden death.

Thrombosis is often the source of stroke, although a stroke caused by thrombosis is less dramatic and severe than one from an embolism or with hemorrhage. Strokes from thrombosis have a better chance for recovery, but some permanent disability usually persists.

A clot in the main vein of a limb produces swelling. For example, a clot in a main vein of the leg, deep in the upper calf, will cause a swelling of the foot and ankle and probably most of the leg below the obstruction. The amount of harm done depends on what area the artery

supplies and whether or not there are alternative routes for the blood. If there is no alternative route, all the living cells which compose the part supplied will die. The effect is exactly the same as that of an embolism or of complete blocking and obliteration of the artery by progressive hardening and narrowing.

Thrombosis is treated by certain anticoagulants, including heparin, dicumarol, and others, and in some cases surgery is employed to remove clots and help restore the flow of blood to the affected parts. Anticoagulants together with proper massage and exercise have been particularly effective for patients with swollen legs due to thrombophlebitis when infection is not a complicating factor. In some cases of varicose veins, a thrombus may change into fibrous or scarlike tissue and the inside of the tube is obliterated. In this way a natural cure is sometimes effected. *See also* APOPLEXY, COAGULATION; CORONARY THROMBOSIS; EMBOLISM; and Chapter 12, "Diseases of the Heart"; Chapter 14, "Blood Pressure; Normal, High and Low."

THRUSH, a fungus infection of the mouth in infants and occasionally older persons. White spots form, then become shallow ulcers. Frequently fever and gastrointestinal disturbance are present. The fungus may spread to the buttocks, groin, and other areas of the body.

THUMB SUCKING. In a healthy happy baby, thumb sucking, if practiced in moderation, is normal and may be ignored. The child will discover new amusement with the passage of time. Persistent thumb sucking, authorities claim, may lead to malocclusion of the teeth. If the child ceases sucking his thumb before the age of five, however, this malocclusion has a tendency to cure itself.

To cure a persistent thumb sucker is not easy. Painting the thumb with a bad-tasting medicine or forcing the child to wear a mitten have not been successful methods and are not recommended. The source of the habit lies in some kind of emotional disturbance or sense of insecurity. To cure thumb sucking, therefore, the source of the habit should be found. *See also* CHILD CARE; and Chapter 9, "Child Care and Training."

THYMUS GLAND, a gland located in the chest near the heart. Its functions are not as yet established. This gland has an unusual part in the development of the body. Instead of growing like the rest of the physical structure, the thymus is largest during the first eight or nine months of life and after the second year normally shrinks almost to the point of disappearance and is replaced by other types of tissue.

If the gland does not shrink and its size and activity continue, the results can be serious. Occasionally, especially in infants, the gland enlarges so much that it interferes with circulation and breathing, because of its proximity to the heart and windpipe. X-ray treatment is often beneficial to reduce such an enlargement. Persons may develop thymic enlargement so suddenly, apparently in response to some stress or shock, that death results. This type of growth

occurs in the condition called status lymphaticus, which is rare.

The person whose thymus gland has failed to shrink has a "peaches and cream" complexion and, if male, will probably not have to shave, or infrequently. Such persons seem younger than their actual age. They lack body hair and may be subject to low blood pressure and fatigue.

In premature cessation of functioning of the thymus, aging seems to occur before the usual time, and blood pressure is apt to be high and body hair excessive.

In laboratory experiments in which animals have been administered thymus extract, their growth and development, both sexual and mental, have been precocious even into the second and third generations. However, giantism does not occur.

Investigation of the thymus is still in an early stage. The thymus is apparently implicated with development of the skeleton, the sex glands, and with metabolism of calcium. *See also* GLANDS.

THYROID GLAND. One of the most significant of the endocrine glands, which produce secretions that regulate many basic processes of the body, the thyroid gland lies in the front part of the throat along the windpipe.

The thyroid secretion, thyroxin, is involved in the process of oxidation which occurs within the cells and by which the tissues generate the energy they require. Its importance is indicated by the serious consequences of excessive or deficient amounts of it in the body. A child born with insufficient thyroid activity becomes a cretin, physically under-grown and mentally an idiot. Thyroid deficiency in later life causes physical and mental coarsening and dulling. Excessive thyroid produces general restlessness, speeds up the heart, and may have other untoward effects. Both hyperthyroidism, too much thyroid, and hypothyroidism, too little, can be successfully treated.

The thyroid is susceptible to a variety of diseases, the most common being simple goiter, usually due to a lack of iodine. In Graves' disease, or exophthalmic goiter, over-activity of the thyroid causes a pop-eyed appearance and other serious symptoms. Tumors too, of lesser or greater malignancy, may affect the thyroid. Surgical removal is indicated for most types of thyroid cancer. X-ray and radium treatment and radioactive iodine have also been beneficial in certain cases. A number of infectious and noninfectious diseases of the thyroid also respond well to treatment. *See also* BASAL METABOLISM; CRETINISM; GLANDS; GOITER; HYPOTHYROIDISM; and Chapter 19, "Endocrine Glands."

TIC DOULOUREUX, or trigeminal neuralgia, one of the more common neuralgias or paroxysmal pains, usually beginning in the middle life and occurring more frequently in women. John Fothergill originally described it in 1776 as an intense stabbing pain which strikes one or a combination of three facial branches supplied by the trigeminal or fifth cranial nerve.

The attacks occur without warning, in violent, knifelike darts of pain. The face is twisted in spasms and there is a free flow of tears and saliva. The seizure lasts only a few seconds and may clear up spontaneously, with varying periods of relief. The pain may involve the first or ophthalmic division which includes the forehead and eye, the second division around the nose, or the third or side of the mouth. The second and third branches seem to be more frequently affected. The pain does not spread to the back of the head or across to the other side of the face. The attacks tend to increase in acuteness and extent and as the condition becomes worse the periods of freedom from pain become shorter. The seizures often are influenced by seasonal changes and occur more frequently during spring and fall. Pain may be prompted by touching the affected side of the face, by exposure to cold, washing, eating, drinking, or talking, and emotional tension or fatigue intensify the attack.

Treatment consists largely of measures to relieve individual attacks. Nicotinic acid and trichlorethylene inhalations give temporary relief. Alcohol injections, once widely used, have been discontinued because relief from pain is too often incomplete and the periods of relief between injections tend to become increasingly shorter. Alcohol injections are now given in some clinics before the operation for trigeminal neuralgia in order to accustom the patient to the facial numbness which generally follows the operation. The operation itself is now common and consists in cutting the branch or branches of the trigeminal nerve which carry the pain to the affected area of the face. In those cases in which the eye is involved and the first branch is cut, the patient is given special instruction in care of the eye, since sensation in this area is affected when the nerve is cut and the patient is unable to detect the presence of foreign bodies in the eye.

TINNITUS. *See* NOISE.

TOBACCO, a plant from which the leaf is especially dried, cured, and prepared for chewing or smoking in the form of cigars or cigarettes. Tobacco, especially in the form of cigarettes, is so popular that it takes a place on almost every family budget along with food, clothing, and shelter.

Many disorders of the human body such as respiratory infections, neuralgia, gastrointestinal difficulties, headache, inability to sleep, constipation, diarrhea, heart murmur, and cancer have been attributed to smoking. The cause-and-effect relationship is seldom clear.

Smoking does have a deleterious effect on the blood vessels and the circulation of the blood. A definite relationship has been determined between smoking and Buerger's disease, which is characterized by inflammation of the lining of the blood vessels.

Excessive smoking of cigarettes, according to recent evidence, may possibly be related to cancer of the lung. As yet the results are not completely scientifically established but many serious research investigations are currently being made. To offset the danger phenomena, cigarettes are being manufactured with filters which, with varying degrees, prevent the passage of the harmful ingredients.

TOENAILS. *See* NAILS.

TONGUE, the movable muscular organ attached to the floor of the back of the mouth. Its chief functions are to help with chewing and swallowing food, with taste, and to form sounds in speech.

The taste buds are on the side of the projections, or papillae, which lie across the tongue at the juncture of the mouth and the pharynx. A fold of membrane, the frenum, joins the undersurface of the tip of the tongue to the floor of the mouth. Sometimes the frenum is abnormally short and results in "tongue-tied" speech, which can usually be remedied by a simple operation.

Normally the tongue is pinkish white in color, moist and clean; a tongue that is dry, dark, and furry indicates disease. Among the most common of peculiar sensations that disturb persons is a burning painful tongue. The tongue, like all other tissue of the human body, is connected with the nervous system, and a burning sensation in the tongue is reflected through its nerves. In some cases, a relationship exists between this burning and vitamin deficiency, anemia, lack of iron, or even an allergy, but when no apparent physical cause exists, purely mental reasons are thought to be responsible—for example, a woman in menopause who is worried about developing cancer might experience a burning tongue.

Sometimes the tongue is inflamed through contact with edges of rough teeth, or ill-fitting false teeth. Frequently burning tongue is associated with difficulties of the digestive system. In such cases, the doctor will want to make a complete examination, which includes blood tests as well as checking the digestive system.

In a few instances, burning, and even ulcers, of the tongue have been found to be caused by the fact that different electric potentials have been used to fill teeth on opposite sides of the mouth. In a condition called glossitis, the tongue itself is infected and may have superficial or deep abscesses. The tongue may be subject to cancer or other specific diseases.

Sometimes the surface of the tongue, instead of being smooth, becomes marked by deep furrows and elevations. This condition, called geographic tongue, is not infectious and may be helped by mouthwashes, mild antiseptics, and a diet rich in vitamins and antianemic substances such as iron and liver. Black patches or hairlike projections can also form on the papillae. *See also* GLOSSITIS.

TONSILLECTOMY. *See* TONSILS.

TONSILS, masses of spongy lymphoid tissue located at the sides of the throat in the entrance to the digestive and respiratory tracts. They frequently become infected, with such symptoms as swelling, inflammation, pain, soreness, difficulty in swallowing, enlargement of the glands of the throat, fever, a rapid pulse, and general illness.

The person affected with tonsillitis should be put to bed and the doctor called. Ice packs or hot compresses may be applied about the throat and neck to relieve pain. The doctor will take steps to combat fever. Early administration of drugs, particularly antibiotics, greatly reduces the possi-

bility of serious complications or aftereffects, which can include deafness, kidney disease, rheumatic fever and other heart ailments.

Extraction of diseased and enlarged tonsils and adenoids, which interfere with breathing, is usually beneficial not only in removing a source of infection but also in improving the child's general health, appearance, and disposition. Surgery to remove tonsils is advised in recurrent attacks of tonsillitis accompanied by swelling of the neck glands. The operation, tonsillectomy, is so common and has been so well perfected that complications are exceedingly rare.

In older persons or in the presence of heart disease and other cases in which anesthetic is not possible, tonsils are sometimes treated with radiation by x-ray. X-ray and radium are also occasionally used to treat fragments of tissue that may be left after tonsillectomy and when there is regrowth of secondary adenoidal tissue.

TORTICOLLIS, commonly called wry neck, a spasmodic movement of the neck muscles which causes the head to be pulled toward one side. In some instances, shortening of neck muscles is present at birth or may occur from an injury, but in the majority of cases the origin of this disorder is unknown.

Wry neck begins suddenly without warning. The neck muscles unexpectedly contract and the head is pulled to one side in irregular jerks. It may follow a nervous reaction due to tension, worry, or anxiety. At this stage the movements can be suppressed by the person, but as the condition grows worse the movements recur involuntarily and cannot be controlled.

Psychotherapy has been successfully tried in treatment of some cases. In more stubborn cases, this treatment is combined with a nerve block, a procedure in which the cervical nerves are blocked with procaine or novocaine. Light exercises also help to relax the muscles. Frequent periods of spontaneous relief occur, but the condition generally returns, even after long intervals of relief. Use of collars or casts is not recommended. Medication includes drugs of the belladonna group and sedatives. Surgery has brought only temporary relief at best, and is not widely employed.

TOXEMIA a condition in which the blood contains poisonous products, either those created by the body cells or those due to the action of microorganisms. It is a general infection in which the blood contains toxins but not bacteria.

TRACHEA, or windpipe, a tube about 4½ inches long which leads from the mouth and larynx to the lungs. It is susceptible to infections similar to those that attack any other part of the respiratory system. Inflammation of the trachea produces a hacking metallic cough, especially severe at night. This cough often produces considerable pain, particularly in the lower part of the neck and behind the breastbone. If the inflammation continues unchecked, mucus and sputum are eructed in coughing; and if the germ is streptococcus, pus may also be expectorated.

Treatment for ordinary inflammation of the trachea is rest in bed, warmth and quiet. A vaporizer, usually an electrical device which moistens and vaporizes the air the patient breathes, often brings relief. Medicated oil added to the water which is boiled in the vaporizer also has been found beneficial.

Ordinarily the inflammation will yield to proper treatment. In severe cases, which might often have become chronic in the past, the sulfa drugs or penicillin will usually eradicate the specific infection.

The tube may be obstructed by a physiological process, as in strangling, by a foreign object, or by disease. Surgical operation, tracheotomy, is performed in some instances to correct the condition.

TRACHOMA, a highly contagious chronic disease of the eyelids, caused by a filterable virus. Trachoma was once an almost universal affliction and the most common cause of blindness. It is still widespread in Egypt, India, China, and other Eastern countries where the standards of health and sanitation are low. Trachoma has affected many American Indians and may still be found in the southern mountainous areas of this country.

Trachoma is most contagious in the early stages and is spread by contact with infected persons, insects, or contaminated objects. The eyes become inflamed and congested, tears pour out excessively, and light is painful. Blisters and crusts appear on the upper lids and form scar tissue. Small gritty particles develop on the cornea, and in severe cases vision is so diminished that only light and dark can be distinguished.

Treatment of trachoma requires the care of a specialist. Each stage of the disease, from the first inflammation of the eyes to the development of granulations and finally scar tissue, demands expert handling. Rigorous hygienic measures must be observed to keep the eyes clean at all times. Sulfonamide drugs and antibiotics have made possible control of the spread of trachoma.

TRANQUILIZING DRUGS. See BARBITURATES.

TRENCH FEVER, a mild acute rickettsial infection. During World War I it was a major medical problem. It occurred during World War II also, but on a much smaller scale.

Trench fever is transmitted from person to person by the body louse, and causes headache and fever, vertigo, pain in the back, legs, and eyes. A distinctive rash appears on the chest, back, and abdomen which usually disappears in about twenty-four hours. Convalescence is prolonged. The pain and discomfort can be controlled by drugs prescribed by a physician, and bed rest and hygienic and dietary measures help forestall a relapse.

Prevention of trench fever consists chiefly of delousing methods and sterilization of contaminated articles. The urine and sputum should be disinfected by chemicals or heat to prevent spreading the disease. *See also* RICKETTSIAL DISEASES.

TRENCH MOUTH. *See* VINCENT'S ANGINA.

TRICHINOSIS, a disease caused by eating pork infected by Trichinella spiralis, a slender roundworm that is barely visible to the naked eye. If the worms have not been destroyed by proper cooking, they may develop in the intestines and later invade the muscle tissue, where they produce stiffness and painful swelling.

Tiny cysts, encasing immature worms, are present in contaminated pork. The human digestive process liberates them in the intestines, and they mature within a few days. The developed males fertilize the females, which then burrow into the intestinal wall and subsequently release larvae.

These larvae, carried through the blood circulation, lodge in the muscles, encysting themselves within a shell-like substance that they secrete. There they cause the pain and muscular irritation which are characteristic of the disease. Other symptoms are headache, fever, sore throat, general illness, and painfully swollen eyes. Specific treatment for the disease is not yet known. In time, the tissues of the body surround the organisms and wall them off.

Protection against trichinosis is possible in at least two ways. Since the trichinae cannot survive freezing or more than a certain degree of heat, they can be killed by freezing the meat at 0° F. for twenty-four hours or at 5° F. for twenty days, or by cooking at 140° F. or more for half an hour per pound of meat.

Another method of protecting against trichinosis is to prevent the infection in hogs. A principal source of trichinosis is uncooked garbage fed to hogs. Field-fed and grain-fed hogs have an infection rate of about

.5 per cent, whereas animals fed on garbage which has not been heat-treated to kill trichinae have an infection rate of 5 per cent. Just as infected pork may be rendered safe for human consumption by proper cooking, so may garbage be made safe for pigs.

Epidemics of trichinosis are usually small and localized, and are associated with consumption of contaminated meat which can often be traced to one source. More than a quarter of pork consumed in the United States is processed without the close government supervision which is given in big packing plants and thus much pork offered for sale may harbor live trichinae. Most Americans probably consume contaminated pork at least once a year, but have no ill effects because the meat has been thoroughly cooked. The disease is, of course, more likely to occur when pork and pork products are eaten in a raw or semi-raw condition.

TRIGEMINAL NEURALGIA. See TIC DOULOUREUX.

TUBERCULOSIS, an infectious disease characterized by the production of tubercles, small rounded nodules which may appear on almost any part of the body. It is caused by the germ commonly called the tubercle bacillus, of which there are many varieties.

The past decade has seen tremendous advances in the control and treatment of tuberculosis. The death rate in the United States has dropped from 250 out of every 100,000 persons to rates as low as 5 in many states.

Tuberculosis remains a chronic disease and if healing is not complete, relapse may occur. Although in the acute phases of the disease, the new drugs act quickly to promote healing, treatment of the tuberculous patient may require a long time. The discovery and application of new drugs, like streptomycin, para-amino-salicylic acid, and isoniazid, has virtually revolutionized the management of tuberculosis, and patients can now be treated by a combination of hospital and home care rather than being placed in sanatoriums. The closing of Trudeau at Saranac Lake, New York, was a dramatic indication of the change in approach to the treatment of tuberculosis. However, sanatoriums are still advisable in some cases where hospital and home care is not adequate.

In the past, tuberculosis was seldom suspected until severe coughs with expectoration, followed by loss of weight and night sweats, set in. With modern methods, the disease can be detected long before such serious symptoms have developed. X-ray pictures reveal changes which have occurred in the lung, and mobile units for lung x-rays are now common in many communities. Another method of detecting tuberculosis is the tuberculin test. A small amount of tuberculin, a material containing proteins of the tubercle bacillus, is applied to the skin or in some cases injected between the layers of the skin. A positive skin reaction indicates that the tissues have been sensitized to the tuberculer germ, and that the germs are present and an infection exists somewhere in the body. Occasionally the reactions to the tuberculin test may be doubtful and additional tests, including sputum and smear tests, are necessary. Generally if the test is positive, other tests, such as the bacteriological diagnosis, are given to establish beyond doubt that tuberculosis is present. Tuberculin-positive cases showing chronic lung infection and confirmed by x-ray are usually considered as tuberculous, unless the bacteriological diagnosis indicates otherwise. Certain fungus diseases of the lung precisely imitate tuberculosis.

The germ causing tuberculosis was first described in 1882 by the bacteriologist Robert Koch. A variety of these germs exist, some affecting primarily human beings and others cattle, birds, or cold-blooded animals. The cattle type of germ may infect human beings, usually through the milk of infected cattle, and is largely responsible for tuberculosis of the bones, joints, and lymph glands, especially in children. However, the incidence of tuberculosis in cattle has been reduced to almost the vanishing point since the institution of tuberculin tests for cattle. In other countries, where the control of tuberculous cattle has not been so efficient, the disease continues at a high rate.

Although pulmonary tuberculosis is the most common form, the glands, covering of the brain (meningeal tuberculosis), the spinal fluid, the eye, and many other tissues may be affected. In acute miliary tuberculosis of the generalized type, the tubercle bacilli may be disseminated throughout the organs of the body. Acute active pulmonary tuberculosis, "galloping consumption," may be difficult to diagnose at the onset. It may attack suddenly, with coughing of blood-stained sputum, and in such cases a doctor should be promptly consulted. This form, which was once rapidly fatal, has now yielded to modern drugs. Tuberculosis of the abdominal region, affecting the intestines and other organs, is rare in the United States. One of the most distressing forms, known as Pott's disease, after the British physician who first described it, causes crippling and curvature of the spine. A person may have tuberculosis of the lung and some other form of the disease at the same time.

The cough is the best-known symptom of tuberculosis, and is an indication of infection of the lung by the tubercle bacillus or by some other germ. Any cough that persists for three or four weeks should always be brought to the attention of a physician. The cough is frequently accompanied by expectoration, and in some cases enough destruction of lung tissue has occurred for blood to be expectorated. Furthermore, fluid may pour out into the walls of the chest, an example of the way the body attempts to control infection. Another way the body tries to check the infection is to cover or wall off the infection with scar tissue, a process known as fibrosis.

The tuberculous person is generally sick, loses weight, and feels weak. A slight rise of temperature in the afternoon, or fever and an increase in the pulse rate, may also appear, and night sweats are common.

X-ray examination will reveal the extent of involvement of the lung, and a physical examination of the chest determines any changes that have taken place in its shape or contour and movement. By placing his hands on the chest, the doctor can determine the presence of spasms of the muscles or vibrations associated with the passing of air into or out of the lung. The doctor will also thump the chest and note whether the sound is dull, has increased resonance or a tympanic response. Sounds made by the air passing into the lung, as heard through a stethoscope, indicate any interference with the passage of air, the presence of fluid or solid tissue, or other changes.

The sputum is examined to determine the presence of the tubercle germs, which conclusively point to tuberculosis. The absence of bacteriological evidence does not, however, exclude the disease, because in the earlier stages of the infection the germs may be absent in as many as 35 per cent of cases.

The success of the treatment depends largely on recognition of the disease at the earliest possible moment.

Once the doctor has determined the extent of the tuberculosis, the age of the infection, the portions of tissue involved, and other significant factors, he decides the course of management to be taken, not only medically but also personally with the patient. An understanding and healthy attitude on the part of the patient toward the disease may be a large contributing factor in the effectiveness of the treatment.

Social and economic problems arise in many families when some member develops tuberculosis, and social service departments in hospitals are often of great help in handling them. From a medical point of view, the principle of rest treatment requires as far as possible freedom from anxiety and worry, and by helping to alleviate these, the social service departments can help the physical state of the patient.

Once the diagnosis is established, almost without exception every case of pulmonary tuberculosis is treated with appropriate drugs for at least twelve months, and usually from eighteen to twenty-four months. Combinations of streptomycin, isoniazid, and para-amino-salicylic acid are prescribed in most cases. Bed rest of the sanatorium type is recommended at the onset of treatment in almost every case of active pulmonary tuberculosis, followed by a semiambulatory stage, and then an ambulatory period of limited activity.

Although it was once believed that a high cool dry climate was most conducive for curing tuberculosis, it has now been established that the disease can be treated in any climate. The attention of a competent physician, the services of a good hospital or sanatorium, sufficient rest, good food, and administration of antituberculous drugs and other factors are primarily significant.

Because of the effectiveness of prolonged drug therapy, a combination of home and hospital treatment is recommended whenever possible. The American Trudeau Society has issued the following summary: "The management of tuberculosis today is a complex matter requiring the continuous supervision of a well-trained physician or physicians; the use of complicated laboratory facilities for proper evaluation; and long term, uninterrupted use of appropriate antituberculous drugs; the availability of competent thoracic surgery in many cases; the opportunity for good nursing care and effective long-term physical rest and emotional relaxation; the availability of patient education and the proper proportion of recreation, occupational therapy and medical social service; and the proper facilities for isolation. It is concluded that in the majority of cases this service and treatment can best be offered in a hospital, during at least the acute phases of tuberculosis, and for the latter phases as well unless adequately supervised home care is available."

Reports indicate that good results are being obtained in those communities where the program of hospital and supervised home care is coordinated. Treatment is begun in the hospital and continued through the acute period, usually until cavities are closed, the sputum is negative, and the course of the disease is predictable. Then an appropriate supervised program of home care with continued drug treatment is established.

The employment of artificial pneumothorax for collapse of the lung has been almost completely abandoned, because of the high incidence of serious complications. However, when it is necessary to collapse the lung to rest it, thoracoplasty, an operation on the chest wall in which portions of the ribs are removed, remains an effective procedure.

The use of isoniazid to treat acute miliary tuberculosis and tuberculous meningitis has brought about a spectacular reduction in fatalities, and in some groups the survival is as high as 80 to 100 per cent. In general, tuberculosis affecting parts of the body other than the lung is treated

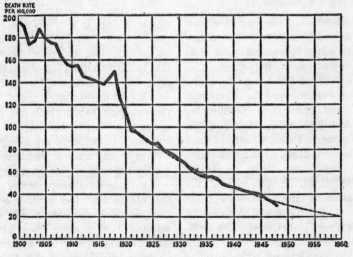

Chart showing decline in tuberculosis mortality in the United States.

with the same drugs as pulmonary tuberculosis.

The extensive knowledge of tuberculosis now available makes its complete prevention an ultimate possibility. Removal of those conditions which lower resistance and make the body more susceptible to tuberculous infection, such as slum areas where health and hygienic standards are low, can greatly decrease the incidence of tuberculosis. A more immediate measure is the detection of tuberculosis through periodic x-ray examination of the chest. Every person should have an x-ray examination of his chest and a general physical examination once a year. Active cases must be isolated, and persons who have been exposed should be particularly watchful. Anyone who has symptoms of tuberculosis—loss of weight and appetite, nausea, persistent fever, persistent cough and expectoration, a prolonged cold or spitting of blood—should immediately consult a doctor.

TULAREMIA, an infectious disease transmitted to man by infected rabbits or other rodents, through their bite or through handling them.

An Arizona physician, Dr. Ancil Martin, first observed the infection in 1907 and traced it to the skinning and dressing of wild rabbits. In 1910, wild game in Tulare County in California were dying by the thousands; two investigators from the U. S. Public Health Service isolated the germ causing the disease, which came to be called tularemia, deriving its name from Tulare County. The medical director of the U. S. Public Health Service, Dr. Edward Francis, made further studies and discovered that human beings contracted the disease from contact with diseased rabbits and, in some rare instances, from bites of ticks and flies.

By far the most common source of infection is contact with the hands with the diseased rabbit. Rabbit meat, thoroughly cooked, is harmless when eaten, since a temperture of 130° F. will kill the germ of tularemia.

When tularemia appears on the body, an ulcerlike sore is usually found at the point where the germs have entered through the skin. This sore ordinarily appears several days after exposure. Following rapidly are headache, aching muscles and joints, weakness, chills, and fever.

The wild rabbit is the animal chiefly infected by tularemia, but the infection has been found in almost every type of small wild animal, including the muskrat, opposum, water rat, and squirrel. Cats and sheep have also been known to be infected.

Persons who handle rabbits for any purpose should wear protective rubber gloves. If they do not, they should wash their hands in a mild antiseptic before and after handling the rabbit. Contact of the rabbit flesh with a scratch, cut, hangnail, or sore should be carefully avoided, and the wrapping paper which has contained the animal burned. If any evidence of swelling or secondary infection around a cut or sore appears, a doctor should be seen promptly.

For those who hunt rabbits, it is well to remember that a rabbit which runs slowly is probably a sick rabbit and best ignored. Any rabbit which a child or dog brings home is likely to have been too sick to run.

In treatment of tularemia, streptomycin is rapidly curative, and other antibiotics including aureomycin, chloromycetin, and terramycin, have been used effectively. Complications, including pneumonia, may arise and require hospitalization, intravenous feeding, and, for serious cases, blood transfusions and oxygen.

TUMOR, literally a lump or swelling, although the term is not used to describe the swelling of normal tissues such as occurs in inflammation or edema, or the enlargement of organs such as the spleen, liver, or kidneys. Specifically a tumor is a mass of cells, resembling ordinary tissue, which develops independently as new growth and serves no useful function. When such newly formed tissue occurs in blood vessels, it is called an angioma; in fatty tissue, a lipoma or fatty tumor; in cartilage, a chondroma. Tumors composed of tissue unlike the host organ may sometimes occur, such as cartilaginous or fatty tumors which develop in a gland— for example, the carotid gland. A malignant tumor, or sarcoma, is composed of fleshy mass derived from connective tissue.

A large class of tumors do not have harmful effects, except as they produce pressure by their growth, and are designated as simple, benign, or innocent. However, a malignant tumor not only exerts pressure on adjoining tissue but actually invades and destroys it, or may disintegrate and produce new tumors in other parts of the body, a condition known as metastasis.

Any lump or swelling should be brought to the attention of a doctor who will diagnose it and determine the necessary treatment. Some tumors may be left undisturbed, whereas others should be removed. *See also* CANCER; CHONDROMA; LIPOMA; METASTASIS; POLYP; SARCOMA; XANTHOMA; and Chapter 17, "Cancer."

TYPHOID FEVER, an acute infection caused by the typhoid bacillus. As late as 1900, typhoid fever was among the most serious of diseases and responsible for numerous deaths each year. Today, although occasional cases still occur, the disease has been practically eliminated and deaths average around 200 a year throughout the United States.

The germ is found in the blood of a person seriously ill with typhoid fever, and in 80 per cent of the cases is also found in the material excreted by the bowels. The germ of typhoid fever is spread through excretions of the body, by contaminated food, clothing, water, and milk. In spite of improved sanitation, methods of treatment, and immunization by vaccination, a primary menace remains, the typhoid carrier, a person who has had the disease and recovered but who continues to propagate the germs and to spread them. Administration of penicillin and removal of the gallbladder of the carrier have helped curb the problem, but many typhoid carriers still exist.

Typhoid fever follows a long and serious course. From three to twenty-one days after the infection, which is known as the incubation period, the germs develop in the body and liberate their poisons. Typhoid fever begins with the usual symptoms of infection, such as headache, pains throughout the body, a feeling of exhaustion, and chills and fever. Frequently nosebleed occurs and almost invariably there is simultaneously a serious disturbance of the bowels, due to the fact that the typhoid germs produce ulcers in the bowels. As the disease progresses, the infected person becomes more and more ill. Clots may form in the blood vessels and rose spots appear on the skin at the end of the first week or beginning of the second. Because of the damage to the bowels, gas forms, causing bloating, and sometimes perforation of the intestines which may produce severe hemorrhage. Occasionally the infection also attacks the nervous system, resulting in not only pain but even delirium.

The doctor in examining the patient with typhoid fever makes his diagnosis on the basis of the history of the case, the nature of the symptoms, and by careful study of the blood. The Widal test of the blood determines, with reasonable certainty, the presence of typhoid fever.

Isolation of typhoid fever patients and good nursing care by an experienced nurse are required. If the illness occurs during the summer when flies are common the sickroom should be screened. The most effective antimicrobial treatment is Chloramphenicol or Chloromycetin, which has induced earlier remission of symptoms and shortened the duration of the illness. Stools and urine of the patient should be disinfected with cresol, formaldehyde, or similar disinfectants. The patient's bed linen and dishes should be sterilized. He must be bathed at least once a day, be

kept clean, and the mouth rinsed after eating to prevent secondary infection. Only a few restrictions in diet are necessary. Nourishing bland foods are given during the early part of the illness, but during convalescence a high-protein, high-calorie diet, containing from 3,000 to 3,500 calories, is recommended.

Typhoid vaccine is highly effective, but not absolutely preventive against typhoid fever. It is administered subcutaneously in three weekly doses by a physician or trained nurse. A booster injection at suitable intervals will maintain a high level of immunity and should be given to persons who because of occupation or travel may be exposed to typhoid-contaminated food or water.

Although areas still exist throughout the world where typhoid fever is a threat, persistent attention to water supplies, pasteurization of milk, disposal of sewage, control of typhoid fever carriers, and general education of the public in hygiene can eliminate the disease entirely. *See also* CARRIERS OF DISEASE.

TYPHUS FEVER, a plague which has occurred in eastern Europe and Asia for centuries, is an infectious disease caused by a rickettsial organism. Other names for it are jail fever, ship fever, camp fever, and louse typhus. It is carried by the body louse or rat flea and an epidemic may arise wherever overcrowding, famine, and poverty prevail. It occurs principally in cold weather and may follow in the wake of war and famine, and spread in slums, concentration camps, asylums, and prisons.

Typhus fever includes three diseases: the epidemic louse-borne typhus, Brill's disease, and murine flea-borne typhus. The three types differ from one another only in the intensity of the symptoms and the severity of the illness and fatality rate.

Epidemic louse-borne typhus is transmitted by the body louse, chiefly in eastern Europe, Asia, and northern Africa. Dried louse feces on clothing or bedding can keep active rickettsial organisms for many months and be a source of contamination. Epidemic typhus is most frequent during winter and spring, when heavier clothing and less frequent bathing create ideal conditions for rapid multiplication of lice.

Symptoms appear about ten days after a person has been bitten by an infected louse. Severe headache, high fever, and aches and pains of the entire body develop. On the third to seventh day, a rash appears, first on the armpits and flanks, then on the trunk and later on the arms and legs. Mental faculties are dulled and prostration is severe. Odor from the mouth is foul and bronchitis and pneumonia often develop. In mild cases recovery is usually rapid, and one attack establishes long immunity.

In the past, the death rate from typhus epidemics was high. In the epidemic of eastern Europe and Russia between 1918 and 1922 thirty million cases occurred, with three million deaths. In Serbia, the mortality rate was between 30 and 80 per cent, and of some 400 doctors who contracted the disease, 126 died. An Egyptian epidemic in 1943 resulted in 40,000 cases and 8,000 deaths.

Brill's disease is a form of typhus found principally among emigrants from countries which have had epidemics of the louse-borne typhus. Though the same rickettsial organism is responsible for both forms of typhus, Brill's disease generally occurs in persons who have had epidemic typhus before emigrating. It is a milder form of typhus and generally is not fatal. Since the specific agent responsible for Brill's disease has not yet been isolated, the means for prevention and control have yet to be developed. Precautions are the same as for typhus.

Murine typhus is a flea-borne disease for which the rat is the breeding animal. Human beings become infected by the bite of an infected flea, or by eating food contaminated by flea feces or rat urine. The disease is not spread by man. It has occurred throughout the United States, but is most common in the Atlantic and Gulf states.

The incubation period is about twelve days, and the symptoms are similar to those of epidemic typhus, but are milder and of shorter duration. The rash is less extensive and fades sooner, and complications are fewer.

Treatment of the typhus fever group consists of good nursing care. Antibiotics have been effective in decreasing the severity of the disease and in controlling its spread.

Prevention of typhus depends largely upon elimination of the animal which breeds the disease and the insect which transmits it. Adult lice are destroyed with DDT, and the eggs are killed by steam sterilization. During World War II, prevention and control of epidemic typhus was one of the great medical accomplishments. Immunization was achieved by means of vaccines given to entire companies of men. Since rats are the primary source of murine typhus, prevention and control involves rat-proofing buildings, especially granaries and storehouses, and eliminating garbage dumps and other conditions conducive to breeding rats. *See also* IMMUNIZATION; RAT CONTROL; RICKETTSIAL DISEASES.

ULCER, any open sore, other than a wound, with an inflamed base. Such a lesion usually occurs in the skin or mucous membrane of some internal organ. Ulcers may result from infection, injury to the blood supply, damage to nerves, or from a wide variety of other cuases. Ulcers require the attention of a physician who will not only endeavor to learn the specific cause but will plan the treatment accordingly. *See* PEPTIC ULCER.

UMBILICUS, or navel, the depressed scar in the median (middle) line of the abdomen, which results from the separation of the umbilical cord in childbirth.

UNDESCENDED TESTES. The development of the testes, or testicles, takes place in the abdominal cavity. Normally they descend into the scrotum soon after birth. If this descent fails to occur, the abnormality is designated as undescended testes.

Undescended testes usually atrophy —that is, waste away. If this occurs in both testes, the person becomes sterile. Undescended testes through

functional failure also hinder proper development of the secondary sex characteristics, such as the beard, the low voice, and the flat chest.

The parents or pediatrician should, therefore, examine the child at an early age to be sure that the testes have descended into the scrotum. Ordinarily the testes can be felt. Rarely it may be possible to press them down gently to the proper position. In cases of any difficulty the advice of a doctor is absolutely essential. If the child is old enough to realize the situation, care should be taken not to arouse his curiosity or create anxiety.

Sometimes surgery is necessary to transplant the testes to their proper position in the scrotum. This operation should, if possible, always be performed before puberty. *See also* REPRODUCTION SYSTEM.

UNDULANT FEVER, known medically as brucellosis, and in different sections of the world as Malta, Mediterranean, Rio Grande, Texas, and goat fever; a remittent febrile disease, caused by infection with Brucella bacteria, named after Bruce, a British physician who first isolated it on Malta. The infection may last weeks or months and during this time the fever rises and falls over periods of several days, and may be severe enough to cause death. Unfamiliar in the United States before 1927, undulant fever has now been reported in every state.

Undulant fever is also found in cattle, sheep, and goats, and human beings may contract the disease from infected animals, although more frequently from infected milk or milk products. Twelve to thirty-six days after exposure, fever and other symptoms are noted. The temperature rises steadily over a period of days, receding temporarily each morning, until a fever of 102° or 103° is reached. It remains at this point for a few days, then steadily drops down, and this cycle may persist for months. Fever periods are accompanied by general malaise, pain, constipation, sweating, and weakness. Undulant fever has occasionally been mistaken for other illnesses with somewhat similar symptoms, such as malaria, typhoid fever, and even tuberculosis.

Until recently, little could be done for the infection, but vaccines now exist which can effectively prevent it, and sulfonamides and antibiotics are helpful in some cases, and other measures, such as heat treatments, have yielded a certain amount of success.

UREMIA, the poisoning which results when the filtering and excretion of wastes from the blood by the kidneys is blocked so that these substances accumulate in the blood. It occurs in acute and chronic forms. The most extreme type is when both kidneys are removed or their excretory channels are blocked. Death then follows in a few days.

An early symptom of uremia is headache, which may be present in annoying severity weeks before other indications of disturbance are perceptible. When the headache is accompanied by restlessness, difficulty in sleeping, nausea, and vomiting, the possibility of uremia definitely exists, and prompt medical attention is imperative.

In its acute form, uremia may attack without warning. A convulsive epileptiform fit followed by coma may be the first manifestation. Sometimes the coma occurs without a fit and in some instances mania seizes the patient. Inflammation of the kidney may occur in children during or after another acute infection, with similar sudden convulsions preceded perhaps by rapid swelling of the tissues and face. The attack may happen so quickly and violently that death ensues. Because of this, doctors watch carefully urine changes in children who have major infections such as pneumonia, acute tonsillitis, or scarlet fever.

In the more slowly developing uremia, the early symptoms are followed by shortness of breath, attendant on accumulation of toxic materials in the body. It is often difficult to distinguish between failing breath due to heart weakness and that accompanying the later stages of kidney disorder. The patient may grow apathetic, drift quietly into unconsciousness, and finally die. Occasionally fluid accumulates, presses upon the lungs, and affects breathing. Similarly fluid may intrude upon the brain and have to be withdrawn by spinal puncture.

In general, treatment of chronic uremia is the same as for chronic nephritis. Acute uremia is often relieved by inducing sweating and by frequent liquid bowel movements, both of which tend to help the body rid itself of excess fluid and liquid wastes. Many uremic patients, with obstructive lesions, are cured by proper treatment, which can include injections of glucose to correct dehydration.

Recent investigation indicates that uremia is probably not the result of accumulating urea in the blood as has been believed for more than a century. In one experiment, the ureters of animals were redirected to empty into the bowel. Some of the urine which would ordinarily be excreted by way of the urinary bladder entered the intestines and part of it was reabsorbed into the blood. Urea in the blood of the animals rose to a remarkable level of fifty times above normal without having any observable effect on them. A tentative conclusion from this experiment is that urea is not toxic enough to bring about the profound and sometimes drastic symptoms found in uremia. *See also* NEPHRITIS.

URETER, a thick-walled muscular tube that passes the urine from the kidney to the bladder. There is one on either side of the pelvis. The ureter acts by a process of contraction or peristalsis that forces urine down the tube in spurts. It is about twelve inches long and about one-fifth of an inch in diameter.

Sometimes a stone may block the ureter and require surgery for its removal. The tube may become twisted or infected, and occasionally it has been ruptured.

Disorders of the ureter or any part of the urinary tract are generally treated by a specialist known as a urologist. When the ureter is affected, x-rays are generally taken, after injection of a substance which causes the ureter to become visible.

URETHRA, the passage from the bladder through which urine is voided. In the male, the urethra is approximately eight inches long, and only an inch and a half in the female. The male urethra begins with a prostatic portion which is surrounded by the prostate gland. It receives ducts through which prostatic secretion and semen are discharged. After a short second part comes the cavernous section which passes through the main body of the penis. It too receives ducts, and recesses emerge from it. Infection of the urethra frequently lodges in these side passages and is difficult to dislodge.

Urethritis, inflammation of the urethra, most frequently the result of gonorrhea, causes a swelling which narrows and partly closes the urethra. The inflammation impedes the flow of urine and the emerging stream may fork or twist. Sometimes the urethra is clogged by a kidney stone or a foreign body which may have to be removed surgically.

Stricture of the urethra requires regular stretching with an instrument designed for the purpose, but sometimes surgical treatment may be needed to open the passage. A stricture of long duration can react on the kidneys and ureters and on the bladder too, causing it to dilate and enlarge abnormally.

The urethra may be ruptured by a severe blow or by an accident, causing urine to escape into nearby tissues.

The female urethra is broader than that of the male and is subject to greater dilatation. Urethral carbuncles are small swellings peculiar to women, and if they do not give any discomfort are best left untouched. If they become tender and painful during urination, they can be removed surgically.

URINATION, technically termed micturition, the passing of urine from the body by the kidneys. A complicated muscular action is involved. The wall of the bladder and another related muscle are contracted. Then a circular muscle around the neck of the bladder which keeps it shut and holds back the urine at all other times is released. The nervous regulation of urination is through a center in the spinal cord. Thus, even an unconscious person can urinate. Complete interruption of urination will bring death in a few days. The spinal center, however, is controlled by the brain, whether during sleeping or waking. Three or four times a day is a normal interval for micturition and ordinarily it is not necessary at night.

Many factors may increase the frequency of urination—for instance, pregnancy, and cold weather. Since less moisture is lost from the skin during cold weather, a greater excretory load is thrown on the urinary system. Other factors may be excitement; inflammation or irritation of the kidney, bladder, or urinary passage; or a growth or presence of a stone within them. In addition, excessive urine may occur in diabetes and nephritis, and acid or other irritants be present in the urine itself.

Diminution of the flow of urine occurs when the prostate gland is enlarged, thus causing contraction of the urethra, the urinary passage leading to the exterior. Complete cessa-

tion may be due to feebleness of the bladder or to an obstruction or interruption of the kidneys' normal formation of urine.

Partially or wholly uncontrolled urination may also arise from several factors. The bladder may have reached its capacity and be unable to hold more, or nervous disorders may induce or permit involuntary urination. Apoplectic or epileptic fits as well as unconsciousness may affect micturition, and sometimes the brain loses its power to regulate the special spinal center.

Occasionally a sense of need to release urine develops when actually the bladder is empty. This condition, dysuria, may come from irritation of the urinary tract or from nervous sources in locomotor ataxia, a disease of the spinal cord. *See also* BED WETTING; BLADDER, URINARY; DIURESIS.

URINE, the watery fluid excreted from the blood by the kidneys, stored in the bladder, and discharged through the urethra. In health, urine is amber-colored and contains urea, inorganic salts, pigments, and other end-products of the metabolism of both protein and minerals in the system. Urine has a somewhat aromatic odor and when it stands for some time ammonia is produced, which is easily recognized by its odor.

The daily quantity of urine may vary in health. In cold weather it may be increased and conversely decreased in hot weather when perspiration removes a large amount of waste products. The quantity is also affected by certain diseases. In diabetes, pints of urine may be excreted each day. In fevers and acute nephritis, urinary output may be greatly lessened. If urine has an ammoniacal odor when excreted, it has undergone decomposition, as occurs in chronic inflammation of the bladder. In diabetes the odor may resemble that of new-mown hay. In certain diseases and disorders, it is essential to determine the quantity of both normal and abnormal constituents of urine, particularly urea. A diminution of urea occurs in nephritis and other disorders. Albumin in urine may be indicative of nephritis or another disorder, but sometimes, as in albuminuria, the cause is physiological. In diabetes the urine is tested to determine the amount of sugar, and another test indicates whether or not blood is present.

The acidity of urine is increased by an ample amount of meat in the diet; large amounts of vegetables make it alkaline. In dyspepsia, when copious amounts of soda are taken, it may also be quite alkaline.

Specific gravity is also tested in diabetes and in diabetes mellitus it is considerably raised. In diabetes insipidus or cirrhosis of the kidney, however, it is quite low. *See also* ALBUMINURIA; HEMATURIA.

UTERUS, a hollow, pear-shaped organ in the female pelvis commonly known as the womb. Within the uterus, the unborn child develops and grows for nine months, nourished by the blood from the mother's body. In the nonpregnant woman, the uterus is about three inches long, but during pregnancy its elastic wall stretches. It returns to normal size after delivery. The uterus is sus-pended in the pelvis by ligaments and opens into the vagina by means of the cervix, a small hollow fibrous tubelike structure situated at the bottom of the uterus. The cervix is a protective passage which shields the rest of the uterus, especially during pregnancy. At delivery it distends to permit expulsion of the fetus. The uterus is a muscular organ, but its lining is a soft glandular material known as endometrium. Bleeding at menstruation comes from this lining. The ovaries are near the uterus, on each side, but do not connect with it. Eggs from the ovary reach the uterus by passing from the top through two armlike projections known as the Fallopian or uterine tubes.

The uterus is prone to infection, especially after childbirth or criminal abortion. Occasionally severe inflammation after abortion may result in permanent sterility, because of destruction of the uterine lining.

Cancer of the uterus occurs most frequently in older women. The symptoms include bleeding, usually between periods or after menopause. Bleeding may occur from less serious sources, such as fibroid growths in the uterine wall. The doctor can usually make the diagnosis by removing tissue from the uterus for examination. This is done by scraping the lining of the uterus. In this procedure sometimes referred to as "D and C," the cervix is dilated and the uterus scraped or curetted. *See also* CANCER; CERVIX; HYSTERECTOMY; and Chapter 17, "Cancer."

URTICARIA. *See* HIVES.

UVULA, the small fleshy conical mass which hangs from the middle of the soft palate in the rear of the mouth. It seldom becomes infected or disturbed.

VACCINATION, inoculation with a preparation containing disease germs or viruses for prevention of ailments caused by these organisms.

When the germs are grown from secretions or blood taken from a patient, so that it contains the strain of organisms responsible for the disease, the vaccine is called autogenous. Usually a vaccine contains killed germs, but sometimes living organisms are used, or a mixed vaccine of a variety of germs or viruses. A vaccine containing several strains of the influenza virus is used to prevent epidemic influenza. The Salk vaccine, which has been widely and effectively employed in immunization for poliomyelitis, is an example of a killed virus. *See also* IMMUNIZATION; VIRUSES; and Chapter 7, "The Process of Infectious Diseases and Immunization of Children"; Chapter 23, "The Neuromuscular and Neurological Disabilities."

VAGINA, the female genital passage or canal which extends from the outer sex organs, or vulva, to the uterus. It consists of muscular tissue which is highly elastic. Inflammation of the vagina occurs in certain venereal infections, such as gonorrhea, or it may be a complication of some other infectious disease, such as scarlet fever or measles. Vaginal discharge is commonly known as leukorrhea or the whites. Vaginismus is a painful spasmodic contraction of the muscles at the entrance to the vagina. *See also* DOUCHE; FISTULA; LEUCORRHEA; and Chapter 11, "Feminine Hygiene."

VARICOSE VEINS, veins which become dilated so that they project in lumpy fashion above the surface of the skin. They are caused by a breakdown of the valves which ordinarily serve to maintain a continuous flow of blood to the heart. These valves cease to function properly, and the blood tends to accumulate at intervals, causing the appearance described.

Varicose veins appear most frequently in the legs, for in this area the blood is required to climb almost straight up on its way to the heart. For the same reason, varicose veins, or hemorrhoids, often develop in the lower part of the bowels.

People who suffer most frequently from varicose veins are those whose blood, for some reason, is failing to circulate in a normal manner. Fat people are susceptible and also pregnant women. After the birth of a child, the interference with normal circulation may terminate. By that time, however, the valves have been broken, and once broken do not repair themselves.

Varicose veins are dangerous because dilation leads to clotting of the blood and therefore to secondary infection.

Occasionally varicosity of the veins can be prevented by proper attention to clothing. The habitual wearing of tight belts or tight garters, for example, should be avoided.

The treatment varies with the patient. Small varicose veins are sometimes emptied of blood and then filled with a fluid which causes the walls of the vein to grow together. In treating the legs, the physician may block off a large vessel in the upper part of the thigh, and so prevent the downward flow of blood into veins which might otherwise become dilated. In some cases this condition can be controlled by the wearing of elastic bandages or stockings.

The current treatment of varicose veins is surgical removal, by stripping and segmental excision. This has largely replaced injection in severe cases; mild cases are generally left untreated. *See also* HEMORRHOIDS.

VEINS, vessels that return blood to the heart, as opposed to arteries which carry blood away from the heart. A vein has a structure like that of an artery, except that the three coats of a vein are thin and inelastic as compared with those of an artery. Many veins, especially those of the lower limbs, are provided with valves which open out when the blood tries to flow backward.

The blood in veins is a dark purplish color, except the blood of the pulmonary veins which is red. It is purified blood carried from the lungs to the heart. All the venous blood from the rest of the body is poured into the heart through two large veins, the vena cava.

Veins generally follow the same course as arteries and many are named after the arteries they accompany.

A wound of the vein is ordinarily less dangerous than a wound of an artery, because the bleeding can be controlled more easily. However, a wound of one of the large veins in the neck or in the armpit is dangerous not only because bleeding may be profuse but also because air may enter the vein and form an embolus, or obstruction. Breathlessness and discomfort may ensue, followed by death within a few seconds if the embolism reaches the lung.

Varicose veins are dilated, hardened, and twisted. Inflammation of a vein that is septic, affected by general reaction of certain bacteria, or simple is phlebitis. *See also* HEMORRHOIDS; PHLEBITIS; THROMBOSIS; VARICOSE VEINS; WOUNDS.

VENEREAL DISEASE. See separate entries for the five venereal diseases, CHANCROID; GONORRHEA; GRANULOMA INGUINALE; LYMPHOGRANULOMA VENEREUM; SYPHILIS.

VENTILATION refers to the circulation or movement of fresh air through rooms and other areas such as halls and stairwells. It is also the process of supplying fresh air or of purifying air.

In natural ventilation, air from an open window, door, or other opening circulates throughout the rooms. If air is forced in or drawn out by a fan or similar apparatus, such as is used in air-conditioning and heating systems, it is described as artificial ventilation.

Good ventilation involves keeping the air free from dust, smoke, odors, and gases. Under normal circumstances, correct use of doors or windows provides a good supply of fresh air. Proper heating and provision of sufficient moisture in the air should be considered. A comfortable house temperature varies in summer from 70° to 85° F. and in winter from 68° to 70,° with sufficient moisture in the air to produce a relative humidity of 30 to 60 per cent.

Investigations which studied the relationship between ventilation and occurrence of the common cold among school children revealed that colds were less frequent in naturally ventilated rooms than in those artificially ventilated. Of course, it is not possible to naturally ventilate many places, such as theaters and large office buildings; and for the person who suffers from hay fever, air conditioning has the advantage of keeping the air free of spores and dust.

VERMIFORM APPENDIX. Vermiform means worm-shaped, and vermiform appendix designates the worm-shaped tube or sac extending from the cecum. The vermiform appendix is commonly referred to simply as appendix. *See also* APPENDICITIS.

VERTEBRA, one of a number of small movable bones which make up the spinal column or backbone. Each vertebra is an irregular bone, the parts of which are: the body, the neural arch through which runs the spinal cord; the spinous process, which is the tip that can be seen or felt by running a finger up and down the spine; and the lateral projections or transverse processes, which provide attachment points for the ligaments and muscles of the back.

The vertebrae have different functions and are described according to location. The seven cervical vertebrae constitute the neck; the twelve thoracic vertebrae form the chest region; and the five movable lumbar vertebrae are found in the middle of the lower back. The sacrum contains five vertebrae, fused together, and the coccyx consists of four vertebrae united as one bone at the end of the spine.

The vertebral joints have cartilage on their adjoining surfaces; and an intervertebral disc, composed also of plates of cartilage, lies between each of two movable vertebrae.

Various disorders involve the vertebrae and vertebral discs. Mechanical imperfections may affect the sacrum and the fifth lumbar vertebra. At the joining site, the nerves may become the seat of low back pain. Spondylolisthesis, also known as swayback, affects the stability of the lower spine, and a slipped disc or injury may affect the intervertebral disc, also causing low back pain. Fractures or protrusions may also occur in connection with intervertebral discs. Tuberculosis of the spine or calcification can implicate or even destroy the discs. *See also* DISC; SLIPPED DISC; SPINAL CORD; SPINE; SPONDYLOLISTHESIS.

VERTIGO. When a person has the sensation that the outside world is revolving around him, or that he is moving in space, he has vertigo. There are various causes for vertigo. For example, a common type occurs when a person looks down from a height or up at a height. Other types are epileptic vertigo and intestinal vertigo. Vertigo is not the same as dizziness or giddiness, which designates a feeling of disturbed relation to the surroundings.

VINCENT'S ANGINA, variously known as trench mouth, Borrelia, and ulcerative stomatitis, an infection of the mouth and throat due to a peculiar spiral organism. It was first described in 1898 by Jean H. Vincent, a French physician, and since then the germ has been known as Vincent's organism. Apparently the infection is found only in man. Infants or adults who have lost their teeth are seldom affected.

In Vincent's angina, sores or ulcers occur on the lining of the cheeks and gums, sometimes also on the tonsils and in the back of the throat. The ulcers may become so large as to incapacitate the infected person. A typical unpleasant mouth odor accompanies the ailment. While the disease often begins with local symptoms, headache and a general feeling of illness may also be present. Pain in swallowing, membrane in the mouth and in the throat are characteristic. Because of this membrane, the disease was once often mistaken for diphtheria.

Vincent's angina is easily spread to other persons through kissing and through contaminated articles such as towels and eating utensils. Cases have been reported in which it has been spread by improperly sterilized dental instruments. An infected child should not go to school until he is cured, although isolation in the home is not necessary.

Prevention of Vincent's angina demands constant watchfulness of the condition of the mouth, teeth, and gums. Persistent bleeding of the gums, the appearance of an unpleasant odor, or occurrence of ulcers in the mouth demands consultation with a dentist or physician. Control of the infection is much easier in the early stages than later when the condition has become chronic.

Poor teeth and negligence of mouth hygiene are the prime causes of Vincent's angina. Conditions such as scurvy, diabetes, lead or bismuth poisoning, and syphilis may produce ulcers and damage to the mouth and gums, with Vincent's angina as a secondary condition.

The infection is treated according to the symptoms. Crystalline penicillin has proved beneficial, and solutions of hydrogen peroxide or perborate of soda are soothing as a mouthwash and of aid in destroying the Vincent's organism. In some instances, injections of arsenical preparations directly into the veins are beneficial. Care, however, is imperative, because of danger of chemical burns of the tender gums and lining of the cheeks.

VIRUSES, the smallest and most elusive of the infectious agents, have been established as causative of more than fifty different infectious diseases of man. All forms of life may be affected by virus infection—animals, plants, birds, and insects, and even bacteria, are subject to injury and disintegration by viruses, known as bacteriophages.

Viruses are so infinitesimally small that they can pass through porcelain filters which hold back ordinary bacteria, though the larger viruses pass through with difficulty. Most of them can be seen only through a powerful electron microscope. Viruses are composed of tiny particles and differ from each other in total size, structure, and stability, from the smallest organism, responsible for foot-and-mouth disease and poliomyelitis, to the largest, which causes parrot infection or psittacosis and which can be seen with an ordinary microscope to resemble the larger bacteria. The shapes vary from the spherical head and long tail of the bacteriophage to the sphere of the influenza virus and the cube of the smallpox virus.

Viruses thrive in the presence of living cells, becoming an intimate part of living body tissues which they damage, and are parasites, completely dependent for their existence upon this close intracellular association. They multiply only in young susceptible living cells and cannot be grown in artificial media unless living cells are present. This has made it difficult to study their growth habits, or to prepare vaccines for preventive treatment.

Each virus shows its specific type of action only upon certain tissues. For example, the virus of rabies does not become active in the body until it reaches the tissues of the nerves and brain. Different viruses which attack the human body are classified according to the part of the body for which they have an affinity. Dermatropic viruses affect the skin; pneumotropic viruses involve the lungs; neurotropic viruses attack nervous tissue; and viscerotropic viruses harm the internal organs or viscera. Among the more familiar diseases caused by viruses are the common cold, measles, German measles, chickenpox, mumps, rabies, poliomyelitis, influenza, encephalitis, smallpox, and yellow fever. A number of other ailments, among them the so-called "virus pneumonia," glandular fever, and epidemic nausea and vomiting, have also been attributed to viral infections.

Virus diseases are conveyed in a variety of ways. The common cold, measles, smallpox, chickenpox, and influenza are probably transmitted by direct contact, as well as by airborne droplets of nasal and salivary secretions. Rabies is carried through the bite or wound produced by an infected animal. Mosquitoes, fleas, ticks, and other insects are carriers, as in yellow fever and in some of the encephalitic infections. Rarely have viral infections been spread by contaminated water or food, although transmission of infectious hepatitis has been traced to water, as well as milk, in some instances.

The fact that the virus becomes an intimate part of the cells of the body has made treatment of viral infections more difficult. Those substances which have thus far been found capable of destroying virus can, unfortunately, also damage body tissues and are too toxic for practical use. Some of the newer antibiotics, such as aureomycin, terramycin, and chloromycetin, have proved effective in treatment of psittacosis and trachoma. The antibiotics may have some value in treatment of measles, chickenpox, and influenza, if not directly upon the virus, at least in combatting any secondary invasion by bacteria, which often occurs in viral infections and aggravates the condition.

Until now, the most encouraging efforts to combat virus infections have been directed toward the establishment of immunity to viral diseases. Immunity is the ability of living tissue to resist and overcome infection. One way of acquiring immunity to a viral disease is to have had that infection. Measles, chickenpox, smallpox, and a few other viral diseases confer a lasting immunity. Immunity for flu, cold, and herpes simplex or fever blisters has not yet been found.

Immunity may be produced artificially by two means. First is the introduction into the body of a vaccine. This substance is composed of weakened viruses which have been submitted to a chemical or other process and are called attenuated viruses. While the virus can still produce diseases in the body, this ability has been materially weakened. However, the vaccine stimulates development in the body of antibodies, a process known as vaccination or active immunization, and in general it induces a high degree of immunity and tends to be lasting.

The second means of producing an immunity is by injection of an immune serum, gamma globulin, or the blood serum of an immune animal or man. Production of immunity by this method is called passive immunization because the person involved does not take an active part in the development of resistance to the disease, but rather receives into his body a substance already containing the essential antibodies. Passive immunity is temporary.

The use of gamma globulin in measles, provided it is given early in the incubation period, has been successful in modifying the severity of that disease. It has also been helpful during the early stages of infectious hepatitis. In poliomyelitis, gamma globulin has been used in children in an attempt to prevent the disease or at least to avert the paralytic complications. The work of Dr. Jonas Salk of the University of Pittsburgh Medical School and his associates has led to the historic development of a polio vaccine that furnishes active immunization—that is, the vaccine causes the body to set up its own defenses against the disease. This is the type of immunization that has overcome smallpox, diphtheria, and whooping cough. *See also* INFECTIONS; INFECTIOUS DISEASES; IMMUNITY; IMMUNIZATION; POLIOMYELITIS; VACCINATION; and Chapter 7, "The Process of Infectious Diseases and Immunization of Children"; Chapter 23, "The Neuromuscular and Neurological Disabilities."

VITAMINS, substances which are found in foods in minute quantities and which are indispensable to the normal functioning of the body. When they are deficient or lacking in the diet, or lost through cooking or processing, certain specific disorders, known as deficiency diseases, occur. About seventeen vitamins are known, and deficiencies of about half of them are definitely causative of disease in human beings. The seventeen vitamins are: vitamins A, C or ascorbic acid, D, E, K, P, and the members of the B complex group, including B_1 or thiamine, B_2 or vitamin G or riboflavin, nicotinic acid or niacin, B_6 or pyroxidine, pantothenic acid, biotin, folic acid, B_{12}, choline, inositol and para-aminobenzoic acid.

Vitamin A is manufactured in the body from carotene, which is found in fish liver oil, green vegetables, egg yolk, butter, and many orange- or yellow-colored foods. One of the first signs of a vitamin A deficiency is night blindness, reduced capacity of the eye to adapt to the dark. A characteristic disease of the eye, usually called xerophthalmia, results from this deficiency, and a thickening of the skin, hyperkeratosis. Vitamin A deficiency usually occurs in persons who subsist largely on a starchy diet, but disturbances of the intestinal tract which prevent effective absorption of vitamin A can also cause it, as well as conditions of pregnancy, infancy, and lactation, when the need for vitamin A increases. If a generous serving of a yellow or green leafy vegetable cannot be included in the daily diet, a teaspoon of fish liver oil instead insures an adequate supply of vitamin A.

B vitamins are found naturally in vegetables and grains, meat and milk. Each vitamin in this group has a particular function to perform in the complicated metabolism of the body. Part of these vitamins are destroyed by cooking or processing, but generous portions of vegetables and grains in the diet provide adequate amounts.

Thiamine or vitamin B_1 deficiencies, beriberi, result most frequently from diets composed largely of refined or polished grain, as in the Orient. Beriberi is quite rare in the United States.

Thiamine is also useful to correct and prevent the loss of appetite that accompanies many forms of digestive disorder. Frequently conditions are noted in which thiamine, although taken into the body, is not properly absorbed. For example, in case of

vomiting, when the person must be fed by tubes, when a paralysis of the muscles associated with swallowing is present, or in the case of excessive alcoholism, it may be imperative to inject extra amounts of thiamine directly into the body. Other conditions in which extra thiamine is required are excessive action of the thyroid gland, fever, or vigorous muscular activities, which use more thiamine than is ordinarily available.

Most symptoms of thiamine deficiency disappear when the vitamin in pure form in combination with other vitamins is administered. Yeast, whole-grain cereals, liver and pork are good sources of thiamine.

Vitamin B_2, riboflavin, deficiencies are found most frequently among persons who live on diets largely composed of starches, and the deficiency is common in the southeastern United States, the West Indies, the Orient, and parts of Africa and India.

Symptoms of riboflavin deficiency may be weakness and disturbances of the vision, skin, tongue, mouth, lips, and face. To correct the deficiency, foods high in riboflavin, such as liver, egg, milk and whole-grain cereals, must be added to the diet. In treating acute cases, pure riboflavin alone is seldom effective, since, as in most deficiency conditions, more than a single vitamin is lacking.

An inadequate amount of nicotinic acid, or niacin, in the diet can cause pellagra, which occurs in most areas of the world, and was once the major form of acute vitamin deficiency in the United States, especially prevalent in the South. Discovery that niacin is a specific in treatment of pellagra was a major step toward combatting this widespread deficiency. Niacin helps to correct the condition and to cure the symptoms which involve the skin, digestion, and nervous system. Until the discovery that nicotinic acid could cure pellagra, two-thirds of all patients died from the condition. Today the death rate is low. In acute cases of pellagra, the vitamin is given in high-level doses. Meat, particularly liver, wholegrain cereals, and peanuts are good sources of niacin.

Cobalt is a chief chemical ingredient of vitamin B_{12}, which has a blood-stimulating activity, similar to that of the anti-anemic factor of liver. It is therefore especially valuable in treating pernicious anemia and sprue, as well as anemia resulting from its deficiency. Although inadequate diets are occasionally responsible for deficiencies of vitamin B_{12} and folic acid, more often the deficiency is caused by some impairment in absorption or utilization of the vitamin in the body.

Other vitamins of the B complex group are vitamin B_6, pantothenic acid, biotin, choline, inositol, and para-aminobenzoic acid. A deficiency of vitamin B_6 can cause neuritis, skin eruptions and sore tongue, nervousness and depression. It is widely employed in the treatment of nausea and vomiting in pregnant women.

Ascorbic acid, vitamin C, the anti-scurvy vitamin, is found abundantly in citrus fruits and juices, tomatoes, potatoes, and leafy vegetables. This vitamin is responsible for the manufacture by the body of the material which cements teeth into position. An infant with a vitamin C deficiency is likely to suffer from fever, diarrhea, loss of weight, vomiting, and have a generally low resistance and probably intestinal bleeding. In children, the bones may be malformed. Most of the symptoms of the deficiency disappear rapidly when the vitamin is administered. All fresh fruits and vegetables contain some vitamin C and to prevent recurrence of the deficiency the diet must include these foods.

Vitamin D, or ergosterol, is manufactured in the body from a combination of chemically related substances, and is essential for the formation and growth of bones and teeth and for the utilization of calcium and phosphorus in the body. It is often called the sunshine vitamin because of the abundance supplied by the sun through its action on the skin, and the person who gets enough sunshine each day receives sufficient amounts of vitamin D.

Vitamin D deficiency causes rickets in children, and in adults it results in improper utilization of calcium in the bones and produces a condition known as osteomalacia. These disorders can be corrected by adequate amounts of calcium and vitamin D. Cod liver oil, vitamin D concentrates, and sunshine or ultraviolet irradiation are effective in promoting a rapid improvement in rickets. Other good sources of vitamin D are eggs, salmon and tuna fish, and milk.

Vitamin E is found abundantly in wheat germ oil, and in adequate amounts in liver, eggs, whole-grain cereals, and lettuce. Experiments with animals have indicated that a deficiency of vitamin E may be associated with sterility and miscarriages; however, it has not been determined whether or not vitamin E deficiencies occur in human beings.

Vitamin K has significant antihemorrhagic properties, and deficiencies of it usually involve the clotting of blood. It is useful in treating obstructive jaundice, hemorrhage which results in certain intestinal disorders, and in hemorrhagic conditions affecting newborn infants. In treating coronary thrombosis, vitamin K together with the drug dicumarol is also of value, since dicumarol affects the action of vitamin K and consequently the clotting of blood. Green vegetables are rich in this vitamin.

Also known as hesperedin, vitamin P is found in the rind of citrus fruits. Whether a deficiency of vitamin P can exist has not yet been determined. The vitamin has been used in connection with vitamin C in cases of abnormal bleeding.

The significance of vitamins cannot be overemphasized, and certain basic foods should appear in the diet each day, notably milk, meat, green leafy vegetables, citrus fruits, and wholegrain products. If the diet furnishes adequate quantities of vitamins, vitamin supplements are not necessary for the average person. A doctor should be consulted if any deficiency exists.

See also NUTRITION; and Chapter 4, "Diet and Health."

VITILIGO, a pigmentary disorder in which the coloring matter disappears in spots from the skin. These spots then appear white, in contrast to the normal coloring of the rest of the skin. Sometimes this condition is an indirect result of another disease of the skin, but usually it occurs without apparent cause.

Vitiligo occurs commonly among Negroes. While not generally considered dangerous, it is often badly disfiguring. This disease sometimes disappears spontaneously.

In about 15 per cent of the cases of vitiligo, repigmentation can be induced by a drug derived from an Egyptian plant called Ammi majus, together with treatment by exposure to sunlight or artificial ultraviolet rays. This must be prescribed by a physician. Persons who have been so treated have relatively small areas of depigmentation when the spots have been present less than five years.

If 80 per cent of the skin surface is depigmented, it is often practical to extend the condition to the entire body by treating the skin with a special compound. The hair and eyes are not affected as in albinism.

VOCAL CORDS. *See* LARYNGITIS; LARYNX.

VOICE BOX. *See* LARYNX.

VOMITING, the forceful ejection of the contents of the stomach through the mouth. The possible causes are innumerable. Vomiting by a person who is seasick is probably caused by a disturbance in the organs of balance. Vomiting may be set off by a severe pain, such as a sharp blow to the abdomen. Psychological factors related to the senses may also produce vomiting, such as an unpleasant smell, a displeasing sight, or even an unkind remark.

When vomiting is imminent, certain nerves are stimulated and a valve in the lower part of the stomach, customarily employed to pass food to the bowels, is then automatically closed. Following this, a chain of waves passes through the wall of the stomach, moving not downward as usual but upward. The person inhales deeply and the climax is a powerful contraction of both the diaphragm and stomach. Whatever happens to be in the stomach is then thrown through the esophagus and out of the mouth. Vomiting may happen so suddenly that some of the material emerges through the nose.

While vomiting is not a disease, it is often a symptom of illness. If vomiting persists, or the matter ejected has traces of blood, a doctor should be consulted to locate and treat the cause.

VULVA, the external sexual organs of the female.

Inflammation of the vulva or vulvitis may result from infection, but often is associated with various skin disorders. In children and in obese women, acute vulvitis results from uncleanliness and from constant irritation. It is characterized by redness, swelling, burning, irritation, and sometimes by itching which may spread to the surrounding areas. The treatment depends on the cause.

In leukoplakia, white thickened areas of the skin are found, usually in the region of the clitoris, labia, or perineum. This condition may also be accompanied by itching. Proper medication is needed promptly to cure these conditions.

In the rare cases of cancer of the vulva, leukoplakia is often the fore-runner. Early diagnosis is essential for a successful treatment by x-ray, radium, surgery, or combinations of these methods.

WASSERMANN TEST, a test used to determine whether or not a person has syphilis. Only a modification of the original test is now used. The test was named after the German physician August von Wassermann. Various modifications, such as the Kahn test, the Eagle test, and the Hinton test, are also used.

In the test, the blood serum and sometimes the cerebrospinal fluid are examined. A positive reaction indicates the presence of syphilis. Tests are also made at frequent intervals during the course of the disease, to determine its progress and the effectiveness of treatment. *See also* KAHN TEST.

WATER, the chemical combination of hydrogen and oxygen, H_2O. Two-thirds of the weight of the body is water and about 75 per cent of the protoplasm, the material surrounding the nuclei of the cells. Water is essential to life and is found in large proportion in most foods. In the body, water transports food elements to the cells. It is removed from the body as waste by the action of the kidneys and the urinary system, the sweat glands, the lungs, and the bowels.

Insufficient production of certain types of hormones in the glands results in a disturbance of the distribution of water and salt in the body. This disturbance is reflected by an excessive loss of water in the urine, a condition known as diuresis, which results in dehydration of the body.

Water may be a carrier of disease-producing bacteria, notably bacteria causing typhoid, cholera, and dysentery. When a dependable municipal water supply does not exist, the individual must insure the purity of his own water. Boiling the water to destroy disease-producing organisms is often the simplest method. Aeration and filtering with charcoal help to remove undesirable tastes and odors. Chlorine tablets can be dissolved in water to purify it, and home filter systems that utilize sand beds several feet thick through which the water passes are also effective.

Spring water should be used only after the spring has been cleaned and the water tested for bacteria. Shallow wells must be walled and a good pumping system installed. Deep well water is generally pure but its source and purity must be tested and expert advice on sanitation sought. Cisterns should be screened against mosquitoes and the water boiled or purified in some way before it is used. Proper sewage disposal is always necessary to safeguard the purity of any water supply system, whether public or private. *See also* FLUORIDATION.

WEN, a sac formed in the skin when the sebum, the fatty material excreted by the skin's sebaceous or oil glands, is obstructed and cannot escape to the skin surface normally. Physicians call such a sac a sebaceous cyst. If not removed, the material within the sac or cyst interacts with the blood and changes from a rather solid mass to one that is semifluid, and may develop an offensive odor.

Since a wen may continue to grow as long as the blockage continues and infection does not occur, it may reach the size of a golf ball or even larger. With a minimum of surgery a doctor can drain the material from the cyst and eliminate the blockage which caused it.

If, however, infection has occurred, merely cutting an opening for drainage is insufficient. Sebaceous matter will continue to be secreted by the inner wall of the sac which will harden, collect, and repeat the initial process. Removal of the entire internal wall of the cyst by surgery may be essential to prevent recurrence of an infected wen.

WHITE BLOOD CELLS. *See* BLOOD; and Chapter 13, "Diseases of the Blood."

WHITFIELD'S OINTMENT, a widely used preparation compounded of salicylic and benzoic acids and petrolatum. The mixture is useful as a fungicide following mechanical removal of the nail in ringworm of the nail, and also in other fungus infections of the skin such as "athlete's foot." Whitfield's ointment is quite strong and should be used with care. It should not be applied to acutely inflamed oozing lesions of the skin, and is best reserved for use in older, scaly lesions.

WHOOPING COUGH, or pertussis, a disease characterized by a convulsive cough, and infecting the mucous membrane of the respiratory system. The cough leaves the patient out of breath and the resultant deep inhalation produces the whooping sound.

The disease is not a trivial affliction of childhood. Coupled with a secondary infection, such as bronchopneumonia, whooping cough can be fatal, especially in young children or the aged. The most frequent victims, however, are children under five.

During the first ten days of this disease, the incubation period, the child exhibits the symptoms of an ordinary cold. The cough, however, does not improve. The second stage begins with the onset of the whooping sound. During a coughing spell the face may grow scarlet while the facial veins swell and tears appear in the eyes. The cough may be followed by vomiting.

Whooping cough is caused by the germ Hemophilus pertussis. To ascertain the presence of this germ, modern science requires the child to cough on a special culture plate on which the germs are then examined. The same test may be used as a proof that the child is finally free of the germ and no longer needs to be isolated. This is the primary purpose of the test. Diagnosis, as well as pronouncement of cure, may be determined by other means. A blood test may be made, since one of the characteristics of whooping cough is an increase in the number of single-nucleus white blood cells. However, the whooping sound in itself is a fairly reliable guide for a doctor.

The prevention of whooping cough primarily involves immunization which is now accomplished by a series of injections which combine immunity against diphtheria and tetanus as well. Only infants and children need to be injected.

If a child develops whooping cough, isolation of the child is necessary, chiefly to prevent secondary infection in the child and exposure of other children. In some cases of children under two or three years of age, antibiotics are used, but older children generally recover without the use of drugs. If convulsions occur, as sometimes happens, the doctor may place the child in an oxygen tent and sedative drugs such as phenobarbital may be given. Treatment requires complete rest as well as constant protection of the patient's lungs from atmospheric irritants such as tobacco smoke or cold drafts of air. The inhalation of steam is sometimes advised, as well as certain drugs which relieve the severity of the coughing attacks. If coughing places a great strain on the stomach muscles, a rubber binder may be worn around that area. It is better to praise the child for coughing less than to pity him for coughing more. Commiseration is not the best medicine.

Finally, special attention should be given to the patient's diet, particularly to that of children, who are susceptible to vomiting and therefore to undernourishment. Generally speaking, the child requires nutritious food which is also easy to digest. The best time for meals is approximately a quarter of an hour after a coughing spell. The child should eat in small amounts, perhaps several times a day. To feed him a large amount of food at any one time is likely to stimulate coughing, whereupon the food which has been eaten will be regurgitated.

Starchy foods—bread, pastries,

and potatoes—should be avoided, as well as any dry and crumbly foods which might tickle the throat and produce a cough. Vegetable soup is recommended, and also meat in small amounts, provided that it is carefully chopped or strained. Fresh fruit juices and plenty of plain drinking water are also to be given. *See also* Chapter 7, "The Process of Infectious Diseases and Immunization of children."

WILM'S TUMOR, a malignant growth that affects the kidneys of children, usually under six years of age. It may grow to great size and cause the child's abdomen to protrude. Sometimes the doctor can feel the tumor with his fingers before such symptoms as pain or blood in the urine appear. Other symptoms are weakness and vomiting.

Removal of the affected kidney followed by radiation is the best means of curing this condition. If the tumor is large, it may be necessary first to treat it with radiation, then follow with surgery and postoperative radiation.

WOMB. *See* UTERUS.

WORMS. Several types of worms live parasitically in the human body, usually in some part of the digestive tract. Although the United States has relatively high sanitation and hygienic standards, various kinds of worm infestation are common in some areas. A study of children in the District of Columbia, for example, revealed that 35 to 65 per cent of certain groups had pinworm infestation, and another study reported that 50 to 60 per cent of children in different parts of the southern United States had intestinal worms.

Some worms attain remarkable size, such as the beef tapeworm which may reach a length of fifteen feet; whereas others, such as the worm which causes trichinosis, are so thin and small that they are barely visible to the naked eye. Often worms are present in the bowels without causing any serious symptoms. However, sometimes they may produce general and far-reaching disturbances.

Pinworm. The pinworm is easily the most widely distributed of worms which live as parasites in human hosts. Known also as the seat or threadworm, it exists only in the form of a human parasite. The adult worm, which is white, may be as long as half an inch down to a quarter of that size. Infestation occurs when worm eggs are taken into the body. They may enter through the mouth from fingers which have touched some contaminated surface, or may be inhaled, for the eggs are so small and light that they can float in the air. From the mouth the eggs pass to the small intestine where they hatch and begin a life cycle that takes about two months. They mature in the intestine and eventually mating occurs. The males then leave the body of the host, but the females migrate to the large bowel where the eggs develop. Finally, when the eggs are ready to be deposited for hatching, the female passes out of the body through the lower end of the digestive tract, leaving behind several thousand eggs on the skin surface just outside the anal opening.

The itching in and around the affected areas is usually the most disturbing symptom of pinworm infestation. In females, the worms sometimes travel to the genital area. The eggs may be widely distributed in the bed, bedclothes, pajamas, and other clothing. When the person scratches the affected area, the worms get under the fingernails and the infection process begins again. Pinworms sometimes become so troublesome that they affect appetite and thus cause loss of weight.

Scrupulous cleanliness is absolutely necessary in the elimination of pinworm, and a daily bath is essential. Since the eggs, the source of infection and reinfection, are distributed so widely and so easily, the entire family should be placed under the doctor's care at the same time, so that reinfection does not pass constantly from infected to uninfected persons.

The drugs used against pinworm can be given only by a doctor's prescription and under his care. Enemas with a chemical called hexylresorcinol are given; a dyestuff, gentian violet, may be given internally; and antiseptic ointments for affected external areas may be prescribed by the doctor. The amount and manner of application of these remedies will vary with each case and must always be determined by the doctor.

Roundworm. After the pinworm, the parasite which most frequently infests the human body is the giant intestinal roundworm, scientifically known as Ascaris lumbricoides. The female reaches a length of ten to fifteen inches and the male is about half that size. Like the pinworm, it lives in the digestive tract. Surveys have shown that around the Gulf of Mexico, on the south Atlantic coast, and through the Appalachians about 40 per cent of the children in early grades of school are affected, particularly those in mining camps and rural areas. In the North, the incidence is far less and a check made in Detroit, Michigan, indicated that only 2 per cent of the children were infested.

Normally the symptoms of roundworm infestation are not serious, except that sometimes, particularly when another illness is present, sensitivities resembling those of an allergy may appear. If, however, the affected person becomes ill enough to develop a fever, or if he is treated with drugs, the worms may migrate within the body to places quite remote from their usual habitation. They may appear in the nose, mouth, and have even entered and blocked the appendix, the bile duct, and the Eustachian tubes which connect the throat and the inner ear. If for no other reason, this makes it obviously desirable to rid the body of these parasites.

The worms live within the intestine, where in a single day the females produce as many as 200,000 eggs, a million and a half each week. Once outside the body of the host, these eggs are ready to hatch in from two to four weeks. On the surface of the ground and in moist shaded spots they can and do survive in this state for months. When the eggs are taken into the human body, almost always because of lack of simple sanitary precautions, they pass first to the small intestine where they hatch. The larvae burrow through the intestinal wall, reach the liver, and finally pass to the lungs. From the lungs they are coughed up into the mouth, swallowed again, and are returned to the intestines where they remain. The total period of development is from four to six weeks and the worm may live in the body for another six months.

Although the consequences of infestation are not particularly alarming, the possible secondary effects are such that the condition should be eliminated. Here again, treatment is strictly the responsibility of a doctor. Hexylresorcinol has been found to be especially effective against the giant roundworm. The stomach is first emptied of its contents by purgation and abstinence from food for at least twelve hours. After the drug is given, the person must not eat for another five hours or more, and only semifluid foods are recommended for the next five hours. At the end of twenty-four hours, a cathartic is taken to wash all residual material from the bowel. Ordinarily one such treatment satisfactorily disposes of worms.

Hookworm. Infestation by hookworm, necator americanus, presents a more serious situation than that of the pinworm or roundworm. The hookworm does specific and substantial damage within the body. In extreme cases it may permanently disable a person or even bring about death. There are still sizable areas of the United States where it is a real public health problem, notably the whole coastal area from North Carolina through the eastern Gulf shore of Texas and as far inland as part of the Appalachians.

The organism itself is about the size of the pinworm, a little less than half an inch long, and the female is slightly larger than the male. The most serious damage that the hookworm does is to fasten itself by its teeth to the bowel wall and secrete a poisonous fluid which at the same time dilates the small blood vessels there and prevents coagulation of the blood. The worm feeds by drawing blood, of which it uses only a small amount for its own nourishment, letting the remainder pass through its system, relatively unaffected, and then out with the digestive waste of the host. When the number of parasitic worms is large, the person will suffer from anemia, weakness, and lassitude. Although his appetite may be increased, he usually loses interest in activity, his face is dull and his hair lusterless. If left untreated, the condition may in time cause invalidism or even death.

This worm may have other adverse effects on the human body, as it makes its way from the surface inward by a route much more complex than that of the roundworm. The female hookworm lays from 6,000 to 15,000 eggs daily and these pass from an infected human being to the ground. Most infested persons have picked up the worms by exposure to infected soil. The larvae penetrate the skin and produce, first of all, a severe local condition on the skin called "ground itch." At the point of entry, they penetrate a blood vessel and are carried in the blood stream to the lungs. Within the lungs they break out in the open space, climb the bronchial tubes to the throat and are swallowed, and eventually reach the small intestine where the adult worm finally develops. Here the females begin to lay eggs and when these appear in the person's excretions the developmental process of the worm is completed. The cycle takes about six weeks from the time the larvae penetrate the skin. During passage through the lungs, the larvae may induce a bronchial inflammation accompanied by fever.

Fortunately hookworm is easily diagnosed and treated. Examination of the patient's bowel waste by the doctor will readily reveal the eggs. A number of remedies which will eradicate the worms from the digestive tract, including hexylresorcinol, tetrachlorethylene, and oil of chemopodium, are effective. All of these drugs are toxic and must be administered only by a physician.

In areas where hookworm is most prevalent, it is possible to avoid infestation by taking simple precautions. Shoes should always be worn, and excrement should be disposed of in such a way that the larvae from the excreted eggs are not scattered about. This can easily be done by providing places for disposal that are sufficiently deep, since the larvae cannot climb vertically to any considerable height.

Tapeworm. Of several types and sizes, tapeworms are among the most common intestinal worms which invade human beings. They vary in size from the beef tapeworm, which can reach a length of fifteen feet, to the dwarf tapeworm which never measures more than a few centimeters. More than thirty species affect human beings, but only six are really common.

Tapeworms are not actually single worms, but are in fact colonies of worms. The first segment serves as the head and other members are separate and hitched to each other, end to end. Each of these individual segments, called proglottids, contains little more than the required equipment of sexual reproduction, since feeding by absorption of predigested nutriment from the host eliminates the need for digestive apparatus. Fertilization may be between a male and female element of a single proglottid or between one proglottid and the next. Fertilized eggs remain within the worm and eventually the proglottid breaks off and is passed to the outside with the waste material.

The most common way in which human beings are infested by tapeworm is by eating the meat of animals that have eaten either the fertilized eggs or a discharged proglottid, then incubated the eggs in their intestine where later the tapeworm larvae develop and finally invade the muscle tissue. The same sequence of development may ensue with the beef tapeworm when cattle have been pastured where there is contaminated human excrement. If beef from such cattle is consumed either raw or partially cooked, the live worm may be taken into the person's body. The beef tapeworm reaches fifteen feet in length and the numbers of its separate parts may be as many as 2,000, of which approximately the lower half will at any one time be bearers of fertilized eggs.

The life history of the pork tapeworm is essentially the same, with some biological variations. Its maximum growth is usually ten feet and the number of parts about 1,000. Infestation is from eating improperly cooked meat from hogs which have consumed infected human sewage. This type is infrequent in the United States but common in Mexico, parts of Latin America, and in some areas of Asia.

The fish tapeworm, with somewhat more substantial differences, experiences the same life cycle within a fish as the other types. This worm does not release whole pregnant proglottids but mature individual eggs which discharge embryos capable of swimming. They enter the water through infected human waste. The embryos are eaten by water fleas and the water fleas by fish. The fish become infected and, if eaten raw, will transmit the infection to man. Sometimes there is an intermediate stage, in which the infected fish is eaten by a larger fish which in turn becomes human food and transmits the infestation. A few areas of fish tapeworm infestation have been found in the United States, but it occurs more frequently in Europe.

Dwarf tapeworms, which measure less than an inch, affect children more often than adults. Dog and rat tapeworms, while of some medical interest, are so rare as to be of little concern to laymen.

Several effective substances are available which can be used by the physician to rid the host of tapeworms. As in the other treatments, the person must abstain from food for a day or a few days while taking the drug. Recovery of the top end of the worm from the bowel waste usually is considered to constitute elimination of the worms. A person who has a tapeworm may have only a few mild symptoms or he may have more severe attacks. The condition often begins with diarrhea, which then alternates with constipation. False hunger pains are characteristic, although the appetite may sometimes diminish. The person loses weight and secondary anemia appears, and still later symptoms may disappear entirely. The victim of beef tapeworm is likely to experience discomfort when the proglottids pass through the rectum. In every case, the diagnosis can be made easily and with certainty by examination of the excrement.

WOUNDS. Any injury that breaks the skin, mucous membrane, or inner surface of the tissues of the body is a wound. Although fractures and bruises are wounds, the term usually is applied to the following:

Cut or incision, a slash or slit in the skin caused by a sharp cutting object, such as a razor blade. This type of wound bleeds profusely, since all the blood vessels are cleanly severed. There is usually little tissue damage, and less danger from infection than in other wounds. A deep cut may possibly sever tendons and nerves.

Laceration or torn wound, an irregular tearing of the tissue by a rough or blunt or jagged-edged object. A laceration might result from a fall against an angular object or piece of machinery. Bleeding is usually not severe, as the blood vessels are irregularly torn, but danger of infection exists because bleeding is often slight and body tissues are damaged at the edge of the wound.

Puncture and stab wound, caused by a penetrating object, such as a nail, bullet, or splinter. Unless a large blood vessel is injured, puncture wounds do not bleed profusely. They are especially liable to infection, since they are difficult to clean.

Abrasion, rubbing off or scraping of skin or mucous membrane, commonly called "floor burn" or "mat burn" although not a true burn. They usually cover a wide surface and so are easily infected.

Severe bleeding or hemorrhage and infection are two dangers to be considered with wounds. If a wound is bleeding profusely, the first step is to attempt to control the bleeding. Bleeding may be from a vein, an artery, or both. When an artery is cut, the blood spurts out. Blood from a cut vein comes in a steady flow, since the blood is under much lower pressure than arterial blood.

Venous bleeding is easier to control than arterial bleeding. Pressure should be applied to the edges of the wound until a compress can be obtained. Usually venous bleeding can be stopped by placing a compress over the wound and bandaging it snugly. If necessary, hand pressure firmly applied directly on the compress will help a clot to form. The injured area should be elevated, unless a fracture accompanies the wound.

In arterial bleeding, if someone is present who has knowledge of the pressure points of the body, this method of controlling hemorrhage is first attempted. A pressure point is some point between the wound and heart where the main artery of the injured area lies close to a bone; hand or finger pressure against the bone may stop bleeding. A dressing or

other material is pressed firmly against the wound. If the bleeding stops, the dressing should be bandaged into position and left undisturbed.

If the firmly pressed gauze dressing does not stop bleeding, a tourniquet may be necessary. *Since a tourniquet cuts off the total blood supply to the area, it is applied only when other methods fail.* In the absence of a ready-made tourniquet, a rolled handkerchief, belt, or other substitute may be used. Anything which would cut the skin, such as wire or cord, should not be used. If circulation is stopped for too long, there is danger of gangrene, and so the tourniquet should never be left in place for more than an hour.

In all cases of serious hemorrhage, the injured person should be kept lying down and quiet, since movement might disturb the blood clot. He should be treated for shock, which is nearly always present, and a doctor called.

Most cases of serious infection and blood poisoning develop from a seemingly insignificant wound which has not been correctly treated. Since danger of infection is present any time the skin is broken, even the smallest wound should receive proper attention. In cases of severe bleeding, the first step is, of course, to control the hemorrhage. Infection is characterized by heat, pain, swelling, redness, and often pus formation, and if these symptoms are present in a wound a doctor should be consulted. Minor wounds can be treated with various antiseptic preparations, such as tincture of iodine, metaphen, merthiolate, boric acid, and others, and then covered with a clean snug bandage or compress. If the wound is more serious, only the bandage should be applied and the cleansing and disinfection of the wound done by a doctor, since amateur efforts can cause serious damage.

XANTHOMA, flat yellow tumor which may develop on the surface of the skin. Xanthomas are caused by the deposit of a fatty substance which the body has failed to dispose of in the normal manner. Most frequently they are seen in the vicinity of the eyes, especially on the inner part of the lower lid. A surgeon can remove these "yellow spots," as they are sometimes called, with relative ease, leaving only slightly visible scars. Xanthomas may tend to recur, but are seldom cancerous. *See also* TUMOR.

XERODERMA, a disorder in which the skin becomes rough and dry, and sometimes discolored, with fine scaly shedding.

XEROPHTHALMIA, a disease in which a severe dryness of the eye occurs, resulting from a deficiency of vitamin A. The cornea becomes clouded and inflamed; ulcers of the cornea may develop. Permanent blindness may result in the advanced stages of this disease if it is not promptly and properly treated. The administration of vitamin A is effective for this condition.

XEROSIS, a disease in which abnormal dryness of the skin caused by vitamin A deficiency is a symp-

tom. This condition may be corrected by taking liver oil extracts and making sure that the diet includes enough leafy green and yellow vegetables, as well as egg yolks, butter, or vitamin A-enriched margarine.

XEROSTOMA, decreased salivary flow; it is a symptom which arises from a number of causes rather than a disease. In many instances it is temporary, as in fever or in a state of fear or anxiety. Atropine, a drug often administered to patients before a surgical operation, may produce a dry feeling in the mouth.

In chronic cases, lack of saliva may cause the mouth to become rough and dry, and painful cracks and fissures which bleed easily may develop. A stone in the duct of the salivary glands may cause obstruction, swelling, and pain that will interfere with the intake of food and predispose the gland to infection. Surgery is the only means then of removing the stones.

X-RAYS, radiation produced by the vacuum tube, similar to light but of much shorter wave length and possessing special penetrating and tissue-ionizing power. First announced in December 1895 by the German physicist Wilhelm Konrad Roentgen, the x-ray has since become one of the most important adjuncts in the practice of medicine and surgery.

One of the chief uses of the x-ray continues to be for the diagnosis of broken bones. Today pictures are made from different angles so that the exact relationship of the broken bones to the tissues may be determined.

An x-ray of the skull shows the

presence of disease of the bone, sometimes the presence of a tumor or changes in the blood vessels in the brain.

It is also now possible by the use of accessory materials to visualize various organs and tissues. These substances include various dyes which may be taken into the body and which localize in certain organs and tissues. Then by the use of the x-ray these tissues and organs are made visible. One dye substance is used in taking x-rays of the gallbladder; others are used for the kidney and urinary bladder; still others for the female genital system or the spinal column. A substance called lipiodol may be injected into the lungs or sinuses to make them visible. For the investigation of the alimentary tract an opaque meal of barium is given and the progress of the meal along the intestinal tract is studied to detect ulcers and obstructions. A barium enema is given to study the large intestine and other organs in the lower abdominal region.

By the use of the x-ray the exact size of the heart may be determined. The x-ray is also used in the treatment of disease, particularly in the treatment of tumors, conditions affecting the skin, inflammations of various kinds, and for a wide variety of purposes where radiation therapy is called for.

Since the introduction of x-ray equipment innumerable improvements have been made. Portable apparatus is now available that can be taken directly to a patient's bedside. One of the most important developments in the use of the x-ray on a mass scale has been the introduction of mobile units as a means of taking chest films of school children and of the general public in order to determine the presence of tuberculosis and cancer of the lung. *See also* RADIATION.

YAWS, also called frambesia, pian, bubos, and leishmaniasis, a disease caused by a spiral microorganism, the treponema pertenue, related to the treponema pallidum, the agent of syphilis. Yaws is rarely found in the United States but is a disease of tropical regions, especially where sanitation is poor. Raspberry-colored growths on various parts of the body, especially the face, feet, legs, hands, and around the external genitals are characteristic signs. The growths may join to form large masses and may become ulcerated.

YEAST. In the compressed form with a starchy or absorbent base, yeast is used medically because of its richness in the water-soluble vitamins, including thiamine, riboflavin, pyroxidine, nicotinic acid, and pantothenic acid. Dried yeast or brewer's yeast is frequently fortified with vitamins of the B complex group.

YELLOW FEVER, an acute infectious disease caused by a filterable virus which is transmitted by the bite of an infected mosquito, aëdes aegypti, in whose system the virus lives and breeds. The illness strikes suddenly, usually three to six days after the mosquito bite. The face becomes flushed and swollen, the eyes suffused, the lips and tongue a bright red, and a high fever appears, with pain in the head and back, and a feeling of extreme exhaustion. In two or three days, the temperature drops below normal, the pulse slows down, and the skin grows cold and assumes the yellow jaundiced hue, which gives the disease its name. A characteristic "black vomit" occurs, indicating internal bleeding. As the patient recovers, the temperature returns to normal, generally by the seventh or eighth day, and convalescence begins, leading to rapid, complete recovery. Complications are rare, and one attack gives lifelong immunity.

Until the twentieth century, large areas of Central and South America were considered uninhabitable because of the disastrous effects of yellow fever. A considerable portion of the population along the southern Atlantic and Gulf seaboard was wiped out in one of the yellow fever epidemics. The first indication that the disease was transmitted by the bite of a mosquito came from Dr. Carlos Finlay, a Cuban, in 1881. Two decades later, Dr. Walter Reed, an American army surgeon, proved that yellow fever was transmitted solely by the bite of an infected mosquito. This led to such effective mosquito control that today yellow fever has been eradicated in the Canal Zone as well as in Cuba. Similar success has followed wherever effective antimosquito measures have been practiced. Studies later showed that yellow fever is also present in the jungles of South America and Africa. It is found in monkeys and possibly in other jungle animals. Native people are also affected by the germ, which is probably transmitted to human beings by several varieties of mosquito.

International health authorities have concerned themselves with preventing the spread of yellow fever into urban communities. In 1951, the Nobel Prize was awarded to Dr. Max Theiler of the Rockefeller Foundation for his development of a vaccine, "17-B," for yellow fever. The vaccine was given to more than 8,000,000 members of the armed forces during World War II.

The greatest precautions are taken to prevent introduction of infected mosquitoes onto airplanes and ships. Crews are vaccinated against the disease and ships are fumigated. Persons who are infected are isolated in a screen-protected room for at least the first four days after development of symptoms of yellow fever. The United States Public Health Service, the World Health Organization, and quarantine agencies all over the world are constantly alert to the threat of mosquito disease carriers. Breeding places are sprayed with DDT or oil to kill the larvae, and such measures in recent years have kept the spread of yellow fever at a minimum.

YELLOW JAUNDICE. *See* JAUNDICE.

ZINC, a metallic element which occurs naturally as silicate and carbonate and is known as calamine in these forms. The uses of zinc in medicine are chiefly as a component of zinc chloride and zinc oxide and similar preparations used in treating the skin. These are combined with ointments and dusting powders.

A poisonous compound of zinc

and phosphorous is used as an ingredient of rat poison.

ZYGOMA, that part of the temple bone of the skull that lies beneath the cheek; it is also known as the zygomatic arch. Some of the muscles involved in mastication of food are attached to it. It is sometimes involved in fracture of the skull.

ZYME, a word derived from the Greek, means ferment. Many different forms of ferment are used in medicine—for example, to dissolve secretions. The zymogenic cells of the stomach are those which secrete pepsin, which is useful in digesting the protein foods.

INDEX

Gullet. *See:* Esophagus
Gums, 682–3
Guthrie, Samuel, 429
Gynecology, 683
Gynecomastia, 683

Habit spasm, 683
Hair, 683–5
  and baldness, 459–60, 684
  bezoars, 222
  bleaching, 685
  care of, 24
  dandruff, 25
  depilatory, 597
  dryness, 24
  excessive growth due to adrenal
      glands, 285
  fine, in pregnancy, 71
  gray and white, 685
  growth of, 683
  in ill health, 24
  lotions for women, 25
  number, 684
  pubic, 122
  structure, 683
  superfluous, 299, 685
  underarm, 122
  undesirable, 137
  washing of, 684
Hair remover. *See:* Depilatory
Halitosis, 685–6
Hallucinations, 321, 685
Halsted, Dr. William S., 429
Hammon, Dr. William McD., 332
Hand-Schuller-Christian disease, 686
Hangnail, 788
Hansen's disease. *See:* Leprosy
Hardening of the arteries. *See:* Ar-
    teriosclerosis
Harelip, 686
Hart, F. Leslie, 462
Hashish. *See:* Marihuana
Haverhill fever. *See:* Rat-bite fever
Hay fever, 308, 686–7
Hazards of cold, 687–8
Headache, 688–90
  migraine, 625, 774–5
Head banging, head rolling, 690
Head injuries, 690–1
Head injury, first aid, 397
Health, good food habits for, 30
  meaning of, 1–7
  mental, defined, 314
  normal, defined, 1

Hearing, deaf-mutism, 590
  deafness, 591–2
  hardness of. *See:* Deafness, Ear,
      Otosclerosis
Heart, 691–4
  angina pectoris, 431
  anomalies, 93
  arteriosclerosis, 150
  bacterial endocarditis, 145
  beats, 2, 20, 143
  blocking of, 579–81
  blood samples, 9
  cardiac defect, 93
  catheters, 9
  coarctation of aorta, 95
  complications in congenital dis-
      ease, 104
  congenital disease, in children, 93–
      107
  congenital disorders, symptoms,
      100
  congenitally defective, 93, 146–7
  coronary artery disease, 150
  digitalis, 607–8
  diphtheria, 115
  diseases, 142–54
  electrocardiograph, 620
  emotions affect, 144, 151
  endocarditis, bacterial, 458–9
  exercise, 152
  failure, *illus.*, 693
  fatigue a symptom of trouble, 145
  fibrillation, 657
  function, 143
  high blood pressure, 157, 486
  hypertension, 173
  impulse, measurement, 20
  interatrial septal defect, 97
  lung machine, 99
  malformations, 93
  murmur, 100, 144
  muscle enlarged by hypotension,
      151
  myocardium, 93
  neuroses, cardiac, 152
  normal, *illus.*, 95, 691
  obesity a handicap, 152
  old age, 154
  palpitation, 144
  patent ductus arteriosus, 96
  pericarditis, 818
  phonocardiogram, 101
  radio diagnosis, 9
  rheumatic, 147

Travelers Insurance Co., 13
Trench fever, 923
Trench mouth. *See:* Vincent's angina
Trichomonas intestinalis, 248
Trichinosis, 59, 247, 923–4
Tridione, 633
Trigeminal neuralgia. *See:* Tic douloureux
Tropical diseases
  amebiasis, 422
  bilharziasis, 472
  blackwater fever, 477
  Chagas' disease, 530
  chromoblastomycosis, 558
  dengue, 594
  dysentery, 614
  elephantiasis, 620
  filariasis, 658–9
  jungle rot, 736–7
  kala-azar, 737
  Leishmaniasis, 744
  madura foot, 758
  malaria, 758–9
  trachoma, 923–4
  yaws, 956
  yellow fever, 956–7
Tuberculosis, 924–8
  anemia in, 160
  of bladder, 479
  death rate, 3
  gastritis in, 225
  hypotension in, 174
  kidneys, 739
  laryngeal, 743
  occupational disease, 58
  philanthropic organization for, 14
  and pleurisy, 827
  stomatitis, tuberculous, 213
Tularemia, 928–9
Tumors, 195, 929. *See also:* Cancer
  adenoma, 411
  adrenal medulla, 283
  in aged, 356
  in bladder, 480
  blood pressure, high, in relation to,
    486
  Boeck's sarcoid, 496
  cancerous, 514
  chondroma, 556
  fibroma, 657
  glioma, 679
  hemangioma, 696
  cause of hypoglycemia, 281
  intestinal, 240
  lipoma, 750

ovarian, 807
parathyroid glands, 280
polyps, 834
sarcoma, 871
thyroid gland (goiter), 679–80
Wilm's tumor, 949
in womb, 69
xanthoma, 955
Tunnel diseases, occupational hazard,
  60
Turpentine poisoning, 57, 832
"Twilight sleep," 78
Typhoid fever, 929–30
  rarity of cases, 4
Typhus, 81, 930–1

Ulcer, 932. *See also:* Peptic ulcer,
  Stomach ulcer
  duodenal, pain after eating, 227
  eyeball, ulcerated, in rosacea, 301
  ulceration of tongue, 214
  ulcerative stomatitis, 153
Ultraviolet rays, body needs, 43
  in psoriasis, treatment of, 303
  virus, killed by, 189
Umbilical cord, 77
Umbilicus, 932
Unconsciousness, first aid in, 398
Undernutrition. *See:* Malnutrition
Undulant fever, 59, 932–3
United Nations Scientific Committee
  on the Effects of Atomic Radia-
  tion, 854
U. S. Public Health Service, 339, 340,
  413, 461, 613, 815
University of Michigan, and polio
  tests, 333
Unsaturated fats, cholesterol and, 6
Urbach, Dr. Fred, 459
Uremia, 933–4
Ureter, 934
Urethra, 934–5
Uric acid, in gout, 346
Urination, 935
  and bed wetting, 467–8
  frequency of, in diabetes insipidus,
    601
Urine, 935–6
  albumin in, 790
  and albuminuria, 417
  blood in, 696
  and melanuria, 769
Urologist, 10
Urticaria. *See:* Hives